NURSING OUTCOMES

The State of the Science

Edited by

Diane M. Doran, PhD, RN, FCAHS

Professor

Scientific Director, Nursing Health Services Research Unit

Nurse Senior Researcher, Ontario Ministry of Health and Long-Term Care

Lawrence S. Bloomberg Faculty of Nursing

University of Toronto

Toronto, Ontario, Canada

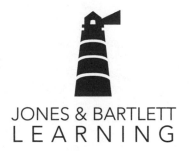

JONES & BARTLETT
LEARNING

D0911823

World Headquarters
Jones & Bartlett Learning
40 Tall Pine Drive
Sudbury, MA 01776
978-443-5000
info@jblearning.com
www.jblearning.com

Jones & Bartlett Learning Canada
6339 Ormindale Way
Mississauga, Ontario L5V 1J2
Canada

Jones & Bartlett Learning International
Barb House, Barb Mews
London W6 7PA
United Kingdom

Jones & Bartlett Learning books and products are available through most bookstores and online booksellers. To contact Jones & Bartlett Learning directly, call 800-832-0034, fax 978-443-8000, or visit our website, www.jblearning.com.

Substantial discounts on bulk quantities of Jones & Bartlett Learning publications are available to corporations, professional associations, and other qualified organizations. For details and specific discount information, contact the special sales department at Jones & Bartlett Learning via the above contact information or send an email to specialsales@jblearning.com.

The authors, editor, and publisher have made every effort to provide accurate information. However, they are not responsible for errors, omissions, or for any outcomes related to the use of the contents of this book and take no responsibility for the use of the products and procedures described. Treatments and side effects described in this book may not be applicable to all people; likewise, some people may require a dose or experience a side effect that is not described herein. Drugs and medical devices are discussed that may have limited availability controlled by the Food and Drug Administration (FDA) for use only in a research study or clinical trial. Research, clinical practice, and government regulations often change the accepted standard in this field. When consideration is being given to use of any drug in the clinical setting, the health care provider or reader is responsible for determining FDA status of the drug, reading the package insert, and reviewing prescribing information for the most up-to-date recommendations on dose, precautions, and contraindications, and determining the appropriate usage for the product. This is especially important in the case of drugs that are new or seldom used.

Production Credits

Publisher: Kevin Sullivan
Acquisitions Editor: Amy Sibley
Associate Editor: Patricia Donnelly
Editorial Assistant: Rachel Shuster
Associate Production Editor: Lisa Cerrone
Marketing Manager: Rebecca Wasley

V.P., Manufacturing and Inventory Control: Therese Connell
Composition: Spoke & Wheel
Cover Image: © Kateryna Larina/ShutterStock, Inc.
Printing and Binding: Courier Stoughton
Cover Printing: Courier Stoughton

Library of Congress Cataloging-in-Publication Data

Nursing outcomes : the state of the science / edited by Diane M. Doran. — 2nd ed.
    p. ; cm.
  Rev. ed. of: Nursing-sensitive outcomes. c2003.
  Includes bibliographical references and index.
  ISBN 978-0-7637-8325-9 (pbk.)
  1. Nursing—Standards. 2. Nursing—Quality control. 3. Outcome assessment (Medical care) I. Doran, Diane. II. Nursing-sensitive outcomes.
  [DNLM: 1. Nursing Care—standards. 2. Treatment Outcome. WY 100 N9735 2011]
  RT85.5.N869 2011
  610.73—dc22

            2010016873

6048
Printed in the United States of America
14 13 12 11 10   10 9 8 7 6 5 4 3 2 1

Contents

7 Psychological Distress as a Nurse-Sensitive Outcome
Doris Howell   285

8 Patient Satisfaction as a Nurse-Sensitive Outcome
Heather K. Spence Laschinger, Stephanie Gilbert, and Lesley Smith   359

9 Mortality Rate as a Nurse-Sensitive Outcome
Ann E. Tourangeau   409

IO   Healthcare Utilization
Sean P. Clarke   **439**

II   Nursing Minimum Data Sets
*Manal Kleib, Anne Sales, Diane M. Doran, Claire Mallette,
and Deborah White*   **487**

Preface

The measurement of outcomes continues to become a more prominent and relevant issue in the delivery of health care as healthcare organizations focus on pressing issues relating to cost efficiency, quality of care, effectiveness of care, and organizational performance. All practitioners, in every dimension of the health field, are being challenged to find ways to demonstrate that the care they provide leads to improved outcomes for patients. To do so, practitioners are attempting to identify relevant outcomes that can be linked in a meaningful way to their practice. Among the many determinations confronting the rapidly developing field of patient outcomes research are: what outcomes to include, where and when to measure those outcomes, how nursing-centric to be, how to move to database construction, and how to benefit front-line clinicians through real-time outcomes feedback and evidence-based practice. The fundamental issue of what to include as an outcome is dependent on the strength of primary research that examines relationships between the myriad of possible effects of nursing care on patients (Pringle & Doran, 2003).

There are now several major international nursing initiatives that are shaping the direction of policy and practice related to nursing-sensitive outcomes measurement. For example, in Ontario, Canada, Health Outcomes for Better Information and Care (HOBIC), funded by the Ontario Ministry of Health and Long-Term Care, is focused on the collection of nursing-sensitive patient outcomes information across four health sectors: acute care, home care, long-term care, and chronic hospital care (Pringle & White, 2002). The Ontario data are collected electronically at the point of care when nurses complete patient assessments. HOBIC introduces a systematic, structured language to admission and discharge assessments of patients receiving acute care and to admission, quarterly (if condition changes), and discharge assessments of patients receiving complex continuing care, long-term care, or home care.

In the United States, several initiatives are aimed at identifying outcomes sensitive to and relevant to nursing practice. For example, the National Database of Nursing Quality Indicators (NDNQI), a national nursing database that healthcare organizations voluntary subscribe to, provides quarterly and annual reporting of structure, process, and outcome indicators to evaluate nursing care at the unit level (Kurtzman & Corrigan, 2007). The initial set of indicators used in establishing that database was selected based on feasibility testing (American Nurses

Association, 1995). These indicators included falls, falls with injury, nursing care hours per patient day, skill mix, pressure ulcer prevalence, and hospital-acquired pressure ulcer prevalence. In another initiative, the Quality Health Outcomes Model developed by the American Academy of Nursing Expert Panel on Quality Health Care, the following five outcome categories expected to be sensitive to nursing care inputs were delineated: achievement of appropriate self-care, demonstration of health-promoting behaviors, health-related quality of life, perception of being well cared for, and symptom management to criterion (Mitchell, Armstrong, Simpson, & Lentz, 1989; Mitchell & Lang, 2004).

In the United Kingdom, outcomes research has demonstrated the impact of variation in nurse staffing and mortality outcomes (Rafferty et al., 2007). Globally, there is interest in broadening the range of nursing-sensitive outcomes being considered in nursing research to include positive patient outcomes, as evidenced by the perspective of international experts from 10 countries (Van den Heede, Clarke, Sermeus, Vleugels, & Aiken, 2007). The next major breakthrough in outcomes research will be harnessing the potential of outcomes measurement to directly benefit patient care and to inform health policy and health human resource planning at local and national levels.

The literature on nursing-sensitive outcomes is expanding. The first edition of this book was published in 2003 (Doran, 2003). Since that time, there has been exponential growth in literature examining a variety of nurse-sensitive outcomes. It is important now to update the literature review that was published in 2003 to capitalize on new evidence. Specifically, the state of the science on nursing-sensitive outcomes needs to be reappraised to take into account studies that have been conducted post-2003. Furthermore, new outcomes have been introduced into the vernacular on nurse-sensitive outcomes, and new outcome measures have now been tested in empirical studies. These new outcomes and new approaches to measurement need to be appraised in light of more recent evidence. It is important to appraise the sensitivity of new measures to nursing variables so that decisions can be made about which instruments are appropriate for measuring nursing-sensitive patient outcomes in various practice settings.

The authors of this book offer a synthesis of the state of the science on nursing-sensitive outcomes. Specifically, the book provides a critical review and analysis of the literature on outcomes that are considered to be indicators of nursing care effectiveness. The authors of the first chapter discuss the importance of building knowledge about nursing-sensitive outcomes for policy, practice, and research. That chapter concludes with a discussion of the specific objectives and methodology for the critical review. In the following nine chapters, the quality of the evidence linking functional, self-care, symptom control, pain control, psychological distress, patient safety, healthcare utilization, mortality, and patient satisfaction is critically examined. A separate chapter is dedicated to a review of the evidence for pain as an outcome of nursing care because of the centrality of pain management to processes of nursing care. The most important distinction between this second edition of the book and the first edition is the introduction of three new chapters on nursing-sensitive outcomes: specifically, chapters on psychological distress, healthcare utilization, and mortality. These new chapters address important gaps that were identified in the previous review and offer new insights into conceptualizing outcomes of nursing care.

The primary goal of this second edition is to present a synthesis of the previous review and update this review with new empirical evidence. The book presents a comprehensive and critical analysis of the evidence concerning nursing-sensitive outcomes by reviewing the conceptual and empirical literature. Each chapter includes a concept analysis of the outcome concept, and defining characteristics are identified and a conceptual definition is proposed. Factors that influence the outcome concept are discussed, as are the consequences for clients' health and well-being. The strength of the evidence is reviewed concerning the sensitivity of the outcome concept to nursing structure variables and nursing processes or interventions. A secondary goal of the book is to review the various methods and tools used to measure the outcome concepts and to review critically the evidence of their reliability, validity, and sensitivity to nursing structure and process variables.

This book will be of particular interest to graduate and undergraduate students who are interested in the state of the science on nursing-sensitive outcomes and their measurement. It will serve as a valuable resource to master's and doctoral students who are developing the methodology for their graduate research. Researchers will also value the book because it not only offers a comprehensive synthesis of the literature, but also critically reviews the quality of the evidence and provides direction for the selection of outcome variables and approaches to measurement. The book will be valuable as well to policy makers and decision makers who are building clinical databases for quality monitoring and quality improvement.

Diane M. Doran, PhD, RN, FCAHS
Editor

REFERENCES

American Nurses Association. (1995). *Nursing report card for acute care.* Washington, DC: American Nurses Publishing.

Doran, D. M. (2003). *Nursing-sensitive outcomes: State of the science.* Sudbury, MA: Jones and Bartlett Publishers.

Kurtzman, E. T., & Corrigan, J. M. (2007). Measuring the contribution of nursing to quality, patient safety, and health care outcomes. *Policy, Politics and Nursing Practice, 8*(1), 20–36.

Mitchell, P. H., Armstrong, S., Simpson, T. F., & Lentz, M. (1989) American Association of Critical-Care Nurses demonstration project: Profile of excellence in critical care nursing. *Heart and Lung, 18,* 219–237.

Mitchell, P. H., & Lang, N. M. (2004) Framing the problem of measuring and improving health-care quality: Has the Quality Outcomes Model been useful? *Medical Care, 42*, II-4–II-11.

Pringle, D. M., & Doran, D. M. (2003). Patient outcomes as an accountability. In D. Doran (Ed.), *Nursing-sensitive outcomes: State of the science* (pp. 1–25). Sudbury, MA: Jones and Bartlett Publishers.

Pringle, D. M., & White, P. (2002). Happenings. Nursing matters: The Nursing and Health Outcomes Project of the Ontario Ministry of Health and Long-Term Care. *Canadian Journal of Nursing Research, 33*, 115–121.

Rafferty, A. M., Clarke, S. P., Coles, J., Ball, J., James, P., McKee, M., et al. (2007) Outcomes of variation in hospital nurse staffing in English hospitals: Cross-sectional analysis of survey data and discharge records. *International Journal of Nursing Studies, 44*, 175–182.

Van den Heede, K., Clarke, S. P., Sermeus, W., Vleugels, A., & Aiken, L. H. (2007) International experts' perspective on the state of the nurse staffing and patient outcomes literature. *Journal of Nursing Scholarship, 39*, 290–297.

Acknowledgments

The first edition of this book was based on work funded by the Ministry of Health and Long-Term Care, Ontario, Canada, in response to a request for a critical analysis of the literature on nursing-sensitive outcomes and approaches to their measurement. The opinions, results, and conclusions are those of the authors; no endorsement by the Ministry of Health and Long-Term Care is intended or should be inferred.

The authors would like to thank Barbara Bauer for her role in directing the copyediting of the first edition, and Jenny Lau for her role in searching the literature and for providing the copyediting of the second edition. The assistance of Verna Cheung in compiling the literature reviewed on healthcare utilization and her assistance in summarizing this literature are gratefully acknowledged.

Contributors

Sean P. Clarke, PhD, RN, FAAN
Lawrence S. Bloomberg Faculty
  of Nursing
University of Toronto
Peter Munk Cardiac Centre
University Health Network
Toronto, Ontario, Canada

Diane M. Doran, PhD, RN, FCAHS
Professor
Scientific Director, Nursing Health
  Services Research Unit
Nurse Senior Researcher, Ontario
  Ministry of Health and Long-Term Care
Lawrence S. Bloomberg Faculty of
  Nursing
University of Toronto
Toronto, Ontario, Canada

Stephanie Gilbert, MS
Halifax, Nova Scotia, Canada

Linda McGillis Hall, PhD, RN, FAAN
Professor, Senior Career Scientist
Associate Dean of Research & External
  Relations
Lawrence Bloomberg Faculty of Nursing
University of Toronto
Toronto, Ontario, Canada

Doris Howell, PhD, RN
Princess Margaret Hospital
Toronto, Ontario, Canada

Manal Kleib, MSN, RN
Faculty of Nursing
University of Alberta
Edmonton, Alberta, Canada

Michelle Lalonde, MN, RN
Lawrence S. Bloomberg Faculty
  of Nursing
University of Toronto
Toronto, Ontario, Canada

Heather K. Spence Laschinger, PhD, RN
Arthur Labatt Family School of Nursing
University of Western Ontario
London, Ontario, Canada

Claire Mallette, PhD, RN
Director of Nursing Education,
  Placement, & Development
University Health Network
Toronto, Ontario, Canada

Michael McGillion, PhD, RN
University of Toronto
Toronto, Ontario, Canada

Dorothy Pringle, PhD, RN, OC
Toronto, Ontario, Canada

Anne Sales, PhD, RN
Professor, Canada Research Chair in
  Interdisciplinary Healthcare Teams
Faculty of Nursing
University of Alberta
Edmonton, Alberta, Canada

Souraya Sidani, PhD, RN
School of Nursing
Ryerson University
Toronto, Ontario, Canada

Lesley Smith, BSN, RN
Arthur Labatt Family School of Nursing
University of Western Ontario
London, Ontario, Canada

Ann E. Tourangeau, PhD, RN
Lawrence S. Bloomberg Faculty
  of Nursing
Faculty of Nursing
University of Toronto
Toronto, Ontario, Canada

Judy Watt-Watson, PhD, RN
Lawrence S. Bloomberg Faculty
  of Nursing
University of Toronto
Toronto, Ontario, Canada

Deborah White, PhD, RN
Associate Dean of Research
Faculty of Nursing
University of Calgary
Calgary, Alberta, Canada

Peggy White, MN, RN
Program Manager
Health Outcomes for Better Information
  and Care
National Project Director
Canadian Health Outcomes for Better
  Information and Care Project
Ontario, Canada

Patient Outcomes as an Accountability

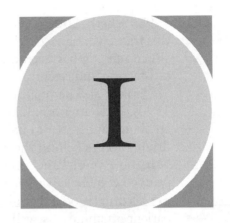

Diane M. Doran
Dorothy Pringle

INTRODUCTION

Outcomes have been of interest to health science researchers for decades. The earliest work concentrated on the outcomes of medical and nursing practice. Nurse researchers were interested in the effects of specific nursing interventions on such things as patient symptoms (with pain being of particular interest), patient sense of well-being, and rapidity of recovery. Physicians examined the effects on patients of new surgical techniques in contrast to existing ones, and drug companies invested billions of dollars in testing whether new drugs improve patient symptoms when compared with either no treatment or currently available ones. The increasing prominence of the randomized controlled trial as the research design of choice for testing many new interventions has accelerated the identification of outcomes. This research, accumulated over 50 years, has produced a rich legacy of information on a wide range of patient outcomes, including their definitions and measurement.

Donabedian's now classic framework of structure, process, and outcomes proposed in 1966 introduced outcomes to the lexicon of health service researchers (Donabedian, 1966). His interest was in identifying factors in healthcare organizations that affected quality of patient care. Hospital structures and processes were the focus of most of the early research based on this framework, but more recent work has moved to a focus on outcomes (Mitchell, Ferketich, & Jennings,

1998; Scherb, 2002). The outcomes that dominate the research emanating from this framework are cost, length of stay, patient mortality, and patient satisfaction. When nursing has been the focus of studies, outcomes have included nurses' job satisfaction and retention rates (Aiken, Sochalski, & Lake, 1997).

Aiken and her colleagues (Aiken et al., 1997) noted that up until the mid-1990s, little attention had been paid to the relationship between organizational attributes and patient outcomes. This picture is rapidly changing, and one of the driving forces behind the change is the work done by the American Academy of Nursing Expert Panel on Quality Health Care. When preparing in 1994 for a planned conference on the relevance of outcomes to nursing, this group developed a conceptual model that linked patient outcomes to organizational structures and patient attributes, as well as to healthcare interventions (Mitchell et al., 1998). The group entertained a revolutionary idea. Perhaps interventions did not directly affect outcomes but rather worked through one of the systems in which the individual is embedded: the physiologic system of the individual, organizational systems, or groups (Mitchell, 2001). The resultant Quality Health Outcomes Model integrated functional, social, psychological, and physical/physiologic factors along with patients' experiences, in contrast to the exclusively physiological outcomes that were the usual indicators of care. Five outcomes were proposed: achievement of appropriate self-care, demonstration of health-promoting behaviors, health-related quality of life, patient perception of being well cared for, and symptom management to criteria (Mitchell et al., 1998).

A conference on outcome measures and care delivery systems, to which health services researchers, insurance company representatives, and nurse researchers were invited, was held in 1996 in Washington, D.C., under the sponsorship of the American Academy of Nursing and the Agency for Health Care Policy and Research. The proceedings from this conference were reported in *Medical Care Supplement, 35*(11). Participants heard and debated papers that summarized the state of knowledge on each of the outcomes of interest. They also explored theoretical and methodological issues involved in linking organizations and outcomes. This conference and the planning that preceded it have had a profound influence on nursing's approach to the study of nursing-sensitive patient outcomes. No longer were mortality and length of stay the only considerations when examining how patients fared in an encounter with the healthcare system.

The Quality Health Outcomes Model deliberately provides a multidisciplinary view of the relationship between patient outcomes and the healthcare system (Mitchell, 2001). Irvine, Sidani, and McGillis Hall (1998) developed an equally deliberate but nurse-specific model that was subsequently tested (Doran et al., 2002). In this model, the nurses' independent, dependent, and interdependent roles are treated as the processes linking the nurse, organizational, and patient structures, and patient outcomes and team functioning. The patient outcomes of interest are symptom control, freedom from complications, functional status/self-care, knowledge of disease and treatment, and satisfaction with care and costs.

Aiken et al. (1997) developed a theoretical framework based on the premise that organizational models that provide nurses with substantial autonomy and more control of resources at the unit level and encourage better relations between nurses and physicians will result in better patient outcomes, including higher satisfaction and reduced complications and mortality. This team is particularly interested in understanding the relationship between nurses and patient mortality. A number of studies have shown correlations between better nursing staffing ratios and lower patient mortality (Aiken, Smith, & Lake, 1994; Al-Hader & Wan, 1991; Hartz et al., 1989; Shortell & Hughes, 1988; Tourangeau et al., 2007; Van Servellen & Schultz, 1999), but why this occurs is poorly understood (Aiken et al., 1997). The concept of "failure to rescue" that Silber and his colleagues at the University of Pennsylvania originally proposed to explain medical effectiveness (Silber, Williams, Krakauer, & Schwartz, 1992) has been coopted by Aiken and her team as a potential explanatory factor in nursing. Failure to rescue means that patients die subsequent to complications from their condition but would have had a chance to recover if the complications had been detected and treated in time (Silber et al., 1992). In nursing, this situation may result when insufficient registered nurses are available to monitor patients and intervene when something goes wrong (Aiken et al., 1997). The concept of failure to rescue has now been applied in a number of clinical contexts (e.g., Beaulieu, 2009; Friese & Aiken, 2008; Kutney-Lee & Aiken, 2008; Silber et al., 2009). However the relationship between nurse staffing and failure to rescue is not consistent in nursing research (Van den Heede et al., 2009). Nevertheless, these three models/frameworks, among others, provide a strong basis for testing relationships between a variety of organizational structures; nursing interventions and processes; and patient, nurse, and organizational outcomes.

Categorizing Patient Outcomes

Many nursing-sensitive patient outcomes have been examined over the last 15 years of research on the topic, and a number of typologies exist to categorize them. Lohr (1985) proposed a list of six categories based on the continuum of care: mortality, adverse events and complications during hospitalization, inadequate recovery, prolongation of the medical problem, decline in health status, and decline in quality of life. Clearly, they are all negative in orientation and do not provide for the possibility that patients might benefit from their healthcare episode. Using a different approach, Hegyvary (1991) suggested four categories of outcome assessment from the patients', providers', and purchasers' perspectives: (a) clinical (patients' responses to interventions), (b) functional (improvement or decline in physical functioning), (c) financial (cost and length of stay), and (d) perceptual (patient satisfaction with care received and persons providing the care).

Jennings, Staggers, and Brosch (1999) reviewed the nursing, medical, and health services research literature from 1974 forward to locate all indicators of outcomes. These were classified as patient focused, provider focused, or organization focused. The patient-focused category was further subdivided into diagnosis-focused and holistically focused outcomes. Examples of the diagnosis-specific outcomes are laboratory values, Apgar scores, and vital signs. The holistically oriented outcomes include health status, health-related quality of life, patient satisfaction ratings, assessments of patient knowledge, and symptom management. Care provider-focused outcomes include complication rates, appropriate use of medications, provider profiling, and, when a family caregiver is involved, a measure of caregiver burden. Adverse events such as falls, deaths, and unplanned readmission are categorized as organization-focused outcomes. Jennings et al. (1999) recommended that a battery of outcomes include both diagnostic and holistic outcomes, using rationale supplied by Guyatt, Feeny, and Patrick (1993).

Although derived and categorized very differently, there is considerable overlap in the actual outcomes recommended by Hegyvary (1991) and Jennings et al. (1999). When the various classification systems and the outcomes included in them are integrated, it is possible to propose a simple three-class system: adverse events, patient well-being, and patient satisfaction. The adverse events include nosocomial infections such as those occurring in the bloodstream or urinary tract, pneumonia, falls, medical complications such as gastrointestinal (GI) bleeding, deep vein thrombosis (DVT) and shock, skin breakdown, and unanticipated death. Outcomes that can be classified as patient well-being include functional status, ability to perform self-care, control of symptoms, performance of health-promoting activities, and health-related quality of life. Patient satisfaction is a subjective rating of nursing care received and can include assessments of the nurses providing the care, the way symptoms were managed, and any education received.

Van den Heede, Clarke, Sermeus, Vleugels, and Aiken (2007) conducted a Delphi survey of international experts' perspectives on the state of the nurse staffing and patient outcomes literature. A total of 24 researchers and 8 nurse administrators from 10 countries participated in the survey. At the end of the second Delphi survey round, the predefined level of consensus (85%) was reached for 32 patient outcomes. The highest consensus levels regarding sensitivity to nurse staffing variables were found for patient satisfaction, pain, symptom management, aspiration pneumonia, postoperative complications, hospital-acquired pneumonia, and medication error. In follow-up, Van den Heede et al. (2009) conducted a study of nurse staffing and patient outcomes in Belgian acute hospitals using 10 of the 32 indicators suggested by the Delphi panel. They included one safety measure (pressure ulcer), three complication measures (deep venous thrombosis, shock or cardiac arrest, postoperative respiratory failure), five infection measures (postoperative complications, urinary tract infection, hospital-acquired pneumonia, ventilator-associated pneumonia, and hospital-acquired sepsis), in-hospital mortality, and failure to rescue. No significant association was found among the acuity-adjusted nursing hours per patient day, proportion of registered nurses with a bachelor's degree, and patient outcomes. The authors, however, concluded that the "absence of association between hospital-level nurse staffing measures and patient outcomes should not be inferred as implying that nurse staffing does not have an impact on patient outcomes in Belgian hospitals" (p. 928). They suggested that "to better understand the dynamics of the nurse staffing and patient outcome relationship in acute hospitals, further analyses (i.e., nursing unit level analyses) of these and other outcomes are recommended" (p. 928).

Bostick, Rantz, Flesner, and Riggs (2006) conducted a systematic review of studies of staffing and quality in nursing homes. Eighty-seven research articles and government documents published from 1975 to 2003 were reviewed. They concluded that there is a proven association between higher total staffing level (especially licensed staff) and improved quality of care. Functional ability, pressure ulcers, and weight loss were identified as the most sensitive quality outcomes linked to staffing.

Dall, Chen, Seifert, Maddox, and Hogan (2009) synthesized findings from the literature on the relationship between registered nurse staffing levels and nursing-sensitive patient outcomes in acute care hospitals. They used hospital discharge data to estimate incidence and cost of these patient outcomes together with productivity measures and determined that as nurse staffing levels increase, patient risk of nosocomial complications and hospital length of stay decrease, resulting in medical cost savings, improved national productivity, and lives saved.

Kane, Shamliyan, Mueller, Duval, and Wilt (2007) conducted a systematic review and meta-analysis of the literature related to registered nurse (RN) staffing levels and patient outcomes. They reported that increased RN staffing was associated with lower hospital-related mortality in intensive care units (ICUs), in surgical patients, and in medical patients. An increase of 1 RN per patient day was associated with a decreased odds ratio of hospital-acquired pneumonia, unplanned extubation, respiratory failure, and cardiac arrest in ICUs, and a lower risk of failure to rescue in surgical patients. Length of stay was shorter, by 24% in ICUs and by 31% in surgical patients.

Major Nursing Research Efforts on Outcomes

It is possible to identify five major research initiatives developed in the 1990s that examined the linkages between selected nursing components of organizations and a variety of patient outcomes. These are the American Nurses Association (ANA) Patient Safety and Nursing Quality Initiative, the Harvard School of Public Health Study, the Kaiser Permanente Medical Care Program Northern California

Region (KPNCR) Project, the Nursing Staff Mix Outcomes Study in Ontario, and an international study under the overall leadership of Aiken that explored the failure-to-rescue phenomenon (Aiken et al., 2001).

The ANA study is an excellent example of the use of adverse events as outcomes. A central database was constructed using information supplied by 200 acute care hospitals participating in the studies; at the same time, nine individual state nursing organizations focused on outcomes of specific interest to them. Patient diagnostic-related groups (DRGs) that were conceptually related to nursing were included, and the New York State nursing intensity weights were used to adjust for complexity across patients. The five outcomes included were urinary tract infections (UTIs), postoperative infections, pneumonias, pressure ulcers, and length of stay. The analyses showed a significant statistical relationship between all five outcomes and nursing staffing, that is, overall increased number of nurses and/or increased numbers of registered nurses as part of the nursing staff (American Nurses Association [ANA], 2000; Lichtig, Knauf, & Milholland, 1999; Rowell, 2001).

Another study that focused on complications as outcomes was conducted by the Harvard School of Public Health (Needleman, Buerhaus, Mattke, Stewart, & Zelevinsky, 2002). Using administrative data from 799 hospitals in 11 American states, they measured length of stay and 12 adverse outcomes: UTIs, pressure ulcers, hospital-acquired pneumonias, shock or cardiac arrest, upper GI bleeding, hospital-acquired sepsis, DVT, central nervous system complications, in-hospital death, wound infection, pulmonary failure, and metabolic derangement. When death resulted from pneumonia, shock, upper GI bleeding, sepsis, or DVT, it was treated as failure to rescue. Significant statistical relationships were found between a higher proportion of hours of care by RNs and a larger number of hours of care by RNs, and some of the adverse outcomes, among them lower rates of UTIs, pneumonia, and failure to rescue (Needleman et al.).

Aiken and a large team of associates (Aiken et al., 2001) from five countries (United States, Canada, Germany, England, and Scotland) examined the effects that nurse staffing, other organizational features in hospitals, and nurses' job satisfaction had on patient outcomes of mortality and failure to rescue. Patient discharge data from 713 hospitals were included; 45,300 nurses completed surveys on their perceptions of their workloads, their satisfaction with their jobs, their intention to remain in their positions, relationships between nurses and management, and their views of the adequacy of the care provided on their units. Hospitals that rated highly in the level of staffing as reported by the nurse survey had lower mortality rates and lower rates of failure to rescue (Jackson, Chiarello, Gaynes, & Gerberding, 2002).

Lush (2001) and her colleagues at the Kaiser Permanente Medical Care Program Northern California Region undertook a project that contrasted in several ways with the three projects just described. Rather than adverse events, the patient outcomes they focused on included functional status, healthcare engagement (both knowledge and involvement in care), and mental and social well-being. Included in the latter were fear, anxiety, individual coping, altered role performance, family/caregiver role strain, and family coping. After some experience with this set of outcomes, the group decided to collect additional information about skin breakdown, symptom distress, nosocomial infections, and UTIs (Lush, 2001). Another difference resulted from the fact that Kaiser Permanente is a health system, and patients receiving home care, ambulatory care, and acute hospital care were included. Finally, this project was not conducted as a research study. Rather, a database was being established that would allow Kaiser Permanente to benchmark best practices, that is, the practice patterns associated with better patient outcomes, shortest length of stay, and lowest costs (Crawford, Taylor, Seipert, & Lush, 1996; Ditmyer et al. (1998). Using this database, the organization was able to identify differing patterns of care across various elements of its service delivery system and to match these against readmissions, number of provider visits after hospital discharges, and the number of visits to the ER (Lush, 2001).

The fifth project was conducted in all 17 teaching hospitals in Ontario, Canada. A total of 2,046 patients admitted to hospitals with a select number of diagnoses and 1,116 nurses who cared for them participated in this Nursing Staff Mix Outcomes Study (NSMOS), which was developed in response to the major restructuring efforts taking place across the province. The mix of skills in nursing staff was being changed, and nonprofessional workers were introduced to the hospital environment for the first time (McGillis Hall et al., 2003). Consequently, there was an interest in knowing the impact of these changes on the nurses, the system, and the patients. The patient outcomes selected were a combination of patient well-being, patient satisfaction, and adverse events. Included among the first two outcomes were functional status and pain control, and among the latter, falls, medication errors, wound infections, and UTIs. This group also investigated the social costs to patients of their hospital episode: the number of days of lost income, the number of days postdischarge that were required to return to gainful employment, whether they were able to return to their previous position of work or to a modified one, and caregiver burden. Nurses in the study reported their levels of job stress, role tension, and job satisfaction. Higher proportions of regulated workers—that is, RNs and registered practical nurses (RPNs)—in the staff mix were associated with better patient functional, social, and pain outcomes at discharge, but not at the 6-week follow-up (McGillis Hall et al., 2003), and better safety outcomes (McGillis Hall, Doran, & Pink, 2004).

The latter two projects come reasonably close to operationalizing the Quality Health Outcomes Model (Mitchell et al., 1998) in their inclusion of most of the five recommended types of outcomes. The one exception is a direct measure of patient quality of life. Neither project team incorporated this into its range of patient outcomes, perhaps because of the conceptual and measurement difficulties inherent in doing so (Anderson & Burckhardt, 1999; Harrison, Juniper, & Mitchell-DiCenso, 1996).

Since these early studies, numerous studies have been conducted in the United States (Aiken, Clarke, Sloane, Lake, & Cheney, 2008; Silber et al., 1992; Stone et al., 2007), Canada (Tourangeau, 2003; Tourangeau et al., 2007), and elsewhere (Van den Heede et al., 2009) that explore the relationship between nursing variables, such as staff mix and/or RN per patient day, and patient outcomes. With the exception of Van den Heede et al. (2009), these studies have demonstrated a relationship between adverse patient outcomes or failure to rescue, and nurse staffing. In comparison, there is a dearth of studies that involve large national databases and examine the relationship between nursing variables and well-being outcomes (e.g., Cohen, Gorenberg, & Schroeder, 2000; Doran et al., 2006; Horn, Buerhaus, Bergstrom, & Smout, 2005; McGillis Hall et al., 2003). With the advent of large-scale outcome initiatives such as Health Outcomes for Better Information and Care (HOBIC) (Pringle & White, 2002), the interRAI suite of tools for inpatient psychiatry (Hirdes et al., 2002), home care (Hirdes et al., 2004, 1999), and long-term care (Hirdes, Frijters, & Teare, 2003), there will be opportunities to address this gap in knowledge.

HOBIC is an initiative funded by the Ontario provincial government that focuses on the collection of a set of patient outcomes sensitive to nursing care in acute care, long-term care, home care, and chronic care settings. The outcomes data, consisting of patients' functional health, symptoms (pain, dyspnea, fatigue, nausea), pressure ulcers, falls, and therapeutic self-care (patients' knowledge of their health situation, resources available to them, and their ability to manage their medications and treatments), are collected electronically at the point of care when nurses complete patient assessments. Valid and reliable scales are used to assess patients' status on the HOBIC outcomes on admission and discharge assessments of patients receiving acute care and short-term home care. The HOBIC outcomes are assessed on admission, quarterly, and if the patient's condition changes for those receiving chronic care, long-term care, or chronic home care. The HOBIC system has been designed to benefit patients, decision makers, and researchers. Two databases exist, one live and accessible only by nurses and administrators in the organization submitting the information, and a second that contains deidentified data for researchers and policy makers. HOBIC information is used by nurses to monitor the impact of care and ensure, for example, that patients are prepared for discharge. For managers and senior nursing executives, HOBIC data are aggregated at the unit and institution level and provided in monthly reports that inform quality improvement initiatives, performance monitoring, and resource allocation; in addition, they provide valuable information about how their organization is managing patient outcomes. For researchers, HOBIC data provide an opportunity to investigate the impact of health human resource utilization, quality work environments, and nursing practice on patient health outcomes.

The structured and systematic language used in HOBIC is approved by the Ontario Health Informatics Standards Council for use in clinical information systems. This allows the database to be linked to other provincial and national databases, extending the research opportunities for its use. The Canadian Nurses Association was founded to extend the value of HOBIC through an initiative called Canadian HOBIC (C-HOBIC). It included the mapping of HOBIC to the standardized clinical reference terminology of nursing, the International Classification for Nursing Practice (ICNP). HOBIC outcomes data can be shared with clinical information systems in other healthcare organizations and across healthcare sectors in Ontario and will be included in the electronic health record. In addition, the collection of HOBIC outcomes electronically was extended to two other provinces, Saskatchewan and Manitoba.

Issues in Outcomes Research

Among the many issues confronting the rapidly developing field of patient outcomes research are what outcomes to include, how to measure them, where and when to measure them, how nursing centric to be, and how to move to database construction. Establishing databases such as HOBIC that house information about nursing's contribution to patient care and patient outcomes known to be reflective of that contribution is critical if we are to further our understanding of how to use nursing resources to their best effect. It is simply too expensive and not sufficiently comprehensive to rely on individual research studies that involve the primary collection of data to answer all of nursing's and the healthcare system's questions about what nursing-related factors lead to better patient outcomes. Among these factors are skill mix and configuration of nursing personnel; staffing levels; assignment patterns (primary, functional, or team); shift patterns; levels of nursing education, experience, and expertise; ratios of full- and part-time nurses; level and type of nursing leadership available centrally and on the units; cohesion and communication among the nursing staff and between nurses and physicians; the implementation of clinical care maps for all patients with selected diagnoses; and the interrelationships of these factors.

Databases that capture the care of all patients in a given hospital, region, or system provide a huge resource both in terms of the number of patients and the amount of information about those patients. The sheer size of this resource cannot be duplicated in primary research efforts. This is important because huge numbers of patients may be needed to examine relationships between nursing factors and subgroups of patients who share certain characteristics. For example, in some research that has already been undertaken, different relationships have been found for medical patients versus surgical patients, and for patients sharing similar diagnoses (diagnostic-related groups [DRGs] in the United States and case mix groups [CMGs] in Canada) when compared with other groups (Lichtig et al., 1999; McGillis Hall et al., 2003; Needleman et al., 2002). However, database establishment is complex (Hegyvary, 1991; Jones, 1993), and "getting it wrong" in terms of what variables are included and what is omitted can be very expensive in terms of cost of nurses' time for assessments and recording information, abstracting the information from the patients' charts, and entering it into the database. If information that is not related to outcomes is collected, it becomes an expensive irrelevancy. Alternatively, if something that is highly relevant is omitted from the model that guides the data collection, it is expensive in terms of what questions cannot be asked and answered. In order for databases that house information relevant to nursing to be established for a region or a healthcare system, there must be consensus among nurses regarding (a) what inputs, processes, and outcomes to include, (b) how to define and measure them, and (c) the timing of their measurement, recording, and abstraction. As important as these dimensions of database establishment are, they are matched by the technical dimensions of the availability of electronic systems, the location of and access to the databases for research, and the security systems that must be in place to ensure that patient privacy is protected.

The issue of what to include as an outcome is dependent on the strength of primary research that examines relationships between the myriad of possible effects of nursing care on patients. At least four factors influence this research: (a) the availability of theoretical explanations to link various nursing inputs and processes to outcomes, (b) the need for access to large samples to detect relationships that may be subtle or exist only between subgroups of patients and nursing factors, (c) the ease of accessing these large samples, and (d) appropriate measures that are congruent with the theory supporting the research and that have demonstrated reliability and validity. These are difficult criteria to achieve. There is still little theory linking patient outcomes and antecedent nursing factors. Most of the patient outcomes included in models are empirically rather than theoretically derived and then tested (Mitchell & Shortell, 1997). Failure to rescue (Aiken et al., 1997; Silber et al., 1992) is an exception because it is a theory that links nursing and adverse patient outcomes, specifically mortality. As such, it is of particular interest. However, it is still in the early days of its theoretical life. Some small-scale research studies that demonstrate a statistically significant relationship between a variety of hospital-acquired infections and these adverse outcomes have now been replicated in several large-scale studies using clinical databases as the sources of data. However, in the failure to rescue research to date, the researchers have taken quite different approaches in how they have tested for the phenomenon. Aiken and her team followed Silber et al.'s (1992) approach and defined failure to rescue as the percentage of patients who died relative to the number who either had a complication and died, or died without complication. Needleman et al. (2002) defined failure to rescue as in-hospital death from six specific complications. Significant statistical relationships were found between some of these complications and nursing factors, suggesting that the theory may have explanatory potential and should be further tested. It will be interesting to see how the definition of failure to rescue evolves with further testing.

A concern with adverse outcomes has dominated outcomes research, as exemplified by three of the five projects described in this chapter. One reason for this is their accessibility. Patient complications are recorded on their charts and abstracted into clinical databases. This process allows the researchers to include thousands of patients without the expense and complexity of contacting all of them and eliciting information from them directly. Similarly, records are kept of adverse events such as patient falls, medication errors, and skin breakdown, making this information reasonably easy to retrieve. However, these types of events are plagued by definitional problems. For example, in some institutions, a fall is not recorded unless the patient sustains an injury, whereas in others, a fall is any situation that results in a patient unintentionally arriving on the floor. Mark and Burleson (1995) examined the consistency with which five adverse events were measured across 16 hospitals in 10 states, and the availability of this information. Information was available on medication errors and patient falls but not on nosocomial infections, decubitus ulcers, and unplanned readmissions. However, the descriptions of what constituted a fall and a medication error differed from one hospital to another, and the location of the data varied (for example, on patients' charts, in incident reports, and in quality assurance reports) across even these two outcomes. When more than one institution is involved and hospital discharge records or administrative databases are the sources of data, it is imperative that common definitions across the institutions are assured.

When measuring an outcome of interest requires a scale, as with all research, issues of validity and reliability are highly relevant. A good example of this is found in the work of the Kaiser Permanente group, which elected to construct its own 14-item instrument, the Health Status Outcomes Dimensions, to measure all the outcomes of interest. They refined it until they were satisfied with its reliability and validity and then used it as the basis for assessment and subsequent database development (Lush, Henry, Foote, & Jones, 1997; Ditmyer et al., 1998). In the NSMOS, the investigator group chose to use established instruments to measure all the outcomes of interest. These included the Functional Independence Measure (FIM) and the Medical Outcome Study SF-36 to measure functional status in medical and surgical patients, and the Inventory of Functional Status after Childbirth (IFSAC) to measure the same outcome in obstetrical patients. To assess the effect of illness on role performance across all patient groups, they used the Functional Status II (R). The Brief Pain Inventory-Short Form (BPI-SF) was used to measure the severity of pain and how it affects patients' functioning, and the Caregiver Load Scale was used to assess caregiver burden (McGillis Hall et al., 2003).

There is merit to using established scales if they exist and are valid for assessing the outcomes of interest. This practice is recommended for all research, but it may be a particularly important principle when databases to house outcomes are being created. When established scales are used, results from analyzing the databases can be compared with benchmarks where they exist. Many more explanations may be generated and questions raised when the outcomes of the population represented in the database can be compared with similar and different populations represented in other studies.

Another issue in outcomes research is timing: When should measurements be taken and with what frequency (Hegyvary, 1991; Jones, 1993)? These questions cannot be answered in a vacuum, but are dependent on the nature of the outcome of interest. Furthermore, if the outcomes are to be housed in databases, then the number of times an outcome will be abstracted over a specific time period must be established. For example, if the outcome of interest is falls, then a summary score of all falls experienced during an episode of care may be sufficient. If functional status is the outcome, assessments on admission and discharge from hospital and/ or home care may provide sufficient information for comparisons. However, if the outcome of interest is pain control, a number of assessments of pain at predetermined intervals may have to be established and a decision made as to how many of these will be abstracted for the purposes of research of database housing. When database development is the objective, it is important that the measurement be useful to staff nurses in their ongoing assessment of, and delivery of care to, patients, as well as to the capture of the outcome for the database.

Should nursing develop nursing-specific models and select outcomes whenever possible that are unique to nursing? It is hard to find support for a nursing-centric approach to the study of outcomes; rather, the importance of acknowledging the multidisciplinary nature of health care is emphasized, as is the need to select outcomes that reflect the contributions of the team of providers, as opposed to a discipline within the team (Crawford et al., 1996; Jennings et al., 1999; Jones, 1993; Mitchell et al., 1998). Frankly, it is difficult to identify any outcome that nursing can claim as uniquely reflective of its contribution alone. Selecting outcomes to which many providers can claim partial contribution is more efficient and realistic than seeking nursing-specific variables. Although the Nursing Role Effectiveness Model (Irvine et al., 1998) seeks to represent nursing's unique contribution to patient outcomes, the outcomes themselves are not unique to nursing. They include symptom control, functional status, and self-care knowledge; although evidence links all of them to nursing inputs and processes (Irvine et al.), other disciplines also make contributions to their achievement. Also, there is likely to be more trust across disciplines if established instruments that are recognized by a number of disciplines are used to measure outcomes.

Why Study Outcomes?

Mitchell (2001) searched Medline from 1978 to 1989 using *outcomes* as a key word; no references were elicited. But when the same exercise was undertaken for the years 1997–2000, more than 700 citations were listed. Why have outcomes generated so much interest in the nursing and health services research communities over the last decade? The explanation seems to be accountability. Outcomes are "in" because accountability has become an important expectation of the healthcare system, and they provide evidence for accountability exercises. All components of the healthcare system are now asked to demonstrate their value, whereas their value was taken for granted in the decades preceding the 1990s. Nursing has had little to offer in terms of "hard" evidence when asked to demonstrate that nurses make a difference to patient care. Consequently, over the last decade, there has been increasing activity to fill this gap by identifying outcomes that demonstrate that nurses do make a difference to patients and their experience of illness. The next major breakthrough will be establishing databases that will house these outcomes collected from all patients who receive the services of nursing personnel within a designated system or healthcare sector. These databases can then serve as the source of data for research studies with policy and practice implications. For example, if the research shows that patients achieve better outcomes when specific proportions of registered nurses are present to care for them or when specific organizational structures are in place, the foundations for policy recommendations are laid (Sovie & Jawad, 2001). If other research demonstrates that patients are leaving hospitals or home care programs with insufficient understanding of their health condition to care for themselves safely, the practice implications are obvious.

There is no guarantee that having evidence demonstrating nursing's direct effect on how well patients achieve outcomes that are important to their recovery from illness and to the financial well-being of the healthcare system will influence how nursing is valued, respected, and heard in political and administrative circles. However, we have years of experience indicating that not having this evidence is seriously damaging nursing as a profession and eroding the quality of care available to society.

Purpose of This Review of the State of Science on Nursing-Sensitive Outcomes

In order to establish the databases that will house outcomes from all patients who receive the services of nursing personnel, we need an evidence-based understanding of which outcomes have demonstrated sensitivity to nursing care. In addition, we need evidence on which to make decisions about how to measure these outcomes in a valid and reliable manner. This book seeks to address this need by critically reviewing the state of the evidence on nursing-sensitive outcomes and approaches to their measurement. The outcomes included in this review were selected based on the theoretical/conceptual work undertaken to categorize nursing-sensitive patient outcomes and on the recommendations of members of the Nursing and Health Outcomes Task Force, Ministry of Health and Long-Term Care, Ontario.

The outcomes included in the original review published in 2003 by Doran were functional status, self-care, symptom management, patient safety, and patient satisfaction. This revised text includes three new outcome concepts—psychological distress, healthcare utilization, and mortality. The goal of the analysis is to provide sound information for building a clinical database to document the quality and effectiveness of nursing care in acute, community or home, and long-term care settings.

The specific objectives of this literature analysis are:

- To identify the essential characteristics or attributes defining each outcome concept. This objective was critical for developing a clear conceptual definition of the concepts.
- To determine the extent to which each outcome has demonstrated sensitivity to nursing care. This was accomplished by examining structure and process variables that influence or contribute to the achievement of the functional, symptom, safety, and perceptual outcomes within acute, community, and long-term care settings.
- To identify the instruments that have been used to measure each outcome concept in acute, community, and long-term care settings.
- To review the content of the instruments and assess their congruence/consistency with the essential attributes of each outcome concept (i.e., to determine the content validity of the instruments).
- To critically review the instruments for reliability, validity, responsiveness to change, and sensitivity to nursing care.

FRAMEWORK

The literature review on nursing-sensitive outcomes was guided by two frameworks: (a) the Nursing Role Effectiveness Model (Irvine et al., 1998), which was used as a guide to identify the structure, process, and outcome variables to be included in the review, and (b) a measurement framework (Sidani & Irvine, 1998), which informed and structured the review of the psychometric properties and clinical utility of the instruments measuring the outcomes of interest. The selection of organizational and nursing variables for study was also informed by the work of Mitchell and Shortell (1997), the recent systematic reviews by Bostick et al. (2006), Dall et al. (2009), Kane et al. (2007), and the Delphi study by Van den Heede et al. (2007). An overview of the frameworks is presented in this section.

The Nursing Role Effectiveness Model

The Nursing Role Effectiveness Model was developed by Irvine et al. (1998) to identify the contribution of nurses' roles to outcome achievement. The model is based on the structure-process-outcome model of quality care (Donabedian, 1980). It has been reformulated based on empirical testing (Doran et al., 2006, 2002) (see **FIGURE 1-1**).

The structure component consists of nurses, patients, and organizational variables that influence the processes and outcomes of care. Nurse variables entail professional characteristics such as experience, knowledge, and skill levels, which can influence the quality of nursing care. Patient variables include personal and health- or illness-related characteristics, such as age, type and severity of illness, and comorbidities, that affect either the delivery of care or the achievement of outcomes. Organizational variables focus on staffing and nursing assignment patterns, which directly affect the delivery of nursing care.

The process component consists of the nurses' independent, medical care-related, and interdependent roles. The independent role concerns functions and activities initiated by professional nurses. They refer to autonomous actions initiated by the nurse in response to the patients' problems; they do not require a physician's order. The medical care-related role concerns functions and activities initiated by nurses in response to a medical order. They include the nurse's clinical judgment, implementation of medically directed care, and evaluation of the patient's response to the care. The interdependent role concerns functions and

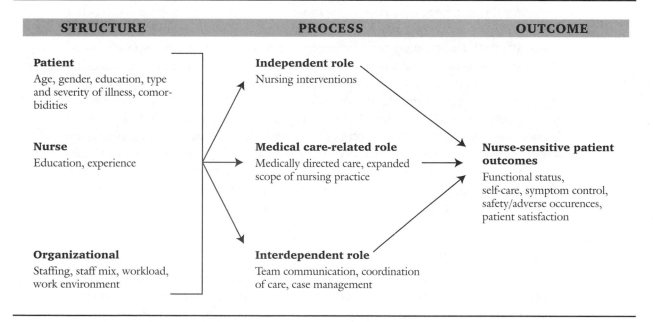

FIGURE 1-1   The nursing role effectiveness model.

Source: Reprinted from Nursing Economic$, 1998, Volume 16, Number 2, pp. 58-64, 87. Reprinted with permission of the publisher, Jannetti Publications, Inc., East Holly Avenue, Box 56, Pitman, NJ 08071-0056; (856) 256-2300; FAX (856) 589-7463; Web site: www.nursingeconomics.net ; For a sample copy of the journal, please contact the publisher.

activities in which nurses engage that are shared by other members of the health-care team. They include activities such as interdisciplinary team communication, care coordination, and health system maintenance and improvement.

The outcome component consists of nursing-sensitive patient outcomes. These are classified into six categories: (a) prevention of complications like injury or noso-comial infections, (b) clinical outcomes such as symptom control, (c) knowledge of the disease, its treatment, and management of side effects, (d) functional health outcomes such as physical, social, cognitive, mental functioning, and self-care abilities, (e) satisfaction with care, and (f) cost.

Irvine et al. (1998) proposed that the structure variables influence the process and outcome variables and that the process affects the outcome variables. They supported the propositions with empirical evidence synthesized from the litera-ture (Irvine et al.) and with an empirical validation of the proposed relationships in acute care settings (Doran et al., 2006, 2002).

Mitchell and Shortell (1997)

Mitchell and Shortell (1997) reviewed the state of the science with respect to morbidity, mortality, and adverse effects as outcomes indicative of variations in organizational variables in care delivery systems. Of the 81 research papers they included in the review, they noted that most research relating mortality and other adverse outcomes to organizational variables has been conducted in acute care hospitals, with these outcome indictors linked more frequently to organizational structures than to organizational or clinical processes. They further noted that there is support in some studies, but not in others, that nursing surveillance, qual-ity of working environment, and quality of interaction with other professionals distinguish hospitals with lower mortality and complications from those with higher rates of these adverse effects. They concluded that adverse events may be a more sensitive marker of differences in organizational quality in acute care hos-pitals and long-term care settings than risk-adjusted mortality outcome, and they challenged researchers to go beyond mortality, morbidity, and adverse events in evaluating the linkage between the organization of care and outcomes.

Recent Reviews

Since the Mitchell and Shortell (1997) review, several more recent reviews have capitalized on the growing literature on nurse staffing and patient outcomes. Some of these reviews were discussed earlier in this chapter, and the findings are summarized here. Bostick et al. (2006) concluded that there is a proven associa-tion between higher total staffing level (especially licensed staff) and improved quality of care in nursing homes. Functional ability, pressure ulcers, and weight loss were identified as the most sensitive quality outcomes linked to staffing in this setting. Dall et al. (2009) concluded that as nurse staffing levels increase in acute care settings, patient risk of nosocomial complications and hospital length of stay decrease, resulting in medical cost savings. In their review, Kane et al. (2007) concluded that increased RN staffing is associated with lower hospital-related mortality in ICUs, in surgical patients, and in medical patients. Taken together, there is good evidence that nurse staffing variables are important structural variables related to patient outcomes. However, this more recent literature demonstrates that the gap observed by Mitchell and Shortell in 1997 regarding the effect of nursing process and organizational process variables on patient outcomes still exists and is an area for further study.

The Nursing Role Effectiveness Model and these systematic reviews guided the selection of variables to be included in the review of the state of the science on nursing-sensitive outcomes. The following structure and process variables that influence the functional, self-care, symptom, safety, and perceptual outcomes of interest were examined:

Structure variables:
- Nurse variables: Education and position, which are often reported in published articles, were used as "proxy" indicators of nurses' knowledge and skill levels.
- Patient variables: Age, gender, and type of illness are frequently reported in published articles. Accumulating evidence is showing that these characteristics influence the patients' responses to some nursing interventions, particularly psychoeducational interventions (Brown, 1992; Hentinen, 1986; Sidani, 1994; Sidani & Braden, 1998).
- Organizational variables: Staffing and staff mix is a variable that has been extensively investigated recently and was found to affect the quality of communication with patients (Doran et al., 2002), adverse occurrences in the hospital (Dall et al., 2009; Needleman et al., 2002), mortality outcome (Kane et al., 2007), and patient satisfaction with care (Lengacher et al., 1996). Evidence is growing that the environment in which nurses work influences the quality of their practice and patient outcome achievement (Aiken et al., 1994; McGillis Hall et al., 2003).

Process variables:
- Nursing independent role functions: Patient education is, by far, the independent nursing activity that has been most commonly investigated in acute, community, and long-term care settings, as evidenced by the number of published meta-analytic studies conducted to synthesize the literature and/or to estimate its effects on various outcomes (e.g., Brown, 1992; Devine & Cook, 1986; Hathaway, 1986). Patient education is usually focused on self-care and symptom management strategies. Doran

et al. (2006) have demonstrated relationships between nursing interventions documented in the healthcare record and patients' functional health outcome.

- Nursing medical care-related role functions: Nurses are assuming direct medical care-related activities with the development of advanced practice roles, such as nurse practitioner (Aiken et al., 1993; Garrard et al., 1990). Furthermore, some practice settings are experimenting with nurse-led inpatient units as a way to provide cost-effective care for less resource-intensive patient populations (Griffiths et al., 2001).
- Nursing interdependent role functions: Coordination of discharge planning and nurse-led case management are two examples of the interdependent functions assumed by nurses in acute, community, and long-term care settings. Their impact on clinical and functional patient outcomes (e.g., Braden, Mishel, Longman, & Burns, 1989; Piette, Weinberger, & McPhee, 2000) has been investigated less frequently than their impact on perceptual outcomes (e.g., Moher, Weinberg, Hanlon, & Runnalls, 1992; Naylor et al., 1999).

Outcome variables:
- Clinical outcomes: Symptom control has been extensively investigated in postsurgical patients, with a particular focus on pain control (Tuman et al., 1991) and in oncology inpatient and outpatient settings (Smith, Holcombe, & Stullenbarger, 1994).
- Functional outcomes: Physical and psychosocial functioning and self-care abilities were outcomes of concern for patients with chronic and acute illness (Doran et al., 2006, 2002; Gillette & Jenko, 1991).
- Patient safety outcomes: These have been the foci of nursing report cards (ANA, 1995, 1996, 1997, 2000; Pierce, 1997) and studies involving secondary databases (Needleman et al., 2002).
- Perceptual outcomes: Satisfaction with nursing care has been examined in a multitude of studies investigating nursing care delivery models (ANA, 1997; Gillette & Jenko, 1991; Lang & Marek, 1990).

Measurement Framework

This literature review and analysis is aimed at providing information that will guide the development of a database for monitoring outcomes of nursing care. Building this database rests on the availability of standardized measures of the outcomes that have the ability to collect accurate data with minimal error. Instruments that have been used to measure the outcomes of interest were identified, and their ability to obtain valid data was critically analyzed. The following framework guided the critical review of the outcome measures. The framework was based on the premise that for an instrument to be useful in accurately measuring or monitoring outcomes, it should demonstrate acceptable reliability, validity, responsiveness, and clinical utility.

Reliability

Reliability refers to the dependability of measurement. It concerns the extent to which measurements are consistent and reproducible across items, individuals, or occasions; that is, it introduces minimal error. Three types of reliability can be assessed:

- Internal consistency: the degree to which the items comprising the instrument are interrelated and able to measure a single concept or domain/dimension of a concept with minimal error. Internal consistency is most commonly assessed with the Cronbach's alpha coefficient (Streiner & Norman, 1995). It is based on the average correlations among the items. An alpha coefficient value of .70 is considered the minimal acceptable level of internal consistency for newly developed instruments, and .80 is the minimum for established instruments (Nunnally, 1978).
- Stability or test-retest: the degree to which the instrument reproduces similar scores for the same individuals when measured at different occasions. Stability is frequently evaluated with a correlation coefficient. A coefficient > 0.70 indicates an acceptable level of stability (Streiner & Norman, 1995).
- Equivalence or interrater: the degree of agreement between raters/observers. It is examined using any of the following statistical tests: percent of agreement among the raters, Cohen's Kappa coefficient, Pearson's correlation coefficient, or intraclass correlation coefficient. A coefficient value ≥ .80 indicates acceptable interrater reliability.

Validity

Validity is concerned with whether an instrument measures what it is supposed to measure; that is, it should accurately reflect all the domains and dimensions of the concept. Different types of validity can be assessed:

- Content validity: the degree to which the content of the items comprising the instrument covers all the domains of the concept it is supposed to measure. It is evaluated by having experts or judges rate the extent to which the items capture all the domains and the relevance of the items' content to their corresponding domain. A content validity index ≥ .80 represents an acceptable level of agreement among the experts, which supports content validity (Lynn, 1986).
- Criterion or concurrent validity: the correspondence between a measure and a criterion (i.e., another instrument measuring the same concept) administered at the same or different points in time. This type of validity is assessed by computing a correlation coefficient or by conducting sensitivity and specificity analyses. A correlation coefficient ≥ .50 and sensitivity

and specificity values ≥ 90% provide empirical support for an instrument's criterion or concurrent validity (Beutler, Wakefield, & Williams, 1994).

- Construct validity: assesses whether a measure is related to other variables in a way that is consistent with theoretically derived predictions. It is evaluated in one of two ways. The first way is to examine the difference in the mean score on the measure between two groups of individuals known to differ on the concept of interest, using a t test or F ratio. A statistically significant difference supports the construct validity of the measure. The second way to evaluate construct validity is to examine the correlation coefficients between the measure of the concept of interest and the measures of related concepts. Statistically significant correlations between the measures of the hypothesized direction and magnitude provide evidence of construct validity (Waltz, Strickland, & Lenz, 1991).

Responsiveness

Responsiveness refers to the instrument's sensitivity to changes in the level of the concept being measured. Evidence for responsiveness includes significant differences in the mean scores obtained at different points in time, such as before and after treatment. The evidence for responsiveness is strengthened when changes in the scores are correlated with other indicators of change, such as clinically assessed changes. No specific criteria indicating responsiveness are well established (Guyatt, Deyo, Charlson, Levine, & Mitchell, 1989).

Clinical Utility

Instruments to be used by clinicians in their everyday practice must be useful. To be clinically useful, an instrument needs to be simple; that is, it does not take much time to complete, it is easy to use or does not require a special technique or extensive training to administer, it is easy to score, and the scores are easy to interpret (Corcoran & Fischer, 1987; Sidani & Irvine, 1998). Although there are no well-defined criteria for evaluating clinical utility, the following information was reported for the instruments: number of items comprising it, amount of time to complete it, and availability of cutoff scores or normative values that could be used as a reference for interpreting the obtained scores (i.e., determining clinically meaningful categories for classifying patients).

METHODOLOGY FOR CONDUCTING THE LITERATURE REVIEW

The literature review was conducted through a series of consecutive steps. Three general categories of references were included—theoretical (or conceptual), systematic reviews, and empirical—in order to address all the objectives set for the review. Theoretical/conceptual references discussed a perspective of how the clinical, functional, safety, or perceptual outcomes are viewed. That is, they presented theoretical and/or operational definitions of the outcomes. The definitions identify the essential characteristics of the outcome concept and point to its domains and indicators. Systematic reviews provided a synthesis of the state of the evidence concerning the relationship between nurse or organizational structural variables, nurse or organizational process variables, and an outcome concept. Empirical articles reported the results of descriptive-correlation or experimental studies that examined the relationships among structure, process, and outcome variables; assessed the psychometric properties of outcome measures; or evaluated the effectiveness of nursing interventions in achieving the desired outcomes.

Step 1: Literature Search

The first step of the literature review consisted of identifying conceptual and empirical references that discussed or investigated the clinical, functional, and perceptual outcomes of interest in acute, community, and long-term care settings. The literature search involved four strategies:

- A comprehensive list was generated of relevant articles, book chapters, books, or other documents that the research team members accumulated through their involvement in previous work on any of the structure, process, or outcome variables of interest to this review.
- A computerized literature search was conducted to update and obtain a comprehensive list of references on the variables of interest in the acute, community, and long-term care patient populations. The following computerized literature databases were used in this step: CINHAL, HEALTH PLANNING, MEDLINE, CANCERLIT, SOCIOFILE, and PSYCHLIT. The Virginia Henderson library, an electronic database that holds reports of completed and in-progress research studies, dissertations, and conference presentations, was also checked for additional references.
- The literature search strategy entailed using specific key words relevant to the outcomes under review. Examples include *functional status*, nausea, *fatigue*, pain, and *self-care*. These specific key words were paired with common key words that were used for each search. The following common key words were used: *nursing-sensitive patient outcomes*, nursing interventions, *nursing care*, quality of nursing care, *nursing outcomes*, patient, and *quality of care*.
- The references reported within the articles, in particular those reporting the results of meta-analytic studies or integrative literature reviews/syntheses (e.g., Heater, Becker, & Olson, 1986; Smith et al., 1994), were traced to identify additional references.

Step 2: Literature Selection

The references identified were included in the literature review if they met the following criteria.

For theoretical/conceptual references:

- They discussed the definition and the domains/dimensions of the functional, self-care, symptom, safety, and patient satisfaction outcome concepts of interest.
- They presented the findings of a concept analysis or literature review performed to identify the essential characteristics, domains, and dimensions, as well as the empirical indicators or manifestations, of the outcome concepts of interest.
- They reported the results of a qualitative study conducted to explore the understanding or perception of the functional, self-care, symptom, safety, or satisfaction outcomes in acute, community, or long-term care settings.

For empirical references:

- They described the development of an instrument used to measure the outcomes of interest in patients in acute, community, or long-term care settings.
- They reported the results of testing the psychometric properties of the instrument in the patient populations of interest.
- They described the instrument in detail and discussed its clinical utility and its applicability or use in practice settings.
- They reported the results of studies that examined the relationships among the structure, process, and outcome variables selected for this review (as identified in the framework section).
- They reported the results of studies that examined the effects of interdependent, independent, or medical care-related nursing functions/interventions (as delineated in the framework section) on the functional, self-care, symptom, safety, and satisfaction outcomes in acute, community, or long-term care settings.

Studies with experimental or quasi-experimental designs were included. Including quasi-experimental studies was important for two reasons: (a) it increased the number of references for the comprehensive literature review, particularly studies that were conducted in the context of actual/everyday practice where randomization may not have been feasible or possible, and (b) it provided evidence for determining the extent to which the outcomes are responsive to change. Differences in research designs were accounted for when synthesizing the findings across studies to address the objectives set for this literature review.

Step 3: Literature Compilation

A list of references was generated for each of the functional, self-care, symptom, safety, and patient satisfaction outcomes of interest. Each author assumed primary responsibility for reviewing the literature pertinent to an outcome. A standardized framework and tables for extracting the relevant data were used to promote a consistent approach to the review among all authors. As the editor of the book, Dr. Doran oversaw and coordinated the activities of all members of the team. The results of the critical analysis of the literature are presented in the chapters that follow.

Each chapter provides a discussion of how the particular outcome concept has been conceptualized in the nursing literature. A conceptual definition is proposed based on this evidence. The empirical evidence linking patient outcome to nursing inputs or processes is critically examined. The approaches to measurement are reviewed with regard to the reliability, validity, and sensitivity of the outcome instrument to nursing variables. Recommendations are proposed related to the strength of the evidence concerning the relationship between nursing practice and patient outcomes. Then recommendations are also made about approaches to the measurement of the outcome concept. The chapters conclude with directions for further research.

REFERENCES

Aiken, L. H., Clarke, S. P., Sloane, D. M., Lake, E. T., & Cheney, T. (2008). Effects of hospital care environment on patient mortality and nurse outcomes. *Journal of Nursing Administration, 38*(5), 223–229.

Aiken, L. H., Clarke, S. P., Sloane, D. M., Sochalski, J. A., Busse, R., Clarke, H., et al. (2001, May–June). Nurses' reports on hospital care in five countries. *Health Affairs,* 43–53.

Aiken, L. H., Lake, E. T., Semaan, S., Lehman, H. P., O'Hare, P. A., Cole, C. S., et al. (1993). Nurse practitioner managed care for persons with HIV infection. *Image: Journal of Nursing Scholarship, 25,* 172–177.

Aiken, L. H., Smith, H. L., & Lake, E. T. (1994). Lower medical mortality among a set of hospitals known for good nursing care. *Medical Care, 32,* 171–187.

Aiken, L. H., Sochalski, J., & Lake, E. T. (1997). Studying outcomes of organizational change in health services. *Medical Care, 35*(Suppl.), NS6–NS18.

Al-Hader, A. S., & Wan, T. T. (1991). Modeling organizational determinants of hospital mortality. *Health Services Research, 26,* 303–323.

American Nurses Association. (1995). *Nursing report card for acute care.* Washington, DC: American Nurses Publishing.

American Nurses Association. (1996). *Nursing quality indicators.* Washington, DC: American Nurses Publishing.

American Nurses Association. (1997). *Implementing nursing's report card.* Washington, DC: American Nurses Publishing.

American Nurses Association. (2000). *Nurse staffing and patient outcomes in the inpatient hospital setting*. Washington, DC: American Nurses Publishing.

Anderson, K. L., & Burckhardt, C. S. (1999). Conceptualization and measurement of quality of life as an outcome variable for health care intervention and research. *Journal of Advanced Nursing, 29*, 298–306.

Beaulieu, M. J. (2009). Failure to rescue as a process measure to evaluate fetal safety during labor. *MCN, American Journal of Maternal Child Nursing, 34*, 18–23.

Beutler, L. E., Wakefield, P., & Williams, R. E. (1994). Use of psychological tests/instruments for treatment planning. In M. E. Maruish (Ed.), *The use of psychological testing for treatment planning and outcome assessment* (pp. 55–74). Hillsdale, NJ: Lawrence Erlbaum.

Bostick, J. E., Rantz, M. J., Flesner, M. K., & Riggs, C. J. (2006). Systematic review of studies of staffing and quality in nursing homes. *Journal of the American Medical Directors Association, 7*, 366–376.

Braden, C. J., Mishel, M. H., Longman, A., & Burns, L. R. (1989). *Nurse interventions promoting self-help response to breast cancer*. Washington, DC: National Cancer Institute.

Brown, S. A. (1992). Meta-analysis of diabetes patient education research: Variations in intervention effects across studies. *Research in Nursing and Health, 15*, 409–419.

Cohen, J., Gorenberg, B., & Schroeder, B. (2000). A study of functional status among elders at two academic nursing centers. *Home Care Provider, 5*(3), 108–112.

Corcoran, K., & Fischer, J. (1987). *Measures for clinical practice: A sourcebook*. New York: The Free Press.

Crawford, B. L., Taylor, L. S., Seipert, B. S., & Lush, M. (1996). The imperatives of outcomes analysis: An integration of traditional and nontraditional outcomes measures. *Journal of Nursing Care Quality, 10*(2), 33–40.

Dall, T. M., Chen, Y. J., Seifert, R. F., Maddox, P. J., & Hogan, P. F. (2009). The economic value of professional nursing. *Medical Care, 47*, 97–104.

Devine, E. C., & Cook, T. D. (1986). Clinical and cost-saving effects of psychoeducational interventions with surgical patients: A meta-analysis. *Research in Nursing and Health, 9*, 89–105.

Ditmyer, S., Koepsell, B., Branum, V., Davis, P., Lush, M.T. (1998). Developing a nursing outcomes measurement tool. *Journal of Nursing Administration, 28*, 10–16.

Donabedian, A. (1966). Evaluating the quality of medical care. *Milbank Quarterly, 44*(Suppl.), 166–206.

Donabedian, A. (1980). *Exploration in quality assessment and monitoring: The definition of quality and approaches to its assessment*. Ann Arbor, MI: Health Administration Press.

Doran, D, M. (2003). *Nursing-sensitive outcomes: State of the science*. Sudbury, MA: Jones and Bartlett.

Doran, D. M., Harrison, J. M., Spence-Laschinger, H., Hirdes, J., Rukhom, E., Sidani, S., et al. (2006). The relationship between nursing interventions and outcome achievement in acute care settings. *Research in Nursing and Health, 29*, 61–70.

Doran, D. M., McGillis Hall, L., Sidani, S., O'Brien-Pallas, L., Donner, G., Baker, G. R., et al. (2002). Nursing staff mix and patient outcome achievement: The mediating role of nurse communication. *Journal of International Nursing Perspectives, 1*, 74–83.

Friese, C. R., & Aiken, L. H. (2008). Failure to rescue in the surgical oncology population: Implications for nursing and quality improvement. *Oncology Nursing Forum, 35*, 779–785.

Garrard, J., Kane, R. L., Radosevich, D. M., Skay, C. L., Arnold, S., Kepferle, L., et al. (1990). Impact of geriatric nurse practitioners on nursing-home residents' functional status, satisfaction, and discharge outcomes. *Medical Care, 28*, 271–283.

Gillette, B., & Jenko, M. (1991). Major clinical functions: A unifying framework for measuring outcomes. *Journal of Nursing Care Quality, 6*, 20–24.

Griffiths, P., Harris, R., Richardson, G., Hallett, N., Heard, S., & Wilson-Barnett, J. (2001). Substitution of a nursing-led inpatient unit for acute services: Randomized control trial of outcomes and cost of nursing-led intermediate care. *Age and Aging, 30*, 483–488.

Guyatt, G. H., Deyo, R. A., Charlson, M., Levine, M. N., & Mitchell, A. (1989). Responsiveness and validity in health status measurement: A clarification. *Journal of Clinical Epidemiology, 42*, 403–408.

Guyatt, G. H., Feeny, D. H., & Patrick, D. L. (1993). Measuring health-related quality of life. *Annals of Internal Medicine, 118*, 622–629.

Harrison, M. B., Juniper, E. F., & Mitchell-DiCenso, A. (1996). Quality of life as an outcome measure in nursing research. *Canadian Journal of Nursing Research, 28*(3), 49–68.

Hartz, A. J., Krakauer, H., Kuhn, E. M., Young, M., Jacobsen, S. J., Gay, G., et al. (1989). Hospital characteristics and mortality rates. *New England Journal of Medicine, 321*, 1720–1725.

Hathaway, D. (1986). Effect of preoperative instruction on postoperative outcomes: A meta-analysis. *Nursing Research, 35*, 269–275.

Heater, B. S., Becker, A. K., & Olson, R. K. (1988). Nursing interventions and patient outcomes: A meta-analysis of studies. *Nursing Research, 37*, 303–307.

Hegyvary, S. T. (1991). Issues in outcomes research. *Journal of Nursing Quality Assurance, 5*(2), 1–6.

Hentinen, M. (1986). Teaching and adaptation of patients with myocardial infarction. *International Journal of Nursing Studies, 23*(2), 125–138.

Hirdes, J., Fries, B. E., Morris, J. N., Ikegami, N., Zimmerman, D., Dalby, D. M., et al. (2004). Home care quality indicators (HCQIs) based on the MDS-HC. *The Gerontologist, 44*, 665–679.

Hirdes, J. P., Fries, B. E., Morris, J. N., Steel, K., Mor, V., Frijters, D., et al. (1999). Integrated health information systems based on the RAI/MDS series of assessment instruments. *Healthcare Management Forum, 12*(4), 30–40.

Hirdes, J. P., Frijters, D. H., & Teare, G. F. (2003). The MDS-CHESS scale: A new measure to predict mortality in institutionalized older people. *Journal of the American Geriatrics Society, 51*, 96–100.

Hirdes, J. P., Smith, T. E., Rabinowitz, T., Yamauchi, K., Perez, E., Curtin Telegdi, N., et al. (2002). The Resident Assessment Instrument-Mental Health (RAI-MH): Inter-rater reliability and convergent validity. *Journal of Behavioral Health Services and Research, 29*, 419–432.

Horn, S. D., Buerhaus, P., Bergstrom, N., & Smout, R. J. (2005). RN staffing time and outcomes of long-stay nursing home residents. *American Journal of Nursing, 105*, 58–70.

Irvine, D., Sidani, S., & McGillis Hall, L. (1998). Linking outcomes to nurses' roles in health care. *Nursing Economic$, 16*(2), 58–64, 87.

Jackson, M., Chiarello, L. A., Gaynes, R. P., & Gerberding, J. L. (2002). Nurse staffing and healthcare-associated infections. *Journal of Nursing Administration, 32*, 314–322.

Jennings, B. M., Staggers, N., & Brosch, L. R. (1999). A classification scheme for outcome indicators. *Image: Journal of Nursing Scholarship, 31*, 381–388.

Jones, K. (1993). Outcomes analysis: Methods and issues. *Nursing Economic$, 11*, 145–152.

Kane, R. L., Shamliyan, T. A., Mueller, C., Duval, S., & Wilt, T. J. (2007). The association of registered nurse staffing levels and patient outcomes: Systematic review and meta-analysis. *Medical Care, 45*, 1195–1204.

Kutney-Lee, A., & Aiken, L. H. (2008). Effect of nurse staffing and education on the outcomes of surgical patients with comorbid serious mental illness. *Psychiatric Services, 59,* 1466–1469.

Lang, N. M., & Marek, K. D. (1990). The classification of patient outcomes. *Journal of Professional Nursing, 6,* 153–163.

Lengacher, C. A., Mabe, P. R., Heinenmann, D., VanCott, M. L., Swymer, S., & Kent, K. (1996). Effects of the PIPC model on outcome measures of productivity and costs. *Nursing Economics, 14,* 205–212.

Lichtig, L. K., Knauf, R. A., & Milholland, D. K. (1999). Some impacts of nursing on acute hospital outcomes. *Journal of Nursing Administration, 29*(2), 25–33.

Lohr, K. N. (1985). *Impact of Medicare prospective payment on the quality of medical care: A research agenda.* Santa Monica, CA: Rand.

Lush, M. (2001). Continuity across sectors. In *Invitational Symposium, Nursing and Health Outcomes Project, March 15 and 16, 2001, Toronto, Ontario, Canada.*

Lush, M. T., Henry, S. B., Foote, K., & Jones, D. L. (1997). Developing a generic health status measure for use in a computer-based outcomes infrastructure. In U. Gerdin, M. Tallberg, & P. Wainwright (Eds.), *Nursing informatics* (pp. 229–234). Amsterdam: IOS Press.

Lynn, M. R. (1986). Determination and quantification of content validity. *Nursing Research, 35,* 382–385.

Mark, B. A., & Burleson, D. L. (1995). Measurement of patient outcomes. *Journal of Nursing Administration, 25*(4), 52–59.

McGillis Hall, L., Doran, D., Baker, G. R., Pink, G., Sidani, S., O'Brien Pallas, L., et al. (2003). Nurse staffing models as predictors of patient outcomes. *Medical Care, 41,* 1096–1109.

McGillis Hall, L., Doran, D., & Pink, G. (2004). Nurse staffing models, nursing hours and patient safety outcomes. *Journal of Nursing Administration, 34,* 41–45.

Mitchell, P. (2001). The evolving world of outcomes. In *Invitational Symposium, Nursing and Health Outcomes Project, March 15 and 16, 2001, Toronto, Ontario, Canada.*

Mitchell, P. H., Ferketich, S., & Jennings, B. M. (1998). Quality health outcomes model. *Image: Journal of Nursing Scholarship, 30,* 43–46.

Mitchell, P. H., & Shortell, S. M. (1997). Adverse outcomes and variations in organization of care delivery. *Medical Care, 35*(Suppl.), NS19–NS32.

Moher, D., Weinberg, A., Hanlon, R., & Runnalls, K. (1992). Effects of a medical team coordinator on length of hospital stay. *Canadian Medical Association Journal, 146,* 511–515.

Naylor, M. D., Brooten, D., Campbell, R., Jacobson, B. S., Mezey, M. D., Pauly, M. V., et al. (1999). Discharge planning and home follow up by advanced practice nurses reduced hospital readmissions of elderly patients. *Journal of the American Medical Association, 281,* 613–620.

Needleman, J., Buerhaus, P., Mattke, S., Stewart, M., & Zelevinsky, K. (2002). Nurse-staffing levels and the quality of care in hospitals. *New England Journal of Medicine, 346,* 1715–1722.

Nunnally, J. C. (1978). *Introduction to psychological measurement.* New York: McGraw-Hill.

Pierce, S. F. (1997). Nurse-sensitive health care outcomes in acute care settings: An integrative analysis of the literature. *Journal of Nursing Quality, 11*(4), 60–72.

Piette, J. D., Weinberger, M., & McPhee, S. J. (2000). The effect of automated calls with telephone nurse follow-up on patient-centered outcomes of diabetes care. A randomized, controlled trial. *Medical Care, 38,* 218–230.

Pringle, D. M., & White, P. (2002). Happenings. Nursing matters: The Nursing and Health Outcomes Project of the Ontario Ministry of Health and Long-Term Care. *Canadian Journal of Nursing Research, 33,* 115–121.

Rowell, P. A. (2001). ANA study on nursing-sensitive outcomes. In *Invitational Symposium, Nursing and health Outcomes Project, March 15 and 16, 2001, Toronto, Ontario, Canada.*

Scherb, C. A. (2002). Outcomes research: Making a difference in practice. *Outcomes Management, 6,* 22–26.

Shortell, S., & Hughes, E. (1988). The effects of regulation, competition, and ownership on hospital rates among hospital inpatients. *New England Journal of Medicine, 318,* 1100–1107.

Sidani, S. (1994). *Empirical testing of a conceptual model to evaluate psychoeducational interventions.* Unpublished doctoral dissertation, University of Arizona, Tucson.

Sidani, S., & Braden, C. J. (1998). *Evaluating nursing interventions. A theory-driven approach.* Thousand Oaks, CA: Sage.

Sidani, S., & Irvine, D. (1998, June). *Defining and operationalizing clinical utility of instruments.* Paper presented at the Nursing Research Conference, Edmonton, Alberta, Canada.

Silber, J. H., Rosenbaum, P. R., Romano, P. S., Rosen, A. K., Wang, Y., Teng, Y., et al. (2009). Hospital teaching intensity, patient race, and surgical outcomes. *Archives of Surgery, 144,* 113–120.

Silber, J. H., Williams, S. V., Krakauer, H., & Schwartz, J. S. (1992). Hospital and patient characteristics associated with death after surgery: A study of adverse occurrence and failure to rescue. *Medical Care, 30,* 615–629.

Smith, M. C., Holcombe, J. K., & Stullenbarger, E. (1994). A meta-analysis of intervention effectiveness for symptom management in oncology nursing research. *Oncology Nursing Forum, 21,* 1201–1210.

Sovie, M. D., & Jawad, A. (2001). Hospital restructuring and its impact on outcomes: Nursing staff regulations are premature. *Journal of Nursing Administration, 31,* 588–600.

Stone, P. W., Mooney-Kane, C., Larson, E. L., Horan, T., Glance, L. G., Zwanziger, J., et al. (2007). Nurse working conditions and patient safety outcomes. *Medical Care, 45*(6), 571–578.

Streiner, D. L., & Norman, G. R. (1995). *Health measurement scales. A practical guide to their development and use* (2nd ed.). Oxford, England: Oxford University Press.

Tourangeau, A. E. (2003). Modeling the determinants of mortality for hospitalized patients. *International Nursing Perspectives, 3*(1), 37–48.

Tourangeau, A. E., Doran, D. M., McGillis Hall, L., O'Brien Pallas, L. L., Pringle, D., Tu, J. V. et al. (2007). Impact of hospital care on 30-day mortality for acute medical patients. *Journal of Advanced Nursing, 57*(1), 32–44.

Tuman, K., McCarthy, R., March, R., Delaria, G., Patel, R., & Ivankovich, A. (1991). Effects of epidural anesthesia and analgesia on coagulation and outcome after vascular surgery. *Anesthesia Analgesia, 73,* 696–704.

Van den Heede, K., Clarke, S. P., Sermeus, W., Vleugels, A., & Aiken, L. H. (2007). International experts' perspectives on the state of the nurse staffing and patient outcomes literature. *Journal of Nursing Scholarship, 39,* 290–297.

Van den Heede, K., Sermeus, W., Diya, L., Clarke, S. P., Lesaffre, E., Vleugels, A., et al. (2009). Nurse staffing and patient outcomes in Belgian acute hospitals: cross-sectional analysis of administrative data. *International Journal of Nursing Studies, 46,* 928–939.

Van Servellen, G., & Schultz, M. A. (1999). Demystifying the influence of hospital characteristics on inpatient mortality rates. *Journal of Nursing Administration, 29*(4), 39–47.

Waltz, C. F., Strickland, O. L., & Lenz, E. R. (1991). *Measurement in nursing research* (2nd ed.). Philadelphia: F. A. Davis.

Functional Status

Diane Doran

INTRODUCTION

"Functional health status has emerged as an important patient outcome because (a) it captures patients' perceptions of their day-to-day functioning and (b) it adds another perspective to more traditional outcomes such as adverse occurrences and physiological clinical data" (Ramler, Kraus, Pringle Specht, & Titler, 1996, p. 72). Maintaining and enhancing the individual's ability to achieve functional independence in personal care, mobility, and social activities has been identified as a goal of nursing in many of the nursing theoretical frameworks (e.g., Olson, 2001; Orem, 1980; Roy & Roberts, 1981). Furthermore, it has been included as a concept in most of the outcome classifications for nursing (Gillette & Jenko, 1991; M. Johnson & Maas, 1997) and has been suggested as a relevant outcome of care for staff nurses (Brown & Grimes, 1995; Irvine, Sidani, & McGillis Hall, 1998; Kline Leidy, 1994; Pringle & White, 2002; Van den Heede, Clarke, Sermeus, Vleugels, & Aiken, 2007) and advanced practice nurses (Mill Barrell, Irving Merwin, & Poster, 1997). Several empirical studies have demonstrated that nursing interventions can have an effect on functional status outcomes (Brown & Grimes, 1995; Doran, et al., 2006, "Nursing-Sensitive Outcomes"; Doran, McGillis Hall, et al., 2002; McCorkle et al., 1989). In a meta-analysis examining the effect of nursing interventions on patient outcomes, Heater, Becker, and Olson (1988) reported a mean effect size of 0.63 for behavioral outcomes and 0.54 for

29

psychosocial outcomes. Both types of outcomes reflect aspects of human functioning. A Delphi study of international experts' perspectives on the state of nurse staffing and patient outcomes literature reached 85% consensus that functional status is a nursing-sensitive outcome (Van den Heede et al., 2007).

Doran conducted a critical review of the literature examining the relationship between nursing and patients' functional status outcomes in 2003 and concluded that there is evidence from both experimental and quasi-experimental studies that functional status is sensitive to nursing intervention; however, the evidence was not conclusive. Stronger associations between functional status outcomes and nursing variables were observed in the quasi-experimental studies than in the randomized controlled trials. Furthermore, the strength of relationship between nursing variables and functional status outcomes varied depending on the approach to measurement. More specifically, the strongest association was observed in studies in which functional status was operationalized as activities of daily living (ADLs) and assessed with the Katz Activities of Daily Living Scale (S. Katz & Akpom, 1976). It is timely to update this systematic review of the functional status literature for several reasons. First, the strength of the evidence needs to be reappraised to take into account studies conducted post-2003. Second, a variety of functional status measures have been used in the empirical literature, and they should be reappraised in light of more recent evidence. It is important to appraise the sensitivity of new measures to nursing variables so that decisions can be made about which instruments are appropriate for measuring functional status in different practice settings.

This chapter provides a synthesis of the findings from the previous review reported by Doran (2003) and the findings from the updated literature review conducted post-2003. In this chapter, the way in which functional status has been conceptualized as an outcome of nursing care is examined, and then a conceptual definition of functional status is proposed based on this evidence. The empirical evidence linking patients' functional status outcomes to nursing inputs or process is critically examined. The approaches to measurement are reviewed with regard to the reliability, validity, and sensitivity of the functional status instrument to nursing variables. Recommendations are proposed related to the strength of the evidence concerning the relationship between nursing practice and functional health outcomes, and approaches to the measurement of functional status. The chapter concludes with directions for further research.

The methodology used to identify the relevant literature, as well as the criteria for the literature selection and systematic review, was discussed in Chapter 1. A systematic search of the nursing and health databases was conducted for the years 2003–2009. Three general categories of references were examined in appraising functional status as an outcome of nursing care: theoretical or conceptual, empirical, and systematic reviews/ meta-analyses. The key words used in the search included: *function, functioning, functional ability, functional capacity, functional status, functional performance, physical function, functional assessment, activities of daily living, independent living,* and *functional health status.* These search terms were selected because functional status is the degree of functional ability, and researchers usually have assessed functional status or functional ability with measures of ADLs, instrumental activities of daily living (IADLs), functional performance, and physical performance (Gu & Conn, 2008). The search was conducted by a reference librarian. After eliminating duplicate citation of sources across the databases, the search yielded a total of 62 new sources. Thirty-six of these sources met the criteria for inclusion in the literature review. These sources were reviewed, and the findings were integrated with those from the previous review that had included 75 empirical and conceptual papers, yielding a total of 111 papers that were included in this current review. Although the focus of the search was nursing-relevant literature, in some instances, nonnursing sources were included when these sources addressed key conceptual and/or methodological issues pertinent to our addressing the objectives of the study.

THEORETICAL BACKGROUND: DEFINITION OF THE CONCEPT

Knight (2000) published a paper on two concepts, cognitive ability and functional status, that offered a very nice overview of the development of functional status as a concept. She noted that in the early literature, discussion of functional status focused on an individual's ability to engage in ADLs such as bathing, dressing, feeding, and motor performance (Knight). In the middle to late 1980s, as providers became more focused on shorter hospital stays and outcomes that reflected an individual's ability to live at home, measures began to emerge that addressed usual daily activities other than ADLs (Knight). Functional status became a descriptor for IADLs such as shopping, cooking, and cleaning. In addition, functional status was used to describe broad functioning in major aspects of living such as the social, occupational, and psychological (Knight). According to Knight, Moinpour, McCorkle, and Saunders (1988) proposed one of the earliest comprehensive definitions of functional status in nursing. They defined functional status measurement as "any systematic attempt to measure the level at which a person is functioning in a variety of areas, such as physical health, quality of self-maintenance, quality of role activities, intellectual status, social activity, attitude toward the world and toward self, and emotional status" (cited in Knight, 2000, p. 1463).

In her conceptual analysis, Knight (2000) noted that the conceptualization of functional status must include cognitive, behavioral, and psychological dimensions. The behavioral dimension typically has been operationally defined as performance of ADLs and IADLs. Knight suggested that the psychological dimension might include components such as mood, affect, and motivation. The cognitive dimension might include components such as attention, concentration, memory, and problem solving. Fawcett, Tulman, and Samarel (1995) identified a psychological and social dimension to functional status. The psychological element of function included mental, cognitive, emotional, and spiritual activities. The social element included activities associated with roles taken on at various stages of development, as well as activities associated with interpersonal relationships (Fawcett et al., 1995).

Cooley (1998) defined functional status as the individual's actual performance of normal day-to-day role activities. These included performance of (a) basic ADLs, such as bathing, dressing, eating, and walking, and (b) carrying out role responsibilities both in and out of the house, such as cleaning, cooking, shopping, and working. Richmond, McCorkle, Tulman, and Fawcett (1997) defined the term *function* as how people perform activities that are relevant to them.

Many terms have been used interchangeably in the literature to refer to functional status. Among them are *function,* functioning, *functional ability,* functional capacity, *functional status,* functional performance, *physical function,* impairment, *handicap,* functional assessment, *activities of daily living,* health status, and *quality of life* (Fawcett et al., 1995; Richmond et al., 1997). Ouellet and Rush (1996), for example, conducted a qualitative study of nurses' perceptions of client mobility that yielded results very similar to those of studies in which functional status had been conceptualized. Nurses in their study described mobility as having three dimensions: physical, cognitive, and social. The physical dimension was expressed as movement of the body, performance of ADLs, and performance of IADLs. Nurses defined mobility as "the ability...to move...either by walking or by moving a joint.... Ability to move through space from point A to point B" (p. 570). Under categories related to ADLs or self-care, nurses included references to instrumental activities, such as, "Can they use the phone, do they do their own affairs, do they do their banking...can they make out their grocery list, can they phone the grocery store, can they order..." (p. 571). The social dimension was described by the nurses as movement of an affiliative nature that enables one to initiate and maintain contact with others through social events and activities. The cognitive dimension was defined as movement of the mind that seeks to keep it active. Cognitive mobility was reflected in such references as keeping up, stimulating the mind, and having an active mind. Critical qualities of mobility emerged from the qualitative data. These included ease of movement, independence, and safety. In a more recent study, Bourret, Bernick, Cott, and Kontos (2002) investigated the meaning of mobility for residents and staff in long-term care facilities. The qualitative results indicated that "the dimensions of mobility for residents included not only the independent performance of physical tasks and activities of daily living, but also the ability to get out of bed and get around the institution on one's own" (p. 342). Independence was an important defining characteristic of mobility.

Wang (2004) conducted a concept analysis of functional status, using the Walker and Avant (1994) concept analysis guidelines. She identified three critical attributes of functional status that appear consistently in the literature: activities that people do in the normal course of their lives to meet basic needs, fulfill usual roles, and maintain their health and well-being. The first two attributes are consistent with the view of functional status as encompassing ADLs and IADLs. Wang concluded that functional status "can best be represented by actual activities performed in various aspects of life, which include personal care, ambulation, household activity, recreational activity, and community participation" (p. 461).

The way in which functional status has been operationally defined within the nursing literature reflects its multidimensional nature. Functional status outcomes have included ADLs (Chang, Hancock, Hickman, Glasson, & Davidson, 2007; Doran et al., 2006, "The Relationship"; Dorman Marek, Popejoy, Petroski, & Rantz, 2006; Horn, Buerhaus, Bergstrom, & Smout, 2005; Schein, Gagnon, Chan, Morin, & Grondines, 2005), physical and social functioning (Bruggink-André de la Porte et al., 2007; Lang & Clinton, 1984; Latour et al., 2006; Peri et al., 2008), role functioning (Naylor, Munro, & Brooten, 1991), cognitive and mental functioning (Aydelotte, 1962; Naylor et al.; Waltz & Strickland, 1988), continence and mobility (M. Johnson & Maas, 1997; Kerse et al., 2008; McCormick, 1991), self-care (Gillette & Jenko, 1991), and home functioning (Lang & Marek, 1990).

Several theorists have drawn a distinction between functional status and functional ability (Knight, 2000; Richmond et al., 1997). For them, functional ability refers to the actual or potential capacity to perform biological, psychological, and social activities normally expected of an individual at a particular age and developmental stage (Knight; Richmond et al.). Functional status or functional performance refers to individuals' actual performance of activities and tasks associated with their current life roles (Wang, 2004). These include basic, instrumental, and advanced ADLs (e.g., working, traveling, engaging in hobbies, and participating in social and religious groups; Richmond et al.).

Kline Leidy (1994) offered an analytic framework for understanding the concept of functional status. She defined it as

> a multidimensional concept characterizing one's ability to provide for the necessities of life; that is, those activities people do in the normal course of their lives to meet basic needs, fulfill usual roles, and maintain their health and well-being. . . . Necessities include, but are not limited to, physical, psychological, social, and spiritual needs that are socially influenced and individually determined. (p. 197)

Furthermore, Kline Leidy (1994) suggested that functional status has four dimensions: capacity, performance, reserve, and capacity utilization. Functional capacity refers to "one's maximum potential to perform those activities people do in the normal course of their lives to meet basic needs, fulfill usual roles, and maintain their health and well-being" (p. 198). She defined functional performance as "the physical, psychological, social, occupational, and spiritual activities that people actually do in the normal course of their lives to meet basic needs, fulfill usual roles, and maintain their health and well-being" (p. 198). These activities are the outcome of individual choice, subject to the limits imposed by capacity. The physical component of functional performance consists of activities motivated by personal bodily needs, that is, ADLs such as dressing, eating, and bathing, and IADLs that enable meeting those needs (Kline Leidy). Kline Leidy suggested that the psychological component consists of activities involving mental health and personal growth, including hobbies or favorite pastimes, such as music, reading, or gardening, and sharing personal concerns with another. The social component includes activities involving interaction with the community and family, such as attending parties or organizational meetings, visiting friends, or phoning relatives. Work activities are included in occupational task performance. The spiritual component encompasses those activities involved in developing spiritual perspective, including devotional activities, meditation, attendance at religious ceremonies or worship services, or volunteer work (Kline Leidy).

According to Kline Leidy (1994), functional reserve is defined as "the difference between capacity and performance, one's functional latency or dormant abilities that can be called upon in time of perceived need" (p. 199). Functional capacity utilization refers to "the extent to which functional potential is called upon in the selected level of performance" (p. 199).

In summary, the early definitions of functional status were narrower in their defining characteristics than what is reflected in the recent literature. Theorists in the literature reviewed in this chapter recognized that functional status includes the basic and instrumental activities of daily living, as well as social, work-related, and spiritual dimensions. Moreover, they considered it important to distinguish the term *functional ability, which encompasses the capacity to perform, from* functional status, which refers to the actual performance of an activity or behavior. The latter is more often the focus of interest when functional status is investigated as an outcome of nursing care.

CONCEPTUAL DEFINITION

Based on the theoretical review, functional status is viewed as a multidimensional construct that consists of, at least, behavioral (e.g., performance of activities of daily living), psychological (e.g., mood), cognitive (e.g., attention, concentration), and social (e.g., activities associated with roles at various stages of development) components. A distinction is made between functional status, the actual performance of an activity, and functional ability, the capacity to perform a given function or activity (Knight, 2000).

FACTORS THAT INFLUENCE FUNCTIONAL STATUS

Individuals' performance of ADLs, work, social, and family role activities is influenced by internal, external, and cultural factors (Fawcett et al., 1995). The individual's health status, attitude, and demographic characteristics are some of the internal influences on functional status (Bourret et al., 2002; Fawcett et al., 1995; Tulman & Fawcett, 1990). For example, functioning is influenced by a positive attitude (Bourret et al.), physical energy (Tulman & Fawcett), and the existence of "acute illness (e.g., pneumonia) and chronic illnesses (e.g., diabetes, cancer, and bipolar disease)" (Fawcett et al., p. 53). The normative beliefs and values that govern role expectations and behavior are examples of the cultural determinants of functional status (Fawcett et al.). The physical characteristics of the environment and access to mobility aids such as canes and wheelchairs are examples of external factors that influence functional status (Bourret et al.). Other external influences include social supports that individuals have in their environment and financial resources (Fawcett et al.; Zemore & Shepel, 1989). Studies have shown that 30–60% of older people develop new dependencies in ADLs during a hospital stay (Hoogerduijn, Schuurmans, Duijnstee, de Rooij, & Grypdonck, 2006). A systematic review of predictors of functional decline among older hospitalized patients found that risk of decline was predicted by age, lower functional status on admission, cognitive impairment, preadmission disability in IADLs, depression, and length of hospital stay (Hoogerduijn et al.). These internal, external, and cultural factors need to be taken into consideration when assessing functional status. Furthermore, when planning and evaluating a nursing intervention, it is important to consider the role of these factors in affecting outcome achievement.

ISSUES IN ASSESSING FUNCTIONAL STATUS

Several important issues concerning the assessment of functional status emerged from the review of the literature. These included: (a) who should assess functional status, (b) what constitutes good outcomes with regard to functional status, (c) how one controls for the impact of aids, adaptations, and helpers (Kaufert, 1983), (d) how one controls for situational variation and motivation factors (Kaufert), (e) whether one should control for the patient's role expectation in the performance of certain functions (Kaufert), (f) what the advantages and disadvantages are of ADL versus IADL scales to measure functional status (Rubenstein, Schairer, Wieland, & Kane, 1984), and (g) whether one can use secondary sources to assess functional status.

Whose Perspective Should Be Considered When Functional Status Is Assessed?

Clinicians and patients often have differing perspectives of the patients' functional ability, with the latter being more optimistic in their view than the clinicians. Reiley et al. (1996) found that nurses' predictions about patients' functional status 2 months after discharge were significantly more pessimistic than warranted. The nurses often overestimated the functional disability of their patients. Rubenstein et al. (1984) found that patients rated themselves higher on ADL and IADL items than nurses, who in turn rated patients higher than a community proxy, such as a spouse or child. The items most likely to show incongruence between the patient and the nurse were ambulation, dressing, bathing, and grooming.

What Constitutes a Good Outcome with Regard to Functional Status?

Although improvements in functional status constitute a good outcome for many patient populations, this is not the case for all of them. Hirdes and Carpenter (1997) noted that for the frail elderly, if restoration of complete independence is not possible, preventing decline and maintaining a stable level of function could be indicative of a successful intervention. In the case of inevitable decline, it may be reasonable to focus on slowing its rate. Moreover, it may not be possible to affect all aspects of functioning, but optimizing specific areas (e.g., cognition) and avoiding pain may have a profound effect on well-being (Hirdes & Carpenter).

How Does One Control for the Impact of Aids, Adaptations, and Helpers?

Kaufert (1983) observed that not all approaches to the assessment of functional status account for the fact that some individuals may successfully use an assistive device or helper, without which they could not attain the same level of function. One approach to control for variation in the effect of the use of aids and helpers is to develop more complex systems for summarizing functional status that also control for the level of difficulty encountered and for consistency of performance (Kaufert, 1983).

How Does One Control for Situational Variation and Motivation Factors?

Situational factors may influence functional performance and thus be a source of variation in performance ratings. Kaufert (1983) also noted that "subjects being assessed by clinicians who are directly involved in their treatment, for example, may attempt to maximize secondary gains by over- or under-representing their level of disability. Additionally, validity comparisons must distinguish between a subject's potential physical ability to perform a function and his actual performance" (p. 264). To minimize the impact of volitional factors, many indices ask, "Do you perform a function?" not "Are you able to perform the function?" (p. 264). Kaufert suggested that "to minimize situational variation, alternate measurement should be made in similar situations" (p. 264).

Whether One Should Control for the Patient's Role Expectation in the Performance of Certain Functions

Cultural expectations about the roles of men and women are important to consider when assessing functional status outcomes (Kaufert, 1983). Furthermore, it is important to establish whether the individual activities being assessed are relevant to the independent functioning of the population being studied or treated (Kaufert).

The Advantages and Disadvantages of ADL versus IADL Measures

The behavioral component of functional status has been measured with ADL and IADL scales. Rubenstein et al. (1984) argued that IADL scales possess several limitations not shared by ADL scales. These include a lack of Guttman scalability, a greater sensitivity of score to variations in mood and emotional health, a greater difficulty in measuring IADLs in institutional settings, and an overemphasis on traditional women's tasks (such as cooking, cleaning, and laundering; Rubenstein et al.). Confirming the lack of sensitivity of IADL items in institutional settings, Meissner, Andolsek, Mears, and Fletcher (1989) found significant improvements on Katz's ADL items between admission and discharge for patients admitted to a dedicated geriatric unit with specialized nursing, but no significant change over time in the instrumental activities of daily living items.

Assessing Functional Status Based on Secondary Sources

One approach to assessing outcomes, including functional status outcomes, is through using data from secondary sources, such as the patient record. This method is economical and unobtrusive because it capitalizes on data that have already been collected for another purpose and does not burden the patient with additional data collection. Burns et al. (1992) evaluated the congruence between self-report and a medical record-derived measure of functional status. Data were collected on 2,504 patients over 65 years of age who were discharged from the hospital alive. A personal interview conducted before hospital discharge recorded the patient's self-reported ability to perform ADLs. Medical record abstraction was used to determine ability to perform the same ADLs. The amount of missing medical record functional status data varied by function, from 20% for bathing to 50% for dressing. Within each function, the amount of missing information was least for patients with a hip fracture and most for patients with chronic obstructive lung disease and congestive heart failure. Overall, the medical record tended to document less dependence than patients reported. On dressing, for example, the medical record contained documentation that 40% of the total population was dependent, but 73% of the population reported themselves as dependent (Burns et al.). Sensitivity of the medical record ranged from 48% for dressing to 68% for transferring. Specificity ranged from 64% for bathing to 83% for feeding. Patients consistently reported more dependencies than were documented in the medical record (Burns et al.).

In summary, a number of issues need to be considered when assessing functional status. The research evidence suggests that patients have a different view of their functional ability than clinicians. Therefore, it is important to clarify whose perspective is the focus of assessment. Second, maintaining functional performance or slowing the rate of decline may be a good outcome for some populations, such as older persons. Third, instruments used to assess functional status should account for the level of difficulty encountered in the activity and the ability to perform with physical aids. Furthermore, instruments assessing functional status need to be sensitive to cultural norms and role expectations for different patient populations. ADL measures are probably more sensitive to functional status change in the institutional setting than IADL measures. To date, there is not good evidence that functional status can be reliably and validly assessed from secondary sources.

EVIDENCE CONCERNING THE RELATIONSHIP BETWEEN NURSING AND PATIENTS' FUNCTIONAL STATUS OUTCOMES

Two types of evidence were considered in assessing the strength of association between functional status outcomes and nursing variables: evidence from systematic review or meta-analyses and evidence from empirical studies. Each is reviewed next, starting with evidence from systematic reviews.

Systematic Reviews

Thompson, Lang, and Annells (2008) conducted a systematic review of the effectiveness of in-home community nurse-led interventions for the mental health of older persons. The review considered randomized controlled trials, quasi-experimental studies, and qualitative studies. Nine studies met the inclusion criteria, of which one was a randomized controlled trial. The authors included studies that assessed the effect of nursing interventions on mental health functioning. They confined their focus to interventions provided by registered nurses who were generalists and employed by an organization providing home-based health care. Interventions of interest were those carried out in a patient's home and that specifically intended to facilitate the mental health of the patient. Three nurse-led interventions were reported as having some benefit for mental health outcomes: individualized management plans, total quality management (TQM) approach, and the PATCH model intervention (i.e., a nurse-based outreach program for identifying and treating psychiatric illness in the elderly). Each of these interventions was embedded in interdisciplinary collaboration. The findings of this review were modest with regard to the impact of community nursing interventions on mental health functioning. Weaknesses in study designs made it difficult to draw strong conclusions.

Huss, Stuck, Rubenstein, Egger, and Cough-Gorr (2008) conducted a systematic review and meta-analysis of studies investigating the effectiveness of preventive home visit programs for community-dwelling older adults. Although they did not differentiate nursing home visits from other provider visits, the paper is included in this chapter because it is one of the only meta-analyses of interventions for functional health outcomes found and because nurses are the dominant providers of home care visits. Trial results of functional decline were heterogeneous—with trials overall having little effect on functional decline—with a combined odds ratio (OR) of 0.89 (95% confidence interval [CI], 0.76–1.03). However, studies that included a clinical examination in the initial home visit showed a beneficial effect on functional status decline with an OR of 0.64 (95% CI, 0.48–0.87).

Doucette (2005) conducted a review of the literature to determine whether nursing-led inpatient units are more effective than usual inpatient care in preparing patients for discharge. Eight randomized controlled trials, two quasi-randomized controlled trials, and one controlled before-after study met the inclusion criteria. The outcomes assessed included functional status at discharge. At discharge, patients who received care in a nursing-led unit had better functional status outcomes than patients receiving care on general ward units (six studies). A similar review was conducted by Griffiths et al. (2001). Griffiths et al. reviewed nine randomized or quasi-randomized controlled trials. The mean age of patients in all studies was over 70 years. The nursing-led units were associated with reduced odds of discharge to institutional care (OR 0.44, 95% CI 0.22–0.89) and better functional status at discharge (standardized mean difference 0.37, 95% CI 0.20–0.54).

Bostick, Rantz, Flesner, and Riggs (2006) conducted a systematic review of studies of staffing and quality in nursing homes. The review encompassed a total of 87 citations/research articles published in English from 1975 to 2003. The authors concluded that functional ability, pressure ulcers, and weight loss are the most sensitive outcome indicators linked to nurse staffing.

Latour et al. (2007) conducted a systematic review of literature investigating nurse-led case management for ambulatory complex patients in general healthcare settings. Only 2 studies of the 10 reviewed measured functional status as an outcome. The authors concluded that there was no evidence that nursing case management has a positive effect on the functional status of patients.

A fourth systematic review and meta-analysis by Gu and Conn (2008) assessed the effects of exercise interventions on functional status in older adults. Modest but statistically significant effects were found for functional performance and physical performance but not for ADL. However, in this review, it is not possible to differentiate exercise interventions provided by nurses from those provided by other care providers.

In summary, evidence from systematic reviews and meta-analyses supports the view that functional status is a nursing-sensitive outcome. Nurse-led inpatient units have been associated with slower functional decline and reduced odds of discharge to institutional care. Nurse staffing variables in long-term settings have been associated with reduced functional decline. Community nursing interventions have been associated with improvements in mental health functioning; however, this conclusion is based on findings from studies of variable methodology design quality.

Empirical Studies

Fifty-four empirical studies were identified and are reviewed in **TABLE 2-1**. Thirty-nine of these studies evaluated a nursing intervention in which functional status was an outcome measure. The other 14 studies described the development and/or testing of a functional status instrument that was used within a nursing context or that described the relationship between nurse staffing variables and functional status outcomes.

Of the 54 empirical studies reviewed, 21 were published prior to 2000, and 35 studies were published in 2000 or later. The mean age of participants in the studies ranged from 39 to 84 (median = 70 years). Sample size varied from 14 to 1,376 participants. Seventeen studies had a sample size of less than 100, whereas five studies had a sample size of over 1,000 participants. Twenty of the studies were conducted in an acute care hospital setting, 12 in a community setting, 5 in a long-term care or residential care setting, 1 in a rehabilitation setting, 9 in an outpatient setting, and 3 in a primary care setting, and 3 involved both hospital and community settings. Five of the studies conducted in the acute care setting are relevant for long-term patient populations because in each case, the studies examined the effectiveness of dedicated geriatric beds or care for postacute older patient populations.

TABLE 2-1 Studies Investigating the Relationship Between Nursing Variables and Functional Status

Author/ date	Design	Sample characteristics/ setting	Definition of the outcome concept	Intervention being evaluated/ nursing variable being evaluated	Results	Limitations
Aiken et al. (1993)	Prospective cohort	Patient with HIV infection N = 87 (RR = 84%); university outpatient setting; (The NP group had more women)	Symptom occurrence (author developed) & self-care management (author developed); functional status (Medical Outcome Study Short Form, SF-36)	Nurse practitioner managed care vs. physician care	NP patients reported significantly more symptoms (even after controlling for gender); NP patients reported poor health status; no significant difference between cohorts in the SF-36 subscales.	No information about the reliability and validity of the symptom and self-care instruments.
Alexy & Elnitsky (1998)	Case control pretest/ posttest; baseline assessment and then 12–15 postbaseline assessment	Recipients of mobile health unit (n = 190); project's home visit component (n = 32) N = 222	Functional status (Katz, α .89); health status (two self-report questions); IOWA Self-Assessment Inventory [economic resources (α .90), anxiety/ depression (α .84), physical health (α .68), alienation (α .83), mobility (α .83), cognitive status (α .79), social support (α .80)]; nutrition screening (α .40); Geriatric Depression Scale (Yesavage et al., 1983)	Community-based mobile health unit; clients participated in the project from 5 to 28 months (mean = 14.8), with a mean number of visits of 7.9; staffed by family nurse practitioner (FNP), MSCN nurse, and two FNP students	There was a significant decline between the baseline and follow-up measures for the ADL scale (in the areas of continence and bathing) ($t = 2.83, p < .005$; mean 15.76 to 15.68 for community group; 12.75 to 11.21 for home group). There was a significant decline in the IADL scores; community 13 vs. 12.70; home 7 versus 6.40; $t = 2.61$, $p < .01$).	Impossible to rule out a Hawthorne effect because of lack of a true control group; small number in the home visit sample.

Note. ADLs = activities of daily living; IADLs = instrumental activities of daily living; MD = medical doctor; MDS = minimum data set; MDS-HC = minimum data set for home care; RR = sample response rate; RCT = randomized control trial.

(continues)

TABLE 2-1 Studies Investigating the Relationship Between Nursing Variables and Functional Status (continued)

Author/date	Design	Sample characteristics/setting	Definition of the outcome concept	Intervention being evaluated/nursing variable being evaluated	Results	Limitations
Barr Mazzuca et al. (1997)	RCT; prospective data collection over five times at 8-week intervals for 32 weeks	Community setting; adults, insulin dependent; N = 22 (RR not stated); age range 49–83	Dietary adherence and weight; foot care (King, 1978); blood glucose monitoring; diabetes knowledge [Michigan Diabetes Research Training Center]; self-care behaviors (The Self-Care Behaviors Questionnaire; Mendenhall, 1991); functional health status (SF-36; α .69 to .89)	Community health nursing by senior undergraduate nursing students	No significant difference over time in the health status measures.	Small sample may have resulted in lack of power to test for significant change over time.
Boockvar, Brodie, & Lachs (2000)	Descriptive	409-bed nursing home; three floors; all daytime nursing assistants rated residents; all residents were observed (n = 74)	Illness Warning Instrument based on behavioral changes	No intervention	Primary outcome was acute illness (researcher went on rounds with nurses weekly to identify episodes of acute illness). Criteria for illness were limited to physical exam and lab tests. A resident for whom one or more of the five acute changes were endorsed was 4.1 times more likely to develop an illness within the next 7 days than a resident for whom no change was endorsed. The final instrument had a sensitivity of 53%, a positive predictive value of 17%, and a negative predictive value of 96%.	Testing limited to one setting.

Bruggink-André de la Porte et al. (2007)	RCT; prospective baseline, 3 months, 12 months	Netherlands Heart failure clinic; $N = 240$ (RR=51%); Intervention ($n =118$), control ($n =1220$; mean age 71 years)	Health status (quality of life): SF-36	Physician- and nurse-directed follow-up heart failure clinic	At 3 months, no significant difference in total scores SF-36. Greater change in SF-36 score for intervention compared with control group at 12 month follow-up ($p = .02$).	No reported results for SF-36 subscales; no reliability for the total score.
Chan, Mackenzie, Tin-Fu, & Leung (2000)	Pretest/ posttest, RCT	Hong Kong 80% diagnosis of schizophrenia; mean age = 39. $N = 62$; 31 in the experimental and control group, respectively	Clinical and functional status: Brief Psychiatric Rating Scale (BPRS); Specific Level of Functioning Scale (SLOF, α reported .80); Risser Client Satisfaction	Newly developed model for nurse case management vs. conventional care by case managers	Clients in the experimental group showed more improvement on the BPRS in areas such as tension, suspiciousness, hallucinatory behavior, and thought disturbance; experimental group showed better improvement in SLOF personal care skills, interpersonal relationships, social acceptability, and community living skills. Significant difference between experimental and control subjects on the Risser scale for time to listen and talk to clients and feeling secure when being cared for by NCM.	
Chang et al. (2007)	Pretest/ posttest	Australia Acutely ill older adults (≥ 65 years); $N = 348$; 232 preimplementation and 116 patients postimplementation	Activities of daily living: Barthel Activity of Daily Living Index (Mahoney & Barthel, 1965)	Nursing-led age-care-specific ward	There was a significant difference between preintervention and postintervention patient groups on Barthel ADL scores ($p < .01$). Intervention patients were more independent in ADLs than preintervention patients. Intervention patients also had significantly higher improvements in ADL scores at discharge compared with preintervention patients.	Nonrandom-ized. No control for history or differences in patient charac-teristics.

Note. ADLs = activities of daily living; IADLs = instrumental activities of daily living; MD = medical doctor; MDS = minimum data set; MDS-HC = minimum data set for home care; RR = sample response rate; RCT = randomized control trial.

(continues)

TABLE 2-1 Studies Investigating the Relationship Between Nursing Variables and Functional Status (continued)

Author/date	Design	Sample characteristics/setting	Definition of the outcome concept	Intervention being evaluated/nursing variable being evaluated	Results	Limitations
Cohen et al. (2000)	Prospective, single-cohort design: 6-month and 1-year intervals	Community setting; elderly clients receiving services from nurses; *n* = 68; mean age = 81.5; 79% women	Functional status is defined as the ability to perform and adapt to the environment; OARS	Nurse-managed centers (NMCs; neighborhood center & apartment building); services include assessment, medication review, safety counseling, symptom and illness management, and personal care	There were no changes in scores among the total sample for any subscale of the OARS.	
Dalton (2001)	Case study	Community clients receiving cardiac disease management; *N* = 51; subsample (*n* = 40) used to examine outcomes post-hospital discharge	Functional status (OASIS)	Cardiac disease management home care program	Improvement in the level of functioning was reflected in all the functional status indicators.	Small sample size; lack of a control group; no information about statistical significance provided.
Doran et al., (2006), "Nursing-Sensitive Outcomes"; Doran et al. (2006), "The Relationship"	Longitudinal descriptive design; outcome data collected at admission and discharge	Canada Hospitalized adults *N* = 574 (RR = 88%); complete data on 471. Mean age 63 years; female 51%	Functional status: ADLs assessed with MDS	Nursing interventions assessed through chart audit using the Nursing Intervention Classification (NIC)	Significant relationship (*p* < .05) between nursing interventions involving exercise promotion, positioning, and self-care assistance, and ADL outcomes.	

(continues)

Doran, McGillis Hall, et al. (2002)	Longitudinal	Canada Medical-surgical patients in 19 teaching hospitals; staff nurses (n = 1,085, RR = 97%); patients (n = 835, RR = 87%); 74 units	Ability to engage in ADLs and mobility assessed with Functional Independent Measure (FIM) instrument (α .87 Time 1, .88 Time 2)	Nurse staff mix (proportion of RN/RPN staffing); nurse communication (Shortell et al. 1991)	The proportion of RN staffing, nurse experience, and effectiveness of nurses' communication had positive effects on patients' functional independence at discharge.
Doran, Sidani, et al. (2002)	Cross-sectional	Canada Medical-surgical patients in one teaching hospital; patients (n = 372, RR = 73%); nurses (n = 245, RR = 35%); 26 units	Functional status: ability to resume usual ADLs; therapeutic self-care ability	Educational preparation of nurses; staff mix; quality of nursing care (Shortell et al., 1991; α .94); quality of nurse communication (Shortell et al.; α .85) and coordination of care (Shortell et al.; α .77); nurse role tension (Lyons, α .78); and autonomy (Hackman & Oldham, α .71).	Quality of nursing care was positively related to higher levels of therapeutic self-care and functional status at hospital discharge.
Dorman Marek et al. (2006)	Comparative, longitudinal design; 6- and 12-month follow-up	USA Older adults (> 64 years) in nurse-led community-based long-term care program (n = 55); control (n = 30) were older adults receiving community-based care without nurse-led coordination	Functional health outcomes: OASIS; ADLs, incontinence, cognitive performance, depression, pressure ulcers assessed with MDS	Nurse-led coordination in community-based long-term care	At 12 months, the intervention group scored better than the comparison group in the outcomes of pain, dyspnea, and ADLs.

Note. ADLs = activities of daily living; IADLs = instrumental activities of daily living; MD = medical doctor; MDS = minimum data set; MDS-HC = minimum data set for home care; RR = sample response rate; RCT = randomized control trial.

TABLE 2-1 Studies Investigating the Relationship Between Nursing Variables and Functional Status (continued)

Author/date	Design	Sample characteristics/setting	Definition of the outcome concept	Intervention being evaluated/nursing variable being evaluated	Results	Limitations
Fawcett & Tulman (1990)	Cross-sectional	Hospital and home setting; Mothers of newborns	Functional status defined as "the degree to which new role responsibilities and usual role activities are performed" (Inventory of Functional Status after Childbirth [IFSAC])	No intervention	Content validity of the IFSAC instrument established at 96.7%; construct validity supported by relative independence of the subscales with correlations ranging from 0.01 to 0.53.	
Gagnon et al. (1999)	RCT; baseline data; 10-month follow-up	Frail elders; intervention ($n = 212$); control (usual care, $n = 215$); setting: university hospital and two community health centers	Quality of life (SF-36); Client Satisfaction Questionnaire; ADLs and IADLs (Older Americans Resource & Services Multidimensional Functional Assessment [OARS]); hospital admissions and emergency room visits	Nurse case management providing in-hospital and outpatient services over a 10-month period	There were no significant differences between elders in the interventions and control group in SF-36 physical functioning, role physical, bodily pain, general health, vitality, social functioning, role emotional, or mental health. No differences in OARS functional ability or satisfaction with care. Greater average number of ED visits in the NCM group.	
Garrard et al. (1990)	Quasi-experimental; baseline, 3-, 6-, and 12-month assessments	Nursing homes: five with NP and five without; two cohorts (long stay, new admission); $N = 848$ (RR 43% by 12 months); 64% female; mean age = 80.24 in admission cohort, 82 in long-stay cohort	Satisfaction (author developed); mental status (derived from Short Portable Mental Status Questionnaire); functional status (author developed)	Geriatric nurse practitioners	For the new admission cohort, residents on nongeriatric NP units improved in functional status more than NP units. There was no significant change in functional status scores for the long-stay cohort, except for affect, with greater improvement in the non-NP units.	Differences between the nursing homes other than having NPs could have confounded the study results; limited psychometric testing of the functional status measure.

Study	Design	Setting/Sample	Functional Status Measure	Intervention	Findings	Limitations
Griffiths (1996); Griffiths et al. (2000, 2001)	RCT; T1 = 24 h of referral and 48 h prior to discharge	Hospital setting; inpatients; N = 112 (RR = 84.2%); mean age = 77; 37% male	Functional independence (Barthel Index); N = 153 (RR = 76.62%)	Nurse-led intermediate care unit *vs.* usual care unit	There were no statistically significant differences between the treatment and control groups in functional independence at discharge, although the difference was large and in favor of the nurse-led unit (73 compared with 53).	It is impossible to rule out the Hawthorne effect or other confounding variables because of the absence of a control group; no information about the reliability of the modified Barthel Index in this study.
Hamilton & Lyon (1995)	Quasi-experimental; one-group pretest/posttest	Hospital setting; geriatric; N = 74; 54% women; mean age = 81	Functional status was defined as the person's ability to carry out ADLs (Modified Barthel Index); mental status was defined as cognitive function in areas of orientation, attention, memory, and language (Mini-Mental State)	CNS-provided clinical support for nurses on a medical unit with six dedicated geriatric beds and where nurses practiced modular nursing	There was significant improvement in functional ability on all items of the Barthel Index between admission and discharge from the unit.	
Harrell et al. (1989)	Cross-sectional	Hospital; two medical units; N = 150; age 65–93 (mean = 74)	Functional status (Katz Activities of Daily Living)	Nursing diagnoses gathered through retrospective chart review following discharge	Those patients who improved in functional status from admission to discharge had the most number of nursing diagnoses. Predictors of functional status at discharge included Katz score at admission and nursing diagnosis of moving.	Small sample size; testing limited to one setting involving only two patient care units.
Heafey et al. (1994)	Descriptive, retrospective review of charts	Hospital and home; subjects with lower extremity amputation (N = 96); 58.3 % males; mean age = 60, for males = 60, for females = 68	Safety awareness and functional ability (Safety Assessment and Functional Evaluation [SAFE] tool, developed in-hospital)	Rehabilitation following lower extremity amputation	Patients demonstrated an improvement in functional status scores from the time of admission to discharge.	No information provided about the psychometric properties of the functional status instrument.

Note. ADLs = activities of daily living; IADLs = instrumental activities of daily living; MD = medical doctor; MDS = minimum data set; MDS-HC = minimum data set for home care; RR = sample response rate; RCT = randomized control trial.

(continues)

TABLE 2-1   Studies Investigating the Relationship Between Nursing Variables and Functional Status (continued)

Author/date	Design	Sample characteristics/setting	Definition of the outcome concept	Intervention being evaluated/nursing variable being evaluated	Results	Limitations
Helberg (1993)	Correlational	Home care patients (N = 367); primarily White; average age = 66	Functional status (OARS; Pfeffer, 1975); Cronbach's alpha .84.	Home care nursing	Physical ADLs at admission correlated with independent discharge status (r = .29), institutionalized (r = −.19), and died (r = −.27; IADLs correlated with independent at discharge (r = 0.31), need for family/community support (r = −0.16), and died (r = −0.19).	
Holzemer & Henry (1992)	Descriptive	Hospital; general medical-surgical units with AIDS patients; N = 74 male patients with HIV-related pneumocystis	Functional status (measured with the Quality Audit Marker); internal consistency, total scale 0.90	Use of a computer-generated vs. manually generated nursing care plan	There were no significant differences in functional status, nutrition/elimination, and social isolation between those patients with the computer-supported care plans and those with the manually generated care plans.	Small sample size; nonrandom sampling procedure.
Horn et al. (2005)	Retrospective design	USA 82 long-term care facilities, N = 1,376 long-term care residents	Functional health status (ADLs): MDS	Nurse staffing time (number of minutes for direct care provided by RNs, LPNs, & CNAs)	More RN direct care time per resident day was associated with less deterioration in the ability to perform ADLs.	
Howard & Reiley (1994)	Correlational	Patients admitted to a medical service of one hospital; N = 87; mean age = 65	Functional status (not explicitly defined): Katz Index	Nursing intensity system (author developed). Interrater reliability range from .82 to .99; Cronbach's alpha in this study for Nursing Intensity = 0.84	Correlation between patient age and Katz (r = .88) and nursing intensity rating (r = .81); there were significant differences in functional status scores between patients admitted from home vs. from rehab, nursing home, or other hospital for the Katz instrument and the Nursing Intensity system.	Small sample size; no information about the psychometric properties of the Katz instrument in this study.

Study	Design	Sample	Measures	Intervention	Findings	Limitations
Irvine et al. (2000)	Correlational; prospective over two points in time	Clients requiring community nursing; average age = 61; 60% female	Functional health status (SF-36); reliability ranged from .76 to .94; quality of life (Quality of Life Profile: Seniors Version [QOLPSV]; Raphael, Smith, Brown, & Renwick, 1995); reliability ranged from .47 to .82	Community nursing visits	There was a significant improvement in health status scores for seven of the subscales of the SF-36 between Time 1 and Time 2. There was a significant improvement in four of the subscales of the QOLPSV over time. The proportion of visits made by an RN was significantly related to change in SF-36 subscales: bodily pain, vitality, and mental health.	Small sample size.
J. E. Johnson, Fieler, Saidel Wlasowicz, Mitchell, & Jones (1997)	Quasi-experimental; control: preintervention; experimental: postintervention; data collected prospectively over four points in time (pretreatment to 1 month posttreatment)	Patients with breast or prostate cancer; $N = 226$ (RR = 77%)	Outcome expectancies (The Life Orientation Test [LOT]); mood (Profile of Mood States [POMS]); reliability ranged from .77 to .83; disruption in usual life activities (Sickness Impact Profile [SIP]); SIP subscales had reliability of .66 to .88 except for the mobility subscale (α .43 to .54)	Nurses were trained to incorporate "self-regulation" theory into their practice	The experimental group, as opposed to the control group, had a 31% reduction in disruption in home management at 4 weeks and a 53% reduction at 1 month posttreatment; In the experimental group, pessimistic patients were more positive than in the control group.	

Note. ADLs = activities of daily living; IADLs = instrumental activities of daily living; MD = medical doctor; MDS = minimum data set; MDS-HC = minimum data set for home care; RR = sample response rate; RCT = randomized control trial.

(continues)

TABLE 2-1   Studies Investigating the Relationship Between Nursing Variables and Functional Status (continued)

Author/date	Design	Sample characteristics/setting	Definition of the outcome concept	Intervention being evaluated/nursing variable being evaluated	Results	Limitations
Kerse et al. (2008)	RCT	Residential care facilities, New Zealand. N = 682 (RR = 83%); control = 352; intervention = 330. 74% female; average age 84	Mobility and function: Timed "up and go" (TUG; Podsialdo & Richardson, 1991); mobility: Elderly Mobility Scale (Smith, 1994); self-reported function: Late Life Function and Disability Questionnaire (Sayers et al., 2004)	Physical activity intervention delivered by gerontology nurse in residential care settings	A significant interaction existed between cognition and group status for the overall scale of the Late Life Function and Disability instrument ($p = 0.024$). For residents with normal cognition, the activity group deteriorated less in overall function (Late Life Function and Disability Instrument, total function component score) in the first 6 months of follow-up. A similar significant interaction ($p = 0.015$) in the lower limb subscale score of the Late Life Function and Disability Instrument showed a maintenance in score in the activity group for those with normal cognition (intervention group score 48.8 at baseline, 48.1 at 6 months, and 47.7 at 12 months; control group 49.5, 45.9, and 46.5) but no differences in the cognitively impaired subgroup.	
Kolt et al. (2007)	RCT	Older community dwelling, low active adults from primary care practices in New Zealand. N = 186; age ≥ 65	Change in physical activity (as measured using the Auckland Heart Study Physical Activity Questionnaire) and quality of life (as measured using the SF-36 over a 12-month period)	Eight telephone counseling sessions	Moderate leisure physical activity increased by 86.8 min/wk more in the intervention group than in the control group ($p = .007$). More participants in the intervention group reached 2.5 hours of moderate or vigorous leisure physical activity per week after 12 months (42% vs. 23%, odds ratio = 2.9, 95% confidence interval = 1.33–6.32, $p = .007$). No differences on SF-36 measures were observed between the groups at 12 months.	

Krichbaum (2007)	RCT; prospective, 12 month follow-up	USA Elders (age > 65 years) with hip fracture postdischarge; N = 33 (RR = 33%); females (n = 73%); average age 78 years	Functional status: Functional Status Index (FSI; Jette et al., 1986)	Gerontology advanced practice nurse postacute care coordination	There was no significant difference between intervention and control groups. Both groups experienced significant improvement in functional status. However the intervention group had better management of ADLs at 3-month follow-up.	Low response rate.
Latour et al. (2006)	RCT, 24 week follow-up	Netherlands Postdischarge N = 208; Intervention (n = 101); control (n = 107); Complete follow-up 121	Quality of life (Functional health): SF-36	Postdischarge nurse-led home-based case management	No significant difference between control and intervention groups on SF-36 subscales at follow-up.	Relatively small sample size.
Legge & Reilly (1980)	Pretest/ posttest	Community setting; cancer patients in U.S.; N = 36; 50% female; 92% White	Functional status (Legge & Reilly, 1980) developed; nurses assessed functional status and classified patients into four categories: dependent, needs assistance, needs supervision, and independent	Home care nursing services	The number of persons "dependent" rose between admission and discharge over 36%.	Instrument not well described; no psychometric information.

(continues)

Note. ADLs = activities of daily living; IADLs = instrumental activities of daily living; MD = medical doctor; MDS = minimum data set; MDS-HC = minimum data set for home care; RR = sample response rate; RCT = randomized control trial.

TABLE 2-1 Studies Investigating the Relationship Between Nursing Variables and Functional Status (continued)

Author/ date	Design	Sample characteristics/ setting	Definition of the outcome concept	Intervention being evaluated/ nursing variable being evaluated	Results	Limitations
Lush et al. (1997)	Prospective	Hospital setting; $N = 125$; adults with total joint replacement ($n = 57$); adults with acute congestive heart failure ($n = 37$); pediatric oncology patients receiving chemotherapy ($n = 31$); study conducted in four medical centers in California	Health Status Outcome Dimensions (HSOD) instrument; dimensions include functional status (α .91), healthcare involvement (α .69), psychosocial well-being (α .77), caregiver status (α .67), and family status (α .83)	Change in functional status following health care; total patient care hours	Significant change in functional status over time (FS scores lowest for joint replacement patients at discharge, lowest for CHF at hospital admission). No significant change for psychological status, family and caregiver status. Significant change over time for healthcare involvement. For the total joint replacement sample, total patient care hours were negatively correlated with functional status at hospital admission ($r = -.39$) and discharge ($r = -.42$), with healthcare involvement at discharge ($r = -.55$), and psychological well-being at admission ($r = -.41$). Patient age correlated with functional status ($r = -.29$), health care involvement ($r = -.32$), and family status ($r = -.39$).	
McCusker et al. (2001)	RCT; T1 and T2 (1 month); T3 (4 month follow-up); intervention ($n = 178$; RR = 82.6%; 155 = 87.1 % at T3); control ($n = 210$; 182 = 86.7% at T2)	Canada Emergency department of four university-affiliated hospitals in Montreal	Functional status (Older American Resource & Services Scale; Geriatric Depression Scale; Caregiver health status (SF-36)	Intervention—brief standardized geriatric nursing assessment	The intervention resulted in a significantly reduced rate of functional decline at 4 months; no significant effect of the intervention on caregiver health status at 4 months.	

Study	Design	Sample/Setting	Functional Measure	Intervention/Focus	Findings	Notes
McGillis Hall et al. (2003)	Longitudinal: admission to hospital, discharge, 6-week follow-up	Canada Adult medical-surgical inpatient; N = 1,811; N = 1,483 at 6 week. Mean age 55 years	Functional health: Functional Independence Index (FIM) (Hamilton et al., 1987); SF-36 (Ware, 1993)	Proportion of regulated staff (registered nurse, registered practical nurse)	Proportion of regulated nursing staff on inpatient medical-surgical units was associated with better FIM score outcomes and better SF-36 social function scores at discharge.	
Meissner et al. (1989)	Descriptive comparative design	Hospital setting; patients older than 70 years (N = 103), mean age = 81	Functional status (Katz Activities of Daily Living); Instrumental Activities of Daily Living (M. P. Lawton & Brody, 1969)	Dedicated geriatric unit with a nurse specialist vs. similar medical unit	Assess independence in six activities: bathing, dressing, toileting, transferring from bed to chair, continence, and feeding. Items rated on a 3-point scale.	
Milisen et al. (2001)	Cohort, prospective	Intervention (n = 60); nonintervention (n = 60); hospital setting in Belgium	Functional status (Katz ADL)	Intervention to enhance the quality of nursing care focused on training in assessment and consultation with specialized nurses	There was no statistically significant difference in functional status between the nonintervention and intervention cohort.	
Mitton et al. (2007)	Prospective mixed methods, pre-post	Canada Home care; N = 37; N = 24 patients after 12 months	Functional Health Status: SF-8	Home care nursing and physician collaborative practice	No change in physical and mental function over time.	Small sample; nonrandomized.
Mock et al. (1994)	RCT	Outpatient setting; women with breast cancer receiving chemotherapy (N = 14); mean age = 44; 93% White	Performance status (Karnofsky Performance Status Scale); 12-minute walking test	Rehabilitation program: walking exercise	Performance of physical activities.	
Mundinger et al. (2000)	RCT	Adult patients; N = 1,316 (RR = 66.4%); mean age = 45.9; 76.8% female; 90.3% Hispanic; community-based primary care clinics	Functional health status (SF-36)	Nurse practitioner vs. physician care.	No difference between NP and MD patients on any scale or summary score at 6 months; significant improvement in health status from baseline to 6-month follow-up for all subscales of the SF-36.	No data provided on the psychometric properties of the SF-36 for this particular sample.

Note. ADLs = activities of daily living; IADLs = instrumental activities of daily living; MD = medical doctor; MDS = minimum data set; MDS-HC = minimum data set for home care; RR = sample response rate; RCT = randomized control trial.

(continues)

TABLE 2-1   Studies Investigating the Relationship Between Nursing Variables and Functional Status (continued)

Author/date	Design	Sample characteristics/setting	Definition of the outcome concept	Intervention being evaluated/nursing variable being evaluated	Results	Limitations
Peri et al. (2008)	RCT	Residential care facilities, New Zealand. $N=149$ (RR=83%); control =352; intervention=330. 74% female; average age 84	Mobility: Elderly Mobility Scale (EMS; Smith, 1994), and the Timed "up and go" score (TUG; Podsialdo & Richardson, 1991); Functional health status: SF-36.	Activity program delivered by a gerontology nurse	There was no difference between groups on mobility measures at any time, nor any measures at 6-month follow-up. In the intervention group, the SF-36 total physical component summary (PCS) score improved at 3 months in comparison with the control group.	Contamination is likely to have affected the 6-month follow-up measures.
Pettersson et al. (1999)	Prospective, single-cohort design	Swedish asthmatics; $N = 32$ (RR = 53%); mean age = 43; 81% female; outpatient clinic	Sickness Impact Profile (SIP)	Nurse-run asthma school	Significant improvement in SIP physical health status subscale only.	No data on the psychometric properties of SIP in this sample; small sample size.
Pugh et al. (2001)	RCT	One community and one teaching hospital; $N = 58$, control ($n = 31$), intervention ($n = 27$)	Quality of life/functional status (SF-36) (All Cronbach's alpha in this study greater than .50). Six-minute walking test	Patient education and nurse case manager discharge planning and 6-month follow-up	There was a trend to greater improvement in SF-36 physical functioning and mental health and 6-minute walk test for the intervention group, but none of the differences was statistically significant.	Small sample size and lack of control for patient risk profile.
Rose, Lawton, Elley, Dowell, & Fenton (2007); B. A. Lawton et al. (2008)	RCT	New Zealand 40–74-year-old physically inactive women recruited from 17 primary care practices. $N = 1089$ (RR = 87%); intervention ($n = 544$), control ($n = 545$); 12-month follow-up ($n = 1008$) (RR = 93%); 24-month follow-up $n = 974$ (RR = 89%)	Quality of life/health status: SF-36 assessed at 12 and 24 months	Nurse-led intervention involving physical activity	SF-36 physical functioning ($p = .03$) and mental health ($p < .05$) scores improved more in intervention compared with control participants, but role physical scores were significantly lower ($p < .01$). More falls ($p < .01$) and injury ($p = .03$) were recorded in the intervention group.	

Rosemann et al. (2007)	RCT	Germany Patients with arthritis, N = 1,021; control (n = 332), intervention 1 (self-management through GP) (n = 345); nurse case management (n = 344)	Quality of life, including functional ability: Arthritis Impact Measurement Scale Short-Form (AIMS2-SF) (Rosemann et al., 2005); physical activity: International Physical Activity Questionnaire (IPAQ; Craig et al., 2003)	Case management of primary practice patients	Nurse case management group had significant increase in lower limb functional ability (p = .05) and social function (p < .001).
Root-mensen et al. (2008)	RCT	Chronic obstructive lung disease outpatient clinic; N = 191 (RR = 91%), intervention (n = 97), control (94); mean age 60.5, female 43%	Health status, including functional health, role functioning: SF-36	Pulmonary nurse-delivered education program	There was no statistically significant difference in SF-36-assessed health outcomes between intervention and control group patients.
Schein et al. (2005)	Longitudinal	Community dwelling elders (≥ 70 years); N = 175	Functional health outcomes: SF-36; and ADL and IADL Older American Resources and Services Multidimensional Functional Assessment questionnaire	Nurse case management	Older people receiving coping interventions demonstrated an increase in IADLs (p < .05); no association with ADLs.	Lack of control of confounding variables.
Shibayama, Kobayashi, Takano, Kadowaki, & Kazuma (2007)	RCT	Japan Non–insulin treated diabetic outpatients; N = 134 (RR = 43%); intervention (n = 67), control (n = 67). 10% attrition at 12 months	Health-related quality of life (including functional status): SF-36	Lifestyle counseling by certified expert nurse	No significant difference between groups in SF-36 scores.	Small sample size; low response rate.

Note. ADLs = activities of daily living; IADLs = instrumental activities of daily living; MD = medical doctor; MDS = minimum data set; MDS-HC = minimum data set for home care; RR = sample response rate; RCT = randomized control trial.

(continues)

TABLE 2-1   Studies Investigating the Relationship Between Nursing Variables and Functional Status (continued)

Author/ date	Design	Sample characteristics/ setting	Definition of the outcome concept	Intervention being evaluated/ nursing variable being evaluated	Results	Limitations
Steiner et al. (2001)	RCT	Britain 1 teaching and 9 community hospitals; $N = 238$ patients; nurse-led unit ($n = 119$) vs. usual care. 6-month follow-up	Physical functioning (Barthel Index)	Nurse-led unit	No difference in functional status at discharge or at 6 month follow-up, between intervention and nonintervention patients.	
Stocker Schneider et al. (2008)	Quasi-experimental, before-after design	Home care $N = 106$; average age 77; 51% male	Functional health: OASIS (Shaughnessy et al, 1998); Nursing Outcome Classification (NOC) (Moorhead, Johnson, Maas, & Swanson, 2007).	Nursing interventions collected at each home care visit using the Nursing Intervention Classification (NIC)	Intraclass correlation/reliability (ICC) for OASIS ranged from 0.27 to 0.63 ($M = 0.48$); the NOC ICC reliability ranged from 0.39 to 0.97 ($M = 0.66$). Neither the OASIS nor the NOC was sensitive to the effects of home health care nursing as measured by intervention intensity. The OASIS was not responsive to clinically discernable change in patient outcomes. The NOC was responsive to patient status change in ADLs ($p < .05$), cardiopulmonary status ($p < .05$), coping ($p < .05$), and illness management behavior ($p < .05$).	

Study	Design	Sample	Measures	Intervention/Variable	Findings	Comments
Suhonen et al. (2007)	Cross-sectional correction design	Finland; $N = 861$ (RR = 84%) predischarged adult patients. Complete data on $N = 687$; female 57%	Health-related quality of life (breathing, mental function, communication, vision, mobility, ADLs, vitality, hearing, eating, elimination, sleeping, distress, discomfort, symptoms, sexual activity, depression): 15D (Sintonen, 2001)	Individualized nursing care: Individualized Care Scale (Suhonen, Välimäki, Katajisto, Leino-Kilpi, & Katajisto, 2004)	A low but significant association was found between individualized nursing care and health-related quality of life (standardized path coefficient = .02, $p < .01$).	
Swan (1998)	Prospective, single-cohort design	Outpatient setting; ambulatory surgical patients ($N = 100$); attrition rate of 26%; mean age = 42.6 ($SD = 12.83$; 63% female; 72% White	Symptom distress (General Symptom Distress Scale [GSDS]; Lalonde, 1987]; Functional Status Questionnaire (FSQ; Jette et al., 1986)	Nurse caring behaviors: The Caring Behaviors Inventory (Wolf, Giardino, Osbourne, & Ambrose, 1994)	Postoperative nurse caring behaviors explained 7-day basic ADLs, mental health, social activity, and 4-day post-op social interaction.	
Walsh et al. (1999)	RCT; nurse-led inpatient care	Hospital setting; postacute medical patients	Barthel Index	Nurse-led inpatient care unit for postacute medical patients	There were no significant differences in the outcome measures, including Barthel scores between patients in the experimental and usual care groups.	No information on psychometric properties of Barthel in this study.
Wanich et al. (1992)	Quasi-experimental; intervention (one unit) vs. control group (two other inpatient units)	Patients aged 70 and older admitted to urban teaching hospital ($N = 235$); mean age = 77	Mini-Mental State Examination; Katz Index of Activities of Daily Living; diagnosis of delirium (psychiatrist)	Nursing intervention based on Orem's Self-Care Deficit Model	More intervention group subjects improved in functional status in comparison with control subjects. Logistic regression indicated that subjects exposed to the intervention were three times as likely to improve in functional status in the hospital as compared with subjects in the control group (odd ratio 3.29).	Full version used in this study.

Note. ADLs = activities of daily living; IADLs = instrumental activities of daily living; MD = medical doctor; MDS = minimum data set; MDS-HC = minimum data set for home care; RR = sample response rate; RCT = randomized control trial.

The first question that arises is the extent to which functional status is a relevant outcome for nursing, as indicated by strong empirical evidence linking nursing variables to functional status outcomes. Nineteen randomized controlled trials examined a nursing intervention in which functional status was included as an outcome variable. Nine of these studies found a significant relationship between nursing intervention and functional status outcome. However, three of these papers were findings from one study of residential care settings in New Zealand (Kerse et al., 2008; B. A. Lawton et al., 2008; Peri et al., 2008). Bruggink-André de la Porte (2007) evaluated the effectiveness of a physician- and nurse-led follow-up heart failure clinic and found a significant difference in functional health outcomes, as assessed by the Medical Outcome Study Short Form (SF-36), between intervention and control subjects. Kerse et al. found significant difference in mobility outcomes between intervention and control cognitively intact residents of a residential care facility in New Zealand following a physical activity intervention delivered by a gerontology nurse. In the same residential care setting in New Zealand, Peri et al. found that a physical activity program delivered by a gerontology nurse resulted in better physical functional health outcomes, assessed with the SF-36, for residents in the intervention group as compared with those in the control group. Also reporting on the same residential care facility, B. A. Lawton et al. reported improved physical and mental health scores for the participants of the physical activity program. Kolt, Schofield, Kerse, Garrett, and Oliver (2007) found that telephone counseling sessions for older adults resulted in an increase in moderate physical activity. McCusker et al. (2001) evaluated the effect of a brief standardized nursing assessment and referral to community services/ follow-up for older people visiting the emergency department. They collected data on ADLs and IADLs using the Older American and Resources Services Scale. Potential confounding variables were controlled for through initial screening and statistical analysis. McCusker et al. found a significantly reduced rate of decline for the older people who received the nursing intervention at a 4-month follow-up. When Chan et al. (2000) evaluated a nurse case management intervention, they found significant differences over time and between the experimental and control groups in outcomes measured by the Brief Psychiatric Rating Scale and the Specific Level of Functioning Scale.

Ten randomized controlled trials found no significant relationship between nursing interventions and functional health outcomes. Barr Mazzuca, Farris, Mendenhall, and Stoupa (1997), who analyzed the effectiveness of community health nursing provided by senior undergraduate nursing students, found no significant difference in functional status scores over time, as measured by the SF-36. Gagnon, Schein, McVey, and Bergman (1999) examined a nurse case management intervention and reported no significant differences in the SF-36 subscales over time and no differences in functional ability, as measured by the Older Americans Resource and Services Questionnaire. Likewise, Pugh, Havens,

Xie, Robinson, and Blaha (2001) found no significant difference in SF-36 sub-scale scores 6 months after elderly persons with heart failure received a targeted educational and nurse case management intervention as compared with persons receiving usual care. Latour et al. (2006) found no difference in SF-36 scores at follow-up between patients receiving postdischarge nurse-led home-based care and those receiving usual care. When Mock et al. (1994) evaluated the effectiveness of a nurse-provided exercise program for women with breast cancer receiving chemotherapy, they found no differences between participants in the experimental and control groups on the Karnofsky Performance Status Scale.

A subset of studies sought to evaluate whether patients predominantly cared for by nurses achieved the same level of outcome as those receiving the usual level of medical care. For instance, Griffiths et al. (2000), who compared the functional status outcomes for patients admitted to a nurse-led intermediate care unit with those for patients admitted to a usual care unit, found no significant difference in functional status outcomes at discharge, as measured by the Barthel Index. Mundinger et al. (2000) reported no difference in SF-36 scores at 6 months follow-up between patients receiving care from primary care nurse practitioners and those receiving care from physicians. Steiner et al. (2001) found no significant difference in the functional health outcomes for postacute patients admitted to a nurse-led inpatient unit compared with patients admitted to usual care. In this study, the authors considered no difference a good outcome because the purpose of the study was to assess whether similar health outcomes could be achieved for postacute patients admitted to a unit where they did not receive the same level of medical coverage as patients on the conventional care units. Walsh, Pickering, and Brooking (1999) found no significant difference in scores on the Barthel Index between postacute medical patients admitted to a nurse-led inpatient unit and similar patients admitted to a conventional medical unit.

In summary, the evidence from randomized controlled trials concerning sensitivity of functional status outcomes to nursing intervention is mixed, with nine trials finding positive evidence of sensitivity to nursing interventions and 10 trials finding negative evidence; however, one of these was underpowered to detect a difference, and in a second, no difference was a positive outcome. There were no apparent methodological or substantive differences between these trials that might explain the conflicting findings. For instance, studies with both positive and negative evidence were conducted in acute care, long-term care, and home care settings and used multidimensional measures of functional status such as the SF-36. There was wide variation in the population types and nursing interventions evaluated, making it difficult to combine results or determine whether such differences could account for the conflicting evidence of sensitivity to nursing variables.

Studies employing quasi-experimental designs are also reviewed in Table 2-1. Researchers in six of these found no significant effects for a nursing intervention/care on functional status outcomes, as measured by the SF-36 (Aiken et al.,

1993), the Older Americans Resource and Services Questionnaire (Cohen, Gorenberg, & Schroeder, 2000), Katz ADL (Milisen et al., 2001), the Quality Audit Marker (Holzemer & Henry, 1992), the OASIS and Nursing Outcome Classification indicators (Stocker Schneider, Barkaukas, & Keenan, 2008), and author-developed instrument (Garrard et al., 1990). However, researchers in eight other studies employing quasi-experimental designs reported significant findings based on a modified Barthel Index (Chang et al., 2007; Hamilton & Lyon, 1995), the Sickness Impact Profile (J. E. Johnson et al., 1997; Pettersson, Gardulf, Nordström, Svanberg-Johnsson, & Bylin, 1999), the Katz Activities of Daily Living Scale (Meissner et al., 1989; Wanich, Sullivan-Marx, Gottlieb, & Johnson, 1992), OASIS (Dorman Marek et al., 2006), and the Jette et al. Functional Status Questionnaire (Swan, 1998). Seven studies employing descriptive and longitudinal designs reported significant relationships between nursing interventions and patients' functional health outcomes (Doran et al., 2006, "Nursing-Sensitive Outcomes"; Doran et al., 2006, "The Relationship"; Doran et al., 2002; Heafey, Golden-Baker, & Mahoney, 1994; Pettersson et al.; Schein et al., 2005; Suhonen, Välimäki, Katajisto, & Leino-Kilpi, 2005).

Another set of studies reviewed in Table 2-1 did not evaluate a nursing intervention, but examined the relationship between functional status outcomes and nursing variables. Harrell, McConnell, Wildman, and Samsa (1989) reported a significant relationship between nursing diagnoses and Katz Activities of Daily Living scores. Patients who improved in functional status from admission to discharge from two medical units had the most number of nursing diagnoses recorded in the medical record when compared with patients who did not improve to the same extent. Howard and Reiley (1994) and Irvine et al. (2000) reported a significant relationship between nursing intensity, and Katz scores and the SF-36 subscale scores, respectively. Irvine et al. also found that the proportion of visits made by a registered nurse was a significant predictor of improvements in SF-36 subscale scores for patients receiving home care nursing services. Lush, Henry, Foote, and Jones (1997) found a significant relationship between total patient care hours and functional status at hospital admission and discharge, as measured by the Health Status Outcomes Dimension. Doran, Sidani, Keatings, and Doidge (2002) noted that functional status scores of medical and surgical patients at hospital discharge were significantly related to the quality of nursing care and the quality of nurse communication. Patients achieved better functional independence at hospital discharge on units where the quality of care was high and where communication among nurses and between nurses and physicians was accurate and timely. Horn et al. (2005) and McGillis Hall et al. (2003) reported a significant relationship between nurse staffing variables and functional health outcomes. Doran, McGillis Hall, et al. (2002) collected data on the functional status outcomes of 835 patients admitted to 19 teaching hospitals in Ontario. Functional status was assessed with the Functional Independent Measure (FIM) instrument at the time of admission to the hospital, at discharge, and again at 6 weeks postdischarge. Patients achieved greater functional independence at hospital discharge on units where nurse communication was timely and accurate and where there was a high proportion of regulated staff (i.e., registered nurses and registered practical nurses).

In summary, a review of the empirical literature provides mounting evidence concerning the impact of nursing variables on functional status outcomes. When the evidence from the most rigorous studies is considered, the findings are equivocal, with as many randomized controlled trials reporting a significant relationship between nursing interventions and patients' functional health outcomes as those that do not. However, because the nursing interventions in these trials varied considerably in design, dose, setting, and patient populations, it is possible that in some cases, the nursing interventions were not strong enough, or properly designed and implemented, to test the impact of nursing on patients' functional health status. The evidence from the quasi-experimental studies and correlational studies offers evidence of a relationship between nursing and patients' functional health status. Significant relationships have been observed between patients' functional health outcomes and (a) nursing interventions documented in the healthcare record (Doran et al., 2006, "Nursing-Sensitive Outcomes"; Doran et al., 2006, "The Relationship"), (b) nurse communication and care coordination (Doran, Sidani, et al., 2002), (c) nursing intensity (Howard & Reiley, 1994; Irvine et al., 2000), (d) proportion of visits made by a home care nurse (Irvine et al., 2000), and (e) nurse staffing variables (Horn et al., 2005; McGillis Hall et al., 2003). Collectively, this evidence supports the argument that functional status is an outcome sensitive to nursing care.

EVIDENCE CONCERNING APPROACHES TO MEASUREMENT

Only those functional status instruments that had been used in a study in which the relationship between the instrument scores and nursing variables was examined were included in this review. Although many functional status instruments exist that may be relevant for assessing outcomes of nursing care, they require evaluation in studies in which their sensitivity to nursing variables can be assessed. Thirteen instruments measuring functional status were identified in the empirical nursing literature. Their characteristics are summarized in **TABLE 2-2**. The names of the instrument and its author are identified. The domains of measurement, number of items, and response format are described. The method of administration is identified, and the evidence of reliability, validity, and sensitivity to nursing variables is summarized.

There are generally two different approaches to functional status assessment. One involves a trained clinician's assessment of clients/patients based on chart

TABLE 2-2   Instruments Measuring Functional Status

Instrument (author)	Target population	Domains (number of items and response format)	Method of administration	Reliability	Validity	Sensitivity to nursing care
Barthel Index (Mahoney & Barthel, 1965)	Chronic patients	Independence in personal care and mobility; two versions: original 10-item version and 15-item version	Completed by health professional from the medical record and observation	Internal consistency 0.87 to 0.92 (McDowell & Newell, 1996).	Concurrent validity, Construct validity (Wade & Hewer, 1987) Predictive validity (McDowell & Newell, 1996)	Sensitive to nursing: Chang et al. (2007); Hamilton & Lyon (1995); No effect: Griffiths et al. (2000); Walsh et al. (1999).
Functional Independence Measure (FIM) (Granger, Hamilton, Keith, Zielezny, & Sherwin, 1986)	Patients of all ages and diagnoses	Domains include self-care, sphincter control, mobility, locomotion, communication, and social cognition; 18 items; scores range from 1 to 7	Completed by clinician based on observation of the patient	Interrater reliability 0.86 to 0.88 (Granger et al., 1990; Hamilton et al., 1987). Doran, McGillis Hall, et al. (2002) reported an internal consistency reliability of 0.87 in a sample of medical-surgical patients.	Content validity Construct validity (Granger et al., 1990)	Changes in the FIM instrument scores were significantly associated with the quality of nurse communication and nurse staff mix (Doran, Sidani, et al., 2002). Proportion of regulated staff was associated with improvement in FIM scores among hospitalized medical surgical patients (McGillis Hall et al., 2003).
Functional Status Questionnaire (Jette et al., 1986)	Ambulatory patients	Ability to perform physical function, psychological function, work performance, social activity, social interaction; 34 items; 4- to 6-point rating scales	Self-administered	Internal consistency of subscales range from 0.64 to 0.82 (Jette & Cleary, cited in McDowell & Newell, 1996).	Construct validity Criterion validity Predictive validity	Sensitivity to change shown with patients undergoing hip replacement (J. N. Katz et al., 1992) and postacute hip fracture patients (Krichbaum, 2007). Sensitive to post-op nurse caring behaviors (Swan, 1998).

Instrument	Population	Description	Administration	Reliability	Validity	Other
Health Status Outcomes Dimension (HSOD) (Kaiser Permanente Northern California) (Lush & Jones, 1995; Lush et al., 1997).	Adult & pediatric versions	Self-care ability/functional status; engagement in health care management; psychological distress; 14 items rated on 4-point scale	Nurse based on patient observation and chart extraction; electronic documentation	No information available.	Content validity	No information.
Index of Independence in Activities of Daily Living (S. Katz & Akpom, 1976)	Elderly and chronically ill populations	Assess independence in six activities: bathing, dressing, toileting, transfer from bed to chair, continence, feeding; items rated on a 3-point scale	Nurse/therapist assesses based on observation	Alexy & Elnitsky (1998) reported internal consistency reliability of 0.89 in nursing study.	Predictive (Åsberg, 1987; Katz, et al., 1992	Association between Katz ADL scores and nursing diagnoses (Harrell et al., 1989); nursing intensity (Howard & Reiley, 1994); and dedicated geriatric nursing care (Meissner et al., 1989).
Inventory of Functional Status After Childbirth (Fawcett & Tulman, 1990; Fawcett, Tulman, & Taylor Myers, 1988)	Postpartum mothers	Measures self-care, household activities, infant care responsibilities, occupational responsibilities, social and community activities after childbirth; 36 items, rated on scale of 1–4	Self-administered	Internal consistency reliability of 0.76. Test-retest reliability of 0.86 (Fawcett & Tulman, 1990).	Content validity (Fawcett & Tulman, 1990) Construct validity (Fawcett & Tulman, 1990)	Sensitivity to change demonstrated in early postpartum period (Fawcett & Tulman, 1990).
Medical Outcome Study-Short Form (SF-36) (Stewart, Hays, & Ware, 1988; Ware, 1993).	Ambulatory	Physical function, mobility, social, mental, general health (36-item and 12-item versions); Likert response format	Self-administered or administered through interview	Internal consistency of 0.76 and higher (Ware, 1993).	Construct Criterion Predictive	Irvine et al. (2000) found sensitivity to community nursing care; Peri et al. (2008) found a relationship between nursing-delivered activity program and improvement in physical function; B. A. Lawton et al. (2008) found sensitivity in community living women 40–74 years old; Hamilton & Hawley (2006) found sensitivity to clinical nurse specialist role.

(continues)

TABLE 2-2   Instruments Measuring Functional Status (continued)

Instrument (author)	Target population	Domains (number of items and response format)	Method of administration	Reliability	Validity	Sensitivity to nursing care
Nursing Outcomes Classification (NOC) tool: Physical Function (M. Johnson & Maas, 1997)	All ages and practice settings	24 outcome category labels related to physical function within which there are subcategory labels; 5-point scale, higher scores more independence	Nurse assessed	No information available.	Content validity	The NOC was not sensitive to the effects of home healthcare nursing as measured by intervention intensity (Stocker Schneider et al., 2008). The NOC was responsive to patient status change in ADLs ($p < .05$) (Stocker Schneider et al., 2008).
Older American Resource and Services Questionnaire (OARS) (Fillenbaum & Smyer, 1981)	Adults, particularly the elderly	Multidimensional functional and service assessment; functional includes ADLs, social, economic, mental and physical health; functional assessment 120 items	Administered by trained interviewer	Interrater reliability and test-retest reliability (McDowell & Newell, 1996).	Criterion validity (Fillenbaum & Smyer, 1981) Predictive validity (Fillenbaum, 1985)	Cohen et al. (2000) found no change in OARS scores over 1 year among elderly clients receiving services from nurse-managed community centers. Gagnon et al. (1999) reported no differences in ADL and IADL scores for clients receiving nurse case management. However, McCusker et al. (2001) and Schein et al. (2005) found sensitivity to change following nursing intervention.
Outcome Assessment Information Set (OASIS) (Shaughnessy et al., 1998)	Clients receiving home care services	General health, physical assessment, ADLs, IADLs; approximately 79 questions with subquestions	Completed by nurse/rater based on chart audit, client interview, nurse interview, and observation	No published information found.	Content validity (Shaughnessy et al., 1998)	Dalton (2001) described the use of OASIS for evaluating a cardiac disease management program and found OASIS data useful in the description of the patients. Nurse-led community intervention led to significant improvement in ADL scores (Dorman Marek et al., 2006).

Instrument	Population	Domains/Items	Method	Reliability	Validity	Comments
Quality Audit Marker (Holzemer et al., 1991; Holzemer & Henry, 1992)	Initially individuals with AIDS, although applicable to all populations	Three domains—functional status, nutrition/elimination, and social isolation; 17 items	Completed on the bases of chart audit, client interview, and observation	Cronbach's alpha of 0.90 for total scale (Holzemer & Henry, 1992).	Construct validity through factor analysis (Holzemer & Henry, 1992)	No information found.
Resident Assessment Instrument (RAI)/Minimum Data Set (Hirdes et al., 1999).	Long-term care, home care, acute care, mental health, and postacute are under development.	Activities of daily living; instrumental activities of daily living include bowel and bladder function, communication, vision, and cognitive function	Chart extraction, client assessment, and interview	Good interrater reliability; reliability across cultural group is under investigation (Hirdes et al., 1999).	Face, content, covergent, and criterion validity. Some evidence of predictive validity in relation to falls (Hirdes et al., 1999)	ADL subscales were significantly related to nursing interventions documented in the healthcare record (Doran et al., 2006, "Nursing-Sensitive Outcomes"; Doran et al., 2006, "The Relationship").
Sickness Impact Profile (Bergner, Bobbitt, Carter, & Gilson, 1981)	Adults experiencing an illness	Measures health status in 12 categories—ambulation, mobility, body care and movement, social interaction, communication, alertness behavior, emotion, sleep and rest, eating, home management, recreation, and work; 136 items	Interview or self-administered	Test-retest reliability (DeBruin, De Witte, Stevens, & Diederiks, 1992; McDowell & Newell, 1996). Internal consistency (0.84–0.91) (Bergner, Bobbitt, Carter, & Gilson, 1981).	Extensive validity testing has been undertaken. Concurrent validity (Bergner et al., 1981), criterion (DeBruin et al., 1992), construct validity (Bergner et al., 1981).	J. E. Johnson et al. (1997) found change in the home maintenance subscale following a training program for nurses but no change in other subscales.

abstraction, observation, and patient interview. This approach is favored by systems designed for outcome tracking and for collecting administrative data because it does not rely on self-report and therefore can be used to assess patients of varying levels of cognitive ability, limitation, and language competence. Other advantages to this approach are that it is minimally intrusive for patients and family members, and it can be completed by clinicians as part of the routine process of patient care and documentation.

Five instruments of this type were included in this review. The Nursing Outcomes Classification tool (NOC) (M. Johnson & Maas, 1997) was counted in this category. Indicators for the NOC are under development, and pilot testing is being conducted in a number of practice settings. There are 24 category labels related to physical function, within which there are subcategory labels. Although a significant amount of work has been done to establish the content validity of the NOC indicators (M. Johnson & Maas), there is limited information available about the reliability and construct validity of the functional status subscales. Stocker Schneider et al. (2008) found that the NOC was not sensitive to the effects of home healthcare nursing intervention intensity. However, these authors observed that the NOC was responsive to patient status change in ADLs. The Health Status Outcomes Dimension (HSOD) (Lush et al., 1997; Lush & Jones, 1995) and the Quality Audit Marker (Holzemer, Janson-Bjerklie, Brown, & Henry, 1991) are two other outcome assessment tools that were specifically developed to evaluate the quality and outcomes of nursing care. The HSOD is designed to track outcomes across the continuum of care and includes a number of functional status indicators. The functional status indicators have demonstrated sensitivity to change over time in adult medical and surgical patients and pediatric patients. The Quality Audit Marker was originally designed for use with an AIDS population but is applicable to other patient populations. Both tools have had limited testing in different practice settings, and there is no published information about their sensitivity to changes in patients' functional health outcomes following nursing interventions. The Outcome Assessment Set (Shaughnessy, Crisler, & Schlenker, 1998) was developed to assess service needs and the outcomes of clients receiving home care services. It has good evidence of reliability and validity; however, evidence of sensitivity to nursing intervention is mixed, with two studies demonstrating sensitivity (Dalton, 2001; Dorman et al., 2006) and one study finding no sensitivity (Stocker Schneider et al., 2008). Hamilton, Granger, Sherwin, Zielezny, and Tashman (1987) developed the Functional Independence Measure instrument to assess functional health outcomes for patients of all ages and diagnoses. It has been used extensively in rehabilitation populations with good evidence of reliability, validity, and sensitivity to change (McDowell & Newell, 1996). Doran, McGillis Hall, et al. (2002) used the FIM instrument to assess functional health outcomes of medical and surgical patients admitted to 19 acute care teaching hospitals in Ontario. They found the FIM instrument sensitive to several nursing variables, including variation in nursing staff mix across the hospital units and variations in the quality of nursing care (Doran, McGillis Hall, et al.). The proportion of regulated staff was associated with improvement in FIM scores in another study (McGillis Hall et al., 2003), and nursing contact time increased exponentially as FIM-assessed disability increased (Heinemann et al., 1997).

The Resident Assessment Instrument (RAI) is a series of instruments that involves person-specific assessment in which data are recorded on a Minimum Data Set (MDS) form (Hawes et al., 1997; Hirdes et al., 1999). The MDS functional status indicators include cognitive items, ADLs, and IADLs. The RAI series of instruments has been developed for nursing homes and home care settings (Hirdes et al.). Acute care, mental health, and postacute care series have also been developed or have undergone initial psychometric testing (Hirdes et al.). The reliability and validity of the MDS long-term care version has been confirmed in multiple studies (Casten, Powell-Lawton, Parmelee, & Kleban, 1998; Frederiksen, Tariot, & Jonghe, 1996; Hartmaier et al., 1995; Hawes et al., 1995; Hirdes et al.). The functional status subscale of the MDS was found to be sensitive to nursing variables in two studies (Doran et al., 2006, "Nursing-Sensitive Outcomes"; Doran et al., 2006, "The Relationship"; Horn et al., 2005).

The other approach to assessing functional status is the use of a self-report questionnaire, which is completed by the patient or through an interview guide. This approach is evidently favored in the research literature; the majority of empirical studies reviewed here that investigated functional status in relationship to nursing care used a structured instrument, based on patients' self-report, to measure functional status outcomes: (a) 16 used the SF-36 (e.g., Aiken et al., 1993; Barr Mazzuca et al., 1997; Gagnon et al., 1999; Irvine et al., 2000; Mundinger et al., 2000); (b) 6 used the Katz Activities of Daily Living Scale (Alexy & Elnitsky, 1998; Harrell et al., 1989; Howard & Reiley, 1994; Meissner et al., 1989; Milisen et al., 2001; Wanich et al., 1992); (c) 4 used the Older Americans Resource and Services Questionnaire (Cohen et al., 2000; Gagnon et al., 1999; Helberg, 1993; McCusker et al., 2001); (d) 5 used the Barthel Index (Chang et al., 2007; Griffiths et al., 2000; Hamilton & Lyon, 1995; Steiner et al., 2001; Walsh et al., 1999); (e) 2 used the Sickness Impact Profile (J. E. Johnson et al., 1997; Pettersson et al., 1999); (f) 1 used the Inventory of Functional Status After Child Birth (Fawcett & Tulman, 1990); (g) 2 used the Jette Functional Status Questionnaire (Krichbaum, 2007; Swan, 1998); (h) 1 used the Late Life Function and Disability Questionnaire (Kerse et al., 2008; Peri et al., 2008); (i) 1 used the Auckland Heart Study Physical Activity Questionnaire (Kolt et al., 2007); and (j) 1 used the SF-8 (Mitton, O'Neil, Simpson, Hoppins, & Harcus, 2007). Commenting on a measure's sensitivity is difficult when evidence is derived from only one or two studies. Therefore, the review is limited to those instruments that were used in multiple studies.

Five of the six studies that used the Katz Activities of Daily Living Scale found sensitivity to nursing practice variables. Two of the five studies using the Barthel Index demonstrated sensitivity to nursing variables, and two of the four studies using the Older American Resource and Services Questionnaire (OARS) demonstrated sensitivity to nursing variables. The functional status subscale of the MDS was found to be sensitive to nursing variables in two studies (Doran et al., 2006, "Nursing-Sensitive Outcomes"; Doran et al., 2006, "The Relationship"; Horn et al., 2005). Based on this empirical evidence, it would appear that instruments that measure ADLs, such as Katz Activities of Daily Living Scale, MDS, and OARS, are sensitive to nursing variables. The ADL items comprising scales such as the Katz Activities of Daily Living Scale, MDS, OASIS are focused on patients' self-care activities in relation to personal care (e.g., bathing, toileting, dressing) and on mobility (e.g., moving in bed, sitting transfer, standing transfer). These very specific ADLs reflect the foci of nursing care. For many patient populations, it is possible to see changes in these activities within a relatively short period. Think, for example, about the course of clinical and functional recovery for a patient undergoing an uncomplicated surgical intervention, such as a total knee replacement. In the immediate 24-hour postoperative period, the nurse helps the patient to sit in bed and transfer from the bed to the chair. By the next day, the nurse may be assisting the patient to ambulate from the bed to a bathroom or along the hospital corridor. In addition, the nurse reinforces the physiotherapist's instructions and supervises range-of-motion exercises. The nurse begins to gauge nursing care to promote graduated recovery of personal self-care activities so that at the time of hospital discharge to home/community or to a rehabilitation setting, the patient may have made significant progress toward functional independence. The nurse's effective management of postoperative pain will also have an important effect on the patient's clinical and functional recovery. This brief clinical example illustrates the applicability of the kinds of items that comprise ADL scales.

Of the studies employing the SF-36, six found a significant relationship between the SF-36 and nursing variables. The six studies that found sensitivity were primarily conducted in postacute, community-based population (Bruggink-André de la Porte, 2007; Irvine et al., 2000; B. A. Lawton et al., 2008) and long-term care settings (Peri et al., 2008). A hospital-based study by McGillis Hall et al. (2003) found a relationship between nursing skill mix and SF-36 social function outcome.

RECOMMENDATIONS NECESSARY FOR FUTURE RESEARCH

Improvement in functional status outcomes is often identified as an intended goal of nursing care. Indeed, much of nursing practice is devoted to the promotion and restoration of healthy functioning, as evidenced by such grand nursing theories as Orem's Self-Care Deficit Theory (Orem, 1980) and Roy's Adaptation Theory (Roy & Roberts, 1981). Since publishing the earlier edition of this book, new empirical studies have investigated the relationship between nursing intervention and patient functional status outcomes. In addition, several systematic reviews have been conducted on the topic of nursing care and functional status outcomes. These two sources of evidence support the conclusion that functional status is a nursing-sensitive patient outcome.

Two approaches to measuring functional status warrant evaluation: one based on a trained clinician's assessment, and the other on patient self-report. Yet evidence suggests that the two approaches may not yield comparable results with regard to patients' actual level of functioning (Reiley et al., 1996; Rubenstein et al., 1984). Therefore, research is needed to evaluate the approaches to measurement for different patient populations and practice settings.

A systematic review of the nursing studies indicated that functional status, as measured by activities of daily living, is sensitive to nursing care and that assessment tools such as the Katz Activities of Daily Living Scale and the MDS ADL subscale show promise for detecting change in functional status following nursing intervention. The evidence of sensitivity of instruments measuring the broader domains of functional status, such as social and work role activities, is less conclusive. Further research is needed to evaluate the reliability, validity, and sensitivity of functional status instruments measuring the broader domains of human functioning in different practice settings. For example, there is reason to expect that indicators measuring the domains that reflect IADLs would be more sensitive to nursing in community settings (Irvine et al., 2000) than in institutional settings.

REFERENCES

Aiken, L. H., Lake, E. T., Semaan, S., Lehman, H. P., O'Hare, P. A., Cole, C. S., et al. (1993). Nurse practitioner managed care for persons with HIV infection. *Image: Journal of Nursing Scholarship, 25,* 172–177.

Alexy, B. B., & Elnitsky, C. (1998). Rural mobile health unit: Outcomes. *Public Health Nursing, 15,* 3–11.

Asberg, K. H. (1987). Disability as a predictor of outcomes for the elderly in a department of internal medicine. *Scandinavian Journal of Social Medicine, 15,* 261–265.

Aydelotte, M. (1962). The use of patient welfare as a criterion measure. *Nursing Research, 11,* 10–14.

Barr Mazzuca, K., Farris, N. A., Mendenhall, J., & Stoupa, R. A. (1997). Demonstrating the added value of community nursing for clients with insulin-dependent diabetes. *Journal of Community Health Nursing, 14,* 211–224.

Bergner, M., Bobbitt, R. A., Carter, W. B., & Gilson, B. S. (1981). The sickness impact profile: Development and final revision of a health status measure. *Medical Care, 21,* 787–805.

Boockvar, K., Brodie, H. D., & Lachs, M. (2000). Nursing assistants detect behavioral changes in nursing home residents that precede acute illness: Development and validation of an illness warning instrument. *Journal of the American Geriatric Society, 48,* 1086–1091.

Bostick, J. E., Rantz, M. J., Flesner, M. K., & Riggs, C. J. (2006). Systematic review of studies of staffing and quality in nursing homes. *Journal of the American Medical Directors Association, 7*, 366–376.

Bourret, E. M., Bernick, L. G., Cott, C. A., & Kontos, P. C. (2002). The meaning of mobility for residents and staff in long-term care facilities. *Journal of Advanced Nursing, 37*, 338–345.

Brown, S. A. & Grimes, D. E. (1995). A meta-analysis of nurse practitioners and nurse midwives in primary care. *Nursing Research, 44*(6), 332–339.

Bruggink-André de la Porte, P. W. F., Lok, D. J. A., van Veldhuisen, D. J., van Wijngaarden, J., Cornel, J. H., Zuithoff, N. P. A., et al. (2007). Added value of a physician-and-nurse directed heart failure clinic: results from the Deventer-Alkmaar heart failure study. *Heart, 93*, 819–825.

Burns, R. B., Moskowitz, M. A., Ash, A., Kane, R. L, Finch, M. D., & Bak, S. M. (1992). Self-report versus medical record functional status. *Medical Care, 30*(Suppl.), MS85–MS95.

Casten, R., Powell-Lawton, M., Parmelee, P. A., & Kleban, M. H. (1998). Psychometric characteristics of the Minimum Data Set I: Confirmatory factor analysis. *Journal of the American Geriatrics Society, 46*, 726–735.

Chan, S., Mackenzie, A., Tin-Fu, D., & Leung, J. K. (2000). An evaluation of the implementation of case management in the community psychiatric nursing service. *Journal of Advanced Nursing, 31*, 144–156.

Chang, E., Hancock, K., Hickman, L., Glasson, J., & Davidson, P. (2007). Outcomes of acutely ill older hospitalized patients following implementation of tailored models of care: A repeated measures (pre- and post-intervention) design. *International Journal of Nursing Studies, 44*, 1079–1092.

Cohen, J., Gorenberg, B., & Schroeder, B. (2000). A study of functional status among elders at two academic nursing centers. *Home Care Provider, 5*, 108–112.

Cooley, M. E. (1998). Quality of life in persons with non-small cell lung cancer: A concept analysis. *Cancer Nursing, 21*, 151–161.

Craig, C. L., Marshall, A. L., Sjostrom, M., Bauman, A.E., Booth, M. L., & Ainsworth, B. E. (2003). International physical activity questionnaire: 12-country reliability and validity. *Medicine & Science in Sports & Exercise, 35*, 1381–1395.

Dalton, J. M. (2001). Using OASIS patient outcomes to evaluate a cardiac disease management program: A case study. *Outcomes Management for Nursing Practice, 5*, 167–172.

DeBruin, A. F., De Witte, L. P., Stevens, F., & Diederiks, J. P. (1992). Sickness Impact Profile: The state of the art of a generic functional status measure. *Social Science & Medicine, 35*, 1003–1014.

Doran, D. M. (2003). Functional Status. In D. M. Doran (Ed.), *Nursing-sensitive outcomes: State of the science*. Sudbury, MA: Jones and Bartlett.

Doran, D. M., Harrison, J. M., Spence-Laschinger, H., Hirdes, J., Rukhom, E., Sidani, S., et al. (2006). Nursing-sensitive outcomes data collection in acute care and long-term care settings. *Nursing Research, 55*, S75–S81.

Doran, D. M., Harrison, J. M., Spence-Laschinger, H., Hirdes, J., Rukhom, E., Sidani, S., et al. (2006). The relationship between nursing interventions and outcome achievement in acute care settings. *Research in Nursing and Health, 29*, 61–70.

Doran, D. M., McGillis Hall., L., Sidani, S., O'Brien-Pallas, L., Donner, G., Baker, G. R., et al. (2002). Nursing staff mix and patient outcome achievement: The mediating role of nurse communication. *Journal of International Nursing Perspectives, 1*, 74–83.

Doran, D. M., Sidani, S., Keatings, M., & Doidge, D. (2002). An empirical test of the Nursing Role Effectiveness Model. *Journal of Advanced Nursing, 38*, 29–39.

Dorman Marek, K., Popejoy, L., Petroski, G., & Rantz, M. (2006). Nurse care coordination in community-based long-term care. *Journal of Nursing Scholarship, 38*, 80–86.

Doucette, C. (2005). Review: Patients in nursing-led units are better prepared for discharge than those receiving usual care. *Evidence-Based Nursing, 11*, 20.

Fawcett, J., & Tulman, L. (1990). Building a programme of research from the Roy Adaptation Model of Nursing. *Journal of Advanced Nursing, 15*, 720–725.

Fawcett, J., Tulman, L., & Samarel, N. (1995). Enhancing function in life transitions and serious illness. *Advanced Practice Nursing Quarterly, 1*(3), 50–57.

Fawcett, J., Tulman, L., & Taylor Myers, S. (1988). Development of the inventory of functional status after childbirth. *Journal of Nurse-Midwifery, 33*, 252–260.

Fillenbaum, G. G. (1985). Screening the elderly: A brief instrumental activities of daily living measure. *Journal of the American Geriatric Society, 33*, 698–706.

Fillenbaum, G. G., & Smyer, M. A. (1981). The development, validity, and reliability of the OARS Multidimensional Functional Assessment Questionnaire. *Journal of Gerontology, 36*, 428–434.

Frederiksen, K., Tariot, P., & Jonghe, E. D. (1996). Minimum data set plus (MDS+) scores from five rating scales. *Journal of the American Geriatrics Society, 44*, 305–309.

Gagnon, A. J., Schein, C., McVey, L., & Bergman, H. (1999). Randomized controlled trial of nurse case management of frail older people. *Journal of the American Geriatrics Society, 47*, 1118–1124.

Garrard, J., Kane, R. L., Radosevich, D. M., Skay, C. L., Arnold, S., Kepferle, L., et al. (1990). Impact of geriatric nurse practitioners on nursing-home residents' functional status, satisfaction, and discharge outcomes. *Medical Care, 28*, 271–283.

Gillette, B., & Jenko, M. (1991). Major clinical functions: A unifying framework for measuring outcomes. *Journal of Nursing Care Quality, 6*, 20–24.

Granger, C. V., Cotter, A. C., Hamilton, B. B., Fiedler, R. C., & Hens, M. M. (1990). Functional assessment scales: A study of persons with multiple sclerosis. *Archives of Physical Medicine and Rehabilitation, 71*, 870–875.

Granger, C. V., Hamilton, B. B., Keith, R. A., Zielezny, M., & Sherwin, F. S. (1986). Advances in functional assessment for medical rehabilitation. *Topics in Geriatric Rehabilitation, 1*(3), 59–74.

Griffiths, P. (1996). Clinical outcomes for nurse-led in-patient care. *Nursing Times, 92(9)*, 40–43.

Griffiths, P., Harris, R., Richardson, G., Hallett, N., Heard, S., & Wilson-Barnett, J. (2001). Substitution of a nursing-led inpatient unit for acute services: Randomized control trial of outcomes and cost of nursing-led intermediate care. *Age and Aging, 30*, 483–488.

Griffiths, P., Wilson-Barnett, J., Richardson, G., Spilsbury, K., Miller, F., & Harris, R. (2000). The effectiveness of intermediate care in a nursing-led in-patient unit. *International Journal of Nursing Studies, 37*, 153–161.

Gu, M. O., & Conn, V. S. (2008). Meta-analysis of the effects of exercise interventions on functional status in older adults. *Research in Nursing & Health, 31*, 594–603.

Hackman, J. R., & Oldham, G. R. (1980). *Work redesign*. Reading, MA: Addision-Wesley.

Hamilton, B. B., Granger, C. V., Sherwin, F. S., Zielezny, M., & Tashman, J. S. (1987). A uniform national data system for medical rehabilitation. In M. J. Fuhrer (Ed.), *Rehabilitation outcomes: Analysis and measurement* (pp. 135–147). Baltimore: Paul H. Brooks.

Hamilton, L., & Lyon, P. S. (1995). A nursing-driven program to preserve and restore functional ability in hospitalized elderly patients. *Journal of Nursing Administration, 25*, 30–37.

Harrell, J. S., McConnell, E. S., Wildman, D. S., & Samsa, G. P. (1989). Do nursing diagnoses affect functional status? *Journal of Gerontological Nursing, 15*(10), 13–19.

Hartmaier, S. L., Sloane, P. D., Guess, H. A., Koch, G. G., Mitchell, M., & Phillips, C. D. (1995). Validation of the minimum data set cognitive performance scale: Agreement with the mini-mental state examination. *Journal of Gerontology, 50A*(2), M128–133.

Hawes, C., Morris, J. N, Phillips, C. D., Fries, B. E., Murphy, K., & Mor, V. (1997). Development of the nursing home resident assessment instrument in the USA. *Age and Aging, 26*(Suppl. 2), 19–25.

Hawes, C., Morris, J. N., Phillips, C. D., Mor, V., Fries, B. E., & Nonemaker, S. (1995). Reliability estimates for the minimum data set for nursing home resident assessment and care screening. *The Gerontologist, 35*, 172–178.

Heafey, M. L., Golden-Baker, S. B., & Mahoney, D. W. (1994). Using nursing diagnoses and interventions in an inpatient amputee program. *Rehabilitation Nursing, 19*, 163–168.

Heater, B. S., Becker, A. M., & Olson, R. K. (1988). Nursing interventions and patient outcomes: a meta-analysis of studies. *Nursing Research, 37*, 303–307.

Heinemann, A. W., Kirk, P., Hastie, B. A., Semik, P., Hamilton, B. B., Linacre, J. M., et al. (1997). Relationships between disability measures and nursing effort during medical rehabilitation for patients with traumatic brain and spinal cord injury. *Archives of Physical Medicine & Rehabilitation, 78*, 143–149.

Helberg, J. L. (1993). Patients' status at home care discharge. *Image: Journal of Nursing Scholarship, 25*, 93–99.

Hirdes, J. P., & Carpenter, G. I. (1997). Health outcomes among the frail elderly in communities and institutions: Use of the minimum data set (MDS) to create effective linkages between research and policy. *Canadian Journal on Aging, 23*(Suppl.), 53–69.

Hirdes, J. P., Fries, B. E., Morris, J. N, Steel, K., Mor, V., Frijters, D., et al. (1999). Integrated health information systems based on the RAI/MDS series of instruments. *Healthcare Management Forum, 12*(4), 30–40.

Holzemer, W. L., & Henry, S. (1992). Computer-supported versus manually-generated nursing care plans: A comparison of patient problems, nursing interventions, and AIDS patient outcomes. *Computers in Nursing, 10*, 19–24.

Holzemer, W. L., Janson-Bjerklie, S., Brown, D. S., & Henry, S. B. (1991). The Quality Marker: A measure of outcomes of nursing care. *Communicating Nursing Research, 24*, 201.

Hoogerduijn, J. G., Schuurmans, M. J., Duijnstee, M. S. H., de Rooij, S. E., Grypdonck, M. F. H. (2006). A systematic review of predictors and screening instruments to identify older hospitalized patients at risk for functional decline. *Journal of Clinical Nursing, 16*, 46–57.

Horn, S. D., Buerhaus, P., Bergstrom, N., & Smout, R. J. (2005). RN staffing time and outcomes of long-stay nursing home residents. *American Journal of Nursing, 105*, 58–70.

Howard, E., & Reiley, P. (1994). Use of a nursing intensity system as a measure of patient function. *Applied Nursing Research, 7*, 178–182.

Huss, A., Stuck, A. E., Rubenstein, L. Z., Egger, M., & Cough-Gorr, K. M. (2008). Multidimensional preventive home visit programs for community-dwelling older adults: a systematic review and meta-analysis of randomized controlled trials. *Journal of Gerontology: Medical Sciences, 63A*, 298–307.

Irvine, D. M., O'Brien-Pallas, L., Murray, M., Cockerill, R., Sidani, S., Laurie-Shaw, B., et al. (2000). The reliability and validity of two health status measures for evaluating outcomes of home care nursing. *Research in Nursing and Health, 23*, 43–54.

Irvine, D., Sidani, S., & McGillis Hall, L. (1998). Linking outcomes to nurses' roles in health care. *Nursing Economic$, 16*(2), 87, 58–64.

Jette, A. M., Davies, A. R., Cleary, P. D., Calkins, D. R., Rubenstein, L. V., Finke, A. et al. (1986). The functional status questionnaire: Reliability and validity when used in primary care. *Journal of General Internal Medicine, 1*, 143–149.

Johnson, J. E., Fieler, V. K., Saidel Wlasowicz, G., Mitchell, M. L., & Jones, L. S. (1997). The effects of nursing care guided by self-regulation theory on coping with radiation therapy. *Oncology Nursing Forum, 24*, 1041–1050.

Johnson, M., & Maas, M. (Eds.). (1997). *Nursing outcomes classification (NOC)*. St. Louis, MO: Mosby.

Katz, J. N., Larson, M. G., Phillips, C. B., Fossel, A. H., & Liang, M. H. (1992). Comparative measurement sensitivity of short and longer status instruments. *Medical Care, 30*, 917–925.

Katz, S., & Akpom, C. A. (1976). Index of ADL. *Medical Care, 14*, 116–118.

Kaufert, J. M. (1983). Functional ability indices: Measurement problems in assessing their validity. *Archives of Physical Medicine and Rehabilitation, 64*, 260–267.

Kerse, N., Falloon, K., Moyes, S. A., Hayman, K. J., Dowell, T., Kolt, G. S., et al. (2008). DeLLITE Depression in late life: An intervention trial of exercise. Design and recruitment of a randomized controlled trial. *BMC Geriatrics.* Retrieved from http://www.biomedcentral.com/1471-2318/8/12

Kerse, N., Peri, K., Robinson, E., Wilkinson, T., von Randow, M., Kiata, L., et al. (2008). Does a functional activity programme improve function, quality of life, and falls for residents in long term care? Cluster randomised controlled trial. *British Medical Journal, 337*, 1445–1551.

King, P. A. (1978). Foot assessment of the elderly. *Journal of Gerontological Nursing, 4*(6), 47–52.

Kline Leidy, N. (1994). Functional status and the forward progress of merry-go-rounds: Toward a coherent analytic framework. *Nursing Research, 43*, 196–202.

Knight, M. M. (2000). Cognitive ability and functional status. *Journal of Advanced Nursing, 31*, 1459–1468.

Kolt, G. S., Schofield, G. M., Kerse, N., Garrett, N., & Oliver, M. (2007). Effect of telephone counseling on physical activity for low-active older people in primary care: A randomized, controlled trial. *Journal of the American Geriatrics Society, 55*, 986–992.

Krichbaum, K. (2007). GAPN postacute care coordination improves hip fracture outcomes. *Western Journal of Nursing Research, 29*, 523–544.

Lalonde, B. (1987). The general symptom distress scale: A home care outcome measure. *Quality Review Bulletin, 7*, 243–250.

Lang, N. M., & Clinton, J. E. (1984). Assessment of quality of nursing care. *Annual Review of Nursing Research, 2*, 135–163.

Lang, N. M., & Marek, K. D. (1990). The classification of patient outcomes. *Journal of Professional Nursing, 6*, 39–42.

Latour, C. H. M., De Vos, R., Huyse, F. J., De Jonge, P., Van Gemert, L. A. M., & Stalman, W. A. B. (2006). Effectiveness of post-discharge case management in general medical outpatients: a randomized, controlled trial. *Psychosomatics, 47*, 421–429.

Latour, C. H. M., van der Windt, D. A. W. M., de Jonge, P., Riphagen, I. I., de Vos, R., Huyse, F. J., et al. (2007). Nurse-led case management for ambulatory complex patients in general health care: A systematic review. *Journal of Psychosomatic Research, 62*, 385–395.

Lawton, B. A., Rose, S. B., Elley, C. R., Dowell, A. C., Fenton, A., & Moyes, S. A. (2008). Exercise on prescription for women aged 40–70 recruited through primary care: Two year randomised controlled trial. *British Medical Journal, 337*, 2509.

Lawton, M. P., & Brody, E. M. (1969). Assessment of older people: Self-maintaining and instrumental activities of daily living. *The Gerontologist, 9*, 179–186.

Legge, J. S., & Reilly, B. J. (1980). Assessing the outcomes of cancer patients in a home nursing program. *Cancer Nursing, 3*, 357–363.

Lush, M. T., Henry, S. B., Foote, K., & Jones, D. L. (1997). Developing a generic health status measure for use in a computer-based outcomes infrastructure. In U. Gerdin, M. Tallberg, & P. Wainwright (Eds.), *Nursing informatics* (pp. 229–234). Amsterdam: IOS Press.

Lush, M. T., & Jones, D. L. (1995). Developing an outcome infrastructure for nursing. In *JAMIA Symposium Supplement, SCAMC Proceeding* (pp. 625–629). American Medical Informatics Association. Philadelphia: Hanley and Belfus.

Lyons, T. F. (1971). Role clarity, need for clarity, satisfaction, tension, and withdrawal. *Organizational Behavior and Human Performance, 6*, 99–100.

Mahoney, F. A., & Barthel, D. W. (1965). Functional evaluation: the Barthel index. *Maryland State Medical Journal, 14*, 61–65.

McCorkle, R., Benoliel, J. Q., Donaldson, G., Georgiadou, F., Moinpour, C., & Goodell, B. (1989). A randomized clinical trial of home nursing care for lung cancer patients. *Cancer, 64*, 1375–1382.

McCormick, K. (1991). Future data needs for quality care monitoring, DRG considerations, reimbursement and outcome measurement. *Image, Journal of Nursing Scholarship, 23*(1), 29–32.

McCusker, J. M., Verdon, J., Yousignant, P., de Courval, L.P., Dendukuri, N., & Belzile, E. (2001). Rapid emergency department intervention for older people reduces risk of functional decline: Results of a multicenter randomized trial. *Journal of the American Geriatric Society, 49*, 1272–1281.

McDowell, I., & Newell, C. (1996). *Measuring health. A guide to rating scales and questionnaires* (2nd ed.). New York: Oxford University Press.

McGillis Hall, L., Doran, D. M., Baker, G. R., Pink, G. H., Sidani, S., O'Brien-Pallas, L., et al. (2003). Nurse staffing models as predictors of patient outcomes. *Medical Care, 41*, 1096–1109.

Meissner, P., Andolsek, K., Mears, P. A., & Fletcher, B. (1989). Maximizing the functional status of geriatric patients in an acute community hospital setting. *The Gerontologist, 29*, 524–528.

Mendenhall, J. (1991). Diabetes self-care behaviors assessment. (Unpublished tool).

Milisen, K., Foreman, M. D., Abraham, I. L., De Geest, S., Godderis, J., Vandermeulen, E., et al. (2001). A nurse-led interdisciplinary intervention program for delirium in elderly hip-fracture patients. *Journal of the American Geriatrics Society, 49*, 523–532.

Mill Barrell, L., Irving Merwin, E., & Poster, E. C. (1997). Patient outcomes used by advanced practice psychiatric nurses to evaluate effectiveness of practice. *Archives of Psychiatric Nursing, 11*, 184–197.

Mitton, C., O'Neil, D., Simpson, L., Hoppins, Y., & Harcus, S. (2007). Nurse-physician collaborative partnership: a rural model for the chronically ill. *Canadian Journal of Rural Medicine, 12*, 208–216.

Mock, V., Barton Burke, M., Sheehan, P., Creaton, E. M., Winningham, M. L., McKenney-Tedder, S., et al. (1994). A nursing rehabilitation program for women with breast cancer receiving adjuvant chemotherapy. *Oncology Nursing Forum, 21*, 899–907.

Moorhead, S., Johnson, M., Maas, M., & Swanson, E. (2007). *Nursing outcomes classification (NOC)*. MO: Mosby.

Mundinger, M. O., Kane, R. L., Lenz, E. R., Totten, A. M., Tsai, W. Y., Cleary, P. D., et al. (2000). Primary care outcomes in patients treated by nurse practitioners or physicians. *Journal of the American Medical Association, 283*, 59–68.

Naylor, M. D., Munro, B. H., & Brooten, D. A. (1991). Measuring the effectiveness of nursing practice. *Clinical Nurse Specialist, 5*, 210–215.

Olson, R. S. (2001). Community re-entry after critical illness. *Critical Care Nursing Clinics of North America, 13,* 449–461.

Orem, D. E. (1980). *Nursing: Concepts of practice* (2nd ed.). New York: McGraw-Hill.

Ouellet, L. L., & Rush, K. L. (1996). A study of nurses' perception of client mobility. *Western Journal of Nursing Research, 18,* 565–579.

Peri, K., Kerse, N., Robinson, E., Parsons, M., Parsons, J., & Latham, N. (2008). Does functionally based activity make a difference to health status and mobility? A randomised controlled trial in residential care facilities (The Promoting Independent Living Study; PILS). *Age and Aging, 37,* 57–63.

Pettersson, E., Gardulf, A., Nordström, G., Svanberg-Johnsson, C., & Bylin, G. (1999). Evaluation of a nurse-run asthma school. *International Journal of Nursing Studies, 36,* 145–151.

Pfieffer, E. (Ed). (1975). *Multidimensional functional assessment: The OARS methodology.* Durham, NC: Center for the Study of Aging and Human Development.

Podsialdo, D., & Richardson, S. (1991). The timed "up & go": A test of basic functional mobility for frail elderly persons. *Journal of the American Geriatrics Society, 39,* 142–148.

Pringle, D. M., & White, P. (2002). Happenings. Nursing matters: The Nursing and Health Outcomes Project of the Ontario Ministry of Health and Long-Term Care. *Canadian Journal of Nursing Research, 33,* 115–121.

Pugh, L. C., Haven, D. S., Xie, S., Robinson, J. M., & Blaha, C. (2001). Case management for elderly persons with health failure: The quality of life and cost outcomes. *MEDSURG Nursing, 10,* 71–78.

Ramler, C. L., Kraus, V. L., Pringle Specht, J., & Titler, M. G. (1996). MOS SF-36: Clinical and administrative implications for nurses. In K. Kelly & M. Maas (Eds.), *Outcomes of effective management practice* (pp. 71–93). Thousand Oaks, CA: Sage.

Raphael, D., Smith, T., Brown, I., & Renwick, R. (1995). Development and properties of the short and brief version of the quality of life profile: Senior version. *International Journal of Health Sciences, 6,* 161–168.

Reiley, P., Lezzoni, L. I., Phillips, R., Davis, R. B., Tuchin, L. I., & Calkins, D. (1996). Discharge planning: Comparison of patients' and nurses' perception of patients following hospital discharge. *Image: Journal of Nursing Scholarship, 28,* 143–147.

Richmond, T., McCorkle, R., Tulman, L., & Fawcett, J. (1997). Measuring function. In M. Frank-Stromborg & S. J. Olsen (Eds.), *Instruments for clinical health-care research* (2nd ed., pp. 75–85). Sudbury, MA: Jones and Bartlett.

Rootmensen, G. N., van Keimpema, A. R. J., Looysen, E. E., van der Schaaf, L., de Haan, R. J., & Jansen, H. M. (2008). The effects of additional care by a pulmonary nurse for asthma and COPD patients at a respiratory outpatient clinic: Results from a double blind, randomized clinical trial. *Patient Education Counseling, 70,* 179–186.

Rose, S. B., Lawton, B. A., Elley, C. R., Dowell, A. C., & Fenton, A. J. (2007). The "Women's Lifestyle Study," 2-year randomized controlled trial of physical activity counselling in primary health care: Rationale and study design. *BMC Public Health, 7,* 166.

Rosemann, T., Joos, S., Laux, G., Gensichen, J., & Szecsenyi, J. (2007). Case management of arthritis patients in primary care: A cluster-randomized controlled trial. *Arthritis & Rheumatism, 57,* 1390–1397.

Roy, C., & Roberts, S. L. (1981). *Theory construction in nursing: An adaptation model.* Englewood Cliffs, NJ: Prentice Hall.

Rubenstein, L. Z., Schairer, C., Wieland, G. D., & Kane, R. (1984). Systematic biases in functional status assessment of elderly adults: Effects of different data sources. *Journal of Gerontology, 39,* 686–691.

Sayers, S. P., Jette, A. M., Haley, S. M., Heeren, T. C., Guralnik, J. M., & Fielding, R. A. (2004). Validation of the late-life function and disability instrument. *Journal of the American Geriatrics Society, 52*, 1554–1559.

Schein, C., Gagnon, A. J., Chan, L., Morin, I., & Grondines, J. (2005). The association between specific nurse case management interventions and elder health. *Journal of the American Geriatrics Society, 53*, 597–602.

Shibayama, T., Kobayashi, K., Takano, A., Kadowaki, T., & Kazuma, K. (2007). Effectiveness of lifestyle counseling by certified expert nurse of Japan for non-insulin treated diabetic outpatients: a 1-year randomized controlled trial. *Diabetes Research and Clinical Practice, 76*, 265–268.

Shaughnessy, P. W., Crisler, K. S., & Schlenker, R. E. (1998). Outcome-based quality improvement in home health care: The OASIS indicators. *Home Health Care Management & Practice, 10*(2), 11–19.

Shortell, S. M., Rousseau, D. M., Gilles, R. R., Devers, K. J., & Simon, T. L. (1991). Organizational assessment in intensive care units (ICUs): Construct development, reliability, and validity of the ICU nurse-physician questionnaire. *Medical Care, 29*, 709–726.

Smith, R. (1994). Validation and reliability of the elderly mobility scale. *Physiotherapy, 80*, 745–747.

Steiner, A., Bronagh, W., Pickering, R. M., Wiles, R., Ward, J., & Brooking, J. I. (2001). Therapeutic nursing or unblocking beds? A randomized controlled trial of a post-acute intermediate care unit. *British Medical Journal, 322*, 453–459.

Stewart, A. L., Hays, R. D., & Ware, J. E., Jr. (1988). The MOS Short Form General Health Survey: Reliability and validity in a patient population. *Medical Care, 26*, 724–735.

Stocker Schneider, J., Barkaukas, V., & Keenan, G. (2008). Evaluating home health care nursing outcomes with OASIS and NOC. *Image: Journal of Nursing Scholarship, 40*, 76–82.

Suhonen, R., Välimäki, M., Katajisto, J., & Leino-Kilpi, H. (2007). Provision of individualized care improves hospital patient outcomes: an explanatory model using LISREL. *International Journal of Nursing Studies, 44*, 197–207.

Suhonen, R., Välimäki, M., Katajisto, J., Leino-Kilpi, H., & Katajisto, J. (2004). Testing the individualized care model. *Scandinavian Journal of Caring Sciences, 18*(1), 27–36.

Swan, B. A. (1998). Postoperative nursing care contributions to symptom distress and functional status after ambulatory surgery. *MEDSURG Nursing, 7*, 148–158.

Thompson, P., Lang, L., & Annells, M. (2008). A systematic review of the effectiveness of in-home community nurse led interventions for the mental health of older persons. *Journal of Clinical Nursing, 17*, 1419–1427.

Tulman, L., & Fawcett, J. (1990). Functional status during pregnancy and the postpartum: A framework for research. *Image: Journal of Nursing Scholarship, 22*, 191–194.

Van den Heede, K., Clarke, S. P., Sermeus, W., Vleugels, A., & Aiken, L. (2007). International experts' perspective on the state of the nurse staffing and patient outcomes literature. *Journal of Nursing Scholarship, 39*, 290–297.

Wade, D. T., & Hewer, R. L. (1987). Functional abilities after stroke: Measurement, natural history and prognosis. *Journal of Neurology, Neurosurgery, and Psychiatry, 50*, 177–182.

Walker, L. O., & Avant, K. C. (1994). *Strategies for theory construction in nursing* (3rd ed.). Norwalk, CT: Appleton and Lang.

Walsh, B., Pickering, R. M., & Brooking, J. I. (1999). A randomized controlled trial of nurse-led inpatient care for post-acute medical patients: A pilot study. *Clinical Effectiveness in Nursing, 3*, 88–90.

Waltz, C. F., & Strickland, O. L. (1988). *Measurement of nursing outcomes, volume 1: Measuring client outcomes.* New York: Springer.

Wang, T. J. (2004). Concept analysis of functional status. *International Journal of Nursing Studies, 41*, 457–462.

Wanich, C. K., Sullivan-Marx, E. M., Gottlieb, G. L., & Johnson, J. C. (1992). Functional status outcomes of a nursing intervention in hospitalized elderly. *Image: Journal of Nursing Scholarship, 24*, 201–207.

Ware, J. E. (1993). *SF-36 Health Survey: Manual and interpretation guide.* Boston: New England Medical Center, The Health Institute.

Wolf, Z., Giardino, E., Osbourne, P., & Ambrose, M. (1994). Dimensions of nurse caring. *Image: Journal of Nursing Scholarship, 26*, 107–111.

Yesavage, J. A., Brink, T. L., Rose, T. L., Lum, O., Adey, M., & Leirer, V. O. (1983). Development and validation of a geriatric depression screening scale: A preliminary report. *Journal of Psychiatric Research, 17*, 37–49.

Zemore, R., & Shepel, L. (1989). Effects of breast cancer and mastectomy on emotional support and adjustment. *Social Science and Medicine, 28*, 19–27.

Self-Care

Souraya Sidani

INTRODUCTION

Self-care has become a key dimension of health-related interventions, services, and practices across the continuum of care, which includes primary care, acute care, home care, long-term care, and rehabilitation settings. Self-care is the focus and the outcome of health and nursing care in these settings. Several factors have contributed to the importance of self-care within the health care system: (a) shifting patterns of disease to chronic illnesses prevalent among the aging population, (b) an ideological shift from a cure to a care and health promotion orientation, (c) healthcare economics characterized by limited resources and funds and by an emphasis on cost containment, leading to shorter hospital lengths of stay and to delivery of care on an outpatient basis, and (d) a consumer movement in which individuals are more knowledgeable about health issues and strategies to address these issues, demand increased control of their health and health care and active involvement in health-related decisions and care, and demonstrate a desire and motivation to improve their health, functioning, and well-being (Craddock, Adams, Usui, & Mitchell, 1999; Dodd & Miaskowski, 2000).

As a result of these changes, self-care has been identified as critical for effective health promotion and for successful management of acute and chronic conditions in various healthcare settings. However, self-care has gained the most attention in the management of chronic illness. Chronic illness, such as cancer, asthma, chronic obstructive pulmonary disease (COPD), diabetes, end-stage renal disease, rheumatoid arthritis, and heart disease, places many demands on the patients and the healthcare system. Chronic illnesses impose multiple and new demands on the affected persons. These illnesses are associated with the physical symptoms resulting from the underlying pathophysiology and/or treatment; emotional stresses of coping with and adjusting to the chronic condition; and changes in interpersonal relationships and physical and social functioning (Burks, 1999). With the changes in healthcare orientation and delivery, patients must assume primary responsibility for addressing these demands, carrying out the therapeutic regimen on a long-term basis, and identifying and effectively managing alterations in their condition.

Self-care is a philosophical orientation, as well as a framework, that underpins the design of health-related services and interventions offered to assist patients with chronic illness in different settings in managing their condition and preserving an acceptable level of healthy functioning. Self-care is a key component of chronic care models (Bodenheimer, Wagner, & Grumback, 2002; Wagner et al., 2001), which emphasize patients' empowerment and acquisition of self-management skills (Baker et al., 2005). Self care is the focus and the outcome of health promotion and illness management interventions aimed at improving resolution of health problems or symptoms, physical and psychosocial functioning, and overall health status of patients (Dodd & Miaskowski, 2000). Self-care represents the theoretical foundation for psychoeducational, cognitive, and behavioral interventions. These interventions entail planned learning activities aimed at enhancing patients' capacity to engage in health- and care-related decision making and their ability to perform self-care behaviors necessary to improve the presenting health condition (Grady, 2008; Rootmensen et al., 2008; Sit, Yip, Ko, Gun, & Lee, 2007). The learning activities involve informing patients about their condition and its treatment, and instructing them in (a) self-monitoring and identifying changes in condition and/or functioning, (b) interpreting the meaning and judging the severity of these changes, (c) assessing options for actions to manage these changes, and (d) selecting and performing appropriate actions. The expected goal of psychoeducational and cognitive-behavioral interventions delivered or coordinated by nurses is the proper performance of self-care actions or behaviors. Accordingly, self-care also is considered a nursing-sensitive outcome (Irvine, Sidani, & McGillis Hall, 1998; Johnson & Maas, 1997; Mitchell, Ferketich, & Jennings 1998).

Although self-care is recognized as the theoretical foundation and an outcome of nursing care and has been discussed in a large number of publications, studies that investigated self-care are characterized by theoretical limitations. Research on self-care as the foundation of nursing care falls short of clarifying the essential ingredients that distinguish self-care components from other components comprising nursing interventions (Chodosh et al., 2005; Grady, 2008). Research on self-care as a nursing-sensitive outcome is hampered by a lack of consistent definition of self-care and conceptualization of its dimensions, which results in variability in its operationalization and in a lack of well-established instruments to measure self-care accurately and comprehensively (Dashiff, McCaleb, & Cull, 2006; Padula, 1992). This state of the science precludes meaningful synthesis of the evidence regarding the effectiveness of self-care interventions in promoting patients' performance of self-care actions or behaviors. In addition, it prevents the generation of theories that explain the mechanism through which interventions produce the expected positive outcomes.

This chapter reviews the available literature on self-care as an outcome of nursing care and interventions. The first section provides a conceptual definition of self-care based on a concept analysis that clarifies the concept at the theoretical and operational levels. The second section summarizes the empirical evidence linking nursing interventions to the outcome of self-care. The third section identifies instruments measuring self-care that demonstrated reliability, validity, and sensitivity to change. The last section discusses issues in the measurement of self-care that should be taken into consideration when this outcome is assessed in research or in everyday practice.

SELF-CARE: A CONCEPT ANALYSIS AND DEFINITION

Self-care is a term that appeared in health-related literature in the 1970s (e.g., Levin, 1976). In nursing, Orem (1971, 1985, 1991, 2001) developed and refined a model of self-care. Other scholars derived from this model middle-range theories for describing self-care practices of various patient populations, or adopted and adapted perspectives on self-care that emerged in different health-related disciplines. These differences in the conceptualization of self-care led to diverse conceptual and operational definitions of this outcome.

In Orem's (2001) conceptualization, self-care is represented by two distinct yet interrelated concepts: self-care agency and self-care behavior. Self-care agency refers to the capacity of an individual to engage in self-care behaviors. It denotes the ability to initiate and perform actions directed toward the care of oneself. Self-care agency involves several domains, including: (1) the cognitive domain, that is, knowledge of the health condition and of the cognitive skills necessary to fulfill the self-care action (e.g., decision-making skills), (2) the physical domain, that is, the physical ability to carry out the self-care action, (3) the emotional or psychosocial domain, that is, attitude, values, desire, motivation, and perceived competence in performing the self-care action, and (4) the behavioral domain, which refers to having the necessary skills for performing the self-care behaviors (Burks, 1999; Lantz, Fullerton, & Quayhagen, 1995).

Self-care behavior entails the practice of actions or activities that individuals initiate and perform, within time frames, on their own behalf in the interest of maintaining life, healthy functioning, continued personal development, and well-being (Jenerette & Murdaugh, 2008; Orem, 2001). The domains comprising self-care behavior are defined in relation to the universal, developmental, and health-deviation requisites. Universal requisites are concerned with basic life processes, such as maintaining an adequate intake of air and food, and a balance between activity and rest. Developmental requisites focus on the life cycle changes. Health-deviation requisites are related to changes in health condition that demand actions to manage, control, and prevent them (Kumar, 2007). Examples of these actions are health monitoring, seeking care as needed, and participating in treatment (Orem, 1991).

Orem characterized self-care behaviors as deliberate, purposeful activities that can be learned and performed voluntarily by individuals on the individuals' own behalf. Some nursing scholars focused on self-care behaviors within the context of illness and defined self-care as the performance of specific activities aimed at managing a health problem resulting from illness or its treatment, preventing complications, and maintaining and/or improving health and functioning throughout the acute and/or chronic illness experience (Braden, 1993; Jenerette & Murdaugh, 2008; Kreulen & Braden, 2004). In addition, other scholars conceptualized self-care as a process that permits people to take initiative and responsibility and to function effectively in developing their potential for health (Norris, 1979; Spradley, 1981). As applied to chronic illness, the process consists of recognizing health problems (e.g., symptoms), selecting appropriate activities to manage the problems, performing the selected activities, and evaluating the success of the activities in managing the problems (Grady, 2008). Riegel et al. (2004) distinguished between self-care and self-management. They defined self-care as a naturalistic decision-making process involving the selection and performance of behaviors that maintain physiologic stability, and self-management as the decision-making process initiated in response to symptoms when they occur.

To complement the scholars' conceptualization, three qualitative studies were conducted to investigate the patients' perception of self-care. The results provided the perspectives of those involved in self-care. Patients with chronic illness described self-care as taking care, not harming self, and listening to the body (Leenerts & Megilvy, 2000). Others defined it as a focused set of actions that participants used to enhance their mental and physical health. It entailed a process involving five dimensions: cognitive (i.e., normalizing), attitudinal (i.e., focusing on living), behavioral (i.e., taking care of oneself), interpersonal (i.e., being in relation to others), and existential (i.e., triumphing) (Barroso, 1995). Elderly persons living at home viewed self-care as involving caring for health and illnesses and carrying out activities of daily living. They identified four categories or levels of self-care performance, which they labeled as responsible, formally guided, independent, and abandoned. Responsible self-care implied activity and responsibility in all activities of daily living. Formally guided self-care consisted of regular but uncritical observance of medical instructions and routine performance of daily tasks. Independent self-care was based on the person's desire to listen to his or her internal voice. Helplessness and lack of responsibility characterized abandoned self-care (Backman & Hentinen, 1999).

Essential Attributes of Self-Care

The different conceptualizations of self-care are complementary, providing a comprehensive view of self-care. Self-care refers to the performance of health-related activities or behaviors. The self-care process underlies the performance of activities. The process entails recognition of changes in health condition, assessment of different activities for addressing the changes, selection of the most appropriate activities, performance of the selected activities, and evaluation of the effectiveness of the activities in addressing the changes in health condition. The self-care process and the performance of activities are initiated by the individuals, independently on their own behalf or in collaboration with health care professionals.

Self-care is operationalized as the actual engagement in activities. The specific activities reflective of self-care vary based on the purpose for which they are carried out (e.g., health promotion and maintenance, disease prevention, illness or symptom management), the target population (e.g., children and adults presenting with different actual or potential health problems), and the setting of healthcare or nursing care delivery (e.g., primary, acute, home, and long-term care).

Antecedents of Self-Care

The actual performance of self-care behavior or activity is influenced by a variety of factors. In addition to self-care agency, the factors are classified into five categories: cognitive, psychosocial, physical, demographic, and sociocultural. Self-care agency reflects the person's capacity to perform self-care behavior. Cognitive factors encompass cognitive function, learning skills, memory, problem-solving skills, organizational skills, and knowledge of the condition and self-care behaviors (Jaarsma, Halfens, Senten, Abu-Saad, & Dracup, 1998; Zambrowski, 2008). Psychosocial factors include self-concept, self-esteem, self-discipline, personality traits, perceived self-competence and self-efficacy, motivation, and perception that the behavior to be carried out is efficacious (Horsburgh, Beanlands, Looking-Cusolito, Howe, & Watson, 2000; Jenerette & Murdaugh, 2008; Whetstone & Hansson, 1989). Physical factors involve dexterity, psychomotor skills, functional or movement level, and disability or injury (Gaffney & Moore, 1996; Zambrowski). Demographic factors affecting self-care behavior are age or maturity, gender, education, socioeconomic status, and living arrangement (Dashiff et al., 2006; Gaffney & Moore; Jenerette & Murdaugh). Sociocultural factors entail family system, cultural beliefs and practices, health beliefs and values, social support, and availability of resources (Backman & Hentinen, 1999; Gaffney & Moore; Jenerette & Murdaugh).

The empirical evidence supporting the influence of the mentioned factors is derived from studies that examined the direct association of selected factors with either self-care agency or self-care behavior. A few studies were concerned with the relationship between self-care agency and self-care behavior.

Antecedents of Self-Care Agency

A few studies investigated the association between selected factors and self-care agency in healthy adults and in adults with chronic illness. Gender, age, perceived health status, health locus of control, perceived self-efficacy, learned helplessness, personality traits, and marital status were found to influence self-care agency in healthy and ill adults. Women reported higher levels of self-care agency than men in a sample of healthy adults (Whetstone & Hansson, 1989) and in patients with end-stage renal disease on dialysis (Horsburgh, 1999). Older persons reported higher levels of self-care agency than younger ones in a sample of healthy adults (Whetstone & Hansson) and in patients with end-stage renal disease on dialysis (Horsburgh, 1999). Perceived health status was positively correlated to self-care agency in older patients with end-stage renal disease (Horsburgh et al., 2000). Perceived health locus of control and perceived self-efficacy were positively related to the exercise of self-care agency in patients with hypertension; that is, patients who perceived more control over their health and had higher self-efficacy had higher scores on self-care agency (Chen, 1999). Learned helplessness was negatively related to self-care agency in healthy adults (Nelson McDermott, 1993). Various personality traits were associated with self-care agency in patients with end-stage renal disease. Patients reporting higher levels of consciousness, openness, and extroversion had higher self-care agency scores (Horsburgh, 1999; Horsburgh et al., 2000). Married adults, whether healthy or with end-stage renal disease, had higher self-care agency scores (Horsburgh, 1999).

Antecedents of Self-Care Behavior

The relationships between different factors and performance of self-care behaviors were examined in a large number of studies. The target populations differed across studies and included healthy and ill children, adolescents, and adults. Although similar factors were found to influence self-care behaviors across the age span, pertinent results are synthesized for two cohorts: children/adolescents and adults.

Multiple factors were related to performance of self-care behaviors in children and adolescents. These were: gender, age, health status, socioeconomic status, cultural beliefs and practices, self-concept, and self-care agency. Although gender differences in self-care behavior performance were reported, the direction of the difference varied with the nature of the specific behaviors (McCaleb & Cull, 2000). For instance, female, more so than male, adolescents with type I diabetes engaged in diabetes self-management practices (Dashiff et al., 2006). Older adolescents tended to engage less in self-care practices (Dashiff et al.; McCaleb & Cull; Moore

& Mosher, 1997). Those who reported experiencing some health problems tended to engage less in self-care practices (McCaleb & Cull). Lower socioeconomic status, indicated by participation in a paid lunch program, was associated with increased self-care practices (McCaleb & Edgil, 1994). Church attendance had a positive influence on self-care; that is, healthy adolescents who attended church tended to practice self-care (McCaleb & Cull; McCaleb & Edgil). Ethnicity was also related to self-care behaviors; being White was associated with increased self-care behavior performance by healthy adolescents (Gaffney & Moore, 1996; McCaleb & Edgil; Moore & Mosher) and those with type I diabetes (Dashiff et al.). Self-concept and self-care agency were positively correlated with performance of self-care behavior in healthy adolescents (McCaleb & Edgil; Slusher, 1999).

A variety of demographic, sociocultural, physical, psychosocial, and cognitive factors were reported to be associated with the performance of self-care behaviors in young and old adults. Women engaged in self-care activities more than men in samples of patients with first-time myocardial infarction (MI) (Rodeman, Conn, & Rose, 1995). Older patients with chronic illness (Carroll, 1995; Wang & Lee, 1999) and patients hospitalized for the treatment of acute conditions (Doran et al., 2006) tended to report minimal engagement in self-care behaviors. Increased socioeconomic status was consistently associated with increased performance of self-care behaviors in patients with cancer receiving radiation therapy (Hanucharurnkul, 1989), in elderly women living in rural areas (Wang & Lee), and in healthy older adults (Nicholas, 1993). Social support was positively correlated with self-care behavior performance. This finding was consistent across samples of patients with first-time MI, patients receiving radiation therapy, and elderly women living in rural areas, despite differences in the operationalization of social support measured with established questionnaires (Hanucharurnkul; Rodeman et al.). Living with others was also associated with increased self-care behavior performance in healthy older adults (Nicholas). Being married was related to increased adherence to self-care recommendations in patients with congestive heart failure (Nail, Jones, Greene, Schipper, & Jensen, 1991).

Individuals' health status had an effect on self-care behavior performance, but the effect's direction was inconsistent because of variability in the operationalization of health status across studies. When health status was measured with general perceived health scales, the relationship with self-care behavior was positive; when health status was measured as perceived disability, the relation was negative. Perception of high level of health correlated positively with perceived effectiveness of self-care behaviors undertaken to manage the side effects of chemotherapy (Dodd, Thomas, & Dibble, 1991), and with performance of self-care by elderly women living in rural areas (Wang & Lee, 1999) and by healthy adults (Nicholas, 1993). In contrast, when health state was measured with perceived disability (LeFort, 2000) or with stage of cancer (Hanucharurnkul, 1989), it was associated with decreased self-care behavior performance.

A high level of perceived self-care efficacy was consistently related to increased self-care practices, despite variability in the measurement of these two variables and variability in the target populations, including patients on hemodialysis (Lev & Owen, 1998), patients recovering from cardiovascular surgery (Carroll, 1995), patients with idiographic pain (LeFort, 2000), and patients with congestive heart failure (Ni et al., 1999). Resourcefulness was also associated with increased engagement in self-help behaviors in patients with idiographic pain (LeFort, 2000). Having high levels of perceived self-care agency had a significant positive influence on self-care behaviors performance, as reported by pregnant women (Hart, 1995), older patients with end-stage renal disease (Horsburgh et al., 2000), and patients with advanced heart failure (Jaarsma et al., 2000). In elderly patients on hemodialysis, Badzek, Hines, and Moss (1998) found a significant positive correlation between the patients' educational level and length of time on hemodialysis, and knowledge of self-care activities related to food and fluid restrictions. Similarly, Ni et al. found a positive relationship between knowledge of, and adherence to, self-care recommendations in patients with congestive heart failure. Doran et al. (2006) reported a negative, weak relationship between cognitive function and self-care in hospitalized patients with acute conditions. Patients exhibiting cognitive impairment had low levels of self-care.

Although the number of studies that examined the relationship between self-care behaviors and each specific factor is rather limited, the results are consistent despite differences in target populations and operationalizations of self-care behaviors. The findings provide preliminary evidence supporting the hypothesized influence of antecedent factors on self-care agency and behavior. Accordingly, these factors could be viewed as determinants or risk factors of self-care and should be taken into consideration when designing nursing interventions aimed at promoting self-care and/or when evaluating the impact of nursing interventions and care on the outcome of self-care. Specifically, the antecedent factors represent the characteristics used to tailor interventions or to individualize nursing care. Further, these characteristics should be accounted for when monitoring patients' self-care practices and determining the effectiveness of nursing care in improving self-care behaviors.

Consequences of Self-Care

The performance of self-care behavior is considered beneficial to the individual patient and to the healthcare system. At the individual patient level, self-care behavior is hypothesized to contribute to increased sense of responsibility, control, and autonomy (Skoner, 1994; Slusher, 1999); improved coping with or adjustment to illness (Leveille et al., 1998; Slusher); enhanced recovery from surgery or illness and decreased risk for complications (Badzek et al., 1998; Kimberly, 1997); and achievement of desired outcomes such as increased sense of well-being, symptom control, functioning, and quality of life (Dodd et al., 1991; Slusher).

Only two studies were located that investigated the effects of self-care behaviors on the proposed consequences at the individual patient level. Doran et al. (2006) reported a significant positive association between self-care behavior and functional independence in patients with acute illness; those who engaged in self-care were also able to perform activities of daily living independently. Kreulen and Braden (2004) found that self-care practice predicted changes in health status of women with stage 1 or 2 breast cancer.

The benefits of self-care behavior to the healthcare system appear to be derived from the patients' achievement of intended outcomes. These include decreased rates of hospital readmission (Dunbar, Jacobson, & Deaton, 1998) and health services utilization (Leveille et al., 1998), as well as reduced healthcare costs (Slusher, 1999). No study was located that systematically explored the impact of self-care behavior on the proposed benefits to the healthcare system.

In summary, this concept analysis identified two aspects of self-care: (1) self-care agency, which is defined as the person's perceived ability to engage in self-care, and (2) self-care behavior, which refers to the performance of health-related activities. The aims of these activities encompass the promotion and maintenance of health, prevention of disease, and management of illness or changes in body function. The specific activities performed vary with the aims and the target population. Persons initiate the activities independently or in collaboration with healthcare professionals, guided by the self-care process. The process entails assessment of activities for addressing the presenting health condition and selection and performance of appropriate activities. The engagement in self-care behaviors is affected by different demographic, sociocultural, physical, cognitive, and psychosocial factors and is beneficial to individual patients and the healthcare system.

EMPIRICAL EVIDENCE LINKING SELF-CARE TO NURSING

Self-care is the fundamental principle underlying many health interventions delivered by nurses independently or in collaboration with other health professionals. It is the primary concern and goal of educational, psychological, cognitive, and behavioral treatments offered as separate interventions or as a component in rehabilitation or chronic disease self-management programs. In general, these interventions focus on providing individuals self-care-related knowledge, which is necessary for engaging in the process underlying self-management, and on instructing them in the skills required to perform self-care behavior. Examples of these interventions include the Pro-Self Program (Dodd & Miaskowski, 2000), the Self-Help Intervention (Braden, Mishel, Longman, & Burns, 1993), psychoeducational programs for managing chronic pain (LeFort, Gray-Donald, Rowat, & Jeans, 1998), the Arthritis Self-Management Program (Lorig, Konkol, & Gonzalez, 1987), and chronic disease self-management for diabetes, hypertension

(Grady, 2008), asthma, COPD (Jónsdóttir, 2008; Rootmensen et al., 2008), and heart diseases (Dunagan et al., 2005).

A comprehensive literature search was conducted to identify studies that evaluated the effects of interventions on self-care. The search covered the following computerized databases: CINHAL, HEALTH PLANNING, MEDLINE, CANCERLIT, and PSYCHLIT. The specific keywords used were: *self-care,* self-care agency, *self-care behavior,* self-care practice, *self-care performance, and* self-management, combined with *nursing interventions and outcomes.* A total of 29 studies and 5 systematic reviews were analyzed for this review. The studies evaluated the effectiveness of interventions that nurses provided independently or in collaboration with physicians. The systematic reviews synthesized the evidence related to the effectiveness of self-management programs delivered by nurses and/ or other health professionals in patients with different chronic diseases. Although self-care is a theoretically anticipated outcome of these interventions, few studies have evaluated their effectiveness in achieving self-care.

A total of 23 studies were analyzed for this review. Almost all evaluated the effectiveness of educational or psychoeducational interventions that nurses provided. **TABLE 3-1** summarizes information pertinent to the studies' design, sample, outcome and measures, intervention, and results.

In several studies done prior to 2000, the intervention was based on Orem's model of self-care, in which the nurses' role in promoting self-care is described as supportive–educative. In general, the interventions were educational or psychoeducational in nature; the nurses' functions involved providing patients with the information and resources needed to engage in self-care, and assisting or supporting them in incorporating self-care behaviors into their everyday lives. Recently, the design of single interventions was guided by the theory underlying cognitive-behavioral or motivational therapy, whereas the design of multicomponent programs was guided by the principles underlying chronic disease models. Single interventions consisted of any of the following elements: education about the illness and its treatment and opportunities to practice self-care skills; setting of individual goal and action plan; cognitive reframing; and discussion of factors that facilitate or impede performance of self-care behaviors (e.g., Dunagan et al., 2005; Ismail et al., 2008; Kreulen & Braden, 2004; Sit et al., 2007; Vrijhoef, van Den Bergh, Diederiks, Weemhoff, & Preeuwenberg, 2007). The multicomponent programs involved collaboration between nurses and physicians to promote patients' self-management of their chronic disease. The nurses' functions entailed coordination of patient care; enhancement of patients' participation in goal attainment, self-monitoring, and accessing of community resources; and promotion of adherence to care guidelines by health professionals involved in patient care management (e.g., Baker et al., 2005; Bauer et al., 2006; Rootmensen et al., 2008).

Although self-care is a theoretically anticipated outcome of these interventions and programs, not all studies evaluated their effectiveness in achieving self-care.

TABLE 3-1 Studies Investigating the Relationship Between Nursing Interventions and Self-Care

Author	Design	Setting/ sample	Outcome	Nurse structural variable	Nurse process variable (intervention)	Description of instrument	Results
Gregory (2000)	Quasi-experimental	School $n = 150$ Students with asthma (Grades 3–5)	Strategies for managing asthma signs and symptoms (pharmacological and nonmedical)	None	Education by school nurse	Minimal description of measure; not validated	Students who attended the educational sessions were able to adequately describe reactions to asthma, recognize signs and symptoms, and manage signs and symptoms through medical or nonmedical strategies (e.g., try to calm down, rest or slow down, taking deep breaths) more so than the control group.
Hagopian (1996)	Experimental with posttest only; random assignment to control and experimental groups	Acute care $n = 31$ in control and 38 in experimental Patients being treated with radiation therapy; mean age 53, majority White, female	Radiation side effects profile: report on side effects experienced and use/ effectiveness of self-care strategies	None	Listening to audiotapes discussing side effects and suggested self-care strategies	Outcome measure not validated	Experimental group reported greater use of self-care strategies and a higher level of perceived effectiveness of self-care strategies used.
Watson et al. (1997)	Experimental with pretest and posttest; random assignment to control and experimental groups	Outpatient $n = 27$ in control and 29 in treatment Patients with COPD, smoking history of 10 years, mean age 67 years, more males	Use of medications, respiratory status	None	Patient education about self-medication (given by nurses)	Not applicable	Patients in experimental group showed improvement in self-medication adjustment.

(continues)

TABLE 3-1   Studies Investigating the Relationship Between Nursing Interventions and Self-Care (continued)

Author	Design	Setting/ sample	Outcome	Nurse structural variable	Nurse process variable (intervention)	Description of instrument	Results
Gallefoss & Bakke (1999)	Experimental; posttest; random assignment to control and experimental groups	Outpatient n = 140 Patients with asthma or COPD; majority women	Compliance with medications	None	Patient education on self-management of medications	Minimal description of measure	The odds ratio for having a compliance rate greater than 75% was 2.8 in education group.
Turner et al. (1998)	Experimental; random assignment to 2 experimental groups	Primary care clinic n = 117 Patients with asthma; 53% women	Medication usage and symptom control	None	Experimental group 1: patient education Experimental group 2: self-management plan	Minimal description of measure	Significant decrease in signs and symptoms scores in both groups. Improvement in medications usage as prescribed in both groups.
Hanucharurnkui & Vinya-nguag (1991)	Experimental with blocking on age; posttest; random assignment to control or experimental groups	Acute care n = 40, 20 in each group Patients who underwent pyelolithotomy or nephrolithotomy	Pain experience and ambulation	None	Patient education focusing on postoperative care	None related to self-care	Experimental group reported lower pain severity and distress and greater ambulation than control group.
Williams et al. (1988)	Quasi-experimental with repeated measures; posttest only	Acute care N = 60 Patient undergoing mastectomy or hysterectomy; 72% < 50 years; 65% married; had stage 1 or 2 cancer	Self-care behavior performance (ambulation, exercise, clinic appointment)	None	Patient education pre- and post-op with a focus on self-care activities	Minimal description of measure	Patients in experimental group performed the self-care behaviors earlier and more appropriately than those in the control group.

Dodd (1983)	Experimental with four experimental groups	Acute care $n = 48$, 12 in each group Patients with cancer receiving chemotherapy	Self-care behavior	None	Group 1: drug info Group 2: informational package for symptom management Group 3: combination Group 4: control	Self-care behavior log; content validity maintained	Significant difference among groups on the number of self-care behaviors performed (highest mean for patients who received the informational package).
Jaarsma et al. (2000)	Experimental with repeated measures	Acute care $n = 132$ Patients with advanced heart failure, mean age 72; 60% men	Appraisal of Self-Care Agency Scale, Heart Failure Self-Care Behavior Scale	None	Patient education with a focus on self-care	Both measures of self-care are validated; limited sensitivity to change	No difference in self-care agency at posttest. Significant difference in Self-care behaviors at posttest and follow-up. Significant correlation between self-care behavior and self-care agency (.30) and psychological adjustment of illness (−.25).
Aish (1996)	Experimental with pretest and posttest; random assignment to control and experimental groups	Acute care $n = 104$ Patients hospitalized for myocardial infarction I; mean age 65 years for women and 59 for men	Food habits questionnaire; appraisal of Self-Care Agency Scale	None	Home visit and instructions on diet management	Measure of self-care agency: validated measure of food habits: minimal description	Experimental group showed significant decrease in fat intake and increase in healthy food habits. Positive correlation between self-care agency and food habits.

(continues)

TABLE 3-1 Studies Investigating the Relationship Between Nursing Interventions and Self-Care (continued)

Author	Design	Setting/sample	Outcome	Nurse structural variable	Nurse process variable (intervention)	Description of instrument	Results
LeFort et al. (1998)	Experimental with block on gender; pretest and posttest; random assignment to control and experimental groups	Outpatient $n = 110$, 57 in treatment and 53 in control Patients with idiographic, chronic pain; more women; middle age; mean pain duration 6 years; taking medications	Pain; performance of self-help activities	None	Psychoeducation program focusing on pain management	Measures of pain and self-help activities (Inventory of Adult Role Behaviors): validated	Patients in experimental group reported less pain and more involvement in valued adult role activities.
Hart & Foster (1998)	Secondary data analysis	Outpatient $n = 127$ Pregnant women enrolled in prenatal care, 119 enrolled in childbirth education classes	Self-care agency	None	Childbirth education	Measure of self-care agency (Appraisal of Self-Care Agency Scale): validated	Women who had childbirth education and were primiparous and college educated had higher scores.
Harper (1984)	Experimental with repeated measures; random assignment to control and experimental groups	Outpatient $n = 60$, 30 in each group Women with essential hypertension; mean age 66 years; widowed; had other diseases	Knowledge of medications; self-care behavior	None	Patient education about medications	Measures of both outcomes: not validated	Patients in experimental group had significant increase in knowledge and self-care behavior.

Craddock et al. (1999)	Quasi-experimental	Outpatient $n = 48$, 26 experimental and 22 in control Women with breast cancer receiving chemotherapy; stage 1 or 2; well educated; mean age 49; 65% married	Self-care agency; effectiveness of self-care strategies	None	Patient education and telephone follow-up focusing on management of side effects	Measure of self-care agency: validated Measure of effectiveness of self-care strategies: minimal description	No significant difference between groups on effectiveness of self-care strategies and self-care agency. No significant correlation between self-care agency and effectiveness of self-care strategies.
Albrecht et al. (1993)	Correlational	Patient home $n = 154$ Patients with arthritis; mean age 56; 85% women; 73% White; married	Self-care behaviors	None	Patient education focusing on self-management	Measure of self-care behaviors: not validated	No effect on self-care behavior performance reported, however (B = .20), age (.23) and number of lessons (.18) affected satisfaction with intervention.
Folden (1993)	Quasi-experimental	Outpatient $n = 34$ in control, 34 in experimental Patients with stoke, mean age 75; 74% married; 56% men	Self-care agency; performance of activities of daily living	None	Guided decision-making regarding self-management	Measure of self-care agency: validated	Patients in experimental group increased self-care agency scores and performance of activities of daily living (i.e., walking).
Goeppinger et al. (1995)	Quasi-experimental (1 group)	Patient home $n = 154$ Patients with arthritis at home	Self-care behavior	None	Patient education	Measure of self-care behavior: validated	Patients showed improvement in self-care behavior performance.

(continues)

TABLE 3-1   Studies Investigating the Relationship Between Nursing Interventions and Self-Care (continued)

Author	Design	Setting/ sample	Outcome	Nurse structural variable	Nurse process variable (intervention)	Description of instrument	Results
Rootmensen et al. (2008)	Experimental with pretest and posttest; random assignment to control and experimental groups	Outpatient $n = 94$ in control and 97 in experimental group Patients with asthma or COPD; mean age 60 years; men; low level of education	Knowledge of self-care; performance of inhalation technique; self-management	None	Education provided by pulmonary nurse	Outcome measures derived from other measures; no psychometric properties reported	No between-group differences in all outcomes at posttest.
Sit et al. (2007)	Quasi-experimental with repeated measures	Primary care $n = 70$ in control and 77 in experimental group Patients with minor stroke; mean age 63 years; 50% men; low level of education	Knowledge of self-care; performance of health maintenance behaviors; dietary habits	None	Group sessions focusing on self-management	Outcome measures adapted from similar measures; no psychometric properties reported	Patients in experimental group showed improvement in all outcomes.
Vrijhoef et al. (2007)	Experimental with repeated measures; random assignment to control or experimental groups	Outpatient $n = 83$ in control and 91 in experimental groups Patients with COPD; more men; mean age 64 years	Self-care knowledge and self-care behavior	None	Consultation with nurse focusing on self-care management	Minimal description of outcome measures	Patients in experimental group showed improvement in self-care behaviors; incomplete response to self-care knowledge questionnaire.
Doran et al. (2006)	Nonexperimental, repeated-measure design	Acute care $n = 574$ Patients admitted to medical and surgical units; mean age 63years; 51% women	Self-care	None	Provision of nursing interventions	Measure of self-care: validated	Self-care predicted by age and cognitive function. No relationship between provision of nursing interventions and self-care.

	Design	Sample	Outcome variables		Intervention/Experimental groups	Measures	Results
Ismail et al. (2008)	Experimental with repeated measures; random assignment to control and 2 experimental groups	Primary care; $n = 121$ in control, 117 in experimental group 1, 106 in experimental group 2; Patients with diabetes; mean age 36 years; 60% women	Self-care behaviors	None	Experimental group 1: motivational enhancement therapy; Experimental group 2: motivational enhancement therapy and cognitive behavioral therapy; Both focus on diabetes self-management.	Measure of outcome (diabetes self-care activities): validated	No significant improvement in self-care behaviors observed in both experimental groups.
Kreulen & Braden (2004)	Experimental with repeated measures; random assignment to 3 experimental groups	Outpatient; $n = 307$; Women with breast cancer receiving adjuvant therapy; mean age 55 years	Self-care behaviors	None	Group 1: self-help classes; Group 2: self-help independent study; Group 3: uncertainty management telephone contact	Measures of self-care behaviors: validated	Significant improvement in self-care behaviors in all groups.
Dunagan et al. (2005)	Experimental with repeated measures; random assignment to control or experimental groups	Outpatient; $n = 75$ in control, 76 in experimental; Patients with heart failure; more women; mean age 69 years	Confidence in knowledge and ability to manage illness	None	Nurse administered telephone-based program focused on disease management	Minimal description of measures	No between-group differences in outcomes following intervention.
Baker et al. (2005)	Cross-sectional survey	Outpatient; $n = 781$; Patients with health failure; age > 65 years; 52% women	Knowledge about disease and self-care; Self-management activities	None	Provision of care under the chronic care model; physician-and-nurse teams counseled patients relative to self-management strategies	Minimal description of measures	Patients in experimental group showed improvement in knowledge and in performance of some self-care strategies (monitoring weight).

When examined as an outcome, self-care was operationalized as self-care agency (e.g., Aish, 1996; Hart & Foster, 1998; Jaarsma et al., 2000) or self-care knowledge, which is one aspect of self-care agency (e.g., Baker et al., 2005; Rootmensen et al., 2008; Vrijhoef et al., 2007), and as self-care behavior, that is, performance of self-care activities (e.g., Albrecht et al., 1993; LeFort, 2000; Ismail et al., 2008; Kreulen & Braden, 2004; Sit et al., 2007). The specific aspects of self-care agency and behaviors measured varied across the studies, depending on the focus of the intervention and on the target population. The specific self-care aspects represented were: (1) adherence to prescribed drug regimen, (2) performance of recommended healthy behaviors related to diet, exercise, and stress management, (3) monitoring and management of symptoms, and (4) engagement in activities of daily living and valued role activities such as work and recreation. Recent studies investigated the direct effects of self-care interventions and programs on other outcomes that represented the consequences of self-care identified through the concept analysis. The additional outcomes encompassed clinical indicators of disease (e.g., blood glucose); symptom exacerbation; physical, mental, and social functioning; health-related quality of life; health services utilization; and costs of care.

However, no study examined the indirect effects of self-care interventions and programs on the additional outcomes. As implied in the framework underlying the interventions, achievement of adequate self-care agency and behavior is the mechanism mediating the effects of the interventions on the additional outcomes. This mediating influence is also consistent with the results of the concept analysis indicating that these outcomes are consequences of self-care.

The populations targeted in these studies involved primarily adults presenting with different acute and chronic conditions. These conditions included general and cardiac surgery, cancer, COPD, asthma, heart failure, MI, idiopathic pain, hypertension, arthritis, diabetes, stroke, and mental disorders.

In the overwhelming majority of the studies, the research designs were experimental or quasi-experimental, involving an experimental and a comparison group. These designs are appropriate to address the study purpose, which is to determine the effectiveness of self-care interventions or programs. Few studies used a nonexperimental design, in which data on receipt of self-management, educational interventions, and posttest outcomes were available in a database or gathered as part of daily practice prospectively. Although lack of a comparison group limits causal inference, the results of these studies provide evidence of the extent to which receipt of these interventions is associated with the intended outcomes in the real world (Sidani & Braden, 1998). As such, they complement the findings of experimental and quasi-experimental studies. Most studies assessed the self-care outcome at pretest and posttest; only a few included one or two follow-up posttest measurements. Yet follow-ups are useful for examining changes in self-care behaviors, which are known to require some time to take place and which are needed to demonstrate sustainability of improved self-care behaviors over time.

The sample sizes ranged from 48 to 781. The largest one was reported in a nonexperimental study targeting self-care in patients with heart failure. The rather small sample size observed in most studies is characteristic of experimental or quasi-experimental design. Nonetheless, the demographic and health-related characteristics of the participants were consistent with those of the target population. For instance, most nursing home residents were older women, whereas most patients with heart disease were middle-aged men.

The instruments used to measure the self-care outcome differed. Most were self-report measures that addressed the specific aspects of self-care of concern. For instance, some instruments assessed self-care knowledge, medication compliance, and blood pressure monitoring; others captured engagement in healthy behaviors such as exercise and diet, in addition to adherence to medications and blood glucose monitoring; and still others focused on performance of usual activities and role functions. Further, in some studies, elements of the process underlying self-care were measured with separate items or instruments.

The variability observed in the nature and focus of self-care interventions, self-care outcome of interest, operationalization of self-care, and target population limited the ability to synthesize the results. Therefore, key findings are summarized in point form for different populations and types of interventions.

- Children with asthma who attended educational sessions provided by school nurses were able to adequately describe physical reactions to asthma, recognize symptoms, and manage the symptoms by properly using medications and applying nonmedical strategies such as trying to calm down, resting or slowing down, and taking deep breaths more so than children in the control group (Gregory, 2000).
- Pregnant women who attended childbirth education classes had higher level of self-care agency than those who did not (Hart & Foster, 1998).
- Patients who had surgery and who were instructed in the performance of postoperative exercises and ambulation engaged in these activities earlier and performed them more appropriately than those who received usual care (Hanucharurnkui & Vinya-nguag, 1991; Williams et al., 1988).
- Patients recovering from cardiovascular surgery showed an increased level of knowledge related to self-care strategies following an educational intervention given in individual or group sessions (Barnason & Zimmerman, 1995).
- Patients with cardiac diseases demonstrated improvement in self-care following educational interventions delivered by nurses and a self-management program given by nurses only or in collaboration with physicians. Specifically, patient education did not have a significant impact on self-care agency in patients with heart failure and advanced heart failure; however, its effect on self-care behavior was inconsistent in these two groups of patients. Whereas no differences were observed between patients with heart failure who received education and those who did not

(Jaarsma et al., 1999), patients with advanced heart failure who received education reported improvement in performance of self-care behaviors as compared with those who did not (Jaarsma et al., 2000). Dunagan et al. (2005) reported no significant changes in the perceived confidence in knowledge and ability to manage illness in patients with heart failure assigned to a nurse-administered self-management program; however, the patients showed modest improvement in physical function and decreased health services utilization. Baker et al. (2005) found statistically significant but small effects on self-care knowledge, engagement in self-management activities, and number of hospitalizations of a self-management program delivered by a nurse–physician team to patients with heart failure.

- Patients with cancer receiving adjuvant therapy appear to benefit from self-care interventions. Patients receiving radiation therapy who listened to audiotapes instructing them in self-management of treatment side effects reported more use of self-care activities and a higher level of perceived effectiveness of the self-care activities used than patients in the comparison group did (Hagopian, 1996). Inconsistent findings were observed for the effect of education on self-care behavior in patients with cancer receiving chemotherapy. Patients who received an information package on symptom management (Dodd, 1983) and a behavioral intervention focusing on problem-solving and symptom management skills, cognitive reframing, and belief in self (Braden et al., 1993; Kreulen & Braden, 2004) performed more self-care behaviors than those assigned to the comparison group. In contrast, patient education did not influence performance or perceived effectiveness of self-care activities in managing the side effects of chemotherapy (Craddock et al., 1999).

- Adult patients with asthma or COPD showed (1) appropriate adjustment in medication following instructions by nurses (Gallefoss & Bakke, 1999; Turner, Taylor, Bennett, & Fitzgerald, 1998; Watson et al., 1997) and (2) increased self-care knowledge and self-management behaviors after receiving collaborative pulmonary care from physicians and nurses (Rootmensen et al., 2008) or respiratory care by a nurse (Vrijhoef et al., 2007).

- Patients with hypertension showed appropriate adjustment of medication after instructions by nurses (Harper, 1984).

- Patients with idiographic pain who received a psychoeducational intervention focusing on pain management reported increased performance of valued adult role activities and self-care behaviors more so than did patients in the comparison group (LeFort et al., 1998).

- Persons with diabetes did not demonstrate significant changes in self-care behaviors after implementation of motivational enhancement therapy or motivational enhancement therapy combined with cognitive-behavioral therapy, as delivered by trained nurses (Ismail et al., 2008).

- The effects of patient education on self-care behaviors in patients with arthritis were inconsistent. Although Goeppinger, Macnee, Anderson, Boutaugh, and Stewart (1995) found a significant improvement in self-care behaviors performance, Albrecht et al. (1993) did not.
- Patients with stroke who were provided with guided decision-making showed increased performance of activities of daily living (e.g., walking) compared with those in the comparison group (Folden, 1993). Persons who suffered minor stroke benefited from a community-based education program for stroke prevention. Significant improvement in knowledge, health maintenance behaviors (e.g., blood pressure monitoring), dietary habits (e.g., decreased fat consumption), and seeking care in response to suspected stroke were observed.

Despite variability in the methodological quality of the studies, the results are consistent in supporting the effectiveness of interventions focused on self-management in improving performance of self-care behaviors. This conclusion was comparable with the findings of several meta-analyses that synthesized the effects of educational, psychoeducational, cognitive-behavioral, and self-management programs on self-care behaviors in different patient populations. The literature review identified the following active ingredients for these programs. The active ingredients for educational programs included provision of information on the health condition and self-care strategies, whereas those for psychoeducational programs consisted of provision of information on the health condition and self-care strategies and provision of support for the implementation of self-care strategies in daily life, and for cognitive-behavioral programs were provision of information, teaching self-care skills with opportunities to practice the skills, instructions in problem-solving, and cognitive reframing. Self-management programs consisted of psychoeducational and cognitive-behavioral interventions provided by members of the healthcare team, in addition to facilitating access to medical care based on acceptable guidelines.

Educational, psychoeducational, cognitive-behavioral, and self-management programs demonstrated the following effects:

- Favorable influence on behavioral change related to smoking, alcohol consumption, nutrition and weight control, and breast self-examination in the general population (Mullen et al., 1997).
- Moderate positive effect on self-care behaviors (effect size = .55) in patients with various conditions (McCain & Lynn, 1990).
- Strong positive effect on medication compliance (effect size = .74) in patients with hypertension (Devine & Reifschneider, 1995).
- Strong positive effect on adherence to treatment (effect size = .78), use of PRN medications (effect size = .62), and psychomotor skills related to the use of inhaler (effect size = 1.02) in adults with asthma (Devine, 1996).

- Enhanced appropriate use of medications (Manninkhof et al., 2003) and increased knowledge and self-efficacy related to self-care behaviors (Jónsdóttir, 2008) in patients with COPD.
- Increased practice of desired behaviors (e.g., exercise, relaxation, and joint protection) in patients with arthritis. This favorable effect was reported in 77–91% of the studies reviewed by Hirano, Laurent, and Lorig (1994) and Lorig et al. (1987), respectively.
- Low to moderate effect on self-care behaviors in patients with diabetes (Brown, 1992).
- Improved self-care performance in patients with heart failure (Hamner, 2005).

The empirical evidence clearly indicates improvement in the performance of self-care behaviors following psychoeducational, cognitive-behavioral, and self-management programs delivered by nurses. Consequently, self-care behavior is sensitive to nursing care and is instrumental for achieving intended patient and healthcare outcomes.

INSTRUMENTS MEASURING SELF-CARE

Several instruments have been developed to measure self-care agency and self-care behaviors. **TABLES 3-2** and **3-3** present information on the domains captured by the instruments measuring self-care agency and self-care behavior, respectively, and summarize the evidence supporting their reliability, validity, and sensitivity to change. Differences in the domains of self-care were observed across instruments, owing to differences in the specific self-care behaviors expected of patients with various conditions.

Measures of Self-Care Agency

Five instruments that measure the concept of self-care agency were located (see Table 3-2). They were all based on Orem's conceptualization of self-care. Because self-care agency refers to the person's capability or perceived ability to perform self-care behaviors, patients themselves would be the best persons to judge or rate the self-care agency. This point implies that measures of this concept should be self-administered, which was the case for four of the instruments reviewed. The Appraisal of Self-Care Agency (ASA) Scale has two versions: One is self-administered, and one is completed by a caregiver. The reported discrepancies between the patient's and the nurse's scores on this scale (Halfens, van Alphen, Hasman, & Philipsen, 1998) renders the nurse's assessment of the patient's self-care agency of limited clinical utility and confines it to specific conditions in which the patient is unable to self-report.

TABLE 3-2   Instruments Measuring Self-Care Agency

Instrument (author)	Target population/ practice setting	Domains (number of items and response format)	Method of administration	Reliability	Content validity	Construct validity	Sensitivity to nursing variable
Denyes Self-Care Agency Questionnaire (Denyes, 1980, as cited in Lantz et al., 1995)	Children and adolescents All settings	Domain: Ability to meet universal self-care requisites (psychosocial, cognitive, affective-moral, and physical) Number of items: 34 for adolescent version; 25 for children version Response format: 5-point, Likert-type	Self-administered	Internal consistency: split-half correlation coefficient .80 to .83 in healthy children (Moore, 1995); α coefficient .81 and .92 in healthy adolescents (Slusher, 1999); .84 in young adolescents with diabetes (Dashiff et al., 2006). Stability/test-retest: no data available	No data available	Positive correlation with self-care practice and with health status in children (Moore, 1995); with a measure of self-care practice in healthy adolescents (Slusher, 1999)	No data available
Exercise of Self-Care Agency Scale (Kearny & Fleischer, 1979)	Adults All settings	Domain: personal motivation, knowledge base and information-seeking, active vs. passive response to situations, self-concept or sense of self-worth. Number of items: original version: 43; adapted version for patients with coronary artery bypass graft (CABG): 35 (Carroll, 1995; Chen, 1999); Response format: 5-point Likert-type (*uncharacteristic of me* to *very characteristic of me*)	Self-administered	Internal consistency: split-half correlation .77 to .81 in health adults; α coefficients .77 and .87 in nursing students, healthy adults, elderly women, in patients with hypertension, patients recovering from CABG (Carroll, 1995; Chen, 1999; Kearny & Fleischer, 1979; Wang & Lee, 1999); Stability/test-retest: .77 in healthy adolescents (Moore, 1995); .79 to .94 in various samples of chronically ill patients, pregnant women, and healthy adults (Folden, 1993)	Established by five experts in self-care	Factorial structure: four factors consistent with domains (Chen, 1999); four factors representing self-care abilities, responsibilities, esteem, and evaluation (Whetstone & Hansson, 1989); Concurrent/ construct: positive correlation with self-confidence in adolescents (Moore, 1995)	Change in scores observed following a supportive-educative intervention (Carroll, 1995)

(continues)

TABLE 3-2 Instruments Measuring Self-Care Agency (continued)

Instrument (author)	Target population/ practice setting	Domains (number of items and response format)	Method of administration	Reliability	Content validity	Construct validity	Sensitivity to nursing variable
Appraisal of Self-Care Agency (ASA) Scale (Evers et al., 1986)	Adults All settings	Domains: Ability to perform the self-care behaviors related to eight universal self-care requisites (e.g., maintaining sanitary conditions, managing to be alone, getting enough sleep, taking safety measures, seeking help). Number of items: 24 Response format: 5-point Likert-type (*totally disagree* to *totally agree*)	2 versions: self-administered (ASA-A), and completed by the individual's spouse, significant other, or caregiver (such as nurse) (ASA-B)	Internal consistency: For ASA-A version: α coefficient .76 for pregnant women (Hart, 1995); .80 to .87 for patients with cardiac disease (Jaarsma et al, 1999); .77 in prenatal women (Hart & Foster, 1998); .84 in adults awaiting renal transplant (Horsburgh et al., 2000); .75 in patients with sickle cell disease (Jenerette & Murdaugh, 2008). For the ASA-B version: .77 to .87 for nurses (Soderhamn, Evers, & Hamrin, 1996) Stability/test-retest: .72 in elderly patients who underwent cardiac surgery (Aish, 1996) Interrater reliability: For ASA-B version for nurses caring for patients .64 to .71 (van Achterberg et al., 1991)	Considered relevant by Orem and eight experts in the theory of self-care	Positive correlation with performance of self-care behaviors in pregnant women (Hart, 1995) and in cardiac patients (Jaarsma et al., 2000); convergence of the ASA-A and ASA-B scores. (van Achterberg et al., 1991)	No data available

Perception of Self-Care Agency Questionnaire (Hanson, 1981, as cited in Nelson McDermott, 1993)	Adults All settings	Domain: Orem's (2001) 10 power components Number of items: 53 Response format: 5-point Likert-type (*not at all like me* to *always like me*)	Self-administered	Internal consistency: α .92–.96 in samples of healthy adults (Nelson McDermott, 1993). Stability/test-retest: No data available	Based on Orem's definition of self-care agency; validated by a panel of experts	Factorial structure: five factors (cognitive ability or limitation, motor motivation, repertoire of skills, ability to set priorities, and ability to integrate self-care operations); factorial invariance was not maintained (Nelson McDermott, 1993)	No data available
Self-Care Agency Inventory (Lantz et al., 1995)	Adults All settings	Domain: person's self-care knowledge and self-care actions. Major components: (1) enabling perceptual elements of motivation, values, responsibility, and decision-making; (2) enactment of self-care (cognitive/perceptual, psychosocial/affective, physical functioning); (3) self-care factors (action and knowledge) Number of items: 40 Response format: Each item presents a short situation and is followed by multiple-choice response options reflecting alternatives for self-care action and/or knowledge	Self-administered	Internal consistency: α coefficient .65 in patients and staff in family practice physician offices (Lantz et al., 1995) Stability/test-retest: .83 in a sample of adult persons (Lantz et al., 1995)	Established by two panels of five and of seven professionals with expertise in the area of self-care (CVI .95)	No clear evidence (Lantz et al., 1995)	No data available

TABLE 3-3 Instruments Measuring Self-Care Behavior

Instrument (author)	Target population/ practice setting	Domains; number of items; response format	Method of administration	Reliability	Content validity	Construct validity	Sensitivity to nursing variable
Denyes Self-Care Practice Instrument (Denyes, 1980; as cited in Lantz et al., 1995)	Healthy adolescents	SC actions performed in meeting the universal SC requisites and general SC actions; 17 items; numeric rating scale	Self-administered	ICR: α of .84 in adolescents (McCaleb & Edgil, 1994); .82 to .89 for healthy adolescents (McCaleb & Cull, 2000; Slusher, 1999). TRR: r of .84 in healthy adolescents (McCaleb & Edgil, 1994)	Established	Positive r with SC agency in healthy adolescents (Slusher, 1999)	No data available
Children and Adolescent Self-Care Practice Questionnaire (Moore, 1995)	Children 9–18 years old	Activities that children perform to meet their developmental and universal needs as identified by Orem; 35 items; 5-point Likert-type	Self-administered	ICR: α of .83 in healthy children (Moore, 1995) TRR: no data available	Rated as valid by a panel of seven experts	Factorial structure: 10 factors representing the developmental and universal SC requisites Positive r with SC agency in children (Moore, 1995)	No data available
Children's Self-Care Performance Questionnaire (Moore, 1995; Moore & Mosher, 1997)	Children with cancer	Developmental, universal, and health-deviation SC requisites; 51 items; 5-point Likert-type	Self-administered	ICR: α of .83 for children with cancer (Moore & Mosher, 1997). TRR: no data available	Rated as valid by pediatric oncology nurses	Performance of SC behaviors decreased with increasing age (Moore & Mosher, 1997)	No data available

Instrument	Population	Description	Administration	Reliability	CVI	Validity	Responsiveness
Dependent Care Agent Performance Questionnaire (Moore & Gaffney, 1989)	Caregivers of children, primarily mothers (healthy and having cancer)	SC activities directed toward meeting children's universal, development, and health-deviation needs; 39 items in healthy version, and 55 in children with cancer version; 5-point Likert-type	Self-administered	ICR: α of .99 for healthy caregivers (Gaffney & Moore, 1996); .91–.93 for mothers of children with cancer (Moore & Mosher, 1997) TRR: no data available	Established by panels of experts	For healthy version: low r with social desirability; negative r with child's age (Gaffney & Moore, 1996) For children with cancer version: positive r with children's performance of SC activity (Moore & Mosher, 1997)	No data available
Personal Life Style Questionnaire (Muhlenkamp & Brown, 1983, as cited in Nicholas, 1993)	Healthy older adults	Engagement in health promotion or SC activities; 24 items; 4-point rating scale	Self-administered	ICR: α of .74 to .76 for healthy adults (Nicholas, 1993) TRR: r of .78 and .88 (Nicholas, 1993)	No data available	Positive r with perceived health status in healthy older adults (Nicholas, 1993)	No data available
Self-Care Behaviors Inventory (Goeppinger et al., 1995)	Patients with arthritis	Performance of 16 SC activities (e.g., exercising, relaxation, nutrition, and sleep); 16 items; report number of times each activity was performed in the last 7 days	Self-administered	ICR: α of .75 for patients with arthritis (Goeppinger et al., 1995). TRR: no data available	No data available	No data available	Significant increase in the scores observed following a psychoeducational intervention

Note: r = correlation coefficient; α = Cronbach's alpha coefficient; ADLs = activities of daily living; CABG = coronary artery bypass graft surgery; CVI = content validity index; ICC = intraclass correlation coefficient; ICR = internal consistency reliability; IRR = interrater reliability; SC = self-care; TRR = test-retest reliability; VAS = visual analog scale.

(continues)

TABLE 3-3　Instruments Measuring Self-Care Behavior (continues)

Instrument (author)	Target population/ practice setting	Domains; number of items; response format	Method of administration	Reliability	Content validity	Construct validity	Sensitivity to nursing variable
Self-Care Diary (Nail et al., 1991)	Patients with cancer receiving chemotherapy	Incidence and severity of side effects experienced by patient receiving chemotherapy, and use and perceived effectiveness of SC activities to manage the side effects (Craddock et al., 1999; Nail et al., 1991); 18 items; 6-point rating scale to indicate use and effectiveness of SC activities	Self-administered	ICR: Not applicable TRR: r of .80 in patients with cancer receiving chemotherapy (Nail et al., 1991)	Reviewed by patients, oncology clinical nurse specialists, and physicians (Craddock et al., 1999; Nail et al., 1991)	Positive r between use of SC activities and SC agency in patients with breast cancer (Craddock et al., 1999)	No data available
Hart Prenatal Care Actions Scale (Hart, 1995)	Pregnant women	Areas of prenatal health activities (health supervision, nutrition maintenance, balancing activity and rest, maintenance of social interaction, abstinence from hazards, and knowledge acquisition); 41 items; 5-point Likert-type	Self-administered	ICR: α of .80 (Hart, 1995). TRR: no data available	Established by SC theory experts, childbirth educators, nurses, and pregnant women	Factorial structure: eight factors Positive r with SC agency (Hart, 1995)	No data available

Instrument	Population	Description	Administration	Reliability	Content validity	Construct validity	Responsiveness
Inventory of Adult Role Behaviors (Braden, 1990a; 1990b)	Adults	Ability to perform adult role responsibilities (e.g., involvement in family roles, leisure and recreation, household duties and SC activities); 16 items; VAS	Self-administered	ICR: α > .80 in patients with arthritis, breast cancer, and chronic pain (Braden, 1990a, 1990b; Braden et al., 1993; Kreulen & Braden, 2004; LeFort, 2000) TRR: no data available	Reviewed by experts in the field of SC (Braden, 1990a)	Correlated with theoretically relevant concepts (e.g., disability, sense of well-being, and affect) (Braden, 1990a, 1990b; LeFort, 2000; Sidani, 1994)	Increase in scores following psychoeducational intervention in patients with breast cancer (Kreulen & Braden, 2004; Sidani, 1994) and in patients with pain (LeFort, 2000)
Items (unnamed) developed to measure SC behavior (Jopp et al., 1993)	Older adults after rehabilitation	Performance of ADLs; one item; 3-point rating scale	Not clear	ICR: not applicable TRR: no data available	No data available	No data available	No data available
Jenkins Activity Checklist (Jenkins, 1985, as cited in Carroll, 1995)	Adults	Five categories of ADLs representing SC behaviors (e.g.,; walking, climbing stairs, roles, and relationships); 51 items; three response options (*No, Yes, Not Applicable*)	Self-administered	ICR: α of .53 to .92 for the five subscales, in elderly patients recovering from CABG (Carroll, 1995) TRR: no data available	No data available	No data available	Scores increased following cardiac surgery (Carroll, 1995) No data available relative to nursing variables
Self-Care Behavior Inventory (Albrecht et al., 1993)	Patients with arthritis	No domain specified; 17 items; no clearly defined response format	Self-administered	ICR: α of .75 in patients with arthritis (Albrecht et al., 1993) TRR: no data available	No data available	No data available	No data available

Note: r = correlation coefficient; α = Cronbach's alpha coefficient; ADLs = activities of daily living; CABG = coronary artery bypass graft surgery; CVI = content validity index; ICC = intraclass validity index; ICR = internal consistency reliability; ICR = intraclass correlation coefficient; ICR = internal consistency reliability; IRR = interrater reliability; SC = self-care; TRR = test-retest reliability; VAS = visual analog scale.

(continues)

TABLE 3-3   Instruments Measuring Self-Care Behavior (continues)

Instrument (author)	Target population/ practice setting	Domains; number of items; response format	Method of administration	Reliability	Content validity	Construct validity	Sensitivity to nursing variable
Universal Self-Care Inventory (Gazda, 1986, as cited in Horsburgh, et al., 2000)	Adults	SC behaviors undertaken in response to universal self-care requisites; 10 items; 6-point Likert-type	Self-administered	ICR: α of .78 to .88 in various patient populations (Horsburgh, 1999; Horsburgh et al., 2000) TRR: no data available	Reported to be supported	Reported to be supported	No data available
Heart Failure Self-Care Behavior Scale (Jaarsma et al., 1999)	Patients with heart failure	SC activities that are essential parts of the therapeutic regimen, to be performed (e.g., managing dyspnea and restricting sodium intake); 19 items; Yes-No response format	Self-administered	ICR: α of .62 to .68 in patients with heart failure (Jaarsma et al., 1999; 2000) TRR: No data available	Established by a panel of experts in cardiac care (Jaarsma et al., 1999)	No data available	Increase in scores in patients with heart failure following an educational intervention (Jaarsma et al., 1999, 2000)
Items (unnamed) developed to measure SC behavior (Ni et al., 1999)	Patients with heart failure	Adherence to therapeutic regimen (e.g., medication, sodium intake, and weight monitoring); 8 items; response reflected frequency of performance of SC behaviors	Self-administered	ICR: not applicable TRR: no data available	No data available	Positive *r* with knowledge of therapeutic regimen (Ni et al., 1999)	No data available
Self-Care Behavioral Rating Scale (Harper, 1984)	Patients with hypertension	SC behaviors related to safe self-medication; 12 items; 5-point rating scale	Administered by trained observers	ICR: inter-item *r* of .73 to .74 for the subscales in patients with hypertension (Harper, 1984) TRR: *r* of .94 in patients with hypertension (Harper, 1984) IRR: ICC of .88 to 1.00 (Harper, 1984)	Established by expert nurses	No data available	Increase in scores observed in patients with hypertension, following an educational intervention (Harper, 1984)

Self-Care Burden Scale (Oberst, Hughes, Chang, & McCubbin, 1991)	Adults	Illness and universal SC demands and behaviors; 16 items; 5-point rating scale	Self-administered	ICR: α of .79 to .90 in various patient populations TRR: no data available	Reported to be established	Reported to be established	No data available
Self-Care Assessment Tool (SCAT) (Boss, Barlow, McFarland, & Sasser, 1996)	Patients with spinal cord injury	Eight areas of SC (bathing, nutritional management, medications, mobility, skin management, bladder management, bowel management, and dressing); 8 items; Yes-No response format	Administered by a nurse observer	ICR: no data available TRR: r of .06 to .86 (Boss et al., 1996) IRR: agreement 94-100%, r of .69-.94 (Boss et al., 1996)	Validated by a panel of 10 clinical nurse specialists (CVI .90) (Boss et al., 1996)	Discharge scores accounted for 82% of the variance in scores obtained at 6 months postdischarge (Boss et al., 1996)	No data available
Strategies Used by Patients to Promote Health (Lev & Owen, 1996)	Adults	Self-confidence to perform strategies to promote health; 29 items; 5-point scale	Self-administered	ICR: α of .94-.96 in patients with renal failure on hemodialysis (Lev & Owen, 1998) TRR: no data available	No data available	Factorial structure: four factors (Lev & Owen, 1996) Construct: no data available	Increase in the scores was observed over time (Lev & Owen, 1998) No data available relative to nursing variables
High Intensity Self-Care Needs and Interventions Survey (Robinson & Posner, 1992)	Patients with cancer receiving biologic response modifier therapy	SC interventions performed to manage the side effects of biologic response modifier therapy; unknown number of items; open-ended questions	May be self-administered or administered by healthcare providers	ICR: not applicable TRR: not applicable	No data available	No data available	No data available

Note: r = correlation coefficient; α = Cronbach's alpha coefficient; ADLs = activities of daily living; CABG = coronary artery bypass graft surgery; CVI = content validity index; ICC = intraclass correlation coefficient; ICR = internal consistency reliability; IRR = interrater reliability; SC = self-care; TRR = test-retest reliability; VAS = visual analog scale.

(continues)

TABLE 3-3 Instruments Measuring Self-Care Behavior (continues)

Instrument (author)	Target population/ practice setting	Domains; number of items; response format	Method of administration	Reliability	Content validity	Construct validity	Sensitivity to nursing variable
Self-Care Behavior Log (Dodd, 1982)	Patients with cancer receiving chemotherapy	Initiation of SC behaviors and perception of the effectiveness of the behaviors used to manage the side effects of chemotherapy; no preset number of items: patients asked to identify symptoms and strategies used to manage each symptom; 5-point rating scale to rate effectiveness of SC behaviors	Self-administered	ICR: not applicable TRR: reported to be established	Established by two groups of oncologists and four nurse clinical oncology specialists (Dodd, 1982)	No data available$	Increase in scores following an educational intervention (Dodd, 1983)$
Self-Care Rating Scale (Williams et al., 1988)	Postsurgical patients who underwent either mastectomy or hysterectomy	Performance of SC behaviors to be carried out by patients at home following mastectomy or hysterectomy; 20 items for the mastectomy version, and 12 items for the hysterectomy version; 4-point rating scale	Either self-administered or administered by the nurse	ICR: not applicable TRR: no data available	Two versions developed in consultation with physicians and nurses	No data available	Increase in scores following an educational intervention (Williams et al., 1988)
Self-Care Behavior Questionnaire (Hanucharurnkul, 1989)	Patients with cancer	SC performed by patients with cancer receiving radiation therapy; 41 items; 5-point Likert-type	Self-administered	ICR: α of .87 in patients with head/neck cancer; .86 in patients with cervical cancer TRR: r of .90	Judged as valid by two groups of experts	Positive r with life satisfaction ($r = .63$) in patients with cancer (Hanucharurnkul, 1989)	No data available

Self-Care Assessment Tool (Johannsen, 1992)	Cardiac patients	Ability to seek medical assistance, attend to the effects of the illness, carry out the therapeutic regimen, regulate the deleterious effects of the therapeutic regimen, live with the illness, and modify self-concept (for each domain, the tool assesses the patient's knowledge base, decision, and action); 86 items; checklist format	Administered by the nurse	ICR: no data available. TRR: no data available	Domains reflective of Orem's six health-deviation self-care requisites	No data available	No data available
Self-Care Assessment Tool (SCAT) (McFarland, Sasser, Boss, Dickerson, & Stelling, 1992)	Patients with spinal cord injury	Two domains of SC: cognitive skills (e.g., selecting appropriate action) and functional skills (e.g., bathing, nutritional management, taking medications, mobility); 81 items; three response options (*No, Yes,* and *Not Applicable*).	Administered by the nurse	ICR: no data available. TRR: *r* of .47 to .80 for the cognitive subscale; -.06 to .86 for the functional subscale; and .45 to .69 for the total scale (McFarland et al., 1992) IRR: *r* of .69–.94 for the cognitive subscale; .74–.92 for the functional subscale; and .74–.94 for the total scale	Reviewed by a panel of 10 clinical nurse specialists in spinal cord injury (McFarland et al., 1992	Predictive validity: reported to be supported (.61 for cognitive subscale; .90 for functional subscale; and .82 for total scale) (McFarland et al., 1992)	No data available

Note: r = correlation coefficient; α = Cronbach's alpha coefficient; ADLs = activities of daily living; CABG = coronary artery bypass graft surgery; CVI = content validity index; ICC = intraclass correlation coefficient; ICR = internal consistency reliability; IRR = interrater reliability; SC = self-care; TRR = test-retest reliability; VAS = visual analog scale.

(continues)

TABLE 3-3 Instruments Measuring Self-Care Behavior (continues)

Instrument (author)	Target population/ practice setting	Domains; number of items; response format	Method of administration	Reliability	Content validity	Construct validity	Sensitivity to nursing variable
Measure (unnamed) developed by (Lenihan,1988)	Elderly residents living in noninstitutional settings in the community	Universal SC demands, health deviation SC demands, and medically derived self-care demands; 123 items; response format unclear	No data available	ICR: no data available TRR: no data available	Developed in consultation with experts in the areas of gerontology and geriatrics, health promotion, and self-care	No data available	No data available
Health Behavior Scale (Miller, Wikoff, & McMahon, 1982)	Adults with cardiac disease	Performance of recommended SC behaviors (e.g., diet, medication and exercise, smoking cessation, and stress management); 20 items; 5-point, Likert-type	Self-administered	ICR: α of .82 and .95 TRR: no data available	No data available	No data available	No data available
Self-Care of Older Persons Evaluation (SCOPE) (Dellasega & Clark, 1995)	Older adults in rehabilitation	Universal SC domains (e.g., food, elimination processes, activity and rest; bathing, prevention of hazards; and social interaction); 13 items; 6-point Likert-type	Administered by observer/ healthcare provider	ICR: α of .89 in patients with rehabilitation needs TRR: no data available IRR: complete agreement was accomplished during the training session (Dellasega & Clark, 1995)	Established by a panel of 30 experts	Factorial structure: three factors Construct: no data available	No data available

Instrument	Population	Description	Administration	ICR/TRR	Development	Validity	Additional
Interstitial Cystitis-Self-Care Responses (Webster & Brennan, 1998)	Women with interstitial cystitis	SC related to universal, developmental, and health deviations demands (e.g., hygiene, diet, and use of medications); about 300 items; rating scale from 0 to 3 (to rate frequency of using and effectiveness of SC strategies)	Self-administered	ICR: no data available TRR: no data available	Developed based on the responses of women with interstitial cystitis to open-ended questions	Positive r with adjustment to the illness (Webster & Brennan, 1998)	No data available
Epilepsy Self-Management Scale (DiIorio & Henry, 1995)	Patients with epilepsy; outpatient	Performance of tasks that are helpful in managing seizures (e.g., medication, self-monitoring, stress management, hypnosis, and biofeedback); 26 items; 5-point scale	Self-administered	ICR: α of .81–.86 in persons with epilepsy (DiIorio & Henry, 1995) TRR: no data available	Derived from the literature; CVI 93%	No data available	No data available
Therapeutic Self-Care (Sidani & Irvine, 1999)	Adult patients in acute care settings	Taking medications, recognizing and managing symptoms, carrying out ADLs, and managing changes in health condition; 13 items; 5-point numeric rating scale	Self-administered	ICR: α of .62 to .85 for the subscales; .89 for total scale in patients admitted to cardiac and general medical and surgical units (Doran et al., 2006; Sidani & Irvine, 1999; Sidani et al., 2002) TRR: No data available	Maintained by generating items based on literature review	Factorial structure: four factors, as hypothesized Construct: negative r with age, affect, number of symptoms experienced; positive r with functional status, and perceived health (Doran et al., 2006; Sidani & Irvine, 1999; Sidani et al., 2002)	Correlated with patient education given by nurses in the hospital (Sidani & Irvine, 1999)

Note: r = correlation coefficient; α = Cronbach's alpha coefficient; ADLs = activities of daily living; CABG = coronary artery bypass graft surgery; CVI = content validity index; ICC = intraclass correlation coefficient; ICR = internal consistency reliability; IRR = interrater reliability; SC = self-care; TRR = test-retest reliability; VAS = visual analog scale.

(continues)

TABLE 3-3 Instruments Measuring Self-Care Behavior (continues)

Instrument (author)	Target population/ practice setting	Domains; number of items; response format	Method of administration	Reliability	Content validity	Construct validity	Sensitivity to nursing variable
Health Promoting Lifestyle Profile (Walker, Sechrist, & Pender, 1995, as cited in Acton & Malathum, 2000)	Adults; primary care	Actions that maintain or enhance wellness (e.g. physical activity, nutrition, interpersonal relations, stress management); 52 items; 4-point rating scale	Self-administered	ICR: α of .83–90 for the subscales; .90 for total scale (Acton & Malathum, 2000) TRR: no data available	No data available	No data available	No data available
Items assessing behaviors for control of heart failure (Baker et al., 2005)	Adults with heart failure; outpatient	Behaviors assessed: (1) having a scale to measure weight, (2) eating low-salt foods	Self-administered	No data available	No data available	No data available	No data available
Self-management behaviors (Schmittdiel et al., 2007)	Adults with chronic illness; outpatient	Behaviors assessed: consuming 5 servings of fruits and vegetables; doing tasks needed to manage condition; following regular exercise program; following stress management program; 4-point Likert scale (*strongly disagree to strongly agree*)	Self-administered	No data available	No data available	No data available	Associated with receipt of care that is aligned with chronic care model (Schmittdiel et al., 2007)
Summary of Diabetes Self-Care Activities (Toobert, Hampson, & Glasgow, 2000)	Adults with diabetes; outpatient	Behaviors assessed: diet, exercise, blood sugar testing; number of days in past week behaviors performed; score ranges between 0 and 7	Self-administered				Not sensitive to nursing variables (Ismail et al., 2008)

Items assessing self-health behaviors (Sit et al., 2007)	Adults with minor stroke; primary care	Behaviors assessed: disease self-management (monitor blood pressure, blood sugar, blood lipids; urine testing on sugar and albumin); medication compliance; cigarette and alcohol consumption; exercise; dietary intake	Self-administered	No data available	Items derived or adapted from other measures	No data available	Increase in self-health behaviors following educational program implemented by nurses (Sit et al., 2007)
Questionnaire assessing self-management (Rootmensen et al., 2008)	Adults with asthma or chronic obstructive pulmonary disease; outpatient	Questionnaire consists of scenarios describing exacerbations of conditions and questions on how to act in these situations	Self-administered	No data available	Adapted from a previous measure	No data available	Not sensitive to patient education implemented by nurses (Rootmensen et al., 2008)

Note: r = correlation coefficient; α = Cronbach's alpha coefficient; ADLs = activities of daily living; CABG = coronary artery bypass graft surgery; CVI = content validity index; ICC = intraclass correlation coefficient; ICR = internal consistency reliability; IRR = interrater reliability; SC = self-care; TRR = test-retest reliability; VAS = visual analog scale.

The capabilities captured in the scale varied across the instruments. The Denyes Self-Care Agency Questionnaire (Denyes, 1980, as cited in Lantz et al., 1995) and the ASA Scale measure the person's ability to perform self-care behaviors related to universal needs and demands. The other three scales capture the domains of self-care agency, including the cognitive, physical, emotional, and behavioral abilities needed to perform self-care behaviors. The operationalization of self-care agency in terms of the cognitive, physical, emotional, and behavioral elements is consistent with the conceptualization of self-care agency advanced earlier. It is encompassing because it is applicable to various situations and conditions of health and illness, as well as to the self-care behaviors to be performed.

Two instruments, the Perception of Self-Care Agency and the Self-Care Agency Inventory, were each discussed in one study (Hanson, 1981, as cited in Nelson McDermot, 1993; Lantz et al., 1995). The study was methodological in nature and aimed at assessing the instruments' psychometric properties. The Perception of Self-Care Agency demonstrated acceptable reliability and validity. The Self-Care Agency Inventory had high test-retest reliability but rather low internal consistency reliability; it had acceptable content and concurrent validity. These two measures require further testing before they can be recommended for practice.

The Denyes Self-Care Questionnaire was used in two studies, one involving children (Moore, 1995) and the other involving adolescents (Slusher, 1999). It demonstrated acceptable reliability and validity. However, the number of items comprising it, as described in Table 3-2, may require these populations to spend some effort and time to complete it.

The Exercise of Self-Care Agency was used in seven studies involving various client populations, including healthy adolescents, adults, and older adults, as well as patients with chronic illnesses. The reported results provide adequate evidence supporting its reliability and initial evidence for its validity and sensitivity to change. Its factorial structure seems to be consistent or invariant across samples of individuals residing in North America only (Chen, 1999); differences in factorial structure were reported for individuals residing in Northern Europe (Whetstone & Hansson, 1989). The shorter version, comprising 35 items, requires a short time to complete.

The ASA Scale was used in 11 studies; it was self-administered in nine studies to healthy persons and in two studies to patients with chronic illnesses. The reported reliability coefficients tended to be slightly lower than those reported for the Exercise of Self-Care Agency Scale but were still supportive of its consistency in measuring the concept. The evidence for its validity is contradictory. Although results provided adequate support for its content, convergent, and construct validity, some findings pointed to the possibility of response bias (i.e., acquiescence and social desirability) by patients (Halfens et al., 1998; Horsburgh et al., 2000). Its sensitivity to change was not demonstrated. Its short length (only 24 items) and its translated versions in four languages other than English render it useful in clinical settings serving persons with different cultural backgrounds.

The empirical evidence on the psychometric properties of self-care agency measures is rather limited. Consequently, it is difficult to make any recommendations about which are the most reliable, valid, sensitive to change, and clinically useful measures of self-care agency. All instruments need further testing.

Measures of Self-Care Behavior

A total of 37 instruments measuring self-care behavior have been located (see Table 3-3). The instruments can be grouped into two general categories reflecting the underlying conceptualization of self-care behavior. The first category represents instruments operationalizing the concept of self-care behavior derived from Orem's (2001) model of self-care. These instruments were designed to assess the three domains comprising self-care behavior. Some capture the universal self-care requisites (e.g., Denyes Self-Care Practice Instrument) only, whereas others incorporate elements of developmental and/or health deviations, in addition to universal, requisites (e.g., Dependent Care Agent Performance Questionnaire). The second category includes instruments operationalizing a set of self-care behaviors expected of the target population. These were rather heuristic, developed on the basis of clinical knowledge. They entail specific activities that patients are recommended to perform to maintain or improve their health and/or to manage the presenting condition (e.g., Heart Failure Self-Care Behavior Scale; Self-Care Assessment Tool). Vrijhoef, Diederiks, and Spreeuwenberg (2000) reached similar conclusions in the literature review they conducted to examine the contribution of advanced practice nurses to self-care. They indicated that self-care was assessed in different ways, depending on the activities involved. None of the instruments reviewed was developed to reflect the self-care process underlying the performance of self-care behaviors. As described earlier, the process involves recognition of changes in health condition, assessment of different self-care activities for addressing the changes, selection and performance of appropriate activities, and evaluation of the effectiveness of the activities in addressing the changes. The Therapeutic Self-Care Scale captures some elements of the self-care process: recognition of changes in body function/symptom, knowledge of and implementation of treatments to prevent and/or manage the changes, and implementation of the prescribed therapeutic regimen.

The literature reviewed and clinical experience clearly suggest that the expected self-care behaviors vary across client populations and across healthcare settings. This variability accounts for the large number of pertinent instruments found. Investigators interested in assessing self-care behaviors in a particular situation seemed to have either (a) developed a new instrument to measure those self-care behaviors of primary concern in the study, as was the case for most of the studies reviewed (e.g., Dellasega & Clark, 1995; Harper, 1984), or (b) adapted previously developed instruments in an attempt to enhance the relevance of their content to the target population and setting involved in the study. The adaptation often consisted of generating additional items related to new/different behaviors expected of clients/patients, as illustrated by the work of Moore (1995), Gaffney and Moore (1996), and Moore and Mosher (1997). These authors adapted the original scale to measure self-care behaviors in various groups encompassing healthy children and adolescents and their parents, and children with cancer and their parents.

The variability in the self-care behaviors expected of different populations and across healthcare settings is also associated with variability in the operationalization of the concept. The following patterns were observed:

- Some researchers operationalized self-care behaviors as the performance of usual activities, that is, activities of daily living, instrumental activities of daily living, and adult role behaviors such as involvement in family, recreational, social, and work-related activities. These activities were measured with various instruments, including the following: items developed by Jopp, Carroll, and Waters (1993); the Jenkins Activity Checklist used by Carroll (1995); and the Inventory of Adult Behavior developed by Braden (1990b) and used by LeFort (2000) and Kreulen and Braden (2004). The activities were investigated in community-dwelling adults with chronic illnesses who were recovering from an acute episode or who required long-term management.

- Some investigators operationalized self-care behaviors in terms of activities performed to meet universal self-care demands. These demands encompassed: (a) air, food, and water, (b) elimination processes (bladder and bowel), (c) activity and rest, (d) normalcy (i.e., bathing and grooming), (e) prevention of hazards, and (f) solitude and social interactions. The scales used to measure these behaviors were: (a) the Denyes Self-Care Practice Instrument used by McCaleb and Edgil (1994), Slusher (1999), McCaleb and Cull (2000), and Dashiff et al. (2006); (b) the Children and Adolescent Self-Care Practice Questionnaire and the Dependent Care Agent Questionnaire used by Moore (1995) and Gaffney and Moore (1996); (c) the Universal Self-Care Inventory used by Horsburgh (1999) and Horsburgh et al. (2000); and (d) the Self-Care of Older Persons Evaluation developed by Dellasega and Clark (1995). These instruments have been used in studies involving healthy adolescents and their parents, healthy children, adolescents with type 1 diabetes, elderly patients with rehabilitation needs, and patients with end-stage renal disease who were on dialysis, respectively.

- Other investigators operationalized self-care behaviors in terms of engagement in health promotion activities such as nutrition, exercise, and relaxation. The instruments used in these situations were (a) the Personal Lifestyle Questionnaire used by Nicholas (1993) with healthy older adults;

(b) the Hart Prenatal Care Actions Scale used by Hart (1995) with pregnant women; and (c) Strategies Used by Patients to Promote Health used by Lev and Owen (1996) with patients with renal failure who were on hemodialysis. All patient populations were community-dwelling adults.

- Most investigators operationalized self-care as the performance of activities aimed at maintaining health and managing the presenting problem(s) related to illness. That is, the measures included various combinations of: (a) health maintenance activities such as exercising, nutrition, sleep, and relaxation, (b) activities associated with implementation of the prescribed therapeutic regimen (e.g., taking medications, adhering to dietary or fluid restriction recommendations, skin management, and appointment keeping), and (c) strategies, whether self-initiated or suggested by health care providers, for recognizing and monitoring symptoms or alterations in body functions and for relieving symptoms.

Most instruments reviewed could be classified in this last category. They have been used with patients with chronic illnesses, such as patients with cancer who are receiving therapy; patients with arthritis, cardiac diseases, diabetes, sickle cell disease, and hypertension; patients with injuries requiring long-term rehabilitation (e.g., spinal cord injury); and patients with acute conditions (i.e., admitted for acute medical problems or for surgery). Measurement of self-care behaviors took place in a few instances when the patient was institutionalized but was conducted primarily after discharge or on an outpatient basis (either in a clinic or at home).

The specific self-care behaviors for managing the presenting problem that were measured varied across populations. For instance, those measured for patients with cancer receiving adjuvant therapy related to using strategies for managing the symptoms or side effects of cancer treatment that patients commonly experience (e.g., Dodd et al., 1991; Nail et al., 1991). The self-care behaviors focused on diet modification, weight reduction, exercise, smoking cessation, and stress management for patients with cardiac disease (e.g., Hamner, 2005; Jaarsma et al., 1999; Ni et al., 1999; Rodeman et al., 1995). For patients with hypertension, the self-care behaviors measured related to taking medications as prescribed and communicating concerns about medications to healthcare providers (Harper, 1984). The relevant self-care behaviors for patients with arthritis concerned exercise, saving energy, rest, medication-taking, and using community resources. Patients with diabetes are expected to exhibit the following self-care behaviors: healthy eating, being active, monitoring blood glucose, taking medications, problem-solving, risk reduction (e.g., hypoglycemia), and healthy coping (Dashiff et al., 2006; Zgibor et al., 2007). For patients with acute conditions, the self-care behaviors related to medication-taking, recognizing and managing symptoms or changes in condition, and following prescribed instructions (like post-surgery exercises). Schmittdiel et al. (2007) identified two domains of self-management behaviors that are relevant to patients with different chronic illness, including asthma, diabetes, heart failure, coronary artery disease, and chronic pain: (1) use of self-management services (Web site, health education classes, emotional support group), and (2) performance of self-management behaviors (consuming five servings of fruits and vegetables, doing tasks needed to manage their chronic condition, following a regular exercise program, and following a regular stress management program). These domains and behaviors were derived from relevant elements of the chronic care model.

Through qualitative interviews with patients and nurses, van Agthoven and Plomp (1989) identified two categories of self-care activities required by patients receiving home health care. The first included practical or physical self-care activities related to (a) general care (like washing, dressing, eating/drinking, and bladder/bowel management), (b) nursing activities associated with a therapeutic regimen (e.g., injections), (c) mobility and exercises (e.g., walking, getting in/out of bed), and (d) household duties. The second category referred to psychosocial self-care activities related to accepting illness and managing psychological, family, and/or marital problems.

The observed patterns underscore the importance of assessing self-care behaviors comprehensively but differently, based on the target population. To be consistent with the conceptualization of self-care behaviors presented in the theoretical background section of this review, nurses should address the following domains of self-care behaviors: promoting and maintaining health; recognizing and monitoring changes in functioning; selecting and applying appropriate strategies for managing these changes; and coping with/adjusting to long-term changes. The domains to be assessed could vary with the patient population. For instance, the assessment of self-care behaviors could be confined to those reflective of health promotion/maintenance for healthy persons. All these domains could be assessed in patients presenting with an illness, whether chronic or acute. Although none of the reviewed instruments adequately reflects all these domains, those classified under the fourth category (i.e., those measuring health maintenance and managing the presenting problems) seem to fit for ill individuals.

In addition to covering some, but not all, domains of self-care behaviors, the empirical evidence supporting the psychometric properties of the reviewed instruments is rather limited. This is related to the fact that most instruments were developed for a particular study and have been used in a rather small number of studies, as Vrijhoef et al. (2000) also explained. This state of affairs precludes accumulating sound and adequate evidence of reliability, validity, and sensitivity to change. Nonetheless, the available results indicate that the instruments are consistent in measuring self-care behaviors. The reliability coefficients, which were lower than the criterion of .70 value, do not detract from the measures' internal consistency and stability over time. This is because the observed low values of the Cronbach's alpha coefficients could be explained with minimal variability in the scores, which is anticipated in homogenous groups, and with the nature of the responses, in which the performance of one specific self-care behavior does not necessarily imply performance of another. The observed low values of the test-retest correlation coefficients could be explained by the changes in self-care behavior performance over time and therefore could be indicative of the instruments' sensitivity to change.

The content validity for most instruments was established, as reported by the tool developers or by investigators who used the measures. However, the evidence supporting the construct validity of the measures is limited. Similarly, few instruments demonstrated changes in their respective scores, which provides initial evidence of their sensitivity to change.

This review suggests that the instruments seem promising in assessing the domain and specific self-care behaviors of relevance to respective target patient populations. However, further testing of their psychometric properties is required prior to using them in day-to-day practice.

ISSUES IN THE MEASUREMENT OF SELF-CARE

This review of the literature on self-care raised some issues about measurement of self-care as an outcome that is sensitive to nursing care. The first issue relates to the operationalization of self-care that results from differences in the conceptualization of self-care. The literature has clarified the distinction between the two concepts—self-care agency and self-care behavior—that were suggested as representing self-care. Self-care agency is the perceived capacity to engage in activities aimed at maintaining or improving health, preventing disease, and managing health-related problems. Self-care behavior is the actual performance of these activities. Recently, there has been growing interest in self-care behavior, defined in terms of the process underlying engagement in self-care behavior, as well as the actual performance of specific behaviors. Although no instrument was found that captures the elements of the self-care process, measuring it assists in determining its adequacy and appropriateness, which can potentially explain observed variability in the performance of self-care behavior. Assessing self-care agency, process, and behavior is highly recommended to gain a comprehensive understanding of self-care as an outcome of nursing interventions. However, administering relevant measures may increase response burden, especially in acutely ill and frail elderly persons. The selection of a self-care concept as an outcome of nursing care or interventions should be guided by an understanding of the components comprising nursing practice or by the theory underlying nursing interventions delivered in various healthcare settings (Sidani & Braden, 1998; Sidani, Doran, & Mitchell, 2004). For instance, it may be meaningful to assess the patients' self-care agency when they are institutionalized, and self-care behaviors when they are in outpatient settings. Institutionalization, especially in acute care settings, may preclude patients from initiating or actively undertaking some self-care activities, such as taking medications as prescribed; nonetheless, hospitalized patients need to have the knowledge and ability (i.e., perceived self-care agency) to engage in self-care after discharge. Cognitive-behavioral interventions may focus on instructing and training individuals in skills pertaining to the recognition of changes in functioning; problem-solving by selecting appropriate self-care activities; and implementing the selected activities correctly. Therefore, assessment of the self-care process is useful in determining the effectiveness of these interventions on this immediate outcome that is expected to mediate the impact of the interventions on the ultimate outcome of self-care behavior.

The second measurement issue concerns the content of instruments measuring self-care behavior. The specific question here is whether to use generic or specific measures of self-care behaviors. Generic measures capture self-care behaviors that are relevant to various client populations seen in various practice settings, as illustrated with the self-management measures developed by Schmittdiel et al. (2007) and the Therapeutic Self-Care Scale. This general applicability makes generic measures standard criteria that are useful for evaluating nursing care. Specific measures, in contrast, are adapted to particular patient populations. They tend to be responsive to particular interventions and sensitive to the particular context and condition of the patients receiving the interventions. Using specific measures, however, limits the ability to compare the effectiveness of different interventions delivered to address the same health problem in different patient populations (Guyatt, Feeny, & Patrick, 1993). Therefore, a combination of generic and specific measures is most effective for conducting a comprehensive assessment of self-care (Sidani & Braden, 1998).

The third issue relates to the method of assessing self-care. Self-care agency, as the person's perceived ability to perform self-care behaviors, is a subjective phenomenon. Consequently, patients themselves would be the best persons to judge or rate self-care agency. This observation implies that measures of this concept should be self-administered, as was the case for the instruments reviewed earlier. When patients are not able to self-report (e.g., children), a caregiver or healthcare professional may be needed to assess self-care agency. The results of such assessments should be viewed with caution because of reported discrepancies between the patients' and others' perceptions. Self-care behavior refers to a person's performance of self-care activities. Although patients can report about engaging in these behaviors, the accuracy of their responses may be questionable in light of response bias (Horsburgh, 1999). Having the patients' significant others report on the patients' performance of self-care behaviors provides another source of information to validate the patients' self-report. This strategy is recommended to enhance validity of outcome measurement. However, no instrument that measures self-care behavior and that is completed by the adult patients' significant other was found.

CONCLUSIONS AND RECOMMENDATIONS FOR PRACTICE AND RESEARCH

Self-care is an instrumental outcome that is consistent with nursing perspective and focus on promoting health, functioning, and well-being and is sensitive to nursing interventions and care. The main points of this chapter are summarized as follows:

- Self-care is operationalized as the patients' perceived ability and their actual practice of behaviors aimed at promoting and maintaining health, preventing disease, and managing or treating illness or changes in body function, as well as the process underlying self-care practice.

- Self-care is a critical concept in the current healthcare system, where much of the required treatment and care are provided in outpatient settings. Self-care enables patients, particularly those with chronic illnesses, to monitor and recognize changes in functioning and choose and implement appropriate strategies for managing these changes.

- The performance of self-care behaviors is influenced by cognitive, psychological, physical, demographic, and sociocultural factors. Engagement in self-care is considered beneficial to the patient and the healthcare system. Self-care behavior is believed to reduce the risk of complications; to enhance adjustment to illness, symptom control, and functioning; and, consequently, to improve quality of life and reduce health services utilization.

- Self-care formed the framework guiding the design of specific nursing interventions and multicomponent programs for various patient populations. These focused on providing individuals with information related to their health condition and self-care strategies and on instructing them in the skills necessary to perform self-care. Although limited, empirical evidence indicates that the interventions and programs were effective in improving the participants' self-care-related knowledge and behaviors. The evidence supporting the beneficial effects of these interventions was obtained from primary studies and from several meta-analytic studies.

- The evidence reviewed provides support for the benefits of nursing interventions and programs in enhancing engagement in self-care behaviors. Self-care is considered an outcome that is sensitive to nursing care and that is instrumental for achieving other patient outcomes, such as symptom control, improved functioning, and sense of well-being, and healthcare system outcomes such as service utilization and costs.

- Self-care is relevant to individuals seen across the healthcare continuum (i.e., primary, acute, home, rehabilitation, and long-term care). However, the expected self-care behaviors vary across patient populations and healthcare settings. This variability in the expected self-care behaviors accounts for the large number of pertinent measures found and poses some challenges in its clinical assessment.

- A large number of instruments that measured self-care behaviors was found. Most assess a combination of health maintenance activities and activities associated with implementing the therapeutic regimen or with strategies for managing the presenting health problem. They captured various domains and behaviors of self-care that are relevant to different patient populations in different practice settings. The instruments demonstrated acceptable reliability; however, the evidence supporting their validity is limited.

These points lead to three main recommendations. First, the measurement of self-care should be further refined. Generic measures of self-care that are relevant and applicable to different patient populations require further validation. Generic measures are useful for evaluating the impact of nursing care in general, for comparing the effectiveness of different nursing interventions and programs, and for developing a database. Such generic measures should be complemented with specific ones so that comprehensive assessments of self-care can be conducted for clients seen across healthcare settings. Instruments measuring the process underlying self-care are needed. Refinement of self-care measures is a prerequisite for investigating the outcome's sensitivity to nursing care. The second recommendation concerns the cognitive, physical, demographic, and sociocultural factors that influence perceived ability and the performance of self-care. These factors should be taken into consideration when researchers or healthcare professionals design interventions and programs aimed at promoting self-care, and when they evaluate the effects of nursing care on this outcome. Finally, additional large-scale studies that evaluate the impact of nursing structural variables and care on self-care are needed to strengthen the empirical evidence supporting the sensitivity of self-care to nursing, as well as the benefits of promoting self-care for patients in different healthcare settings.

REFERENCES

Acton, G. J., & Malathum, P. (2000). Basic need status and health-promoting self-care behavior in adults. *Western Journal of Nursing Research, 22,* 796–811.

Aish, A. (1996). A comparison of female and male cardiac patients' responses to nursing care promoting nutritional self-care. *Canadian Journal of Cardiovascular Nursing, 7*(3), 4–13.

Albrecht, M., Goeppinger, J., Anderson, M. K., Boutaugh, M., Macnee, C., & Stewart, K. (1993). The Albrecht nursing model for home healthcare: Predictors of satisfaction with a self-care intervention program. *Journal of Nursing Administration, 1,* 51–54.

Backman, K., & Hentinen, M. (1999). Model for the self-care of home-dwelling elderly. *Journal of Advanced Nursing, 30,* 564–572.

Badzek, L., Hines, S. C., & Moss, A. H. (1998). Inadequate self-care knowledge among elderly hemodialysis patients: Assessing its prevalence and potential causes. *ANNA Journal, 25,* 293–300.

Baker, D. W., Asch, S. M., Keesey, J. W., Brown, J. A., Chan, K. S., Joyce, G. J., et al. (2005). Differences in education, knowledge, self-management activities, and health outcomes for patients with heart failure cared for under the chronic disease model: The improving chronic illness care evaluation. *Journal of Cardiac Failure, 11,* 405–413.

Barnason, S., & Zimmerman, L. (1995). A comparison of patient teaching outcomes among post-operative coronary artery bypass graft (CABG) patients. *Progress in Cardiovascular Nursing, 10*(4), 11–20.

Barroso, J. (1995). Self-care activities of long-term survivors of acquired immunodeficiency syndrome. *Holistic Nursing Practice, 10*(1), 44–53.

Bauer, M. S., McBride, L., Williford, W. O., Glick, H., Kinosian, B., Altshuker, L., et al. (2006). Collaborative care for bipolar disorder: Part II. Impact on clinical outcome, function, and costs. *Psychiatric Services, 57,* 937–945.

Bodenheimer, T., Wagner, E. H., & Grumbach, K. (2002). Improving primary care for patients with chronic illness: The chronic care model, part 2. *Journal of the American Medical Association, 288,* 1909–1914.

Boss, B. J., Barlow, D., McFarland, S. M., & Sasser, L. (1996). A self-care assessment tool (SCAT) for persons with a spinal cord injury: An expanded abstract. *Axon, 17,* 66–67.

Braden, C. J. (1990a). Learned self-help response to chronic illness experience: A test of three alternative learning theories. *Scholarly Inquiry for Nursing Practice, 1*(1), 23–41.

Braden, C. J. (1990b). A test of the self-help model: Learned response to chronic illness experience. *Nursing Research, 39,* 42–47.

Braden, C. J. (1993). Research program on learned response to chronic illness experience: Self-help model. *Holistic Nursing Practice, 8*(1), 38–44.

Braden, C. J., Mishel, M. H., Longman, A., & Burns, L. R. (1993). *Nurse interventions promoting self-help response to breast cancer* (Grant No. NCI 1R01 CA48450–01 A1). Washington, DC: National Cancer Institute.

Brown, S. A. (1992). Meta-analysis of diabetes patient education research: Variations in intervention effects across studies. *Research in Nursing and Health, 15,* 409–419.

Burks, K. J. (1999). A nursing practice model for chronic illness. *Rehabilitation Nursing, 24,* 197–200.

Carroll, D. L. (1995). The importance of self-efficacy expectations in elderly patients recovering from coronary artery bypass surgery. *Heart and Lung, 24,* 50–59.

Chen, Y. M. (1999). Relationships among health locus of control, self-efficacy, and self-care of the elderly with hypertension. *Nursing Research, 7,* 504–516.

Chodosh, J., Morton, S. C., Mojica, W., Maglione, M., Suttorp, M. J., Hilton, L., et al. (2005). Meta-analysis: Chronic disease self-management programs for older adults. *Annals of Internal Medicine, 143,* 427–438.

Craddock, R. B., Adams, P. F., Usui, W. M., & Mitchell, L. (1999). An intervention to increase use and effectiveness of self-care measures for breast cancer chemotherapy patients. *Cancer Nursing, 22,* 312–319.

Dashiff, C. J., McCaleb, A., & Cull, V. (2006). Self-care of young adolescents with type 1 diabetes. *Journal of Pediatric Nursing, 21,* 222–232.

Dellasega, C., & Clark, D. (1995). SCOPE: A practical method for assessing the self-care status of elderly persons. *Rehabilitation Nursing Research, 4,* 128–135.

Devine, E. C. (1996). Meta-analysis of the effects of psychoeducational care in adults with asthma. *Research in Nursing and Health, 19,* 367–376.

Devine, E. C., & Reifschneider, E. (1995). A meta-analysis of the effects of psychoeducational care in adults with hypertension. *Nursing Research, 44,* 237–245.

Dilorio, C., & Henry, M. (1995). Self-management in persons with epilepsy. *Journal of Neuroscience Nursing, 27,* 338–343.

Dodd, M. J. (1982). Chemotherapy knowledge in patients with cancer: Assessment and informational interventions. *Oncology Nursing Forum, 9*(3), 39–44.

Dodd, M. J. (1983). Self-care for side effects in cancer chemotherapy: An assessment of nursing interventions. Part II. *Cancer Nursing, 6,* 63–67.

Dodd, M. J., & Miaskowski, C. (2000). The pro-self program: A self-care intervention program for patients receiving cancer treatment. *Seminars in Oncology Nursing, 16,* 300–308.

Dodd, M. J., Thomas, M. L., & Dibble, S. L. (1991). Self-care for patients experiencing cancer chemotherapy side effects: A concern for home care nurses. *Home Healthcare Nurse, 9*(6), 21–26.

Doran, D., Harrison, M. B., Laschinger, H., Hirdes, J., Rukholm, E., Sidani, S., et al. (2006). Relationship between nursing interventions and outcome achievement in acute care settings. *Research in Nursing and Health, 29,* 61–70.

Dunagan, C., Littenberg, B., Ewald, G. A., Jones, C. A., Emery, V. B., Waterman, B. M., et al. (2005). Randomized trial of a nurse-administered, telephone-based disease management program for patient with heart failure. *Journal of Cardiac Failure, 11,* 358–365.

Dunbar, S. B., Jacobson, L. H., & Deaton, C. (1998). Heart failure: Strategies to enhance patient self-management. *AACN Clinical Issues, 9,* 244–256.

Evers, G. C., Isenberg, M., Philipsen, H., Brouns, G., Holfens, R., & Smets, H. (1986). The appraisal of self-care agency A.S.A.- scale: Research program to test reliability and validity. In S. M. Stinson (Ed.), *Proceedings of the International Nursing Research Conference* (pp. 34–35). Edmonton: University of Alberta, Canada.

Folden, S. L. (1993). Effect of a supportive-educative nursing intervention on older adults' perceptions of self-care after a stroke. *Rehabilitation Nursing, 18,* 162–167.

Gaffney, K. F., & Moore, J. B. (1996). Testing Orem's theory of self-care deficit: Dependent care agent performance for children. *Nursing Science Quarterly, 9,* 160–164.

Gallefoss, F., & Bakke, P. S. (1999). How does patient education and self-management among asthmatics and patients with chronic obstructive pulmonary disease affect medication? *American Journal of Respiratory and Critical Care Medicine, 160,* 2000–2005.

Goeppinger, J., Macnee, C., Anderson, M. K., Boutaugh, M., & Stewart, K. (1995). From research to practice: The effects of the jointly sponsored dissemination of an arthritis self-care nursing intervention. *Applied Nursing Research, 8,* 106–113.

Grady, K. L. (2008). Self-care and quality of life outcomes in heart failure patients. *Journal of Cardiovascular Nursing, 23,* 285–292.

Gregory, E. K. (2000). Empowering students on medication for asthma to be active participants in their care: An exploratory study. *Journal of School Nursing, 16*(1), 20–27.

Guyatt, G. H., Feeny, D. H., & Patrick, D. L. (1993). Measuring health-related quality of life. *Annals of Internal Medicine, 118,* 622–629.

Hagopian, G. A. (1996). The effects of informational audiotapes on knowledge and self-care behaviors of patients undergoing radiation therapy. *Oncology Nursing Forum, 23,* 697–700.

Halfens, R. J. G., van Alphen, A., Hasman, A., & Philipsen, H. (1998). The effect of item observability, clarity and wording on patient/nurse ratings when using the ASA scale. *Scandinavian Journal of Caring Science, 13,* 159–164.

Hamner, J. B. (2005). Posthospitalization nursing interventions in congestive heart failure. *Advances in Nursing Science, 28*, 175–190.

Hanucharurnkui, S., & Vinya-nguag, P. (1991). Effects of promoting patients' participation in self-care on postoperative recovery and satisfaction with care. *Nursing Science Quarterly, 4*, 14–20.

Hanucharurnkul, S. (1989). Predictors of self-care in cancer patients receiving radiotherapy. *Cancer Nursing, 12*, 21–27.

Harper, D. C. (1984). Application of Orem's theoretical constructs to self-care medication behaviors in the elderly. *Advances in Nursing Science, 6*(3), 29–46.

Hart, M. A. (1995). Orem's self-care deficit theory: Research with pregnant women. *Nursing Science Quarterly, 8*, 120–126.

Hart, M. A., & Foster, S. N. (1998). Self-care agency in two groups of pregnant women. *Nursing Science Quarterly, 11*, 167–171.

Hirano, P. C., Laurent, D. D., & Lorig, K. (1994). Arthritis patient education studies, 1987–1991: A review of the literature. *Patient Education and Counseling, 24*, 9–54.

Horsburgh, M. E. (1999). Self-care of well adult Canadians and adult Canadians with end stage renal disease. *International Journal of Nursing Studies, 36*, 443–453.

Horsburgh, M. E., Beanlands, H., Looking-Cusolito, H., Howe, A., & Watson, D. (2000). Personality traits and self-care in adults awaiting renal transplant. *Western Journal of Nursing Research, 22*, 407–437.

Irvine, D., Sidani, S., & McGillis Hall, L. (1998). Linking outcomes to nurses' roles in health care. *Nursing Economics, 16*, 58–64.

Ismail, K., Thomas, S. M., Maissi, E., Chalder, T., Schmidt, U., Bartlett, J., et al. (2008). Motivational enhancement therapy with and without cognitive behavior therapy to treat type I diabetes. A randomized trial. *Annals of Internal Medicine, 149*, 708–719.

Jaarsma, T., Halfens, R., Abu-Saad, H. H., Dracup, K., Gorgels, T., van Ree, J., et al. (1999). Effects of education and support on self-care and resource utilization in patients with heart failure. *European Heart Journal, 20*, 673–682.

Jaarsma, T., Halfens, R., Senten, M., Abu-Saad, H. H., & Dracup, K. (1998). Developing a supportive-educative program for patients with advanced heart failure within Orem's general theory of nursing. *Nursing Science Quarterly, 11*, 79–85.

Jaarsma, T., Halfens, R., Tan, F., Abu-Saad, H. S., Dracup, K., & Diederiks, J. (2000). Self-care and quality of life in patients with advanced heart failure: The effect of a supportive educational intervention. *Heart and Lung, 29*, 319–330.

Jenerette, C. M., & Murdaugh, C. (2008). Testing the theory of self-care management for sickle cell disease. *Research in Nursing & Health, 31*, 355–369.

Johannsen, J. M. (1992). Self-care assessment: Key to teaching and discharge planning. *Dimensions of Critical Care Nursing, 11*, 48–56.

Johnson, M., & Maas, M. (Eds.). (1997). *Nursing Outcomes Classification (NOC)*. St. Louis, MO: Mosby.

Jónsdóttir, H. (2008). Nursing care in the chronic phase of COPD: A call for innovative disciplinary research. *Journal of Clinical Nursing, 17*, 272–290.

Jopp, M., Carroll, M. C., & Waters, L. (1993). Using self-care theory to guide nursing management of the older adult after hospitalization. *Rehabilitation Nursing, 18*, 91–94.

Kearney, B., & Fleischer, B. (1979). Development and testing of an instrument to measure exercise of self-care agency. *Research in Nursing and Health, 2*, 25–34.

Kimberly, O. (1997). Home-taught pediatric asthma program improves outcomes, cuts hospital, physician visits. *Health Care Cost Reengineering Report, 2*(3), 40–43.

Kreulen, G. J., & Braden, C. J. (2004). Model test of the relationship between self-help-promoting nursing interventions and self-care and health status outcomes. *Research in Nursing and Health, 27,* 97–109.

Kumar, C. P. (2007). Application of Orem's self-care deficit theory and standardized nursing languages in a case study of a woman with diabetes. *International Journal of Nursing Terminologies and Classifications, 18,* 103–110.

Lantz, J. M., Fullerton, J., & Quayhagen, M. P. (1995). Perceptual and enactment measurement of self-care. *Advanced Practice Nursing Quarterly, 1,* 29–33.

Leenerts, M. H., & Megilvy, J. K. (2000). Investing in self-care: A midrange theory of self-care grounded in the lived experience of low-income HIV-positive White women. *Advances in Nursing Science, 22*(3), 58–75.

LeFort, S. M. (2000). A test of Braden's self-help model in adults with chronic pain. *Journal of Nursing Scholarship, 32,* 153–160.

LeFort, S. M., Gray-Donald, K., Rowat, K. M., & Jeans, M. E. (1998). Randomized controlled trial of a community-based psychoeducation program for the self-management of chronic pain. *Pain, 74,* 297–306.

Lenihan, A. A. (1988). Identification of self-care behaviors in the elderly: A nursing assessment tool. *Journal of Professional Nursing, 4,* 285–288.

Lev, E. L., & Owen, S. V. (1996). A measure of self-care self-efficacy. *Research in Nursing and Health, 19,* 421–429.

Lev, E. L., & Owen, S. V. (1998). A prospective study of adjustment to hemodialysis. *ANNA Journal, 25,* 495–506.

Leveille, S. G., Wagner, E. H., Davis, C., Grothaus, L., Wallace, J., LoGerfo, M., et al. (1998). Preventing disability and managing chronic illness in frail older adults: A randomized trial of a community-based partnership with primary care. *Journal of the American Geriatrics Society, 46,* 1191–1198.

Levin, L. S. (1976). The layperson as primary care provider. *Public Health Report, 91,* 206–210.

Lorig, K., Konkol, L., & Gonzalez, V. (1987). Arthritis patient education: A review of the literature. *Patient Education & Counseling, 10,* 207–252.

Manninkhof, E., van de Valk, P., van der Palen, J., van Herwaarden, C., Partridge, M. R., & Zielhuis, G. (2003). Self-management education for patients with chronic obstructive pulmonary disease: A systematic review. *Thorax, 58,* 394–398.

McCain, N. L., & Lynn, M. R. (1990). Meta-analysis of a narrative review. Studies evaluating patient teaching. *Western Journal of Nursing Research, 12,* 347–358.

McCaleb, A., & Cull, V. V. (2000). Sociocultural influences and self-care practices of middle adolescents. *Journal of Pediatric Nursing, 15,* 30–35.

McCaleb, A., & Edgil, A. (1994). Self-concept and self-care practices of healthy adolescents. *Journal of Pediatric Nursing, 9,* 233–238.

McFarland, S. M., Sasser, L., Boss, B. J., Dickerson, J. L., & Stelling, J. D. (1992). Self-care assessment tool for spinal cord injured persons. *Science Nursing, 9*(4), 111–116.

Miller, P., Wikoff, R., & McMahon, A. (1982). Development of a health attitude scale. *Nursing Research, 31,* 132–135.

Mitchell, P. H., Ferketich, S., & Jennings, B. M. (1998). Quality health outcomes model. *Image: Journal of Nursing Scholarship, 30,* 43–46.

Moore, J. B. (1995). Measuring the self-care practice of children and adolescents: Instrument development. *Maternal-Child Nursing Journal, 23*(3), 101–108.

Moore, J. B., & Gaffney, K. G. (1989). Development of an instrument to measure mothers' performance of self-care activities for children. *Advances in Nursing Science, 12,* 76–83.

Moore, J. B., & Mosher, R. B. (1997). Adjustment responses of children and their mothers to cancer: Self-care and anxiety. *Oncology Nursing Forum, 24,* 519–525.

Mullen, P. D., Simons-Morton, D. G., Ramirez, G., Frankowski, R. F., Green, L. W., & Mains, D. A. (1997). A meta-analysis of trials evaluating patient education and counseling for three groups of preventive health behaviors. *Patient Education and Counseling, 32,* 157–173.

Nail, L. M., Jones, L. S., Greene, D., Schipper, D. L., & Jensen, R. (1991). Use and perceived efficacy of self-care activities in patients receiving chemotherapy. *Oncology Nursing Forum, 18,* 883–887.

Nelson McDermott, M. A. (1993). Learned helplessness as an interacting variable with self-care agency: Testing a theoretical model. *Nursing Science Quarterly, 6,* 28–38.

Ni, H., Nauman, D., Burgess, D., Wise, K., Crispell, K., & Hershberger, R. E. (1999). Factors influencing knowledge of and adherence to self-care among patients with heart failure. *Archives of Internal Medicine, 159,* 1613–1619.

Nicholas, P. K. (1993). Hardiness, self-care practice, and perceived health status in older adults. *Journal of Advanced Nursing, 18,* 1085–1094.

Norris, C. M. (1979). Self-care. *American Journal of Nursing, 3,* 486–489.

Oberst, M., Hughes, S., Chang, A., & McCubbin, M. (1991). Self-care burden, stress appraisal, and mood among persons receiving radiotherapy. *Cancer Nursing, 14,* 71–78.

Orem, D. E. (1971). *Nursing: Concepts of practice.* New York: McGraw-Hill.

Orem, D. E. (1985). *Nursing: Concepts of practice* (3rd ed.). New York: McGraw-Hill.

Orem, D. E. (1991). *Nursing: Concepts of practice* (5th ed.). St. Louis, MO: Mosby.

Orem, D. (2001). *Nursing concepts of practice* (6th ed.). St Louis, MO: Mosby.

Padula, C. A. (1992). Self-care and the elderly: Review and implications. *Public Health Nursing, 9*(1), 22–28.

Riegel, B., Carlson, B., Moser, D., Sebern, M., Hicks, F. D., & Roland, V. (2004). Psychometric testing of the self-care of heart failure index. *Journal of Cardiac Failure, 10,* 350–360.

Robinson, K. D., & Posner, J. D. (1992). Patterns of self-care needs and interventions related to biologic modifier therapy: Fatigue as a model. *Seminars in Oncology Nursing, 18*(4), 17–22.

Rodeman, B. J., Conn, V. S., & Rose, S. (1995). Myocardial infarction survivors: Social support and self-care behaviors. *Rehabilitation Nursing Research, 4,* 58–63, 71.

Rootmensen, G. N., van Keimpema, A. R. J., Looysen, E. E., van der Shaaf, L., de Haan, R. J., & Jansen, H. M. (2008). The effects of additional care by a pulmonary nurse for asthma and COPD patients at a respiratory outpatient clinic: Results from a double blind, randomized clinical trial. *Patient Education and Counseling, 70,* 179–186.

Schmittdiel, J., Mosen, D. M., Glasgow, R. E., Hibbard, J., Remmers, C., & Bellows, J. (2007). Patient assessment of chronic illness care (PACIC) and improved patient-centered outcomes for chronic conditions. *Journal of General Internal Medicine, 23,* 77–80.

Sidani, S. (1994). *Effects of sedative music on the respiratory status of clients with chronic obstructive airway disease.* Unpublished master's thesis, University of Arizona, Tucson.

Sidani, S., & Braden, C. J. (1998). *Evaluating nursing interventions: A theory-driven approach.* Thousand Oaks, CA: Sage.

Sidani, S., Doran, D. M., & Mitchell, P. H. (2004). A theory-driven approach to evaluating quality of nursing care. *Journal of Nursing Scholarship, 36,* 60–65.

Sidani, S., & Irvine, D. (1999). *Evaluation of the care delivery model and staff mix redesign initiative: The collaborative care study.* Unpublished report.

Sidani, S., Irvine, D., Porter, H., LeFort, S., O'Brien-Pallas, L. L., & Zahn, C. (2002). *Evaluating the impact of nurse practitioners in acute care settings.* Final report, submitted to Canadian Institutes of Health Research.

Sit, J. W. H., Yip, V. Y. B., Ko, S. K. K., Gun, A. P. C., & Lee, J. S. H. (2007). A quasi-experimental study on a community-based stroke prevention programme for clients with minor stroke. *Journal of Clinical Nursing, 16*, 272–281.

Skoner, M. M. (1994). Self-management of urinary incontinence among women 31 to 50 years of age. *Rehabilitation Nursing, 19*, 339–347.

Slusher, I. L. (1999). Self-care agency and self-care practice of adolescents. *Issues in Comprehensive Pediatric Nursing, 22*, 49–58.

Soderhamn, O., Evers, G., & Hamrin, E. (1996). A Swedish version of the Appraisal of Self-Care Agency (ASA) Scale. *Scandinavian Journal of Caring Science, 10*, 3–9.

Spradley, B. W. (1981). *Community health nursing: Concepts and practice.* Boston: Little, Brown.

Toobert, D. J., Hampson, S. E., & Glasgow, R. E. (2000). The summary of diabetes self-care activities measure: Results from 7 studies and a revised scale. *Diabetes Care, 23*, 943–950.

Turner, M. O., Taylor, D., Bennett, R., & Fitzgerald, J. M. (1998). A randomized trial comparing peak expiratory flow and symptom self-management plans for patients with asthma attending a primary care clinic. *American Journal of Respiratory and Critical Care Medicine, 157*, 540–546.

van Achterberg, T., Lorensen, M., Isneberg, M. A., Evers, G. C. M., Levin, E., & Philipsen, H. (1991). The Norwegian, Danish and Dutch version of the Appraisal of Self-Care Agency Scale: Comparing reliability aspects. *Scandinavian Journal of Caring Science, 5*, 101–108.

van Agthoven, W. M., & Plomp, H. N. (1989). The interpretation of self-care: A difference in outlook between clients and home-nurses. *Social Science and Medicine, 29*, 245–252.

Vrijhoef, H. J. M., Diederiks, J. P. M., & Spreeuwenberg, C. (2000). Effects on quality of care for patients with NIDDM or COPD when the specialized nurse has a central role: A literature review. *Patient Education and Counseling, 41*, 243–250.

Vrijhoef, H. J. M., van Den Bergh, J. H. A. M., Diederiks, J. P. M., Weemhoff, I., & Preeuwenberg, C. (2007). Transfer of care for outpatients with stable chronic obstructive pulmonary disease from respiratory care physician to respiratory nurse: A randomized controlled study. *Chronic Illness, 3*, 130–144.

Wagner, E. H., Glasgow, R. E., Davis, C., Bonomi, A., Provost, L., & McCulloch, D. (2001). Quality improvement in chronic illness care: A collaborative approach. *Joint Commission Journal of Quality Improvement, 27*, 63–80.

Wang, H. H., & Lee, I. (1999). A path analysis of self-care of elderly women in a rural area of Southern Taiwan. *Kaohsiung Journal of Medical Science, 15*, 94–103.

Watson, P. B., Town, G. I., Holbrook, N., Dwan, C., Toop, L. J., & Drennan, C. J. (1997). Evaluation of a self-management plan for chronic obstructive pulmonary disease. *European Respiratory Journal, 10*, 1267–1271.

Webster, D. C., & Brennan, T. (1998). Self-care effectiveness and health outcomes in women with interstitial cystitis: Implications for mental health clinicians. *Issues in Mental Health Nursing, 19*, 495–519.

Whetstone, W. R., & Hansson, A. M. O. (1989). Perceptions of self-care in Sweden: A cross-cultural replication. *Journal of Advanced Nursing, 14*, 962–969.

Williams, P. D., Valderrama, D. M., Gloria, M. D., Pascoguin, L. G., Saaveda, L. D., De La Roma, D. T., et al. (1988). Effects of preparation for mastectomy/ hysterectomy on women's post-operative self-care behaviors. *International Journal of Nursing Studies, 25*, 191–206.

Zambrowski, C. (2008). Self-care at the end of life in patients with heart failure. *Journal of Cardiovascular Nursing, 23*, 266–276.

Zgibor, J. C., Peyrot, M., Ruppert, K., Noullet, W., Siminerio, L. M., Peeples, M., et al. (2007). Using the American Association of Diabetes Educators Outcomes System to identify patient behavior change goals and diabetes educator responses. *Diabetes Educator, 33*, 839–842.

Symptom Management

Souraya Sidani

INTRODUCTION

Symptoms play an important role in the health-illness experience. They signal a change in physiological, physical, or psychological functioning that is indicative of an acute alteration in health or an exacerbation of a chronic condition. Whether acute or chronic, the experience of a symptom prompts persons to initiate the self-care process to manage the symptom effectively. Symptom management involves the application of self-care strategies that are medically prescribed or developed by individuals for the purpose of relieving the presenting symptom (Christenbery, 2005). In addition, the experience of a symptom represents the reason for seeking health care (Dodd et al., 2001; O'Neill & Morrow, 2001). Healthcare professionals are expected to assist patients in understanding the meaning of symptoms and work with patients to manage the symptoms effectively. Symptom management is viewed as an essential component of independent and collaborative healthcare and nursing practice (Baker et al., 2005; R. Johnson, 1993). The end result of symptom management, implemented by patients or healthcare professionals, is symptom control. Symptom control refers to the resolution of the presenting symptom, or the attenuation of its level of severity and/or distress.

As implemented by nurses, symptom management entails steps consistent with the nursing process. The symptom management process begins with a comprehensive and accurate assessment of the patient's symptom experience. Assessment is followed by selecting appropriate interventions to relieve the symptom, alleviate its severity or distress, and/or prevent its occurrence or impact. The next steps involve the delivery of selected interventions and the evaluation of their effectiveness in controlling the symptoms (Dodd et al., 2001; Haworth & Dluhy, 2001). Symptom assessment, therefore, forms the foundation for effective management; it guides the selection of interventions and represents the criterion for determining their effectiveness.

This chapter presents an overview of how symptom experience is conceptualized. Issues in symptom measurement are discussed, and instruments for assessing general symptoms are briefly reviewed. The conceptualization, measurement, and sensitivity to nursing care of the following three symptoms are presented: fatigue, nausea and vomiting, and dyspnea. These symptoms were selected based on their reported frequency of occurrence and impact on daily functioning in different patient populations across healthcare settings.

SYMPTOM EXPERIENCE: CONCEPTUALIZATION

A clear understanding of the symptom experience is necessary for accurate management. Knowledge of the critical attributes that characterize symptoms from related concepts is essential for developing instruments and choosing methods for assessing symptoms. Awareness of symptoms' dimensions, antecedents, and consequences points to particular aspects of symptoms amenable to interventions and hence guide the selection of interventions.

Definition

Symptoms refer to (a) sensations or experiences reflecting changes in a person's biopsychosocial functions, (b) a patient's perception of an abnormal physical, emotional, or cognitive state, (c) the perceived indicators of change in normal functioning as experienced by patients, or (d) subjective experience reflecting changes in the biopsychosocial functioning, sensations, or cognition of an individual (Dodd et al., 2001; Henry, Holzemer, Weaver, & Stotts, 1999; Holzemer et al., 1999; Rhodes, McDaniel, & Matthews, 1998; University of California, San Francisco [UCSF] School of Nursing Symptom Management Faculty Group, 1994). These definitions identify the critical attributes that distinguish symptoms from the related concept of signs.

Symptoms reflect alterations in function in any domain of health (e.g., biological, psychological). They are characterized by their subjective nature and are experienced by the individual. Whereas some symptoms are manifested by behavioral indicators (e.g., anxiety, vomiting), others are difficult to measure objectively (e.g., fatigue, dyspnea); they cannot be clearly and/or easily detected by another person, such as a healthcare professional (UCSF Symptom Management Faculty Group, 1994). In contrast, signs refer to objective abnormality, or manifestations indicative of illness or disease that are distinct from the patient's impressions (Rhodes et al., 1998). They can be detected by the patients themselves or by the healthcare professionals (UCSF Symptom Management Faculty Group).

Framework

The framework is derived from available conceptual and empirical literature and presents elements underlying the symptom experience and the response to the experience. The symptom experience is triggered by the subjective perception of changes in function. The sensation is then evaluated for its meaning. The interpretation of the sensation is influenced by several factors and shapes the response to the symptom experience (UCSF Symptom Management Faculty Group, 1994).

The first element of the symptom experience is the subjective perception. Perception of a symptom involves notice of a change from usual feelings or behaviors (Dodd et al., 2001). It is the conscious awareness of alterations in function in any domain of life and the cognitive interpretation of the sensations. The recognition and interpretation of the sensations is affected by a host of factors, including (a) demographic characteristics, such as age and gender, (b) sociocultural variables such as social support, religious or cultural beliefs, and values, (c) psychological factors such as personality traits, cognitive capacity, and perceived life or work stress, and (d) health- or illness-related variables such as presence of illness and perceived health status (Dodd et al., 2001; UCSF Symptom Management Faculty Group, 1994).

There is limited empirical evidence supporting the influence of the mentioned factors on symptom perception. This may be related to the assumption underlying symptom-related research. It is often assumed that symptoms are indicators of disease or treatment rather than an individual experience, as highlighted by Paterson, Canam, Joachim, and Thorne (2003) in the case of fatigue. The results of two studies provide preliminary evidence of the relationship between selected factors and symptom experience. Anastasia and Blevins (1997) reported that very young and elderly patients with cancer receiving chemotherapy on an outpatient basis were the least tolerant of symptoms. Sutcliffe-Chidgey and Holmes (1996) found that patients in palliative care settings did not always perceive the presence of a symptom as a cause of concern.

The second element of the symptom experience consists of evaluating its meaning. Once persons perceive the sensations and recognize the symptom, they evaluate them and assign them a meaning. Specifically, they assess the symptom in terms of severity, frequency, duration, temporal nature, and impact. Severity refers to the intensity or the degree to which the symptom is experienced. Frequency relates to the number of times the symptom is experienced within a specified time period, such as a day or a week. Duration is the length of time over which the symptom is experienced. Temporal nature involves an evaluation of the occurrence of the symptom relative to other events of relevance, such as engagement in an activity or exposure to treatment. Impact relates to the pattern of disability and the distress associated with the symptoms experienced. Disability involves the perceived threat posed by a symptom, such as its danger and disability effect (Dodd et al., 2001; UCSF Symptom Management Faculty Group, 1994). It also entails the extent to which the symptom interferes with the person's physical, psychological, and social functioning. Distress is defined as the degree of physical or psychological discomfort, anguish, or suffering experienced as a result of the symptoms (Hogan, 1997; Rhodes et al., 1998). Persons also assign a meaning to the symptom based on the observed symptom pattern (J. E. Johnson, Fieler, Wlasowicz, Mitchell, & Jones, 1997). Symptoms could represent usual or normal alterations expected as a result of some activities in which the person engaged. For instance, tiredness and breathlessness are anticipated following excessive, high-intensity physical exercise. Symptoms are indicative of changes in the person's functioning or the presence of health problems. They may be the first warning of an impending illness, whether acute or chronic. Symptom experience, therefore, brings the problem to the person's attention. The meaning assigned to symptoms is, again, determined by the same set of demographic, sociocultural, psychological, and health- or illness-related variables mentioned earlier. For instance, Lai, Chan, and Lopez (2007) explored the perception of dyspnea by Chinese patients with terminal lung cancer. Patients described this symptom as very painful, restricting their performance of usual daily activities. They explained that dyspnea results in a negative perception of the self, owing to the burden on family members assisting the patients in activities of daily living. The negative self-perception resulted in feelings of worthlessness and hopelessness, as well as a desire for death.

The third element is the response to the symptom experience. The response is shaped by the interpretation or the meaning assigned to the symptom. As described by the UCSF Symptom Management Faculty Group (1994), the response encompasses physiological, emotional, or behavioral components. The physiological component can be manifested by exacerbation of the symptoms experienced or by the development of physical symptoms reflective of stress. It also can include alterations in functioning (Dodd et al., 2001). The emotional component is reflected by cognitive or affective changes, such as the generation of uncertainty and anxiety. The behavioral component consists of engaging in activities for the purpose of managing or relieving the symptom. The behavioral component represents symptom management, which was introduced earlier in this chapter. The activities that make up symptom management vary with the symptom interpretation. Patients may ignore the symptom; assume a "wait-and-see" attitude; seek advice from laypersons (i.e., family members and friends), from available resources (e.g., the World Wide Web), or from healthcare professionals; use commonly recommended strategies, home remedies, or alternative therapies; and apply self-initiated treatment based on common knowledge (e.g., over-the-counter medications) or previous experience. Briefly, individuals initiate the self-care process and perform self-care behaviors, independently or in collaboration with healthcare professionals, in an attempt to relieve the symptom experienced.

The last element of the symptom experience relates to its consequences. Symptoms experienced with acute conditions may be successfully managed in a rather short period of time, particularly when the cause of the symptom is clearly identified, and appropriate, effective treatment is given. The result is the resolution of the symptoms. Symptoms are commonly experienced with chronic illnesses. With these conditions, symptoms are indicative of changes in health and functioning, or the persistence of the illness. In chronic illness, symptoms not only reflect the pathophysiological alterations characteristic of the disease but are also triggered or exacerbated by medical treatments, such as chemotherapy, radiation therapy, or biological therapy. They form the criteria for monitoring and evaluating the effectiveness of treatment, for modifying treatment dosage, and, in some instances, for discontinuing treatment. In addition, patients with chronic illness "live" with symptoms, which are often debilitating and incapacitating. They are a constant reminder of the illness. Furthermore, symptoms tend to occur with high frequency and intensity toward the end stages of illness, resulting in increased distress and demand for palliative care.

The consequences of uncontrolled symptoms are devastating to the patients, their families, and the healthcare system. Outcomes associated with the symptom experience are conceptualized in terms of the following indicators: symptom status, physical and emotional functioning, comorbidity, mortality, quality of life, and health services use (UCSF Symptom Management Faculty Group, 1994). That is, inadequate symptom management results in worsening of the symptom severity, frequency, and distress, which could not be managed effectively with available strategies. Symptoms experienced with high levels of severity are incapacitating and adversely affect individuals' ability to function as usual, to perform activities of daily living, and to care for themselves. Limited physical ability is associated with emotional distress and restricts the person's engagement in work-related, recreational, and social activities. Ultimately, quality of life is affected. Uncontrolled symptoms may lead to comorbid conditions (such as sleep disruption, discomfort, and decreased energy level) and increased utilization of health services.

The concept of symptom cluster has been recently introduced to refer to the experience of multiple symptoms observed in patients with chronic diseases such as cancer (e.g., Dodd et al., 2005). A cluster is a group of interrelated symptoms that occur concurrently and independently from other symptoms (Kim, McGuire, Tulman, & Barsevick, 2005). The conceptualization of symptom clusters is evolving. The clustering of symptoms is related to either (1) a common underlying biophysiological mechanism responsible for the simultaneous experience of alterations in functions, or (2) a psychobehavioral mechanism, in which the inadequate management of one symptom is associated with the emergence of comorbid symptoms (Cleeland et al., 2003; B-N. Lee et al., 2004; Miaskowski & Aouizerat, 2007; Parker, Kimble, Dunbar, & Clark, 2005). Examples of symptom clusters are pain, sleep disturbance, fatigue, and depression in patients with cancer (Armes, Chalder, Addington-Hall, Richardson, & Hotopf, 2007; Beck, Dudley, & Barsevick, 2005). Symptom clusters have implications for the assessment of symptoms, design of symptom management programs, and evaluation of interventions. Multicomponent interventions may be needed to address a symptom cluster. Also, interventions designed to manage a specific symptom may also be effective in addressing other symptoms that make up a cluster, as reported by Dirksen and Epstein (2008).

The distressing nature and debilitating consequences of individual or clusters of symptoms underscore the importance of adequately managing symptoms. Management involves (a) identifying and recognizing symptoms, (b) appropriately interpreting symptoms, (c) monitoring and evaluating symptoms, (d) selecting strategies to relieve the symptoms experienced and enhance functioning and well-being, and (e) evaluating the effectiveness of these strategies. This description of how to manage symptoms is similar to the nursing process and the process underlying self-care, as discussed in Chapter 3. Self-care or self-management of symptoms should aim at controlling or relieving symptoms. Effective management of symptoms begins with a comprehensive and accurate assessment. Such an assessment is also needed to evaluate the effectiveness of symptom management strategies. However, measuring symptoms presents some issues.

ISSUES IN SYMPTOM MEASUREMENT

The subjective and multidimensional nature of symptoms experienced by various patient populations raises some issues related to the development, validation, and administration of measures. The issues pertaining to instrument development have to do with the selection of terms describing the sensation and of the symptom dimension to assess.

The subjective nature of symptoms poses the challenge of clarifying sensations perceived by the affected persons. For instance, Lai et al. (2007) interviewed Chinese patients with terminal lung cancer to characterize their perception of dyspnea. The investigators reported that most patients were unable to clearly describe the sensation experienced with this symptom. This challenge results in difficulty in identifying descriptors of the sensation and in finding the most appropriate term or terms that accurately capture it in this patient population. To overcome this difficulty, some instrument developers chose to provide both the label of the symptom and a few terms that describe it in common language. For example, "feeling tired" are the terms presented to reflect fatigue, and "feeling sick to the stomach" are words given to reflect nausea. This practice may be of limited effectiveness in diverse populations. The terms may not have comparable meanings and may not be acceptable or relevant to patients of different backgrounds (e.g., cultural, educational, linguistic).

The multidimensional nature of the symptom experience is well recognized at the conceptual and clinical levels. These include occurrence, frequency, duration, severity, distress, and impact; in addition, factors that aggravate and/or alleviate the symptom, and the use and perceived effectiveness of strategies applied to manage the symptom, can be assessed. Covering all these dimensions is essential for an initial or baseline assessment of the symptom (Yancey, Given, White, DeVoss, & Coyle, 1998). It gives a comprehensive picture of the symptom experience and informs planning of individualized care. Conducting a similar assessment at subsequent regular time intervals to determine the effectiveness of nursing care or self-management strategies in relieving the symptom is questionable. In most instances, the symptom dimension or dimensions targeted by health or nursing interventions or self-management strategies are not clearly identified. Assessing all possible dimensions may be useful in detecting changes in intended and unintended dimensions; however, it is time consuming and potentially burdensome to patients. Response burden negatively affects the accuracy and validity of the data. One-item, global measures have been developed to capture one dimension of symptoms. Symptom severity is the dimension most commonly assessed. Although one-item measures demonstrated acceptable validity and are clinically relevant (i.e., easy to administer and interpret in the practice setting), they may not represent all domains (i.e., physical, behavioral, cognitive manifestations) and dimensions of symptoms that are of concern in planning care, individualizing interventions, and evaluating their effectiveness.

The issue related to validation of measures has to do with identifying a criterion for determining the validity of instruments measuring symptoms. The subjective nature of sensations and the private and unique experience of symptoms do not correspond with objective indicators of symptoms. Objective indicators include physiological, physical, or behavioral manifestations that can be detected by healthcare professionals. Physiological indicators of some symptoms did not correlate or converge with the subjective indicators. For instance, oxygen saturation levels, arterial blood gases, respiratory rate, and forced expiratory volume correlate poorly with self-report of dyspnea (O'Rourke, 2007). Similarly, differences were found between patients' and healthcare professionals' ratings of symptoms. Professionals' ratings were often based on their clinical observations. The results of several studies supported the discrepancy in the patients' and professionals' ratings of symptom intensity and distress. Rhodes et al. (1998) found that nurses working in hospice settings overestimated their patients' experiences of symptoms, whereas nurses in other settings underestimated those of their patients, particularly pain and dyspnea. Holzemer et al. (1999) also reported that nurses' ratings of symptoms were consistently shown to underestimate the frequency and intensity of symptoms experienced by patients with HIV disease. Maguire, Walsh, Jeacock, and Kingston (1999) found marked discrepancies between patients with colorectal cancer, their spouses, and their general practitioners in the assessment of breathlessness, pyrexia, nausea and vomiting, and loss of appetite. Justice, Chang, Rabeneck, and Zachin (2001) reported that healthcare providers consistently underestimated the frequency and severity of symptoms experienced by persons with HIV infection. The consistently observed incongruence between patients' and others' ratings of symptoms points to the importance of assessing the patients' perspective and to consider patients' self-report as the "gold standard" for measuring symptoms (Dodd et al., 2001). Therefore, validation of symptom measure should be investigated with strategies other than criterion validity, such as known group comparison.

The administration of self-report measures to capture the subjective symptom experience poses challenges in some patient populations, such as persons with confusion (e.g., hospitalized elders), mild cognitive impairment (e.g., early stage dementia), and difficult communication (e.g., minor stroke). These patients do experience symptoms (such as pain and nausea) but may not be able to recognize accurately the nature of the subjective sensation, report its presence, or rate it on the dimension of interest (such as severity). Two approaches can be used to address these challenges. The first consists of developing observational instruments to assess the behavioral indicators of symptoms, as was done for pain. These can be completed by healthcare professionals for nonverbal patients like those admitted to critical care units. The second approach entails reformulating the items to facilitate completion of the measures by patients having difficulty responding to the items. Fox, Sidani, and Streiner (2007) described strategies to reformulate the items to make it easier for institutionalized older persons with chronic illness to complete them. The strategies are breaking up, rephrasing, and contextualizing items, and using descriptive response options. Participants reported no difficulty responding to the revised items.

GENERAL SYMPTOM MEASURES

Patients with chronic illnesses such as cancer experience different symptoms as a result of the pathophysiological mechanisms underlying the disease and/or the treatments given to remedy the disease. Several instruments were developed to assess symptoms commonly experienced by these patients. The characteristics of these instruments are summarized in **TABLE 4-1**. The instruments were designed to measure a combination of physical (e.g., pain, constipation), psychological (e.g., depression, anxiety), and cognitive (e.g., impaired concentration, confusion) symptoms reported by patients with cancer, patients with HIV, patients in palliative care, and women with premenstrual syndrome. The instruments

TABLE 4-1 Instruments Measuring General Symptoms

Instrument (author)	Target population	Domains; number of items; response format	Method of administration	Reliability	Validity	Sensitivity to change and nursing care
Symptom Distress Scale (Rhodes et al., 1984, 1998)	Patients in hospice care or patients with cancer	Several symptoms (e.g., nausea, pain, anorexia, sleep disturbances, fatigue, difficulty in breathing, coughing, impaired concentration, change in body temperature and in appearance, and restlessness); 31 items; 5-point Likert-type	Self-administered	ICR: No data available TRR: Not applicable	Content: No data available Concurrent/construct: No data available	Sensitivity to change: no data available Sensitivity to nursing: no data available.
Signs and Symptom Checklist for Persons with HIV Disease (SSC-HIV) Holzemer et al. (1999) adapted this checklist from the HIV Assessment Tool (HAT) developed by Nokes, Wheeler, and Kendrew (1994)	Persons with HIV disease	Six clusters of symptoms (fever, fatigue, confusion, nausea/vomiting, psychological distress, shortness of breath, GI discomfort, and diarrhea); 41 items for original version and 26 for reduced version; 3-point Likert scale	Self-administered	ICR: α of .80 for fever, .78 for fatigue, .82 for confusion, .74 for nausea/vomiting, .76 for psychological distress, .75 for shortness of breath, .72 for GI discomfort, and .76 for diarrhea TRR: Not applicable	Content: Validated for its relevance by six clinicians Construct: Subscales correlated with relevant subscales of the MOS-SF-36 (Henry et al., 1999; Holzemer et al., 1999)	Sensitivity to change: Changes in scores observed over time (i.e., fewer symptoms reported on discharge than at admission) Sensitivity to nursing: No data available

α = Cronbach's alpha coefficient; CVI = content validity index; GI = gastrointestinal; ICR = internal consistency reliability; IRR = interrater reliability; r = correlation coefficient; SC = self-care; TRR = test retest reliability.

(continues)

TABLE 4-1   Instruments Measuring General Symptoms (continued)

Instrument (author)	Target population	Domains; number of items; response format	Method of administration	Reliability	Validity	Sensitivity to change and nursing care
Symptom Distress Scale (SDS) (McCorkle & Young, 1978; modified by Munkres, Oberst, & Hughes, 1992, and Sutcliffe-Chidgey & Holmes, 1996)	Patients with cancer	Several symptoms (e.g., pain, fatigue, anorexia, nausea, vomiting, constipation, breathing difficulty, weakness, loss of appetite, mood, and insomnia); 10 items; 5-point numeric rating scale (McCorkle & Young; Sutcliffe-Chidgey) or VAS (Munkres et al., 1992)	Self-administered	ICR: α of .82–.85 in patients with cancer (Munkres et al.; McCorkle & Young) TRR: Not applicable	Content: No information provided Construct: Correlated with affective mood in patients receiving chemotherapy (Munkres et al.); scores differed between patients with cancer with and without metastasis (McCorkle & Young)	Sensitivity to change: No data available Sensitivity to nursing: No data available
Menstrual Symptom Severity List (MSS) (Mitchell et al., 1991, cited by Taylor, 1999)	Women with premenstrual syndrome	Physical, cognitive, behavioral, and mood symptoms; 51 items; 5-point scale	Self-administered	ICR: α > .70 (Taylor) TRR: Not applicable	Content: No data available Construct: Subscales scores consistent with symptoms severity across menstrual cycles (Taylor)	Sensitivity to change: No data available Sensitivity to nursing: No data available
Breast Cancer Prevention Trial Symptom Checklist (Gantz, Day, Ware, Redmond, & Fisher, 1995)	Women with breast cancer receiving adjuvant therapy	Symptoms associated with the menopause and tamoxifen use (e.g., vaginal, hot flashes, urinary symptoms); 43 items; 5-point, Likert-type	Self-administered	ICR: α of .73 for vaginal subscale, .76 for hot flashes subscale, .76 for urinary subscale, and .50 for total scale (Gantz et al., 2000) TRR: Not applicable	Content: No data available Construct: No data available	Sensitivity to change: No data available Sensitivity to nursing: No data available

Measure	Population	Symptoms/Items	Administration	Reliability	Validity	Sensitivity
Support Team Assessment Schedule (STAS) (Higginson & McCarthy, 1989); Edmonton Symptom Assessment System (ESAS) (Bruera et al., 1991); Palliative Care Assessment (PACA), which is a modified version of the STAS (Ellershaw, Peat, & Boys, 1995)	Patients in palliative care	12 core symptoms (pain, mouth discomfort, anorexia, nausea, vomiting, constipation, breathlessness, depression, agitation, confusion, patient psychological distress, and family anxiety); 12 items but varies with version; 4-point rating scale	Self-administered or completed by the healthcare provider based on his or her clinical assessment of the patient's condition	ICR: Not applicable TRR: Not applicable IRR: No data available	Content: Core symptoms selected based on clinicians' input Construct: No data available	Sensitivity to change: No data available Sensitivity to nursing: No data available
Semistructured interview (Maguire et al., 1999)	Terminally ill patients with colorectal cancer	Symptoms of pain, pyrexia, breathlessness, abdominal swelling, constipation, diarrhea, sore mouth, nausea, and vomiting; 9 items; response format not described	Interview by observer	ICR: Not applicable TRR: Not applicable IRR: No data available	Content: No data available Construct: No data available	Sensitivity to change: No data available Sensitivity to nursing: No data available
Symptom Reporting Tool (Tucci & Bartels, 1998)	Patients with cancer	Symptoms of pain, nausea and vomiting, numbness/tingling, and diarrhea; diary/log completed by patients at home; 10-point rating scale to rate symptoms and SC strategies	Self-administered	ICR: Not applicable TRR: Not applicable	Content: No data available Construct: No data available	Sensitivity to change: No data available Sensitivity to nursing: No data available
Symptom Report Form (White, 1992)	Patients with cancer receiving biotherapy	Cluster of symptoms related to cardiovascular condition; dietary intake; fatigue; oral integrity; skin manifestations; flulike syndrome; unclear number of items; 4-point rating scale	Administered by interviewer	ICR: Not applicable TRR: Not applicable IRR: No data available	Content: No data available Construct: No data available	Sensitivity to change: No data available Sensitivity to nursing: No data available

α = Cronbach's alpha coefficient; CVI = content validity index; GI = gastrointestinal; ICR = internal consistency reliability; IRR = interrater reliability; r = correlation coefficient; SC = self-care; TRR = test retest reliability.

(continues)

TABLE 4-1 Instruments Measuring General Symptoms (continued)

Instrument (author)	Target population	Domains; number of items; response format	Method of administration	Reliability	Validity	Sensitivity to change and nursing care
Symptom Control Assessment (SCA) (Benor et al., 1998)	Patients with cancer	Several symptoms (e.g., those related to respiration, fluid and food intake, ADLs, rest and sleep, mobility, hygiene, sociability, bacteriologic and physical safety, pain, anxiety, and sexuality); 16 items; 7-point numeric scale assessing intensity, independence, help, and knowledge	Self-administered or administered by interviewer	ICR: α of .85 for total scale TRR: *r* of .97 for intensity, .90 for independence, .89 for perception of familial help, and .88 for knowledge dimensions IRR: *r* of .90	Content: Reviewed by experts in the field Construct: Patients' and nurses' ratings were almost identical (*r* of .93 to .95 across the items)	Sensitivity to change and to nursing: Changes in scores found for the different dimensions following an educative-supportive nursing intervention
Symptom indexes (J. A. Clark & Talcott, 2001)	Patients with prostate cancer receiving therapy	Symptoms related to urinary incontinence and obstruction, bowel symptoms, and sexual dysfunction	Self-administered	ICR: α of .86 for urinary incontinence, .65 for urinary obstruction, .73 for bowel symptoms, .80 for sexual dysfunction TRR: Not applicable	Content: No data available Construct: Correlated with health-related quality of life	Sensitivity to change: Scores changed over time Sensitivity to nursing: No data available

α = Cronbach's alpha coefficient; CVI = content validity index; GI = gastrointestinal; ICR = internal consistency reliability; IRR = interrater reliability; *r* = correlation coefficient; SC = self-care; TRR = test retest reliability.

measure only one dimension of the symptom experience, with severity or perceived distress being the most frequently assessed. A Likert-type or numeric rating scale was often used to capture varying levels on the dimension of interest.

The instruments have been used in a small number of studies. Examining the internal consistency reliability of these instruments is not highly recommended, which explains the reported lack of evidence to support this type of reliability (Table 4-1). This is related to the fact that patients may experience some, but not necessarily all, of the symptoms listed. However, some instruments comprised subscales, in which the items contained in a subscale capture indicators of the same symptom (e.g., SSC-HIV, Breast Cancer Prevention Trial symptom checklist). In these cases, the internal consistency reliability was evaluated for each subscale and was acceptable (≥ .70) for newly developed measures. There were limited data to support content and construct validity of the instruments. Their sensitivity to change was not extensively tested. Additional research is required before the use of these instruments in practice can be recommended.

In the next sections, the conceptualization, measurement, and sensitivity to nursing care or interventions of the symptoms of fatigue, nausea and vomiting, and dyspnea are discussed. These symptoms are frequently experienced by patients with acute and chronic conditions, seen in primary, acute, and long-term healthcare settings.

FATIGUE

The terms *tiredness*, *fatigue*, and *exhaustion* are often used interchangeably to express varying levels of a subjective sensation characterized by lack of energy and capacity to engage in physical or mental work. Tiredness is reported by any person following heavy or sustained physical or mental work. It is effectively relieved by adequate rest and sleep. Unresolved and severe tiredness presents a warning signal and a cue for seeking health care. This feeling of fatigue is experienced by individuals with acute (e.g., cold, anemia) and chronic (e.g., cancer, depression) conditions and those receiving medical (e.g., chemotherapy) or surgical treatment. Inappropriately managed and persistent severe fatigue leads to the incapacitating feeling of exhaustion (Olson et al., 2008; Ream, 2007).

Fatigue is of concern to healthcare professionals in different healthcare settings. It is reported by a variety of patient populations presenting with physical and psychological conditions. Fatigue is a common manifestation of acute illnesses such as pneumonia, flu, and sinusitis and of the physical stress related to surgical interventions. It is also associated with psychological stress and with alterations in mood, primarily depression. Most commonly, fatigue is experienced by patients with different chronic conditions such as cancer, cardiac disease, chronic obstructive pulmonary disease, end-stage renal disease, HIV/AIDS, and chronic fatigue syndrome. It is reported with some treatment modalities such as chemotherapy and radiation therapy. In addition to its high prevalence, fatigue is a distressing symptom with an adverse impact on patients. It limits the patients' ability to maintain normal functioning; it interferes with performance of daily activities and self-care activities, reduces sense of emotional well-being, disrupts family life and work, and ultimately influences quality of life.

Assisting patients in managing fatigue effectively is an instrumental goal of nursing care. Successful relief of this distressing symptom is necessary to regain and maintain usual physical and psychological functioning, enhance engagement in self-care, and improve quality of life. To be effective in managing fatigue, nursing care should be guided by a clear definition of this symptom and a precise identification of its indicators. It should be based on a comprehensive and systematic assessment of fatigue and on empirical evidence demonstrating the effectiveness of interventions designed to address this symptom.

In the next section, the literature on fatigue is reviewed with the purposes of (a) defining fatigue and identifying its critical attributes and indicators, (b) evaluating the reliability, validity, and sensitivity to change of instruments measuring fatigue, and (c) determining the extent to which fatigue is a symptom that is affected by nursing care and/or interventions. The literature search covered CINAHL, CANCERLIT, and MEDLINE computerized databases. The specific keywords used were: *fatigue*, *tiredness*, *lassitude*, and *exhaustion*; these were combined with *symptom management*, *treatment*, *intervention*, and *nursing care*. Conceptual articles were included if they presented conceptualization of fatigue advanced by nursing scholars. Empirical articles were selected if they reported on the experience of fatigue or on the effectiveness of interventions delivered by nurses to manage fatigue in various patient populations. It is important to note that fatigue has been extensively investigated in patients with cancer.

Conceptualization of Fatigue

The review of conceptual nursing literature pointed to some similarities and differences in the definitions of fatigue that were advanced. There was consistency in characterizing fatigue as a subjective feeling, however, differences were noted in other attributes of this symptom. The differences were related to difficulty in defining, and hence operationalizing, fatigue (Whitehead, 2009); difficulty in differentiating among its antecedents (i.e., contributing factors), manifestations (i.e., indicators), and consequences (i.e., impact); and possible variability in its experience across patient populations. Often, fatigue has been defined in terms of its antecedents and consequences, rather than the nature of the sensation, observed in a particular patient population. For instance, Tsay (2004) defined fatigue in end-stage renal disease as a feeling of tiredness affected by circadian rhythms. Ream (2007) described fatigue experienced by patients in palliative care settings as a subjective, unpleasant symptom characterized by feelings that range from tiredness to exhaustion and that interfere with the persons' ability to function normally. Armes et al. (2007) referred to cancer-related fatigue as a perceived sense of tiredness experienced in relation to cancer or its treatment that interferes with performance of usual functions. In an attempt to clarify the nature of fatigue as experienced by healthy and ill persons, Olson et al. (2008) synthesized the findings of their quantitative and qualitative studies, as well as those reported by others. They identified the following common characteristics of fatigue: difficulty concentrating, anxiety, a gradual decrease in stamina, difficulty sleeping, decreasing control over body processes, and limitation of social interaction. Although grounded in individuals' experience, these features encompass other distinct symptoms such as anxiety and difficulty sleeping, which contribute to fatigue, and states such as limited social interactions, which result from fatigue. This lack of differentiation among the antecedents, manifestations, and consequences of fatigue is due to their well-recognized interrelationships (Winningham, 1995) and to the recently introduced concept of symptom cluster. Fatigue tends to be experienced with other symptoms, including pain, anxiety, depression, and insomnia (Visowsky & Schneider, 2003). The differences in definitions were associated with some variability in the domains and indicators of fatigue. Some authors focused on one domain, primarily physical; others were concerned with attitudinal, sensory, affective, cognitive, and behavioral domains of the symptom. The specific manifestations indicative of each domain were described differently. These differences in the conceptualization account for the large number of instruments developed to measure fatigue (Whitehead, 2009).

In addition to these theoretical definitions, scholars have been interested in examining the patients' accounts of the fatigue experience. This was accomplished through systematic clinical observations (e.g., Piper, 1993; Winningham et al., 1994) and qualitative research studies exploring how patients experience this symptom (Glaus, Crow, & Hammond, 1996; Olson, Krawchuk & Quddusi, 2007). Patients described fatigue as a feeling of being unusually tired, ready to drop, worn out, weary, listless, or pooped; as a sense of weakness, lack of energy, malaise, and lethargy; as inability to concentrate and to think clearly; as decreased physical performance or reduction in activities; and as feeling hampered, having no desire or motivation for work, short-tempered, and edgy. These descriptors provided by patients experiencing fatigue were consistent with those proposed in the theoretical definitions, supporting the clinical utility of this concept (Penrod & Hupcey, 2005).

Essential Attributes

Based on the presented definitions and descriptions, the following attributes are considered characteristic of the symptom of fatigue:

- Fatigue is a subjective feeling that is perceived by the individual. It is self-recognized. It varies in intensity, frequency, and duration.

- Fatigue is expressed in terms of physical, affective or emotional, cognitive, attitudinal, and behavioral experiences.
- Overall, fatigue is characterized as a sense of lack of energy and decreased capacity for physical activity or for physical and mental work.
- The physical experience of fatigue is manifested by feeling tired in the whole body, arms, or legs; feeling weary, listless, or worn out; having no energy; experiencing malaise or discomfort; feeling heaviness in the arms, legs, or eyes; having tremors and/or numbness in the extremities; having eye strain; and experiencing weakness or lack of strength.
- The affective or emotional experience of fatigue is manifested by unpleasant feelings, increased irritability (e.g., short-tempered, edgy), and lack of patience.
- The cognitive experience of fatigue is manifested by difficulty in thinking or the inability to think clearly, decreased attention, inability to concentrate, slowed and impaired perception of environmental stimuli/information, poor judgment, and forgetfulness.
- The attitudinal experience of fatigue is manifested by decreased interest, decreased motivation, apathy, and being indifferent to the surroundings.
- The behavioral experience of fatigue is manifested by feeling able to do only a little, requiring more effort to do things, wanting to lie down, having a strong desire to sleep, and exhibiting changes in general appearance and communication pattern.

Antecedents

Different categories of factors have been suggested as contributing to the experience of fatigue. These categories include physiological, physical, psychosocial, environmental, and innate host factors. The specific factors, within each category, that were proposed to affect fatigue entail the following:

- Physiological factors: These are related to the nature of the illness condition experienced by the individual and/or the treatment received. Illness conditions that result in alterations in fluid and electrolyte balance (e.g., dehydration), accumulation of metabolites (e.g., hydrogen ions), hormone imbalance (e.g., thyroid disorder), and oxygenation (e.g., anemia) are associated with the experience of fatigue (Piper, 1993). The experience and severity of cancer-related fatigue are related to cancer site and stage. Patients with cancer of the lung and of the gastrointestinal, urogenital, and hematologic systems, as well as those having metastasis of cancer, reported high levels of fatigue (Visowsky & Schneider, 2003). Treatment of some illness conditions, whether medical or surgical, leads to fatigue. In particular, cancer adjuvant therapy is associated with the accumulation of toxic waste products contributing to fatigue (A. Richardson, 1995; Visowsky & Schneider).

- Physical factors: These often represent the experience of other symptoms and/or alterations in the patterns of activity, rest, sleep, and fluid and food intake. Examples of these include pain, fever, and diarrhea. The following symptoms were found to initiate or trigger cancer-related fatigue: dyspnea, weight loss, pain, nausea, and sleep disturbances. Physical inactivity, used as a strategy to cope with cancer-related fatigue, is viewed as a factor that perpetuates or maintains this symptom (Ream, 2007). Dirksen and Epstein (2008) reported that insomnia predicted fatigue experienced by breast cancer survivors.
- Psychosocial factors: These are related to increased demands of illness and the need to adapt and adjust to changes in various aspects of life; to the emotional response to illness and/or treatment characterized by anxiety and depression; to ineffective coping strategies used by patients; and to prolonged stress (Berger & Walker, 2001; Olson et al., 2007; Smets, Garssen, Schuster-Uitterhoeve, & De Haes, 1993). Specifically, fatigue was found to correlate with anxiety and depression in patients with cancer (Armes et al., 2007) and end-stage renal disease (Tsay, 2004).
- Environmental or situational factors: These include increased noise, changes in temperature, social and life event patterns, sensory deprivation, and informational overload (Cimprich, 1993; Piper, 1993).
- Innate host factors: These are exemplified with age, sex, and genetic makeup (Piper, 1993).

Although relationships between specific factors—in particular, physical and psychosocial symptoms—have been supported empirically, the exact mechanisms through which the factors affect fatigue are not well understood. Two frameworks have been suggested to explain the observed relationships: the biobehavioral model (Payne, Held, Thorpe, & Shaw, 2008) and the Edmonton Fatigue Framework (Olson et al., 2008). The biobehavioral model proposes dysregulation in hormones produced within the neuro-endocrine system (e.g., cortisol, serotonin) as the mechanism linking fatigue to other symptoms such as sleep disturbance and depression. The Edmonton Fatigue Framework is built on the fatigue adaptation model. It conceptualizes fatigue as the inability to adapt to stressors related to disease and its treatment. Although the frameworks offer alternative views of fatigue and its clustering with other symptoms, additional research is needed to validate the propositions.

Consequences

Fatigue has untoward effects on the patient. The consequences of fatigue that have been identified in the literature include:
- Physical consequences: These consist of decreased performance of physical activity, which yields to limited performance of usual activities (such as

difficulty accomplishing household chores), modification in recreational activities, and engagement in self-care activities (Graydon et al., 1997; Neuberger et al., 2007; Ream, 2007; Visowsky & Schneider, 2003).

- Psychosocial consequences: These include feelings of hopelessness and uncertainty; poor psychological adjustment; loss of employment; decreased engagement in social activities, leading to impaired self-concept, interpersonal relationships, and social isolation (Graydon et al., 1997; Visowsky & Schneider, 2003).
- Cognitive consequences: These involve altered thought processes and decreased performance of mental work (Graydon et al., 1997).

Instruments Measuring Fatigue

A large number of instruments have been used to measure fatigue in studies involving various populations. These are grouped into single-item measures, multiple-item scales capturing one domain of fatigue (i.e., unidimensional), and multiple-item scales capturing more than one domain of fatigue (i.e., multidimensional). **TABLE 4-2** summarizes the characteristics of the three types of measures.

Single-Item Measures

Fatigue has been recognized as a distressing symptom experienced with physical and psychological conditions. The interest in assessing this symptom and in evaluating the effectiveness of interventions in managing it prompted researchers and clinicians to develop single items measuring fatigue. Similar single-item measures have been validated as useful for assessing the perception of other symptoms, such as pain and dyspnea. They capture the individuals' perception of the whole phenomenological experience of the symptom.

In most instances, the single measures were developed for use in particular research studies (Armes et al., 2007; Devlen, Maguire, Phillips, Crowther, & Chambers, 1987; Greenberg, Gary, Mannix, Eisenthal, & Carey, 1993; Greenberg, Sawicka, Eisenthal, & Ross, 1992; Joly et al., 1996; Love, Leventhal, Easterling, & Nerenz, 1989; Morant, 1996; Ream, Richardson, & Alexander-Dann, 2006; A. Richardson & Ream, 1996; Tsay, 2004). Two single-item measures have been used in more than one study: the analogue fatigue scale (AFS) and the Rhoton Fatigue Scale (RFS) (see Table 4-2). These measures often consist of a term reflecting the symptom of fatigue or a descriptor indicative of fatigue. Although the terms or descriptors used capture the global experience of fatigue, they differed across studies and included fatigue, tiredness, weakness, and lack of energy. None has been validated as the most accurate reflection of fatigue from the patients' perspective. The dimension of fatigue assessed also differed and reflected the symptom's severity, perceived distress, and impact on chores, work, or recreational activities (e.g., Ream et al., 2006). The response options consisted of

TABLE 4-2   Instruments Measuring Fatigue

Instrument (author)	Target population/ setting	Domains (number of items and response format)	Method of administration	Reliability	Content validity	Construct validity	Sensitivity to nursing variables
SINGLE ITEMS STANDING ALONE							
Analogue fatigue scale (AFS) (Christensen et al., 1982)	Surgical patients	Domain: Global rating of fatigue, which captures the physical domain Number of items: 1 Response format: Vertical linear analogue scale	Self-administered or administered by clinician	Internal consistency: Not applicable Stability/test-retest: .81 over a 2–4 hour interval in postoperative patients (Christensen et al., 1982)	No data available	Correlated with subjective measures of fatigue (e.g., POMS) in surgical patients (Christensen et al., 1982); correlated with objective measure of fatigue (effort in the cycle ergometer test (Christensen et al., 1982) and with state anxiety (Christensen, Hjortso, Mortensen, Riis-Hansen, & Kehlet, 1986) and pulse rate change during exercise (Christensen, Nygaard, Stage, & Kehlet, 1990)	Responsive to change in level of fatigue observed postoperatively in surgical patients (Christensen et al., 1986; Schroeder & Hill, 1991) No data available relative to nursing variable
Rhoten Fatigue Scale (RFS) (Rhoten, 1982)	Surgical and cancer patients	Domain: Global experience of fatigue, with a primary focus on physical indicator (feeling of tiredness and lack of energy) Number of items: 1 Response format: Horizontal linear analogue scale	Self-administered and administered by clinician	Internal consistency: Not applicable Stability/test-retest: Not applicable	No data available	Correlated with CA 125 (an indicator of tumor response to treatment) in patients with cancer receiving therapy; did not discriminate among individuals with different levels of fatigue, that is, healthy versus cancer patients (Blesch et al., 1991; Pickard-Holley, 1991)	Not able to detect significant change in fatigue during course of chemotherapy in patients with ovarian cancer (Pickard-Holley, 1991) No data available relative to nursing variables
Unnamed items (Ream et al., 2006)	Patients with cancer undergoing chemotherapy	Dimensions: Distress, impact on activity Number of items: 4 Response format: Visual analogue	Self-administered	Not applicable	No data available	Reported to be valid and sensitive to change	Decrease in fatigue following supportive- educational intervention (Ream et al., 2006)

(continues)

TABLE 4-2   Instruments Measuring Fatigue (continued)

Instrument (author)	Target population/ setting	Domains (number of items and response format)	Method of administration	Reliability	Content validity	Construct validity	Sensitivity to nursing variables
UNIDIMENSIONAL SUBSCALES EMBEDDED IN GENERAL INSTRUMENTS							
European Organisation for Research and Treatment of Cancer Quality of Life Questionnaire (EORTC-QLQ) Fatigue subscale (Aaronson et al., 1991)	Patients with cancer; outpatient	Domain: Physical domain of fatigue Number of items: 3 Response format: 4-point rating scale to rate severity of fatigue	Self-administered	Internal consistency: α coefficient > .70 in patients from various countries (Aaronson, Bullinger, & Ahmedzai, 1996) Stability/test-retest: Not applicable	No data available	Correlated with physical functioning, anxiety, depression, and pain in patients with cancer (Aaronson et al., 1996); discriminated different levels of fatigue as experienced by cancer patients with different prognoses (Joly et al., 1996)	Responsive to change over course of chemotherapy (Osoba et al., 1996) No data available relative to nursing variables
Profile of Mood States (POMS) fatigue-inertia subscale (McNair, Lorr, & Droppleman, 1981)	General, healthy population; also used in patients with chronic illness	Domain: Physical domain of fatigue Number of items: 7 Response scale: 5-point Likert-type (*not at all* to *extremely*)	Self-administered	Internal consistency: α coefficients .80–.95 in various patient populations (Bowling, 1995; McNair et al., 1981), patients with cancer (Meek et al., 2000), and women with breast cancer (Dirksen & Epstein, 2008) Stability/test-retest: coefficient .74 in patients with cancer (Meek et al.)	No data available	Correlated with other self-report measures of fatigue (Greenberg et al., 1992) and with mood, pain, and performance status in patients with cancer (Cassileth et al., 1985; Glover, Dibble, Dodd, & Miaskowski, 1995; Jamar, 1989; Meek et al., 2000); discriminated among cancer patients with different levels of fatigue (Gritz, Wellish, & Landsverk, 1988)	Scores changed over course of adjuvant therapy (Meek et al.; Stanton & Snider, 1993) and following cognitive-behavioral interventions for managing insomnia delivered by nurses (Dirksen & Epstein)

Instrument	Population	Domain	Administration	Reliability	Origin/Validity	Correlation	Findings
Functional Assessment of Cancer Therapy fatigue subscale (cited in Godino et al., 2006)	Patients with cancer; outpatient	13 items measure fatigue; higher score reflects low fatigue level	Self-administered	No data reported	No data reported	No data reported	Significant improvement in fatigue score (10 points) following attendance at educational intervention given by nurses (Godino et al.)
UNIDIMENSIONAL, INDEPENDENT INSTRUMENTS OF FATIGUE							
Pearson-Byars Fatigue Feeling Checklist (PBFFCL) (Pearson & Byars, 1956)	Healthy individuals	Domain: Positive aspect (freshness) and negative aspect (tiredness) of fatigue. Number of items: 10. Response format: Respondents indicate if they feel better than, the same as, or worse than the feeling of fatigue described in each item	Self-administered	Internal consistency: α coefficients .82–.97 in patients with cancer (Graydon et al., 1995; Greenberg et al., 1992; Jamar, 1989). Stability/retest: Not applicable	Based on the work of tool developers in examining fatigue in military aircrew (Pearson & Byars)	Correlated with other measures of fatigue (Greenberg et al., 1992)	Scores increased over course of cancer treatment (Graydon et al., 1995; Greenberg et al., 1992). No data available relative to nursing variables
Fatigue Severity Scale (FSS) (Krupp, LaRocca, Muir-Nash, & Steinberg, 1989)	Patients with multiple sclerosis (MS) and systemic lupus erythematosus (SLE)	Domain: Impact of fatigue on daily functioning in these patient populations. Number of items: 9. Response format: 7-point Likert-type (*strongly agree* to *strongly disagree*)	Self-administered	Internal consistency: α coefficients .88 in healthy persons, .81 in patients with MS, .89 in patients with SLE, .95 in rural patients with cancer (Winstead-Fry, 1998). Stability/retest: .84 (Whitehead, 2009)	Development and refinement of items based on theoretical considerations and results of factor analysis	Factorial: One factor (Whitehead, 2009). Correlated with visual analogue scale for fatigue in patients with SLE, MS, and healthy persons; with other measures of fatigue in rural patients with cancer (Winstead-Fry); significant differences in scores between healthy individuals and patients with MS and SLE; correlated with depression (Krupp et al., 1989)	Some changes in scores observed before and after drug therapy for fatigue in patients with MS and SLE (Winstead-Fry). No data available relative to nursing variables

(continues)

TABLE 4-2 Instruments Measuring Fatigue (continued)

Instrument (author)	Target population/setting	Domains (number of items and response format)	Method of administration	Reliability	Content validity	Construct validity	Sensitivity to nursing variables
Composite Measure of Fatigue (Buxton, Frizelle, Parry, Pettigrew, & Hopkins, 1992)	Surgical patients	Domain: Severity of fatigue Number of items: 5 Response format: Semantic differential scale; 7 point	Self-administered	Internal consistency: α > .70 in patients who had elective general surgery Stability/test-retest: correlation coefficient > .70	Maintained by selecting descriptors from the literature	Correlated with other self-report measures of fatigue (visual analogue scale, and Profile of Mood States fatigue subscale); with objective indicators of fatigue (i.e., loss of body weight, cycle ergometer test, handgrip test of muscle strength) (Buxton, Frizelle, Parry, Pettigrew, & Hopkins, 1992)	Increase in scores observed from presurgery to postsurgery, followed by a decrease during the recovery period
Fatigue Questionnaire (FQ) (David et al., 1990)	Healthy individuals in a primary care setting	Domain: Tiredness, need for rest, sleepy or drowsy, difficulty starting doing things, weak, getting tired when concentrating, having enough energy, strength in muscles Number of items: 11 Response format: 4-point Likert-type (*none, same as usual, more than usual,* and *much more than usual*)	Self-administered	Internal consistency: Not assessed Stability/test-retest: Not applicable	No data available	Factorial: Items loaded on one factor Construct: Individuals who reported a brief duration of fatigue had a lower score on the FQ (David et al.)	No data available
Fatigue Outcome Measure (Armes et al., 2007)	Patients with cancer, outpatient	Dimensions: Severity, distress, ability to cope with fatigue, extent to which it is overwhelming, uncontrollable, unpredictable, and abnormal Number of items: 7 Response format: Graphic rating scale; score ranges from 0 to 100	Self-administered	No data available	No data available	No data available	No change in scores following behavioral intervention focused on self-management of fatigue (Armes et al.)

Measure	Population/Setting	Dimension/Domain	Administration	Reliability	Development	Validity	Responsiveness
Brief Fatigue Inventory (BFI) (cited in Whitehead, 2009)	Patients with cancer	Dimension: Severity Number of items: 9 Response format: 11-point Likert scale	Self-administered	Internal consistency: alpha coefficients: .89–.91 Stability/test-retest r: .79–.91	No data available	Factorial: Items loaded on one factor Construct: Correlated with other measures of fatigue (e.g., POMS)	No data available
Rhoten Fatigue Scale (RFS) (cited in Whitehead, 2009)	Patients with cancer	Dimension: Severity Number of items: 1 Response format: 11-point numeric rating scale	Self-administered	No data available	No data available	Correlated with other measures of fatigue (e.g., POMS); did not detect difference in fatigue between healthy patients and patients with cancer	No data available
Schedule of Fatigue and Anergia (SOFA) (cited in Whitehead, 2009)	Healthy population; primary care	Dimension: Severity Number of items: 10 Response format: 5-point Likert scale	Self-administered	No data available	No data available	Detected difference in fatigue level between healthy and ill persons	No data available
MULTIPLE-ITEM, MULTIDIMENSIONAL SCALES							
Fatigue Impact Scale (FIS) (Fisk et al., 1994)	Patients with chronic fatigue syndrome, hypertension, and multiple sclerosis	Domain: Impact of fatigue on quality of life (i.e., cognitive, physical, and psychosocial functioning) Number of items: 40 Response format: 5-point Likert-type (*no problem* to *extreme problem*)	Self-administered	Internal consistency: Alpha coefficients > .87 in patients with chronic fatigue syndrome, hypertension, and multiple sclerosis Stability/test-retest: Not applicable	Generated from existing fatigue questionnaires and from interviews with patients	Significant differences in scores across patient groups (score was highest for patients with chronic fatigue syndrome, followed by those with multiple sclerosis and hypertension); positive correlation with Sickness Impact Profile	No data available
Fatigue Rating Scale (FRS) (Kashiwagi, 1971)	FRS is an observational tool that has been used in Japanese industrial settings	Domain: Weakened activation and weakened motivation Number of items: 20 Response format: Not described	Observation	Internal consistency: No data available Stability/test-retest: No data available Interrater: Not tested	Generated from a self-report measure of fatigue; rated for relevance by healthy individuals	Factorial structure: Items clustered into the two hypothesized dimensions of subjective fatigue feelings Construct: No data available	No data available

(continues)

TABLE 4-2   Instruments Measuring Fatigue (continued)

Instrument (author)	Target population/ setting	Domains (number of items and response format)	Method of admin-istration	Reliability	Content validity	Construct validity	Sensitivity to nursing variables
Fatigue Assess-ment Scale (FAS) (Chalder et al., 1993)	General practice client population	Domain: Physical and mental fatigue Number of items: 14 Response format: Better than usual, no more than usual, worse than usual, and much worse than usual	Self-adminis-tered	Internal con-sistency: α .89 for total scale, .84 for physical subscale, and .82 for men-tal subscale, in patients in gen-eral practice Stability/test-retest: Not applicable	Generated from an exten-sive literature review	Factorial structure: Two-factor solution, as hypothesized Construct: No data available	No data available
Fatigue Assess-ment Instru-ment (FAI) (Schwartz, Jan-dorf, & Krupp, 1993)	Patients with chronic fatigue syn-drome and multiple sclerosis	Domain: Extension of the FSS developed by Krupp et al. (1989); assesses severity of fatigue, consequences of fatigue, and responsive-ness of fatigue to rest/ sleep Number of items: 29 Response format: 7- point Likert scale (*completely disagree* to *completely agree*)	Self-adminis-tered	Internal consis-tency: α coef-ficient .70–.92 for subscales in ill individuals Stability/test-retest: Coef-ficients .29 for the responsive-ness to rest/ sleep subscale, .62 for fatigue consequences, .69 for sever-ity of fatigue subscale, in patients with multiple sclerosis	Items drawn from clinical experience and from patients' responses to interviews	Factorial structure: Items loaded on four factors, as hypothesized Discriminated between patients with chronic illness and healthy individuals	No data available

Lee Fatigue Scale (LFS) (K. Lee, Hicks, & Nino-Murcia, 1991)	Initially developed for use with individuals with sleep disorders. Also used in patients with chronic conditions	Domain: Fatigue and energy Number of items: 18 Response format: 100-mm horizontal visual analogue scale	Self-administered	Internal consistency: α coefficient .91 for fatigue subscale and .94 for energy subscale in individuals in general practice (K. Lee et al.); .94 and .96 in patients with cancer receiving treatment (Meek et al., 2000) Stability/test-retest: Coefficient .47 for fatigue subscale and .77 for energy subscale in patients with cancer receiving treatment (Meek et al.)	No data available	Factorial structure: Two factor, consistent with scale theoretical structure (K. Lee et al.; Meek et al.) Correlation with the POMS-fatigue subscale in general practice patients (K. Lee et al.) and with theoretically relevant mood states (e.g., depression) in patients with cancer (Meek et al.)	Changes in scores observed in patients with cancer during periods of expected high and low levels of fatigue (i.e., around exposure to treatment) (Meek et al.) No data available relative to nursing variables
Fatigue Symptom Checklist (Yoshitake, 1971, 1978)	Healthy individuals	Domain: Drowsiness and dullness (e.g., feeling heavy in the head), difficulty concentrating (e.g., difficulty thinking clearly), and physical discomfort (e.g., back pain) Number of items: 30 Response format: Indicate whether the symptoms were experienced	Self-administered	Internal consistency: No data available Stability/test-retest: No data available	No data available	Difficulty to concentrate subscale scores higher in workers involved in mental work; physical discomfort subscale scores higher in workers involved in physical work; correlated with general measure of general feeling of fatigue	No data available

(continues)

TABLE 4-2   Instruments Measuring Fatigue (continued)

Instrument (author)	Target population/ setting	Domains (number of items and response format)	Method of admin- istration	Reliability	Content validity	Construct validity	Sensitivity to nursing variables
Piper Fatigue Scale (PFS) (Piper, Dodd, Paul, & Weleer, 1989)	Any patient population	Domain: Temporal, affective, sensory, and severity Number of items: 76 in original version; 41 or 24 in revised, shorter versions Response format: 100-mm horizontal visual analogue scale (none and a great deal)	Self-adminis- tered	Internal con- sistency: α coefficients for subscales .69 and .95 and for total scale .85 (Berger & Walker, 2001; Piper, Dodd, Paul, & Weleer, 1989) Stability/test-retest: Not tested	Developed from clinical experience and from pertinent literature; rated as relevant by experts; dimen- sions supported by results of cluster analysis	Correlated with POMS subscales, Fatigue Symp- tom Checklist	Significant improvement in fatigue (and differ- ence between groups) follow- ing acupres- sure delivered by nurses (Tsay, 2004); no changes in fatigue fol- lowing walk- ing program (Payne et al., 2008)
Multidimen- sional Fatigue Inventory (MFI) (Smets, Gars- sen, Bonke, & De Haes, 1995)	Patients with vari- ous chronic conditions	Domain: General fatigue, physical fatigue, mental fatigue, reduced motiva- tion, and reduced activity Number of items: 20 Response format: Five boxes aligned horizon- tally and anchored with *Yes, that is true* and *No, that is not true*	Self-adminis- tered	Internal con- sistency: α coefficients for subscales .53– .94 in patients with can- cer receiving radiotherapy, patients with chronic fatigue syndrome, psy- chology stu- dents, medical students, army recruits, and junior physi- cians (Meek et al., 2000; Smets, Gars- sen, Cull, & de Haes, 1996), and patients with cancer receiving	Derived from a litera- ture review and patient interviews	Factorial structure: Hypothesized five-factor structure supported in various client popula- tions (Meek et al., 2000; Smets et al., 1996) Correlated with visual analogue measuring fatigue and with mea- sures of mood, activities of daily living, and emo- tional distress; discrimi- nated between patients with different levels of fatigue and between medically ill patients and healthy persons expe- riencing fatigue (Meek et al.; Smets et al., 1996)	Significant changes in sub- scales scores between times of high and low fatigue associated with expo- sure to cancer treatment (Meek et al.) Significant improvement in physical fatigue and reduced activ- ity follow- ing behavioral intervention for management of fatigue (Armes et al., 2007) and following

Instrument	Population	Description	Administration	Reliability		Validity	Utility/Responsiveness
				chemotherapy (Molassiotis et al., 2007) Stability/test-retest: .50–.72 (Meek et al.)			acupuncture (Molassiotis et al., 2007)
Multidimensional Assessment of Fatigue (MAF) (Belza, Henke, Yelin, Epstein, & Gillis, 1993)	Patients with arthritis, chronic pulmonary disease, and cancer	Domain: Severity, distress, interference with daily activity, and frequency. Number of items: 16. Response format: 10-point numeric rating scale anchored with *not at all* and *a great deal* is used for the severity, distress, and interference subscales; 4-point scale for the frequency subscale	Self-administered	Internal consistency: α coefficient for total scale .88–.93 in patients with various conditions (Belza, 1995; Belza et al.; Meek et al.); .88 in rural patients with cancer (Winstead-Fry, 1998). Stability/test-retest: Coefficient for total scale .74 and .87	No data available	Factorial structure: Two-factor solution, consistent with hypothesized structure (Meek et al.). Correlated with other measures of fatigue and theoretically relevant concepts such as anxiety and depression (Belza, 1995; Meek et al.; Winstead-Fry)	Changes in scores observed during times of high and low fatigue experienced with cancer therapy (Meek et al.). No data available relative to nursing variables
Fatigue Scale (FS) (cited in Whitehead, 2009)	General population	Domain: Physical and mental fatigue. Number of items: 11. Response format: 4-point Likert scale	Self-administered	Internal consistency: Alpha coefficients: .88–.90. Stability/test-retest: No data available	No data available	Detected differences in fatigue between persons who experienced fatigue and those who did not	No data available
Fatigue Symptom Inventory (FSI) (cited in Whitehead, 2009)	Patients with cancer	Domain/dimension: Severity, duration, and impact of fatigue. Number of items: 13. Response format: 11-point Likert scale	Self-administered	Internal consistency: Alpha coefficients: .93–.95. Stability/test retest *r*: .35–.75	No data available	Correlated with other measures of fatigue (e.g., POMS). Detected differences in fatigue among healthy individuals, patients not on treatment, and patients on treatment	No data available

(continues)

TABLE 4-2   Instruments Measuring Fatigue (continued)

Instrument (author)	Target population/setting	Domains (number of items and response format)	Method of administration	Reliability	Content validity	Construct validity	Sensitivity to nursing variables
Multidimensional Fatigue Symptom Inventory (MFSI) (cited in Whitehead, 2009)	Patients with cancer	Domains: Global, somatic, affective, cognitive, behavioral; Number of items: 83 (original), 30 (short form); Response format: 5-point Likert scale	Self-administered	Internal consistency of sub-scales: Alpha coefficients: .85–.96; Stability/test-retest r: .51–.70	No data available	Correlated with other measures of fatigue (e.g., POMS); Detected differences in fatigue between patients with and without cancer	No data available
Myasthenia Gravis Fatigue Scale (cited in Whitehead, 2009)	Patient with myasthenia gravis	Domain/dimension: Severity, physical, effect on behaviors; Number of items: 26; Response format: 5-point Likert scale	Self-administered	Internal consistency: Alpha coefficients: .89–.93; Stability/test-retest r: .85	No data available	Detected differences in fatigue between healthy adults and patients with myasthenia gravis	No data available
Parkinson's Fatigue Scale (cited in Whitehead, 2009)	Patients with Parkinson's disease	Dimension: Physical, impact of fatigue; Number of items: 16; Response format: 5-point Likert scale	Self-administered	Internal consistency: Alpha coefficients: .62–.98; Stability/test-retest r: .72	No data available	Correlated with other measures of fatigue (e.g., visual analogue scale)	No data available
Schwartz Cancer Fatigue Scale (cited in Whitehead, 2009)	Patients with cancer	Domains: Physical, emotional, cognitive; Number of items: 28; Response format: 5-point Likert scale	Self-administered	Internal consistency: Alpha coefficient: .97; Stability/test-retest: No data available	No data available	Detected difference in fatigue between patients receiving treatment and those not receiving treatment	No data available

100 mm visual analogue scales (VASs) or 11-point (0–10) numeric rating scales. The single-item measures of fatigue have shown acceptable construct validity and sensitivity to change (Armes et al.; Christensen, Bendix, & Kehlet, 1982; Ream et al., 2006).

The advantages of single-item measures relate to their simplicity of use; (a) they can be administered in a very short time period (about 1 minute), which is suitable for fatigued or sick patients; (b) they are easy to administer (that is, they do not require special instructions or training); and (c) they do not need a complex scoring system, and their scores are easy to interpret. The limitations of these measures relate to several points. First, the item provides an overall, global rating of fatigue. Global ratings do not provide information about the specific domain of fatigue that is affected and hence requires remediation. Second, the respondents' answers to a single item may be unreliable, introducing error; thus, it is difficult to evaluate the reliability of one-item scales. Last, the VAS response format may be difficult to use in some patient populations, including children and elders; the VAS reproduction may be inaccurate; and their scoring may be cumbersome, especially if respondents did not precisely follow the instructions for indicating their fatigue level.

Multiple-Item, Unidimensional Instruments

Multiple-item instruments were developed to measure the general perception of fatigue and to overcome the limitation of single-item measures; incorporating multiple items improves the reliability of measurement. A few of these instruments formed subscales embedded within measures of general health condition, whereas others formed separate, independent measures of fatigue.

Unidimensional Subscales Embedded in General Instruments

Unidimensional subscales measuring fatigue have constituted instruments assessing general health condition (e.g., Medical Outcome Study Short Form 36–vitality subscale), health-related quality of life (e.g., Functional Assessment of Cancer Therapy–fatigue subscale), and mood (e.g., Profile of Mood States–Fatigue Inertia). It is beyond the scope of this book to discuss all these subscales in detail. However, three such subscales that were used in nursing studies are included in this review: the European Organisation for Research and Treatment of Cancer Quality of Life Questionnaire (EORTC-QLQ) fatigue subscale, the Functional Assessment of Cancer Therapy (FACT) fatigue subscale, and the Profile of Mood States (POMS) fatigue subscale (Table 4-2).

The three subscales measure the physical domain and the severity dimension of fatigue. The EORTC-QLQ and the FACT are specific to patients with cancer. Their subscales have been used to assess fatigue in this population only. The EORTC-QLQ fatigue subscale has shown acceptable psychometric properties. In contrast, the POMS fatigue subscale has been used to measure this symptom in different populations and demonstrated reliability, validity, and sensitivity to change; it also detected statistically significant and clinically meaningful changes in fatigue in breast cancer survivors who participated in behavioral interventions delivered by nurses for the management of insomnia (Dirksen & Epstein, 2008).

Unidimensional, Independent Measures

Nine unidimensional, independent measures of fatigue are described in Table 4-2. These include the Pearson-Byars Fatigue Feeling Checklist (PBFFCL), the Fatigue Severity Scale (FSS), the Composite Measure of Fatigue, Fatigue Questionnaire (FQ), the Brief Fatigue Inventory (BFI), the Rhoten Fatigue Scale (RFS), the Schedule of Fatigue and Anergia (SOFA), and the Fatigue Outcome Measure. The items constituting most of these unidimensional measures reflect indicators of the physical domain of fatigue. A few capture selected indicators of the cognitive domain of fatigue; for example, the FQ contains an item inquiring about difficulty when concentrating. Consistent with the domain of fatigue reflected, the majority of unidimensional measures assess the severity of the symptom; the FSS assesses the impact of fatigue on the person.

The unidimensional measures were developed, tested, and used in descriptive and experimental studies targeting various patient populations ranging from healthy individuals to patients with different chronic conditions requiring surgical, medical, and/or nonpharmacological interventions. Their psychometric properties were evaluated in a small number of studies; however, they demonstrated adequate reliability, validity, and sensitivity to change. Limited data are available to determine sensitivity to nursing interventions. It is important to note that although the PBFFCL has been used in different patient populations and has shown acceptable psychometric properties, its content may not be relevant in today's social and healthcare systems. Some terms (e.g., *bushed*) are no longer in common use and may not be relevant to persons with diverse cultural and linguistic backgrounds.

Multiple-Item, Multidimensional Scales

A total of 14 multi-item, multidimensional measures appeared in the literature included in this review and are described in Table 4-2. Most have been developed and used in a small number of studies, often confined to the initial study aimed at testing their psychometric properties.

Except for the FRS, the multidimensional measures assess the subjective perception of fatigue, which is consistent with the conceptualization of this symptom. They may cover slightly different domains of fatigue. The physical domain is the most frequently included, followed by mental fatigue, which reflects indicators of the cognitive experience of fatigue discussed earlier. None of the measures captures all domains of fatigue identified in the literature (i.e., physical, affective, cognitive, attitudinal, and behavioral domains). All instruments assess the severity dimension of fatigue. The interest in determining the impact of fatigue on everyday functioning led some scholars to measure this dimension of the fatigue experience as well.

The evidence of the instruments' psychometric properties is based on the results of the initial testing of the tools. Investigators who used the tools in subsequent studies did not report additional testing of their properties. The MFI and PFS are exceptions because they were validated in large samples of various clinical and healthy populations, which improves the precision of the estimates. The instruments showed acceptable initial reliability, validity, and acceptability by different patient populations. However, some may be long, which may increase the response burden for patients who already experience fatigue.

Recommendations for Measuring Fatigue

The decision about which fatigue instrument to use depends on the purpose of the clinical assessment, on the instrument's psychometric properties, and on the characteristics of the patient population. Unidimensional and single-item scales could be used to monitor the severity of fatigue over time and to evaluate how effective nursing interventions are in relieving this symptom. Unidimensional scales offer respondents different descriptors of fatigue, which could be acceptable and best describe the experience of persons with diverse sociocultural backgrounds. A single, global measure of fatigue provides information on the patients' overall perception of the symptom severity, with minimal response burden. Such a measure of fatigue is similar to the one used for assessing pain and other symptoms in clinical practice. Nonetheless, it does not indicate which specific domain of fatigue is affected. Multidimensional measures present an accurate operationalization of fatigue. They are useful for comprehensively assessing the patients' experience of fatigue, which is helpful for planning care, individualizing interventions, and evaluating their effectiveness. Ream (2007) presented guidelines, developed by the National Comprehensive Cancer Network, for the assessment of fatigue in palliative care settings. The guidelines specify 11 indicators of fatigue, which are considered criteria for diagnosing fatigue, and recommend the 11-point (0–10) numeric rating scale to assess the degree to which fatigue is experienced. The guidelines advocate the following cutoff score for the numeric rating scale to determine the level of fatigue severity: 1–3 reflects *mild fatigue;* 4–6 *moderate fatigue, and 7–10 severe fatigue.* These heuristic cutoff scores should be validated empirically prior to their application in the practice setting.

Sensitivity to Nursing Care

The distressing and debilitating experience of fatigue prompted researchers to investigate interventions that could be useful in relieving this symptom. Because fatigue is frequently experienced in patients with chronic conditions, most of the intervention studies were conducted with such patient populations, primarily patients with cancer who were receiving adjuvant therapy. Two types of intervention studies were reported. The first included descriptive studies aimed at identifying strategies initiated and implemented by patients to manage fatigue. The second involved experimental studies concerned with evaluating the effectiveness of interventions delivered by nurses to assist patients in managing fatigue.

Five descriptive studies were found that explored the use of self-initiated strategies to manage cancer-related fatigue. The strategies included the following:

- Alteration of activity and rest pattern, such as resting and napping, taking things easy, modifying usual activities, and walking or exercising.
- Alteration in sleep and wake pattern, such as going to bed early and taking naps during the day.
- Diversional activities, such as listening to relaxation tapes, listening to music, reading, and watching TV.
- Alternative therapies, such as taking homeopathic remedies and acupuncture.
- Social activities, such as engaging in hobbies, going to movies, and having dinner with family and friends.
- Preservation of normality, such as doing housework, going shopping, and cooking (Dodd, 1984; Graydon, Bubela, Irvine, & Vincent, 1995; Jamar, 1989; Nail, Jones, Greene, Schipper, & Jensen, 1991; Ream & Richardson, 1999; A. Richardson & Ream, 1996).

The studies generally found that the self-initiated strategies were moderately effective in relieving fatigue (Graydon et al., 1997).

Mainstream and complementary/alternative interventions were evaluated for their effectiveness in relieving fatigue experienced by patients with chronic conditions, specifically cancer. The mainstream interventions included education, cognitive behavioral therapy, relaxation, energy conservation and activity pacing, and exercise. The complementary/alternative interventions were attention-restoring activities and acupressure/acupuncture. Although different healthcare professionals (e.g., psychologists, exercise therapists) have also examined the effectiveness of some interventions targeting fatigue, those conducted by nurse clinicians and researchers were selected for review. This was done to determine the sensitivity of fatigue, as an outcome, to nursing care. Because the number of nursing-led studies was rather limited, the results were compared with the findings of relevant systematic reviews or meta-analyses in an attempt to strengthen the evidence base supporting the effectiveness of the interventions. The effects of the types of interventions identified above are reviewed next.

- Education: The key element of educational interventions consists of providing patients with information about the meaning and experience of fatigue and about self-care strategies to manage this symptom. The specific topics covered varied slightly across studies; some addressed ways to monitor changes in fatigue, to identify possible triggers, and to change lifestyle, and some added an emotional support component. The mode of delivering the education included (a) distribution of written materials, (b) one-on-one, individualized teaching, and (c) small-group (10) discussion led or facilitated by nurses. Participants were patients with stage 1 or 2 malignant melanoma (Fawzy, 1995; Fawzy et al., 1990); with cancer in different sites (lymphoma, gastrointestinal, lung, colorectal, breast) and due to commence chemotherapy (Ream et al., 2006), and colon or gastric cancer (Godino, Jodar, Duran, Martinez, & Schiaffino, 2006). All studies used a randomized clinical trial (RCT) design; participants in the comparison group received usual care. The sample size ranged from 40 to 103, which was adequate for this type of design and target population. Fatigue was measured with valid self-report instruments at pretest and at least once at posttest. The results were consistent in showing a significant reduction in fatigue severity following implementation of the intervention in the experimental group; however, the between-group differences at posttest were not large enough to be considered clinically meaningful. Lotfi-Jam et al. (2008) reached similar conclusions. Ream (2007) suggested that educational interventions serve to empower patients, encourage adoption of self-care strategies, and help patients live effectively with fatigue more so than relieving this symptom in patients with cancer.

- Cognitive-behavioral therapy: Two studies were found that investigated interventions consistent with the active ingredients of cognitive-behavioral therapy (CBT). One intervention targeted fatigue directly and comprised the following components: discussing the meaning and experience of cancer-related fatigue; monitoring fatigue; goal setting; and activity scheduling. The intervention was given in three 60-minute individual face-to-face sessions at 3–4 weekly intervals. Participants were patients with cancer receiving cytotoxic treatment ($n = 55$) (Armes et al., 2007). The other intervention addressed fatigue indirectly. It consisted of a cognitive-behavioral intervention for managing insomnia in breast cancer survivors ($n = 77$). Its components were sleep education and hygiene, stimulus control instructions, and sleep restriction therapy. The intervention was implemented in six 60–90 minute sessions given once a week over a 6-week period. The first four sessions entailed small-group discussion, and the last two involved individual telephone discussion with the nurse (Dirksen & Epstein, 2008). The effectiveness of these interventions was evaluated in the context of a RCT. Fatigue was measured with reliable and valid self-report instruments before and after treatment. A significant decrease in the level of fatigue was observed in both studies, providing preliminary effectiveness of the interventions. Jacobson,

Donovan, Vadaparampil, and Small (2007) also reported significant effect size for psychological interventions for cancer-related fatigue, and D. Lee, Newell, Ziegler, and Topping (2008) reported similar effects of CBT on fatigue in patients with multiple sclerosis; however, most of the studies included in the review were judged to be of low quality.

- Relaxation: Decker, Cline-Elsen, and Gallagher (1992) examined the impact of stress reduction, given in the form of progressive muscle relaxation and imagery, on fatigue. The design was experimental; patients were randomly assigned to the experimental group (i.e., received muscle relaxation and imagery) or the control group. Patients ($n = 82$) with cancer undergoing curative or palliative radiation therapy were included. Fatigue was measured with the POMS-Fatigue subscale at pretest and posttest. Patients in the experimental group experienced no significant change in the level of fatigue, whereas those in the control group showed a significant increase from pretest to posttest. The results indicate that relaxation training may prevent patients from experiencing worsening levels of fatigue during the course of radiation therapy. Lotfi-Jam et al. (2008) reported inconsistent evidence for the effects of relaxation on fatigue.

- Energy conservation and activity pacing: Ream (2007) summarized the results of two studies that investigated the effects of energy conservation and activity pacing on fatigue experienced by patients with cancer and patients with multiple sclerosis. This strategy for managing fatigue is frequently recommended by nurses (Visowsky & Schneider, 2003). It involved advising patients to set their priorities and restrict activities or pace engagement in physical activities and alternate periods of activity and rest for the purpose of preventing energy depletion. The advice was delivered individually by telephone or in person. The results of these two studies showed that patients perceive energy conservation and activity pacing as acceptable interventions and that the intervention was effective in managing fatigue. Similar favorable effects (i.e., improvement in fatigue) were found in two RCTs investigating energy conservation in patients with cancer and patients with multiple sclerosis that were critically reviewed by C. Smith and Hale (2007).

- Exercise: The effectiveness of exercise in relieving fatigue was examined in four studies involving patients with chronic diseases. The exercise consisted of (a) a program of walking given to women with breast cancer, in combination with a support group throughout the course of chemotherapy (Mock et al., 1994); (b) a 10-week program of walking that targeted patients with cancer who were receiving adjuvant therapy (Graydon et al., 1999); (c) a home-based walking program implemented for 20 minutes four times a week by postmenopausal women with breast cancer who were receiving hormonal therapy (Payne et al., 2008); and (d) low-impact exercise program in which patients with rheumatoid arthritis engaged in

1 hour of exercise three times a week for 12 weeks, either in a class setting or at home (Neuberger et al., 2007). The design was experimental
with repeated measures in three studies, and preexperimental involving
one group with repeated measures in one study (Graydon et al., 1999).
The sample size ranged from 14 to 220. Fatigue was measured with different self-report tools that showed acceptable reliability and validity. Mock
et al. (1994) reported that women with breast cancer who participated
in the walking program experienced less fatigue at program completion
than those assigned to the comparison (usual care) group. Neuberger
et al. found that patients with rheumatoid arthritis who attended the class
sessions performed an amount of exercise comparable with those who
engaged in home-based exercise; however, the class group experienced a
significant reduction in fatigue, whereas the home group did not. Graydon
et al. (1999) and Payne et al. reported no significant changes in fatigue in
patients with cancer who performed the prescribed walking program, over
time. Inconsistent results were also found in two reviews of exercise-based
interventions. Jacobson et al. (2007) concluded that activity-based interventions have a weak effect on cancer-related fatigue. C. Smith and Hale's
(2007) findings indicated that aerobic exercises may not reduce fatigue in
patients with multiple sclerosis and may be beneficial in relieving fatigue
during and following treatment for cancer. Differences in the type, dose,
and context of performing the exercise, in the target population, and
in the measures of fatigue could account for the inconsistent findings
reported in individual studies and systematic reviews. It is important to
note that the attrition rate was rather high in some studies, implying that
exercise may not be well tolerated by patients experiencing fatigue.

- Attention-restoring activities: Cimprich (1993) explored the effects of
  an intervention on attentional fatigue in women who had surgery for
  breast cancer. Women were randomly assigned to the experimental group
  ($n = 16$) or the control group ($n = 16$). Women in the experimental
  group engaged in restorative activities (e.g., walking in nature, gardening)
  for 20–30 minutes three times a week. Attentional capacity was measured
  3, 18, 60, and 90 days postsurgery. Significant improvement in attentional
  capacity was observed in the experimental group over time. However, the
  small sample size and the initial group nonequivalence present threats to
  the validity of conclusions. This intervention was not further investigated
  (Ream, 2007).

- Acupressure/acupuncture: Two RCTs examined the effects of acupres-
  sure/acupuncture on fatigue in patients with end-stage renal disease (Tsay,
  2004) and cancer (Molassiotis, Sylt, & Diggins, 2007). Acupressure/acu-
  puncture is based on the concept of natural balance in Chinese medicine.
  It consists of massaging or applying pressure (acupressure) or stimulating
  (acupuncture) specific body points for the purpose of achieving a balance

of life energy and hence promoting comfort (Tsay). The exact mechanisms underlying its effect on different symptoms such as pain, nausea, and dyspnea are not quite clear; however, it is proposed that acupressure/acupuncture affects the release of neuropeptides and activates the opioid systems (Tsay). Acupressure was more effective than usual care in relieving fatigue experienced by patients with end-stage renal disease treated with hemodialysis ($n = 100$); however, this effect on fatigue was comparable for acupressure and placebo, which entailed sham acupressure (i.e., massage of nonspecific body points) (Tsay). Acupuncture demonstrated significant impact in reducing the severity of fatigue experienced by patients with cancer who completed chemotherapy; the magnitude of the impact was greater for the acupuncture, as compared with acupressure and sham acupressure (Molassiotis et al.). Similar positive effects were reported in the limited number of studies reviewed by C. Smith and Hale (2007).

The results of the studies included in the review provide preliminary evidence of the effectiveness of some nursing interventions in managing fatigue. They suggest that fatigue is potentially responsive to nursing. Additional research is needed to validate the benefits of mainstream and complementary/alternative interventions in patients presenting with different health conditions, sociodemographic backgrounds, and levels of fatigue. In addition, there is a need to identify appropriate dose and format for delivering the interventions in the practice setting.

NAUSEA AND VOMITING

Nausea and vomiting are symptoms that tend to co-occur. They are reported by women in their first trimester of pregnancy and are also experienced in a variety of acute and chronic medical conditions, as well as postsurgery. For instance, nausea and vomiting are experienced with food indigestion, food poisoning, acute inflammation/infection or obstruction of the gastrointestinal system, and some fluid and electrolytes imbalances caused by a disease or dialysis. Nausea and vomiting also have been reported in a few psychological conditions, particularly in patients who use somatization as a coping mechanism. Some patients may experience these symptoms following surgery, depending on the anesthetic agent used.

To gain an understanding of these two symptoms and to identify evidence-based strategies to manage them, a comprehensive literature review was conducted. The literature search covered the following computerized databases: CINAHL, CANCERLIT, and MEDLINE. The key words used in this search were: *nausea, vomiting, anticipatory nausea and vomiting, postoperative nausea and vomiting*, and *emesis*. These terms were also combined with *symptom management, treatment, intervention*, and *nursing care*. The search yielded a rather limited number of studies that investigated these prevalent symptoms. Nausea and vomiting, along with fatigue, have been of primary concern and consequently have been extensively studied in patients with cancer receiving chemotherapy. Therefore, the following discussion draws primarily on the empirical evidence gathered across studies involving patients with cancer receiving chemotherapy. The discussion focuses on (a) defining these symptoms, (b) assessing the psychometric properties and clinical utility of available measures, and (c) determining the extent to which independent nursing interventions that are nonpharmacological in nature are effective in relieving nausea and vomiting.

Conceptualization of Nausea and Vomiting

Only two sources reviewed provided a conceptual definition of nausea and vomiting. Worcester et al. (1991) defined nausea as a "disagreeable feeling experienced in the back of the throat (epigastrium), and generally culminating in vomiting" (p. 54). They suggested that it may be accompanied by pallor, cold and clammy skin, increased salivation, faintness, tachycardia, and diarrhea. De Carvalho, Martins, and dos Santos (2007) characterized nausea as a subjective sensation that is "associated with the conscious recognition of the will or desire to vomit" (p. 163); it may be accompanied by other symptoms such as hypersalivation and tachycardia.

The two sources advanced a similar definition of vomiting. Vomiting refers to an involuntary reflex that causes the forceful oral expulsion of the contents of the stomach or intestines. It is preceded by nausea, rapid and irregular heartbeat, tachypnea, salivation, vertigo, sweating, pallor, and pupil dilation.

In cancer-related literature, three types of chemotherapy-induced nausea and vomiting have been identified. The first is acute nausea and vomiting, which take place within a couple of minutes or 24 hours after chemotherapy is administered. The second is delayed nausea and vomiting, which occur within the period extending from the second to the fifth day after chemotherapy is given. The third type is called anticipatory nausea and vomiting; it is reported by patients before the subsequent cycle of chemotherapy (de Carvalho et al.).

Essential Attributes

The definitions imply that (a) nausea and vomiting tend to cooccur, and nausea usually precedes vomiting; (b) nausea is a subjective sensation felt by the affected individual as the desire to vomit; and (c) vomiting has a rather objective nature that can be detected by another person, in addition to the affected individual; the objective manifestations of vomiting include expulsion of content, pallor, and sweating.

Antecedents

The causes of nausea and vomiting vary with the physiological and/or pathological alterations underlying the condition in which they are experienced. The causative factors could be physical/physiological and/or psychological in nature. For instance, in patients with cancer receiving chemotherapy, several factors have been considered as contributing to nausea and vomiting, including the type, number, and dose of chemotherapeutic agent, and metastasis to the brain or liver. The conditioning effects of the exposure to and receipt of chemotherapy are responsible for anticipatory nausea and vomiting. This latter psychological factor has been described as a "classical" conditioning process; that is, through their association with pharmacologically induced side effects, various stimuli (e.g., smells, thoughts, tastes) become capable of eliciting nausea, vomiting, and intense emotional reactions (Burish, Carey, Krozely, & Greco, 1987; J. Richardson et al., 2007).

Consequences

The consequences of nausea and vomiting are essentially related to nutritional deficits, such as loss of fluid and electrolytes, loss of appetite, and loss of weight. These changes ultimately lead to reduced energy and fatigue, which constrains the person's ability to engage in activities of daily living and in self-care.

Instruments Measuring Nausea and Vomiting

Single, global items have been most frequently used to measure nausea and vomiting in empirical, descriptive-correlational, and experimental studies. In most instances, the items were part of instruments or checklists designed to assess the experience of multiple symptoms, or part of a symptom subscale incorporated in a scale measuring quality of life, as discussed in the first part of this chapter. In a few cases, the single item was used independently.

The term most commonly used to describe nausea in these single items, whether embedded in a multi-item scale or used independently, was *nausea*. It is a word commonly found in laypersons' language and in medical encounters. The items often assessed the perceived severity or intensity of nausea, using Likert-type response options. The response options selected varied across scales and included the following:

- *Mild*, *moderate*, or *severe* in the Sign and Symptom Checklist for Persons with HIV Disease (Holzemer et al., 1999)
- *None* to *severe* in the instruments measuring the symptoms experienced by patients in palliative care settings (Edmonds, Stuttaford, Penny, Lynch, & Chamberlain, 1998)
- A 100-mm horizontal VAS, often used in research with palliative patients (Fainsinger, Miller, Bruera, Hanson, & MacEachern, 1991) and patients with

cancer receiving chemotherapy (Billhult, Bergom & Stener-Victorin, 2007; de Carvalho et al., 2007)

- A 7-point numeric rating scale ranging from *none* to *most of the time* in the Symptom Control Assessment (Benor, Delbar, & Krulik, 1998)
- A 7-point rating scale anchored with *not at all* and *extremely* (Burish et al., 1987; Burish & Jenkins, 1992; Burish, Snyder, & Jenkins, 1991; Carey & Burish, 1987; Lyles, Burish, Krozely, & Oldham, 1982; Vasterling, Jenkins, Tope, & Burish, 1993)

A few scales were designed to assess the distress associated with nausea. The response options used were:

- A 5-point Likert scale in the Symptom Distress Scale (Rhodes, Watson, & Johnson, 1984)
- A 5-point numeric rating scale or a 100-mm horizontal VAS anchored with *not at all* and *very much so* in the original and modified versions of the Symptom Distress Scale (McCorkle & Young, 1978)
- A 10-point linear analog scale with three descriptors ranging from *no change in lifestyle* to *unable to maintain lifestyle* (Tucci & Bartels, 1998)
- A 4-point scale consisting of none; mild, activity not interfered with; moderate, activity interfered with; and severe, bedridden with nausea for more than 2 hours, in the Duke's Descriptive Scale used by Cotanch (1983) and Cotanch and Strum (1987). Grande, Barclay, and Todd (1997) measured the perceived difficulty in controlling nausea with a 5-point scale ranging from *not at all difficult* to *very difficult.*

The term most commonly used to describe vomiting in the single or multi-item scales mentioned earlier was *vomiting*, which is again in common use. The same response options were used to assess the severity and distress of vomiting. The Duke's Descriptive Scale was the exception. The four grades to assess vomiting used in this scale were: (a) no vomiting 24 hours after chemotherapy; (b) mild: vomiting fewer than five times within 24 hours after chemotherapy; (c) moderate: 5–10 times within 24 hours of chemotherapy; and (d) severe: more than 10 times within 24 hours, patient bedridden, possible dehydration (Cotanch, 1983; Cotanch & Strum, 1987). In addition to these dimensions, the frequency of vomiting (i.e., the reported number of vomiting episodes) was assessed in a few instances (e.g., Tucci & Bartels, 1998).

Three multi-item instruments measuring nausea and vomiting were reported in the literature reviewed. Two were used in studies evaluating psychological-behavioral interventions for managing anticipatory nausea and vomiting in patients with cancer who were receiving chemotherapy. These two measures were not used in nursing research; therefore, they will be mentioned only briefly.

The first of these two measures, the Morrow Assessment of Nausea and Vomiting, contains items assessing the frequency, severity, and duration of nausea and vomiting before and after receiving chemotherapy (Morrow, 1982; Morrow & Morrell, 1982). The second instrument, referred to as the Patient Postchemotherapy Nausea and Vomiting Rating Form, was developed by Gard, Edwards, Harris, and McCormack (1988) and modeled after Morrow's assessment form. It contains five items assessing the severity, frequency, and duration of nausea and vomiting with a semantic differential scale anchored with *very mild* and *intolerable*.

The third multi-item instrument, the Rhodes Index of Nausea and Vomiting (INV-Form 2), was reported and published by Worcester et al. (1991). These authors described it as an outcome measure assessing the occurrence of nausea and vomiting and their perceived intensity and distress. Lay terms were used to describe nausea ("sick at my stomach") and vomiting ("throw up"), which represents an advantage over the previously reviewed measures of these symptoms. The instrument consists of eight items. Each item assesses one dimension of a symptom. That is, one item inquires about the frequency, one about the severity, and one about the distress of nausea and vomiting. Two of the items ask about the frequency and distress of retching. Descriptive statements are provided to reflect varying degrees of frequency, severity, and distress, and the respondents are asked to circle the statement that most clearly corresponds to their experience. The scoring method was not described. No additional source describing this measure was found.

The psychometric properties of the single, global items measuring nausea and vomiting were not evaluated or reported in any of the sources included in this review. Although it may be difficult to examine these properties for items incorporated in multi-item instruments, it is possible to examine the validity and sensitivity to change of independent single measures of subjective sensations, as has been reported for single-item indicators of fatigue and dyspnea. Youngblut and Casper (1993) reviewed the psychometric properties of single-item indicators, which are being used increasingly in clinical research to evaluate symptom experience. They concluded that (a) the test-retest reliability of these measures could not be established because of the changing nature of the symptoms experienced; (b) these measures provide a global rating of the phenomenon of interest that has been shown to be valid; and (c) the single, global items were able to detect change over time. Despite these possibilities, single global measures of nausea and vomiting have not been validated. However, they demand minimal burden and time on the part of the respondent to complete, and they have been used in practice. Therefore, they are clinically useful. Providing descriptors of nausea and vomiting in lay terms will further enhance the clinical utility of these measures, ensuring understanding by, and applicability to, various client populations.

The reliability, validity, and sensitivity to change of the multi-item measures of nausea and vomiting have not been reported. These measures address several dimensions of these symptoms; that is, frequency, intensity, and distress, which gives a comprehensive assessment of the symptom experience. Such an assessment may be useful in understanding the symptom experience and in guiding care planning. The Rhodes INV-Form 2 may be of limited clinical relevance because of the length and complexity of the descriptive statements used. It requires the respondents to have an acceptable reading and comprehension ability, to concentrate, and to compare and contrast the statements before selecting the most appropriate response. These abilities may be limited in patients with chronic illness.

Recommendations for Measuring Nausea and Vomiting

From this discussion of the measurement of nausea and vomiting, the use of single, global items assessing the frequency, intensity, and/or distress of these symptoms is recommended for clinical practice. The items should contain lay terms to describe the symptoms and simple numeric scales to quantify the experience (similar to those used to quantify pain). Further validation of these single measures is also needed before their widespread use in everyday practice.

Sensitivity to Nursing Care

A variety of independent nursing interventions have been suggested to relieve nausea and vomiting. Most are based on clinical experience or trial and error, and few have been systematically investigated. In addition to administering antiemetics as prescribed, the following categories of interventions were mentioned for addressing nausea and vomiting experienced by various patient populations:

- Changing the types of food and fluid offered to patients, the amounts taken at any one time, and the frequency of eating (e.g., small frequent meals, dry food, clear fluids)
- Maintaining cleanliness, both personal and environmental
- Encouraging rest periods before and after meals
- Creating pleasant settings around mealtime (e.g., preventing strong odors, exposure to fresh air, involving family members)

Different nonpharmacological interventions have been used to manage chemotherapy-induced nausea and vomiting. Miller and Kearny (2004) presented an overview of behavioral and complementary/alternative interventions in which they summarized the key ingredients characterizing each. The interventions were: relaxation; guided imagery; self-hypnosis; acupressure, acupuncture, or transcutaneous electrical nurse stimulation; biofeedback; cognitive distraction/attentional diversion such as computer games; and music therapy. Miller and

Kearny proposed the following as possible reasons underlying the interventions' usefulness: (1) the nonpharmacological interventions reduce the general feeling of emotional distress experienced by patients receiving chemotherapy, (2) the interventions serve as cognitive distractors, shifting the patients' attention to relaxing images, and (3) the interventions promote a sense of control and reduce the feeling of helplessness. Miller and Kearny identified the advantages of nonpharmacological interventions as being inexpensive, easy to learn, self-performed, and free from side effects. The empirical evidence supporting the effectiveness of these interventions is reviewed next.

- Relaxation: M. C. Smith, Holcombe, and Stullenbarger (1994) synthesized the results of four studies that investigated the effects of relaxation, such as progressive muscle relaxation, on chemotherapy-induced nausea and vomiting. Although the observed effects were positive, implying that relaxation training is effective in relieving these symptoms, the magnitude of the reported effect size (.23–.36) is small, which limits the clinical utility of the intervention. Recently, de Carvalho et al. (2007) tested the effects of progressive muscle relaxation on nausea and vomiting in 30 patients receiving chemotherapy. They found a statistically significant decrease in the perceived severity of nausea and vomiting and in the objective manifestations of these symptoms, specifically blood pressure, pulse, breathing, and body temperature. Participants reported experiencing a sense of wellbeing, sleepiness, and tranquility after treatment. Billhult et al. (2007) examined the effects of skin massage on nausea in women with breast cancer undergoing chemotherapy. Skin massage was given as an adjunct to antiemetic medication during chemotherapy infusion. It consisted of soft strokes to the foot/lower leg or hand/lower arm, in combination with cold-pressed vegetable oil. The results indicated a significant decrease in the severity of nausea, with a mean improvement of 73% in the experimental group, and no significant change in this symptom experience in the comparison group.
- Guided imagery: Sanzero Eller (1999) conducted a systematic review of the effects of guided imagery without relaxation on diverse physical and psychological symptoms in adult patients. She reported the results of six studies in which guided imagery was used to relieve anticipatory nausea and vomiting in patients receiving chemotherapy. Guided imagery was implemented by trained psychologists. In all six studies, the intervention was effective in reducing the aversive impact of nausea and vomiting. Similar results were reported by Van Fleet (2000), who also observed that guided imagery is more effective than relaxation in relieving nausea and vomiting.
- Self-hypnosis: J. Richardson et al. (2007) reported the results of a systematic review of six randomized controlled trials that evaluated the effectiveness of hypnosis in relieving nausea and vomiting experienced with

cancer chemotherapy. The researchers found that five of these six studies involved children and had positive effect, indicating that hypnosis is effective in controlling nausea and vomiting more so than usual treatment. In contrast, one study focused on adult patients and reported nonsignificant effects of hypnosis on nausea and vomiting.

- Acupressure, acupuncture, and electrical stimulation: Ezzo, Streitberger, and Schneider (2006) undertook a Cochrane systematic review to determine the effectiveness of these complementary/alternative treatments in managing nausea and vomiting experienced by three patient populations. In postoperative young (i.e., children) and adult patients, all three methods of stimulating the P6 acupuncture point were effective in reducing nausea and vomiting; the effectiveness was observed when acupressure, acupuncture, and electrical stimulation were compared with sham procedure (i.e., applying stimulation to other points) and to antiemetic medication. In cancer patients, acupressure and electrical stimulation alleviated the experience of acute chemotherapy-induced vomiting, whereas acupuncture was effective in relieving acute chemotherapy-induced nausea. None of the interventions affected delayed nausea and vomiting. In pregnant women, these interventions were more effective than no treatment and sham treatment in decreasing the proportion of women experiencing nausea and vomiting. Ezzo et al. (2009) reviewed 14 trials comparing the same three interventions in cancer patients receiving chemotherapy. The results showed that (1) acupuncture reduced acute vomiting but not the severity of acute nausea, (2) acupressure is effective in lowering the severity of acute nausea but not acute vomiting, and (3) electrical stimulation offered no benefit for these symptoms. The inconsistency in the results of the two systematic reviews pertaining to chemotherapy-induced nausea and vomiting can be partially explained by differences in the operationalization of the outcomes. In the first review, the outcomes were reported in the proportion of participants experiencing the symptoms (Ezzo et al., 2006); in the second review, the frequency and severity dimensions of nausea and vomiting were analyzed.
- Biofeedback, cognitive distraction, and music therapy: The empirical evidence supporting the effects of each intervention is limited to one study, as presented by Miller and Kearny (2004). The studies were led by non-nursing professionals in the period before the year 2000.

An additional complementary/alternative treatment, use of ginger, has gained the interest of the scientific community for managing nausea and vomiting. This interest culminated in the conduct of a meta-analysis. Chaiyakunapruk, Kitikannakorn, Nathisuwan, Leeprakobboon, and Leelasettagool (2006) found that ginger, given 1 hour before induction of anesthesia (administered in small amount), was significantly better than placebo in the prevention of postoperative nausea and vomiting. The investigators explained that ginger's antispasmodic effect is responsible for its impact on these symptoms. They also reported abdominal discomfort as a side effect that was experienced by a small number of patients.

Although the nonpharmacological interventions discussed above were not designed based on nursing theory, they can be, and have been, implemented by trained nurses. Symptom management appeared to be a component of some psychoeducational interventions that nurses delivered to patients with cancer who were receiving adjuvant therapy (e.g., Benor et al., 1998; Dodd, 1983; J. E. Johnson et al., 1997). Symptom distress and the number of symptoms/side effects of chemotherapy or radiation therapy experienced were measured as indicators of the interventions' effectiveness. The results of these studies supported the effectiveness of the interventions in alleviating symptom distress. There is no clear indication of the extent to which psychoeducational interventions addressed strategies to manage nausea and vomiting, nor of how successful they were in relieving these symptoms. However, the instruments used to measure symptom distress have incorporated items assessing nausea and vomiting. Instructing patients about such strategies may be effective in assisting them to manage these symptoms.

The empirical evidence provided in this review indicates that various interventions have shown initial effectiveness in relieving nausea and vomiting, primarily in patients receiving chemotherapy. Although valid, the evidence is not adequate for making any final recommendations as to which interventions delivered by nurses are most effective for which patient population seen in day-to-day practice.

DYSPNEA

The terms *dyspnea* and *breathlessness* have been used interchangeably in the literature despite their description as two symptoms that differ in the nature of the sensation. Dyspnea involves an unpleasant sensation of difficult or labored breathing. It is this uncomfortable feeling that distinguishes dyspnea from breathlessness. Breathlessness is normally experienced as increased breathing by healthy individuals following excessive exercise. It is relieved soon after the activity is stopped and/or with rest (Carrieri & Janson-Bjerklie, 1986). The unpleasant sensation that characterizes dyspnea interferes with the person's ability to carry out any physical activity (Rosser & Guz, 1981) and leads to an emotional response to the symptom that is often characterized by fear and anxiety (D. M. Clark, Salkovskis, & Chalkley, 1985; Dudley, Galse, Jorgenson, & Logan, 1980). Dyspnea requires prompt relief, which makes this symptom one of primary concern to healthcare professionals.

In this section, a review of the conceptualization and the measurement of dyspnea will be followed by a summary of the results of studies that investigated the effectiveness of interventions in managing this symptom, in an attempt to determine the extent to which it is sensitive to nursing care. The studies were identified through a comprehensive literature search. The computerized databases included CINAHL, CANCERLIT, and MEDLINE. The key words used were: *dyspnea*, *breathlessness*, and *shortness of breath*, which were also combined with *symptom management*, *treatment*, *intervention*, and *nursing care*.

Dyspnea can be experienced by patients with various acute conditions, such as pneumonia and injury to the chest. It is, however, most frequently reported by patients with (a) chronic respiratory diseases, such as asthma and chronic obstructive pulmonary diseases; (b) chronic cardiac diseases, such as congestive heart failure; and (c) end-stage lung cancer, lung metastasis, or HIV. Dyspnea has been studied in patients with chronic respiratory diseases, cardiac diseases, and lung cancer. Therefore, the sources included in this review are drawn from this pool of research.

Conceptualization of Dyspnea

As a subjective sensation, dyspnea is conceptualized as involving the actual sensation of shortness of breath, the perception of that sensation, and the individual's reaction to the sensation (Gift, 1990; Mahler, 1990). The actual sensation refers to the awareness of the physiological changes associated with this symptom. These changes include alterations in respiration, specifically in respiratory rate, FEV1, and PsO$_2$ (Van Der Molen, 1995). Perception involves interpreting the sensation experienced. Dyspnea is perceived as an unpleasant and/or uncomfortable sensation. Reaction to the sensation consists of the behavioral and emotional responses exhibited by the person in relation to the symptom. The behavioral responses entail restlessness and changes in position, as well as movement or activity, in an attempt to provide immediate relief to this distressing symptom. The emotional responses most frequently observed are fear and anxiety (Carrieri & Janson-Bjerklie, 1986; Mahler, 1990).

Some objective indicators have been reported to accompany dyspnea, including audible labored breathing, gasping, rapid respiratory rate, irregular respiration, use of accessory muscles, and change in respiratory volumes/spirometry (Worcester et al., 1991). It should be emphasized that no consistent relationship was found between the physiological changes associated with dyspnea and the subjective perception of the symptom. That is, the perceived severity of dyspnea did not correlate with alterations in respiration (O'Rourke, 2007; Van Der Molen, 1995). Accordingly, the subjective perception of dyspnea is of concern.

Essential Attributes

Clinical observations and quantitative and qualitative studies contributed to the identification of the subjective sensations that characterize dyspnea. These include:

- Unpleasant, uncomfortable, even "painful" sensation arising from the chest or lungs
- Difficult, labored breathing
- Inability to get in enough air; needing more air; being out of breath
- Tightness in the chest
- Feeling of suffocation, or smothering (Carrieri & Janson-Bjerklie, 1986; Lai et al., 2007; Mahler, 1990; McCarley, 1999; McCord & Cronin-Stubbs, 1992; Worcester et al., 1991)

Antecedents

The exact mechanisms that cause dyspnea are not clear. However, it is postulated that any increase in ventilatory requirements leading to an increase in respiratory effort contribute to the experience of dyspnea (O'Rourke, 2007). Several factors have been suggested to have an influence on the perception of, and the response and reaction to, this symptom. These antecedent factors have been organized into the following categories:

- Physiological: An increased demand for oxygen; type, duration, and frequency of dyspneic attacks (i.e., the perception of dyspnea may decline with prolonged and repeated exposure to the stimulus triggering the symptom or to repeated experience of the symptom) (Altose, 1985; McCord & Cronin-Stubbs, 1992); exercise, physical activities; and experience of concurrent symptoms such as pain and fatigue (Lai et al., 2007).
- Demographic: Age (i.e., younger persons perceive dyspnea more intensely than older persons) (Gottfried, Altose, Kelson, & Cherniack, 1981; Mahler, 1990); gender (i.e., women were found to report more dyspnea than men, especially among those with asthma); and sociocultural orientation and beliefs, as well as life experiences, which influence the identification and interpretation of sensations and symptoms (Lai et al., 2007; Mahler, 1990; McCord & Cronin-Stubbs, 1992).
- Environmental: Factors such as smoke, pollutants, temperature changes, and stress (Mahler, 1990; McCord & Cronin-Stubbs, 1992).
- Psychological/emotional: Cognitive status and emotional disturbances such as stress, anger, depression, and anxiety. Of these factors, anxiety has been consistently found to relate to dyspnea, creating a vicious circle in which anxiety leads to dyspnea, and dyspnea leads to anxiety (Altose, 1985; D. M. Clark et al., 1985; Gift, 1990; Gift & Cahill, 1990; Gift, Plaut, & Jacox, 1986; Lai et al., 2007; McCarley, 1999; O'Rourke, 2007).

Consequences

The experience of dyspnea is debilitating. It interferes with people's physical, psychological, and social functioning. Difficult breathing causes people to stop the activity in which they were engaged when it was felt. Patients experiencing frequent dyspnea may have to move slowly and therefore limit the amount of physical activity in which they engage in their daily lives. This, along with fatigue experienced in association with dyspnea, affects the patient's ability to perform activities of daily living and self-care (Haas, Salazar-Schicchi, & Axen, 1993; Lai et al., 2007). Dyspnea has a negative impact on psychological function; it results in tension and apprehension or anxiety (D. M. Clark et al., 1985), a negative perception of self, and a feeling of hopelessness (Lai et al.), and depressive symptoms (Wu, Lin, Wu, & Lin, 2007). Alterations in physical and psychological functioning interfere with engagement in social roles and life, potentially leading to isolation (Lai et al.).

In summary, dyspnea is a subjective experience characterized by an unpleasant and/or uncomfortable sensation associated with increased efforts in the act of breathing. It is triggered by physiological, physical, and psychological alterations that increase the respiratory effort, and it negatively impacts all domains of functioning. This distressing and debilitating symptom requires prompt and adequate management.

Instruments Measuring Dyspnea

As described earlier, dyspnea, just like other symptoms (e.g., pain, fatigue, nausea), is a subjective sensation; it is best assessed by self-report measures. However, dyspnea has been investigated and managed clinically by healthcare professionals from different backgrounds. Differences in professional focus led to differences in the approaches used to measure dyspnea. Three general approaches that were reported in the literature—psychophysics, dyspnea and activity, and experience of dyspnea—will be reviewed briefly next.

- Psychophysics: In this approach, a psychophysical technique is used to measure the perceived intensity of a sensation produced by a range of physical stimuli presented with varying intensity. This technique is based on Stevens' power law, which states that the perceived magnitude of the stimulus is a direct function of its actual intensity, implying that changes in stimulus intensity produce proportional changes in perceived magnitude (Killian, 1985; Mahler, 1990; Nield, Kim, & Patel, 1989; Van Der Molen, 1995). Magnitude estimation is one psychophysical technique that has been applied, primarily in laboratory settings, to study the sensation of dyspnea. External resistive loads, with varying intensity, are added. The person is asked to estimate the magnitude of the resistive loads on a rating scale. The scale could range from 0 to 10 (e.g., modified Borg Scale) or from 0 to 100 (e.g., VAS). The relationship between the intensity of the added resistive load and the magnitude of the dyspnea is then examined. The results of psychophysical studies have supported the relationship between perceived dyspnea and airflow obstruction/effort of breathing (e.g., Killian; Mahler et al., 1987; Nield et al., 1989). Although this approach was useful in clarifying the relationship between perceived dyspnea and changes in pulmonary function parameters, its application in everyday nursing practice is of limited clinical utility. Such assessment requires (a) intensive training in the use of equipment, administering tests, and interpreting results; (b) availability of specialized equipment and time to conduct the tests; and (c) willingness and effort on the part of patients. It increases the burden on nurses and patients, especially if it is to be performed on repeated occasions. This approach to assessing dyspnea was not designed for, and has not been used as a means for, evaluating effectiveness of care.

- Dyspnea and activity: In this approach, dyspnea is assessed in relation to physical activity (Brown, 1985). It is often used in rehabilitation to determine the level of activity at which the patient experiences difficulty breathing for diagnostic and evaluative purposes. The assessment is done either retrospectively, by asking the person to indicate the type of activities that induce dyspnea (e.g., Medical Research Council's Questionnaire, Oxygen-Cost Questionnaire, American Thoracic Society Dyspnea Scale, Baseline Dyspnea Index), or prospectively, by asking the person to engage in physical activity and to report about shortness of breath before, during, and/or after its performance. The physical activity often selected is walking at the person's own pace (e.g., 6- or 12-minute walk test, which is frequently used with patients with chronic obstructive pulmonary disease [COPD]). Various self-report scales could be used in this approach to assessing dyspnea; however, the Borg Scale was commonly used. This approach to assessing dyspnea has been used in nursing research. It is also employed in clinical practice, particularly in respiratory care clinics or rehabilitation settings.
- Experience of dyspnea: In this approach, dyspnea as experienced by patients is assessed, regardless of its association with physical activity. The most frequently measured dimensions of dyspnea are its intensity or severity, distress, and its impact. Patients are often asked to rate their current experience (today or the past few days). This approach has been used in research and in clinical practice to explore the patients' view and status and to evaluate the effectiveness of care.

The scales that have been used to identify the activities that induce or that are associated with dyspnea and the instruments that capture the experience of dyspnea will be reviewed separately.

Scales Measuring Activities Associated with Dyspnea

The scales measuring activities associated with dyspnea are: the Modified Medical Research Council's Scale, the Oxygen Cost Diagram Scale, the American Thoracic Society Dyspnea Scale, and the Dyspnea Index (see **TABLE 4-3**). Of these scales, the Medical Research Council's Scale and the Dyspnea Index seem promising as reliable and valid measures of activities associated with the perception of dyspnea. However, they do not assess the perceived severity of this symptom. They could be useful in rehabilitation care. Although they demonstrated initial sensitivity to change, they have not been used extensively in treatment effectiveness research. Their ability to detect changes in dyspnea experience in response to treatment needs further investigation.

Scales Measuring the Experience of Dyspnea

Three scales measuring dyspnea that are described in Table 4-3 are the Modified Borg Scale, the VAS, and the Descriptors of Breathlessness. The Modified Borg Scale and the VAS have been used to assess different dimensions of dyspnea, such as severity or intensity and discomfort or distress. Christenbery (2005) used a numeric rating scale (NRS) to measure the sensory (i.e., intensity) and affective (i.e., distress) dimensions of dyspnea in patients with COPD. The NRS consists of an 11-point scale ranging from 0 to 10, where 0 reflects absence of the dimension being assessed, and 10 reflects the worst, or high level. Christenbery presented preliminary evidence supporting the validity of the dyspnea NRS: It correlated positively and strongly ($r \geq .80$) with the dyspnea VAS before and after ambulation in patients with COPD. In addition to these, two subscales incorporated in multidimensional instruments were found to measure dyspnea: the dyspnea subscale in the Bronchitis-Emphysema Symptom Checklist, or BESC (Kinsman et al., 1983), and a subscale in the Chronic Respiratory Disease Questionnaire, or CRD (Guyatt, Berman, Townsend, Pugsley, & Chambers, 1987). Examples of items in the BESC dyspnea subscale include the following: feel like I need air, hard to breathe, shallow breathing, short of breath, and gasping for breath. These are different subjective descriptors of the sensation of dyspnea, as identified through clinical observations and descriptive studies. Limited data were available about the psychometric properties of the subscales; however, the reviewed evidence supports the reliability and validity of the BESC and provides initial support for those of the CRD (McCord & Cronin-Stubbs, 1992). A measure that contains multiple descriptors of dyspnea is clinically useful if the nature of this symptom varies across patient populations. Further investigation is needed to determine the BESC's and CRD's sensitivity to change.

Several symptom checklists presented earlier in the chapter include items measuring the severity of dyspnea, such as the Signs and Symptoms Checklist–HIV (Holzemer et al., 1999) and the Palliative Care or Support Team Assessment Schedule (Edmonds et al., 1998).

TABLE 4-3   Instruments Measuring Dyspnea

Instrument (author)	Target population/ setting	Domains (number of items and response format)	Method of administration	Reliability	Content validity	Construct validity	Sensitivity to nursing variables
SCALES MEASURING ACTIVITIES ASSOCIATED WITH DYSPNEA							
Modified Medical Research Council's Scale (Fletcher, Elmes, & Wood, 1959)	Patients experiencing dyspnea (e.g., patients with cardiac or pulmonary disorders)	Domain: Incremental grades of breathlessness experienced with physical activities (e.g., hurrying and walking) Number of items: 5 Response format: Grades range from 0 (*not troubled with breathlessness except with strenuous exercise*) to 4 (*too breathless to leave the house or breathless with dressing or undressing*)	Self-administered or administered by an interviewer	Internal consistency: Not applicable Stability/test-retest: No data available Interrater reliability: Acceptable	Derived from previous scales and results of descriptive studies	Correlated weakly to moderately with lung function tests (FVC and FEV1) and moderately with other self-report measures of dyspnea in patients with chronic lung disease (COPD, asthma, cystic fibrosis), interstitial lung disease, and cardiac diseases (Mahler, 1990; Mahler et al., 1987; Mahler & Wells, 1988; Mahler & Harver, 1989)	Grades are too coarse and may not be sensitive to small changes in the level of dyspnea (McCord & Cronin-Stubbs, 1992; Van Der Molen, 1995) No data available relative to nursing variables
Oxygen Cost Diagram Scale (McGavin, Gupta, & McHardy, 1976)	Patients with dyspnea	Domain: Activities representing different levels of perceived oxygen demand (e.g., sleeping, walking, brisk walking uphill) Number of items: 1 Response format: 100 vertical visual analogue scale, anchored with 0 at the bottom	Administered by an interviewer	Internal consistency: Not applicable Stability/test-retest: No data available Interrater: Acceptable	Derived from work done on oxygen uptake during the activity	Correlated with other measures of dyspnea in patients with cardiac and pulmonary diseases	Changes in scores reported with 12-minute walk (Eaton, MacDonald, & Church, 1982; Mahler & Harver, 1989; Mahler et al., 1987; Mahler & Wells, 1988; McCord & Cronin-Stubbs, 1992) No data available relative to nursing variables

American Thoracic Society Dyspnea Scale (cited in Ferris, 1978)	Patients with dyspnea	Domain: Similar in content and format to the Medical Research Council's scale Number of items: 5 Response format: 5-point rating scale	Self-administered or administered by an interviewer	Internal consistency: Not applicable Stability/test-retest: No data available Interrater: No data available	No data available	No data available	No data available
Dyspnea Index (Mahler, Weinberg, Wells, & Feinstein, 1984; modified by Stoller, Ferranti, & Feinstein, 1986)	Patients with dyspnea	Domain: Three dimensions of dyspnea: functional impairment (i.e., degree to which activities of daily living are impaired by dyspnea); magnitude of task (i.e., intensity of activity that provoked dyspnea); and magnitude of effort (i.e., overall effort exerted to perform activities that provoked dyspnea) Number of items: 3 Response format: Two versions: Baseline Dyspnea Index, designed to measure the three dimensions of dyspnea at a single point in time using a 4-point rating scale (*severe* to *unimpaired*), and Transition Dyspnea Index, designed to measure changes in the dimensions of dyspnea from a baseline condition using a 7-point rating scale: −3 (*major deterioration*) to +3 (*major improvement*)	Administered by an observer	Internal consistency: Not applicable Stability/test-retest: No data available Interrater: Acceptable (Mahler & Harver, 1989; Mahler, Matthay, Snyder, Wells, & Loke, 1985; Mahler et al., 1987, 1984; Mahler & Wells, 1988)	Derived from research and clinical experiences	Acceptable validity in patients with cardiac and pulmonary diseases (Mahler & Harver, 1989; Mahler et al., 1984, 1985, 1987; Mahler & Wells, 1988)	Acceptable sensitivity to change (Mahler & Harver, 1989; Mahler et al., 1984, 1985, 1987; Mahler & Wells, 1988) Improvement in dyspnea following self-management program delivered by nurses (Carrieri-Kohlman et al., 2005)

No data available relative to nursing variables

(continues)

TABLE 4-3 Instruments Measuring Dyspnea (continued)

Instrument (author)	Target population/ setting	Domains (number of items and response format)	Method of administration	Reliability	Content validity	Construct validity	Sensitivity to nursing variables
SCALES MEASURING THE EXPERIENCE OF DYSPNEA							
Modified Borg Scale (Borg, 1982)	Patients with dyspnea	Domain: Perceived exertion and effort during exercise; perceived severity of dyspnea Number of items: 1 Response format: Vertical, 11-point rating scale, 0 (*not at all*) to 10 (*maximal*)	Self-administered or administered by an interviewer	Internal consistency: Not applicable Stability/retest: Not reported	Derived from Borg's work with exertion, psychophysiological relationship between the intensity of a physical stimulus and the intensity or magnitude of the perceived sensation	Correlated with FEV1 in patients with asthma; intensity of physical exercise in patients with COPD (Bernsteiner et al., 1994); and in healthy individuals (Killian, 1985)	Change following 12-minute walk test and exercise training in patients with COPD (Goldstein, Gort, Stubbing, Avendano, & Guyatt, 1994; Guyatt et al., 1984) Change in score following listening to soothing music (Sidani, 1991) in patients with COPD
Visual analogue scale (VAS)	Patients with dyspnea	Domain: Severity Number of items: 1 Response format: Horizontal or vertical 100 mm line	Self-administered or administered by an interviewer	Internal consistency: Not applicable Stability/retest: Acceptable in 30 patients with lung cancer (Brown, Carrieri, Janson-Bjerklie, & Dodd, 1986)	Maintained by using lay terms to describe the sensation	Horizontal and vertical correlated highly in patients with asthma (Gift, 1989; Gift et al., 1986); correlated with peak expiratory flow rate (Gift et al., 1986); differed in patients with asthma and patients with COPD, under different levels of obstruction (Gift, 1989)	Sensitivity to change: Not well supported (McCord & Cronin-Stubbs, 1992) Decrease dyspnea following acupressure (Wu et al., 2007)

Descriptors of breathlessness (as cited in McCord & Cronin-Stubbs, 1992)	Tested on healthy adults	Domain: No report found Number of items: 19 Response format: No report found	Self-administered	Internal consistency: Acceptable in healthy adults (McCord & Cronin-Stubbs, 1992) Stability/test-retest: No report found	No data available	Acceptable validity (McCord & Cronin-Stubbs)	No data available

COPD = chronic obstructive pulmonary disease.

Recommendations for Measuring Dyspnea

Of the scales reviewed, the Borg Scale and the vertical VAS have been well validated. They have shown sensitivity to changes in the level of perceived dyspnea, which makes them useful to monitor changes associated with progression of the illness condition or with treatment. They are simple to use with various patient populations, and they are quick and easy to administer in clinical practice. The Borg Scale could be used to assess dyspnea in relation to physical activity in rehabilitation programs, where it has been commonly applied. The vertical VAS could be used to assess this subjective sensation under any condition, such as following treatment. The VAS, in general, has demonstrated ability to detect small changes; however, the reproduction of the 100 mm line should be carefully monitored. Printing and photocopying it may alter its length. The 0–10 NRS is a promising alternative to the 100 mm VAS.

Sensitivity to Nursing Care

The uncomfortable, distressing, and debilitating nature of dyspnea requires prompt relief. In the absence of a clear understanding of the exact mechanisms causing dyspnea, physiological and psychological factors have been well recognized to contribute to dyspnea. This state of knowledge led to the use of different interventions to assist patients in managing this symptom. The interventions encompass those targeting the physiological and those addressing the psychological aspects of the dyspnea experience.

- Physiological interventions: These interventions are subdivided into pharmacological treatments and physical therapies. Pharmacological treatments include (1) bronchodilators and corticosteroids, which showed usefulness in reducing dyspnea experience in patients with COPD and asthma; (2) opioids, whose effectiveness in relieving dyspnea is still controversial; (3) oxygen therapy, which was found to have no impact on dyspnea in the absence of hypoxemia; and (4) anxiolytic, whose use to decrease the distress or anxiety that causes dyspnea is not well substantiated (O'Rourke, 2007). Physical therapies advocated to manage dyspnea include: positioning such as sitting in an upright position; breathing control exercises such as pursed-lips breathing; mechanical therapies (e.g., vibration of respiratory muscles); and rehabilitation (Gift, 1993). Rehabilitation consists of exercise training to increase tolerance for physical activity and teaching patients how to plan activities at a pace that will not precipitate dyspnea. The goal is to maintain engagement in physical, recreational, work, and role-related activities valued by the person. Rehabilitation has been recommended for patients with COPD and cardiac diseases.

- Psychological interventions: These interventions aim at (1) relieving the anxiety associated with dyspnea, (2) altering the person's interpretation of and beliefs about dyspnea, and (3) enhancing self-management of the symptom. Examples of these interventions are relaxation, guided imagery, distraction, and cognitive-behavioral interventions with a focus on promoting self-management.

In addition to the mentioned physiological and psychological interventions, recent literature revealed an interest in complementary/alternative therapies to manage dyspnea. Specifically, acupressure/acupuncture and use of fan/cool air have been investigated for their effects on dyspnea.

Although nurses may be involved in the implementation of any of the specific treatments, they especially have taken initiatives in investigating the effectiveness of psychological interventions. However, only a few published studies were found that were led by nurses. They were concerned with evaluating different interventions, and they used different subjective and objective indicators of dyspnea. This variability precluded integrating results across the studies, which limited the ability to reach meaningful conclusions and recommendations for practice.

Renfroe (1988) examined the effects of progressive muscle relaxation on dyspnea and anxiety in patients with COPD. Patients ($n = 20$) were randomly assigned to an experimental group or a control group. Those in the experimental group were instructed to tense each muscle group for 5–10 seconds while inhaling, then relaxing while exhaling completely. Patients attended four weekly sessions in a laboratory setting, during which they were given the instructions and feedback on their performance. They were asked to practice muscle relaxation once a day, in between sessions. Patients in the control group were instructed to relax in any way they wished. Dyspnea was measured with a VAS. Significant reductions in the level of perceived dyspnea were reported by the experimental group following each session; the reductions were greater in the experimental group than in the control group. Significant decreases in respiratory rate were also observed in the experimental group from the beginning to the end of each session. Similar changes were reported for state anxiety. The experimental control exerted by the investigators was successful in enhancing the internal validity of the study. However, the small sample size and the high rate of refusal to participate (55%) limit the ability to generalize the findings.

Gift, Moore, and Soeken (1992) conducted a randomized clinical trial to determine the effects of progressive muscle relaxation on dyspnea, anxiety, and airway obstruction in patients with COPD. Patients in the experimental group were (a) seated in a comfortable position in the physician's office room, (b) asked, over a total of four sessions, to listen to a prerecorded tape giving them instructions on how to perform progressive muscle relaxation, and (c) asked to practice muscle relaxation at home while listening to the tape. Twenty-six patients completed all the sessions, yielding an attrition rate of 24%. Dyspnea was measured with the VAS, and airway obstruction with the peak expiratory flow rate (PEFR). Significant group x time interaction effects were reported for dyspnea and anxiety and for PEFR. Patients in the experimental group showed a decrease in the perceived level of dyspnea and anxiety and an increase in PEFR over time, more so than the control group. Initial group nonequivalence on anxiety and smoking history, the small sample size, and the observed attrition rate limit the validity of the results.

Moody, Fraser, and Yarandi (1993) evaluated the effectiveness of guided imagery in relieving dyspnea, anxiety, fatigue, and depression, and in enhancing quality of life in patients with chronic bronchitis and emphysema. A one-group design with repeated measures was used. Nineteen patients attended four sessions, one per week. During the sessions, the patients in the group were instructed to close their eyes and imagine a scene described with a standard script. The nature of the scene was not depicted. No significant decrease in dyspnea, anxiety, fatigue, and depression was reported, but some improvement in quality of life was observed over the 4-week intervention period. The lack of a control group and of a clear description of the intervention implementation, as well as the small sample size, presents threats to the validity of the study conclusions.

Use of distraction, in the form of listening to music, was examined in three studies for its effectiveness in relieving dyspnea and improving respiration. The target population in all the studies was patients with COPD. The designs were preexperimental, involving only one group of patients. The samples included a small number of patients (20–36). The music was soothing in two studies (McBride, Graydon, Sidani, & Hall, 1999; Sidani, 1991) and of moderate tempo in one (Thornby, Haas, & Axen, 1995). Dyspnea was measured with the Borg Scale or a VAS. Sidani reported a greater reduction in respiratory rate following 20 minutes of resting while listening to music than following 20 minutes of resting only; no significant decrease in perceived dyspnea, measured with the Borg Scale, was observed. McBride et al. found that listening to music for 20 minutes while sitting down resulted in decreased levels of perceived dyspnea, measured with the VAS, and perceived anxiety. The findings of Thornby et al. indicated that patients undergoing treadmill exercise testing reported lower levels of perceived dyspnea, walked about 25% longer, and performed 53% more work when listening to moderate-tempo music than when listening to gray noise (i.e., hum) or silence during the exercise test. The results of these studies are consistent and point to the potentially beneficial effects of music in alleviating dyspnea and anxiety and in enhancing engagement in physical activity in this patient population. However, most studies were considered pilot tests of this intervention. Further investigation of its effectiveness, with a more rigorous research design, is necessary to develop a sound, relevant knowledge base.

Sassi-Dambron, Eakin, Ries, and Kaplan (1995) evaluated the effectiveness of a treatment program in managing dyspnea in patients with COPD. The program consisted of six weekly group sessions in which the following strategies for coping with dyspnea were discussed and practiced: progressive muscle relaxation, diaphragmatic and pursed-lips breathing, pacing and energy-saving techniques, self-talk and panic control, and stress management. The 89 patients who consented to participate were randomly assigned to the treatment program or to a control condition that consisted of six weekly sessions of general health education. Dyspnea was measured with the VAS and with the Borg Scale, administered before and after a 6-minute walk test. No significant difference in dyspnea was found between the two groups at posttest; however, both groups showed a significant decrease in perceived dyspnea from pre- to posttest. Despite the observed favorable outcome, the results of this study cannot be generalized because of the reported difference in the level of dyspnea between those who dropped out (had more severe dyspnea) and those who completed the study.

Carrieri-Kohlman et al. (2005) evaluated the long-term outcomes of three versions of a dyspnea self-management program. The first version was the dyspnea self-management program (DM); it involved individualized education, a home walking program, and biweekly nurse telephone calls. The second version consisted of all components of the DM program and four sessions of supervised treadmill exercises done once every other week. The third version entailed all components of the DM program and 24 supervised exercise sessions. A total of 115 patients with COPD participated in the randomized trial. Outcome data were collected before, and every 2 months over the 1-year postintervention period. Dyspnea was assessed with the Borg Scale, the Chronic Respiratory Disease Questionnaire, the Baseline Dyspnea Index, and the transitional dyspnea index. Participants in the three groups were comparable at baseline and reported improvement in dyspnea over the 1-year posttest period. Adherence to the home exercise program was not optimal. The results of this study highlight the importance of the exercise component of a dyspnea self-management program.

Wu et al. (2007) reported the results of a randomized trial. The purpose was to test the effects of acupressure in reducing dyspnea and depressive symptoms experienced by patients with COPD. Of the 151 patients who met the study eligibility criteria, 62 (41%) actually enrolled in the study. Dyspnea was measured with a VAS before and after the 16-minute sessions, which were given five times a week over a 4-week period. Significant reduction in dyspnea was observed at posttest in the group that received acupressure. The low enrollment rate limits the generalizability of the findings. O'Rourke (2007) stated that the evidence of the efficacy of acupressure and use of fan/cool air in managing dyspnea is conflicting.

The findings of the studies described earlier indicate the potential benefits of psychological intervention in managing dyspnea. Further research is needed to generate a sound knowledge base about the effectiveness of nursing interventions in relieving this symptom. Until such knowledge is acquired, it is difficult to claim with certainty that dyspnea is sensitive to nursing care.

CONCLUSIONS AND RECOMMENDATIONS

The literature reviewed in this chapter provides evidence supporting the following points:

- Symptoms are subjective sensations that reflect a change in normal functioning. They are experienced by individuals with various health or illness conditions, and they represent the reason for seeking health care across the healthcare continuum.
- Symptoms are experienced, perceived, and reacted to by patients. The process of perceiving, interpreting, and responding to symptoms is individual and is affected by a host of personal, environmental, and health-related variables. These should be accounted for when evaluating the effects of nursing interventions on symptom control.
- Symptoms interfere with the person's physical, psychological, and social functioning. If not managed effectively and controlled, symptoms have a devastating impact on the person, the family, and the healthcare system.
- Nurses are in a good position to assist patients in managing symptoms. This statement is consistent with (a) the caring perspective underlying nursing, (b) the focus of some models or middle-range theories of nursing (e.g., theory of self-care, symptom management model), (c) the emphasis on self-management and active patient participation in care, and (d) clinical observations and informal patient reports explaining that they seek medical care for the diagnosis and treatment of medical problems, and nursing care for assistance in managing day-to-day functioning and symptoms.
- Symptom management is considered an important component of nursing care for different patient populations, but specifically for patients with chronic illness, with the ultimate outcome of relieving or controlling symptoms.
- Various interventions have been applied and evaluated for their effectiveness in managing different symptoms experienced by patients with chronic illness.
- Educational or psychoeducational interventions have been designed to assist patients in adjusting to chronic illness and to provide them with the knowledge and skills to recognize and manage symptoms they may experience. The interventions have addressed multiple physical and psychological symptoms commonly experienced by the target population. They were delivered by nurses and consisted of discussing the patients' symptoms or concerns and the strategies patients could use to manage symptoms. The results indicated that patients who received the psychoeducational interventions reported lower levels of symptom severity at posttest.

The interventions' effects on symptom severity were more prominent at follow-up.

- The effectiveness of various specific nursing interventions in relieving the symptoms of fatigue, nausea and vomiting, and dyspnea was also examined in the sources included in this review. The studies used different designs, ranging from experimental to preexperimental. They included rather small sample sizes. The symptoms were measured with reliable and valid instruments. In general, the results supported the favorable effects of these specific interventions in relieving the severity of symptoms. These findings, however, should be considered with caution because of the possible introduction of bias.

- The evidence reviewed provides initial support for the benefit of nursing interventions in managing symptoms experienced by patients. Symptom control can be considered an outcome that is sensitive to nursing care.

- Symptom control is of utmost importance for patients with chronic illness, and it constitutes a primary focus for nurses providing care to these patients on an inpatient or outpatient basis.

- The symptoms experienced differ across patient populations, based on the nature of the pathophysiological mechanisms underlying the illness condition and on the type of treatment given.

- Effective symptom management begins with a comprehensive assessment of the symptom experience. It encompasses (a) the occurrence of multiple symptoms that are commonly reported by the patient population to which the patient belongs, and (b) the multiple dimensions of each symptom experienced (i.e., severity, frequency, duration, meaning, impact, response, alleviating and aggravating factors, and strategies used). This comprehensive assessment should inquire about the patient's individual perception of the symptom. It can be completed in a structured and systematic manner that involves using symptom checklists developed for specific patient populations, such as the Signs and Symptoms Checklist for Persons with HIV Disease, the Symptom Distress Scale for patients with cancer, or the Support Team Assessment Schedule for patients in palliative care. The checklists measure the symptoms' occurrence and severity.

- Measuring symptoms as outcomes of nursing care is necessary for determining the effectiveness of the care provided in everyday practice. The same checklist used in the initial clinical assessment of symptoms could be used for evaluating the outcome of symptom control.

- The checklists reviewed here have demonstrated initial reliability and validity. Further testing is needed to determine their sensitivity to change and to generate normative values and/or cutoff scores before they can be used in clinical practice.

- Similar checklists will have to be developed for assessing symptoms commonly reported by other patient populations.
- Fatigue, nausea and vomiting, and dyspnea are symptoms reported by many patients. Assessing these symptoms could become an integral part of routine nursing assessment, as is done for pain. Single items with a 10-point numeric rating scale, ranging from 0 (*not at all*) to 10 (*very severe*), are reliable, valid, sensitive, and clinically useful measures of these symptoms.

REFERENCES

Aaronson, K. K., Ahmedzai, S., Bullinger, M., Crabeels, D., Estape, J., Filiberti, A., et al. (1991). The EORTC core quality-of-life questionnaire: Interim results of an international field study. In D. Osoba (Ed.), *Effects of cancer on quality of life* (pp. 416–422). Boca Raton, FL: CRC Press.

Aaronson, K. K., Bullinger, M., & Ahmedzai, S. (1996). A modular approach to quality of life assessment in cancer clinical trials. *Recent Results in Cancer Research, 111*, 231–249.

Altose, M. D. (1985). Assessment and management of breathlessness. *Chest, 88*(Suppl. 2), S77–S82.

Anastasia, P. J., & Blevins, M. C. (1997). Outpatient chemotherapy: Telephone triage for symptom management. *Oncology Nursing Forum, 24*(Suppl. 1), 13–22.

Armes, J., Chalder, T., Addington-Hall, J., Richardson, A., & Hotopf, M. (2007). A randomized controlled trial to evaluate the effectiveness of a brief, behaviorally oriented intervention for cancer-related fatigue. *Cancer, 110*, 1385–1395.

Baker, D. W., Asch, S. M., Keesey, J. W., Brown, J. A., Chan, K. S., Joyce, O., et al. (2005). Differences in education, knowledge, self-management activities, and health outcomes for patients with heart failure cared for under the chronic disease model: The improving chronic illness care evaluation. *Journal of Cardiac Failure, 11*, 405–413.

Beck, S. L., Dudley, W. N., & Barsevick, A. (2005). Pain, sleep disturbance, and fatigue in patients with cancer: Using a mediation model to test a symptom cluster. *Oncology Nursing Forum, 32*(3), E48–E55.

Belza, B. L. (1995). Comparison of self-reported fatigue in rheumatoid arthritis and controls. *Journal of Rheumatology, 22*, 639–643.

Belza, B. L., Henke, C. J., Yelin, E. H., Epstein, W. V., & Gillis, C. L. (1993). Correlates of fatigue in older adults with rheumatoid arthritis. *Nursing Research, 42*, 93–99.

Benor, D. E., Delbar, V., & Krulik, T. (1998). Measuring impact of nursing intervention on cancer patients' ability to control symptoms. *Cancer Nursing, 21*, 320–334.

Berger, A. M., & Walker, S. N. (2001). An explanatory model of fatigue in women receiving adjuvant breast cancer chemotherapy. *Nursing Research, 50*, 42–52.

Bernstein, M. L., Despars, J. A., Singh, N. P., Avalos, K., Stansbury, D. W., & Light, R. W. (1994). Reanalysis of the 12-minute walk in patients with chronic obstructive pulmonary disease. *Chest, 105*, 163–167.

Billhult, A., Bergom, I., & Stener-Victorin, E. (2007). Massage relieves nausea in women with breast cancer who are undergoing chemotherapy. *Journal of Alternative and Complementary Medicine, 13*, 53–57.

Blesch, K. S., Paice, J. A., Wickham, R., Harte, N., Schnoor, D. K., Purl, S., et al. (1991). Correlates of fatigue in people with breast or lung cancer. *Oncology Nursing Forum, 18*, 81–87.

Borg, G. A. V. (1982). Psychophysical bases of perceived exertion. *Medicine and Science in Sports Exercise, 14*, 377–381.

Bowling, A. (1995). *Measuring disease: A review of disease-specific quality of life measurement scales.* Buckingham, England: Open University Press.

Brown, M. L. (1985). Selecting an instrument to measure dyspnea. *Oncology Nursing Forum, 12*(3), 98–100.

Brown, M., Carrieri, V., Janson-Bjerklie, S., & Dodd, M. (1986). Lung cancer and dyspnea: The patient's perception. *Oncology Nursing Forum, 13*(1), 19–24.

Bruera, E., Kuehn, N., Miller, M. J., Selsmar, P., & Macmillan, K. (1991). The Edmonton Symptom Assessment System (ESAS): A simple method for the assessment of palliative care patients. *Journal of Palliative Care, 7*(1), 6–9.

Burish, T. G., Carey, M. P., Krozely, G., & Greco, A. (1987). Conditioned side effects induced by cancer chemotherapy: Prevention through behavioral treatment. *Journal of Consulting and Clinical Psychology, 55*, 42–48.

Burish, T. G., & Jenkins, R. A. (1992). Effectiveness of biofeedback and relaxation training in reducing the side effects of cancer chemotherapy. *Health Psychology, 11*(1), 17–23.

Burish, T. G., Snyder, S. L., & Jenkins, R. A. (1991). Preparing patients for cancer chemotherapy: Effect of coping preparation and relaxation interventions. *Journal of Consulting and Clinical Psychology, 59*, 518–525.

Buxton, L. S., Frizelle, F. A., Parry, B. R., Pettigrew, R. A., & Hopkins, W. G. (1992). Validation of subjective measures of fatigue after elective operations. *European Journal of Surgery, 158*, 393–396.

Carey, M. P., & Burish, T. G. (1987). Providing relaxation training to cancer chemotherapy patients: A comparison of three delivery techniques. *Journal of Consulting and Clinical Psychology, 55*, 732–737.

Carrieri, V., & Janson-Bjerklie, S. (1986). Dyspnea. In V. K. Carrieri, A. M. Lindsey, & C. M. West (Eds.), *Pathophysiological phenomena in nursing: Human responses to illness* (pp. 191–215). Philadelphia: W. B. Saunders.

Carrieri-Kohlman, V., Nguyen, H. Q., Donesky-Cuenco, D., Demir-Deviren, S., Neuhaus, J., & Stulbarg, M. S. (2005). Impact of brief or extended exercise training on the benefit of a dyspnea self-management program in COPD. *Journal of Cardiopulmonary Rehabilitation, 25*, 275–284.

Cassileth, B. R., Lusk, E. J., Bodenheimer, B. J., Farber, J. M., Jochimsen, P., & Morrin-Taylor, B. (1985). Chemotherapeutic toxicity: The relationship between patients' pretreatment expectations and post-treatment results. *American Journal of Clinical Oncology, 8*, 419–425.

Chaiyakunapruk, N., Kitikannakorn, N., Nathisuwan, S., Leeprakobboon, K., & Leelasettagool, C. (2006). The efficacy of ginger for the prevention of postoperative nausea and vomiting: A meta-analysis. *American Journal of Obstetrics and Gynecology, 194*, 95–99.

Chalder, T., Berelowitz, G., Pawlikowska, T., Watss, L., Wessely, S., Wright, D., et al. (1993). Development of a fatigue scale. *Journal of Psychosomatic Research, 37*, 147–153.

Christenbery, T. L. (2005). Dyspnea self-management strategies: Use and effectiveness as reported by patients with chronic obstructive pulmonary disease. *Heart and Lung, 34*, 406–414.

Christensen, T., Bendix, T., & Kehlet, H. (1982). Fatigue and cardiorespiratory function following abdominal surgery. *British Journal of Surgery, 69*, 417–419.

Christensen, T., Hjortso, N. C., Mortensen, E., Riis-Hansen, M., & Kehlet, H. (1986). Fatigue and anxiety in surgical patients. *Acta Psychiatrica Scandinavia, 73*, 76–79.

Christensen, T., Nygaard, E., Stage, J. G., & Kehlet, H. (1990). Skeletal muscle enzyme activities and metabolic substrates during exercise in patients with postoperative fatigue. *British Journal of Surgery, 77*, 312–315.

Cimprich, B. (1993). Development of an intervention to restore attention in cancer patients. *Cancer Nursing, 16*, 83–92.

Clark, D. M., Salkovskis, P. M., & Chalkley, A. J. (1985). Respiratory control as a treatment for panic attacks. *Journal of Behavioral Therapy and Experimental Psychiatry, 16*(1), 23–30.

Clark, J. A., & Talcott, J. A. (2001). Symptom indexes to assess outcomes of treatment for early prostate cancer. *Medical Care, 39*, 1118–1130.

Cleeland, C. S., Bennett, G. J., Dantzer, R., Dougherty, P. M., Dunn, A. J., Meyers, C. A., et al. (2003). Are the symptom of cancer and cancer treatment due to a shared biologic mechanism? *Cancer, 97*, 2919–2925.

Cotanch, P. H. (1983). Relaxation training for control of nausea and vomiting in patients receiving chemotherapy. *Cancer Nursing, 8*, 277–283.

Cotanch, P. H., & Strum, S. (1987). Progressive muscle relaxation as antiemetic therapy for cancer patients. *Oncology Nursing Forum, 14*(1), 33–37.

David, A., Pelosi, A., McDonald, E., Stephens, D., Ledger, D., Rathbone, R., et al. (1990). Tired, weak, or in need of rest: Fatigue among general practice attenders. *British Medical Journal, 301*, 1199–1202.

Decker, T., Cline-Elsen, J., & Gallagher, M. (1992). Relaxation therapy as an adjunct in radiation oncology. *Journal of Clinical Psychology, 48*, 388–393.

de Carvalho, E. C., Martins, F. T. M., & dos Santos, C. B. (2007). A pilot study of a relaxation technique for management of nausea and vomiting in patients receiving cancer chemotherapy. *Cancer Nursing, 30*(2), 163–167.

Devlen, J., Maguire, P., Phillips, P., Crowther, D., & Chambers, H. (1987). Psychological problems associated with diagnosis and treatment of lymphomas: A retrospective study. *British Medical Journal, 295*, 953–954.

Dirksen, S. R., & Epstein, D. R. (2008). Efficacy of an insomnia intervention on fatigue, mood, quality of life in breast cancer survivors. *Journal of Advanced Nursing, 61*, 664–675.

Dodd, M. J. (1983). Self-care for side effects in cancer chemotherapy: An assessment of nursing interventions: Part II. *Cancer Nursing, 6*, 63–67.

Dodd, M. J. (1984). Patterns of self-care in cancer patients receiving radiation therapy. *Oncology Nursing Forum, 11*(3), 23–27.

Dodd, M. J., Cho, M., Cooper, B., Miaskowski, C., Lee, K. A., & Bank, K. (2005). Advancing our knowledge of symptom clusters. *Journal of Supportive Oncology, 3*(6, Suppl. 4), 30–31.

Dodd, M., Janson, S., Facione, N., Fawcett, J., Froelicher, E. S., Humphreys, J., et al. (2001). Advancing the science of symptom management. *Journal of Advanced Nursing, 33*, 668–676.

Dudley, D. C., Galse, E. M., Jorgenson, B. N., & Logan, D. L. (1980). Psychosocial concomitants to rehabilitation in chronic obstructive pulmonary disease: Part I. *Chest, 77*, 544–551.

Eaton, M. L, MacDonald, F. M., & Church, T. R. (1982). Effects of theophylline on breathlessness and exercise tolerance in patients with chronic airflow obstruction. *Chest, 82*, 538–542.

Edmonds, P. M., Stuttaford, J. M., Penny, J., Lynch, A. M., & Chamberlain, J. (1998). Do hospital palliative care teams improve symptom control? Use of a modified STAS as an evaluation tool. *Palliative Medicine, 12*, 345–351.

Ellershaw, J. E., Peat, S. J., & Boys, L. C. (1995). Assessing the effectiveness of a hospital palliative care team. *Palliative Medicine, 9*, 145–152.

Ezzo, J., Richardson, M. A., Vickers, A., Allen, C., Dibble, S., Issell, B. F., et al. (2009). Acupuncture-point stimulation for chemotherapy-induced nausea and vomiting (Review). *The Cochrane Collaboration,* (2), CD002285.

Ezzo, J., Streitberger, K., & Schneider, A. (2006). Cochrane systematic reviews examine P6 acupuncture-point stimulation for nausea and vomiting. *Journal of Alternative and Complementary Medicine, 12,* 489–495.

Fainsinger, R., Miller, M. J., Bruera, E., Hanson, J., & MacEachern, T. (1991). Symptom control during the last week of life on a palliative care unit. *Journal of Palliative Care, 7*(1), 5–11.

Fawzy, N. W. (1995). A psychoeducational nursing intervention to enhance coping and affective state in newly diagnosed malignant melanoma patients. *Cancer Nursing, 18,* 427–438.

Fawzy, F. I., Cousins, N., Fawzy, N. W., Kemeny, M. E., Elashoff, R., & Morton, D. (1990). A structured psychiatric intervention for cancer patients. *Archives of General Psychiatry, 47,* 720–725.

Ferris, B. G. (1978). Epidemiology standardization project (American Thoracic Society). *American Review of Respiratory Disease, 118,* 1–120.

Fisk, J. D., Ritvo, P. G., Ross, L., Haase, D. A., Marrie, T. J., & Schlech, W. F. (1994). Measuring the functional impact of fatigue: Initial validation of the Fatigue Impact Scale. *Clinical Infectious Diseases, 18*(Suppl. 1), S79–S83.

Fletcher, C. M., Elmes, P. C., & Wood, C. H. (1959). The significance of respiratory symptoms and the diagnosis of chronic bronchitis in a working population. *British Medical Journal, 2,* 257–266.

Fox, M. T., Sidani, S., & Streiner, D. (2007). Using standardized survey items with older adults hospitalized for chronic illness. *Research in Nursing and Health, 30,* 468–481.

Gantz, P. A., Day, R., Ware, J. E., Redmond, C., & Fisher, B. (1995). Baseline quality of life assessment in the National Surgical Adjuvant Breast and Bowel Project. *Journal of the National Cancer Institute, 87,* 1372–1382.

Gantz, P. A., Greendale, G. A., Peterson, L., Zibecchi, L., Kahn, B., & Belin, T. R. (2000). Managing menopausal symptoms in breast cancer survivors: Results of a randomized controlled trial. *Journal of the National Cancer Institute, 92,* 1054–1064.

Gard, D., Edwards, P. W., Harris, J., & McCormack, G. (1988). Sensitizing effects of pretreatment measures on cancer chemotherapy nausea and vomiting. *Journal of Consulting and Clinical Psychology, 56,* 80–84.

Gift, A. G. (1989). Validation of a vertical visual analogue scale as a measure of clinical dyspnea. *Rehabilitation Nursing, 14,* 323–325.

Gift, A. G. (1990). Dyspnea. *Nursing Clinics of North America, 25,* 955–965.

Gift, A. G. (1993). Therapies for dyspnea relief. *Holistic Nurse Practice, 7*(2), 57–63.

Gift, A. G., & Cahill, C. A. (1990). Psychophysiologic aspects of dyspnea in chronic obstructive disease: A pilot study. *Heart and Lung, 19,* 252–257.

Gift, A. G., Moore, T., & Soeken, K. (1992). Relaxation to reduce dyspnea and anxiety in COPD patients. *Nursing Research, 41,* 242–246.

Gift, A. G., Plaut, S. M., & Jacox, A. (1986). Psychologic and physiologic factors related to dyspnea in subjects with chronic obstructive pulmonary disease. *Heart and Lung, 15,* 595–601.

Glaus, A., Crow, R., & Hammond, S. (1996). A qualitative study to explore the concept of fatigue/tiredness in cancer patients and in healthy individuals. *European Journal of Cancer Care, 5*(Suppl. 2), 8–23.

Glover, J., Dibble, S. L., Dodd, M. J., & Miaskowski, C. (1995). Mood states of oncology outpatients: Does pain make a difference? *Journal of Pain and Symptom Management, 10,* 120–128.

Godino, C., Jodar, L., Duran, A., Martinez, J., & Schiaffino, A. (2006). Nursing education as an intervention to decrease fatigue perception in oncology patients. *European Journal of Oncology Nursing, 10*, 150–155.

Goldstein, R., Gort, E., Stubbing, D., Avendano, M., & Guyatt, G. (1994). Randomized controlled trial of respiratory rehabilitation. *Lancet, 344*, 1394–1397.

Gottfried, S. B., Altose, M. D., Kelson, S. G., & Cherniack, N. S. (1981). Perception of changes in airflow resistance in obstructive pulmonary disorders. *American Review of Respiratory Disease, 124*, 566–570.

Grande, G. E., Barclay, S. I. G., & Todd, C. J. (1997). Difficulty of symptom control and general practitioners' knowledge of patients' symptoms. *Palliative Medicine, 11*, 399–406.

Graydon, J. E., Bubela, N., Irvine, D., & Vincent, L. (1995). Fatigue-reducing strategies used by patients receiving treatment for cancer. *Cancer Nursing, 18*, 23–28.

Graydon, J. E., Sidani, S., Irvine, D., Vincent, L., Harrison, D., & Bubela, N. (1997). *Literature review on cancer-related fatigue.* Unpublished report, Canadian Association of Nurses in Oncology.

Graydon, J., Vincent, L., Bubela, N., Thorsen, E., Harrison, D., & Sidani, S. (1999). *A physical activity program for cancer-related fatigue.* Unpublished report, Canadian Association of Nurses in Oncology.

Greenberg, D. B., Gary, J. L., Mannix, C. M., Eisenthal, S., & Carey, M. (1993). Treatment-related fatigue and serum interleukin-1 levels in patients during external beam irradiation for prostate cancer. *Journal of Pain and Symptom Management, 8*, 196–200.

Greenberg, D. B., Sawicka, J., Eisenthal, S., & Ross, D. (1992). Fatigue syndrome due to localized radiation. *Journal of Pain and Symptom Management, 7*, 38–45.

Gritz, E. R., Weliish, D. K., & Landsverk, J. A. (1988). Psychological sequelae in long-term survivors of testicular cancer. *Journal of Psychosocial Oncology, 6*(3/4), 41–63.

Guyatt, G., Berman, L., Townsend, M., Pugsley, S., & Chambers, L. (1987). A measure of quality of life for clinical trials in chronic lung disease. *Thorax, 42*, 773–778.

Guyatt, G. H., Pugsley, S., Sullivan, M. J., Thompson, P. J., Berman, L. B., Jones, N. L., et al. (1984). Effect of encouragement on walking test performance. *Thorax, 39*, 818–822.

Haas, F., Salazar-Schicchi, J., & Axen, K. (1993). Desensitization to dyspnea in chronic obstructive pulmonary disease. In R. Casaburi & T. Petty (Eds.), *Principles and practice of pulmonary rehabilitation* (pp. 241–251). Philadelphia: W. B. Saunders.

Haworth, S. K., & Dluhy, N. M. (2001). Holistic symptom management: Modelling the interaction phase. *Journal of Advanced Nursing, 36*, 302–310.

Henry, S. B., Holzemer, W. L., Weaver, K., & Stotts, N. (1999). Quality of life and self-care management strategies of PLWAs with chronic diarrhea. *Journal of the Association of Nurses in AIDS Care, 10*(2), 46–54.

Higginson, I. & McCarthy, M. (1989). Measuring symptoms in terminal cancer. *Palliative Medicine, 3*, 267–274

Hogan, C. M. (1997). Cancer nursing: The art of symptom management. *Oncology Nursing Forum, 24*, 1335–1341.

Holzemer, W. L., Henry, S. B., Nokes, K. M., Corless, I. B., Brown, M. A., Powell-Cope, G. M., et al. (1999). Validation of the Sign and Symptom Checklist for Persons with HIV Disease (SSC-HIV). *Journal of Advanced Nursing, 30*, 1041–1049.

Jacobson, P. B., Donovan, K. A., Vadaparampil, S. T., & Small, B. J. (2007). Systematic review and meta-analysis of psychological and activity-based interventions for cancer-related fatigue. *Health Psychology, 26*, 660–667.

Jamar, S. C. (1989). Fatigue in women receiving chemotherapy for ovarian cancer. In S. G. Funk, E. M. Tornquist, M. T. Champagne, L. A. Copp, & R. A. Wiese (Eds.), *Key aspects of comfort: Management of pain, fatigue, and nausea* (pp. 224–228). New York: Springer.

Johnson, J. E., Fieler, V. K., Wlasowicz, G. S., Mitchell, M. L., & Jones, L. S. (1997). The effects of nursing care guided by self-regulation theory on coping with radiation therapy. *Oncology Nursing Forum, 24*, 1041–1050.

Johnson, R. (1993). Nurse practitioner–patient discourse: Uncovering the voice of nursing in primary care practice. *Scholarly Inquiry for Nursing Practice: An International Journal, 7*, 143–157.

Joly, F., Henry-Amar, M., Arveux, P., Reman, O., Yanguy, A., Peny, A. M., et al. (1996). Late psychosocial sequelae in Hodgkin's disease survivors: A French population-based case-control study. *Journal of Clinical Oncology, 14*, 2444–2453.

Justice, A. C., Chang, C. H., Rabeneck, L., & Zachin, R. (2001). Clinical importance of provider-reported HIV symptoms compared with patient-report. *Medical Care, 39*, 397–408.

Kashiwagi, S. (1971). Psychological rating of human fatigue. *Ergonomics, 14*(1), 17–21.

Killian, K. J. (1985). Objective measurement of breathlessness. *Chest, 88*(Suppl. 2), S84–S90.

Kim, H., McGuire, D. B., Tulman, L., & Barsevick, A. M. (2005). Symptom clusters: Concept analysis and clinical implications for cancer nursing. *Cancer Nursing, 28*(4), 270–282.

Kinsman, R., Yaroush, R., Fernandez, E., Dirks, J., Shocket, M., & Fukuhara, J. (1983). Symptoms and experiences in chronic bronchitis and emphysema. *Chest, 5*, 755–761.

Krupp, L. B., LaRocca, N. G., Muir-Nash, J., & Steinberg, A. D. (1989). The Fatigue Severity Scale: Application to patients with multiple sclerosis and systemic lupus erythematosus. *Archives of Neurology, 46*, 1121–1123.

Lai, Y. L., Chan, C. W. H., & Lopez, V. (2007). Perceptions of dyspnea and helpful interventions during the advanced stage of lung cancer. Chinese patients' perspectives. *Cancer Nursing, 30*(2), E1–E8.

Lee, B-N., Dantzer, R., Langley, K. E., Bennett, G. J., Dougherty, P. M., Dunn, A. J., et al. (2004). A cutokine-based neuroimmunologic mechanism of cancer-related symptoms. *Neuroimmunomodulation, 11*, 279–292.

Lee, D., Newell, R., Ziegler, L., & Topping, A. (2008). Treatment of fatigue in multiple sclerosis: A systematic review of the literature. *International Journal of Nursing Practice, 14*, 81–93.

Lee, K., Hicks, G., & Nino-Murcia, G. (1991). Validity and reliability of a scale to assess fatigue. *Psychiatry Research, 36*, 291–298.

Lotfi-Jam, K., Carey, M., Jefford, M., Schofield, P., Charleson, C., & Aranda, S. (2008). Nonpharmacologic strategies for managing common chemotherapy adverse effects: A systematic review. *Journal of Clinical Oncology, 26*, 5618–5629.

Love, R. R., Leventhal, H., Easterling, D. V., & Nerenz, D. R. (1989). Side effects and emotional distress during cancer chemotherapy. *Cancer, 63*, 604–612.

Lyles, J. N., Burish, T. G., Krozely, M. G., & Oldham, R. K. (1982). Efficacy of relaxation training and guided imagery in reducing the aversiveness of cancer chemotherapy. *Journal of Consulting and Clinical Psychology, 50*, 509–524.

Maguire, P., Walsh, S., Jeacock, J., & Kingston, R. (1999). Physical and psychological needs of patients dying from colo-rectal cancer. *Palliative Medicine, 13*, 45–50.

Mahler, D. A. (Ed.). (1990). *Dyspnea*. Mount Kisco, NY: Futura.

Mahler, D., & Harver, A. (1989). Factor analysis demonstrates independence of dyspnea ratings and physiologic function in obstructive airway disease. *American Review of Respiratory Disease, 139,* A243.

Mahler, D. A., Matthay, R. A., Snyder, P. E., Wells, C. K., & Loke, J. (1985). Sustained-release theophylline reduces dyspnea in nonreversible obstructive airway disease. *American Review of Respiratory Disease, 131,* 22–25.

Mahler, D. A., Rosiello, R. A., Harver, A., Lentine, T., McGovern, J. F., & Daubenspeck, A. (1987). Comparison of clinical dyspnea ratings and psychophysical measurements of respiratory sensation in obstructive airway disease. *American Review of Respiratory Disease, 135,* 1229–1233.

Mahler, D. A., Weinberg, D. H., Wells, C. K., & Feinstein, A. R. (1984). The measurement of dyspnea. *Chest, 85,* 751–757.

Mahler, D., & Wells, C. (1988). Evaluation of clinical methods for rating dyspnea. *Chest, 93,* 580–586.

McBride, S., Graydon, J., Sidani, S., & Hall, L. (1999). The therapeutic use of music for dyspnea and anxiety in patients with COPD who live at home. *Journal of Holistic Nursing, 17,* 229–250.

McCarley, C. (1999). A model of chronic dyspnea. *Image: Journal of Nursing Scholarship, 31,* 231–236.

McCord, M., & Cronin-Stubbs, D. (1992). Operationalizing dyspnea: Focus on measurement. *Heart and Lung, 21,* 167–179.

McCorkle, R., & Young, K. (1978). Development of a symptom distress scale. *Cancer Nursing, 5,* 373–378.

McGavin, C. R., Gupta, S. P., & McHardy, G. J. R. (1976). Twelve-minute walking test for assessing disability in chronic bronchitis. *British Medical Journal, 1,* 822–823.

McNair, D. M., Lorr, M., & Droppleman, I. F. (1981). *Profile of Mood States.* San Diego, CA: Educational and Industrial Testing Service.

Meek, P. M., Nail, L. M., Barsevick, A., Schwartz, A. L., Stephen, S., Whitmer, K., et al. (2000). Psychometric testing of fatigue instruments for use with cancer patients. *Nursing Research, 49,* 181–190.

Miaskowski, C., & Aouizerat, B. E. (2007). Is there a biological basis for the clustering of symptoms? *Seminars in Oncology Nursing, 23*(2), 99–105.

Miller, M., & Kearny, N. (2004). Chemotherapy-related nausea and vomiting: Past reflections, present practice and future management. *European Journal of Cancer Care, 13,* 71–81.

Mock, V., Burke, M. B., Sheehan, P., Creaton, E. M., Winningham, M. L., McKenny-Tedder, S., et al. (1994). A nursing rehabilitation program for women with breast cancer receiving adjuvant chemotherapy. *Oncology Nursing Forum, 21,* 899–907.

Molassiotis, A., Sylt, P., & Diggins, H. (2007). The management of cancer-related fatigue after chemotherapy with acupuncture and acupressure: A randomized controlled trial. *Complementary Therapy in Medicine, 15,* 228–237.

Moody, L. E., Fraser, M., & Yarandi, H. (1993). Effects of guided imagery in patients with chronic bronchitis and emphysema. *Clinical Nursing Research, 2,* 478–486.

Morant, R. (1996). Asthenia: An important symptom in cancer patients. *Cancer Treatment Reviews, 22*(Suppl. A), 117–122.

Morrow, G. R. (1982). Prevalence and correlates of anticipatory nausea and vomiting in chemotherapy patients. *Journal of the National Cancer Institute, 68,* 585–588.

Morrow, G. R., & Morrell, C. (1982). Behavioral treatment for the anticipatory nausea and vomiting induced by cancer chemotherapy. *New England Journal of Medicine, 307,* 1476–1480.

Munkres, A., Oberst, M. T., & Hughes, S. H. (1992). Appraisal of illness, symptom distress, self-care burden, and mood states in patients receiving chemotherapy for initial and recurrent cancer. *Oncology Nursing Forum, 19*, 1201–1209.

Nail, L. M., Jones, L. S., Greene, D., Schipper, D. L., & Jensen, R. (1991). Use and perceived efficacy of self-care activities in patients receiving chemotherapy. *Oncology Nursing Forum, 18*, 883–887.

Neuberger, G. B., Aaronson, L. S., Gajewski, B., Embretson, S. E., Coyle, P. E., Loudron, J. K., et al. (2007). Predictors of exercise and effects of exercise on symptom, function, aerobic fitness, and disease outcomes of rheumatoid arthritis. *Arthritis and Rheumatism, 57*, 943–952.

Nield, M., Kim, M. J., & Patel, M. (1989). Use of magnitude estimation for estimating the parameters of dyspnea. *Nursing Research, 38*, 77–80.

Nokes, K., Wheeler, K., & Kendrew, J. (1994). Development of an HIV assessment tool. *Image: The Journal of Nursing Scholarship, 26*, 133–138.

Olson, K., Krawchuk, A., & Quddusi, T. (2007). Fatigue in individuals with advanced cancer in active treatment and palliative settings. *Cancer Nursing, 30*(4), E1–E10.

Olson, K., Turner, A. R., Courneya, K. S., Field, C., Man, G., Cree, M., et al. (2008). Possible links between behavioral and physiological indices of tiredness, fatigue, and exhaustion in advanced cancer. *Support Care Cancer, 16*, 241–249.

O'Neill, E. S., & Morrow, L. L. (2001). The symptom experience of women with chronic illness. *Journal of Advanced Nursing, 33*, 257–268.

O'Rourke, M. E. (2007). Clinical dilemma: Dyspnea. *Seminars in Oncology Nursing, 23*, 225–231.

Osoba, D., Zee, B., Warr, D., Kaizer, L., Latreille, J., & Pater, J. (1996). Quality of life studies in chemotherapy-induced emesis. *Oncology, 53*(Suppl. 1), 92–95.

Parker, K. P., Kimble, L. P., Dunbar, S. B., & Clark, P. C. (2005). Symptom interactions as mechanisms underlying symptom pairs and clusters. *Journal of Nursing Scholarship, 37*, 209–215.

Paterson, B., Canam, C., Joachim, G., & Thorne, S. (2003). Embedded assumption in qualitative studies of fatigue. *Western Journal of Nursing Research, 25*, 119–133.

Payne, J. K., Held, J., Thorpe, J., & Shaw, H. (2008). Effect of exercise on biomarkers, fatigue, sleep disturbances, and depressive symptoms in older women with breast cancer hormonal therapy. *Oncology Nursing Forum, 35*, 635–642.

Pearson, R. G., & Byars, G. E. (1956). *The development and validation of a checklist for measuring subjective fatigue.* Randolph Air Force Base, TX: School of Aviation Medicine.

Penrod, J., & Hupcey, J. E. (2005). Enhancing methodological clarity: Principle-based concept analysis. *Journal of Advanced Nursing, 50*, 403–409.

Pickard-Holley, S. (1991). Fatigue in cancer patients: A descriptive study. *Cancer Nursing, 14*, 13–19.

Piper, B. F. (1993). Fatigue. In V. K. Carrieri-Kolman, A. M. Lindsey, & C. M. West (Eds.), *Pathophysiological phenomena in nursing: Human responses to illness* (2nd ed., pp. 279–302). Philadelphia: Saunders.

Piper, B. F., Dodd, M. L., Paul, S. M., & Weleer, S. (1989). The development of an instrument to measure the subjective dimension of fatigue. In S. G. Funk, E. M. Tornquist, M. T. Champagne, L. A. Copp, & R. A. Wiese (Eds.), *Key aspects of comfort management of pain, fatigue, and nausea* (pp. 199–208). New York: Springer.

Ream, E. (2007). Fatigue in patients receiving palliative care. *Nursing Standard, 21*(28), 49–56.

Ream, E., & Richardson, A. (1999). From theory to practice: Designing interventions to reduce fatigue in patients with cancer. *Oncology Nursing Forum, 26*, 1295–1305.

Ream, E., Richardson, A., & Alexander-Dann, C. (2006). Supportive intervention for fatigue in patients undergoing chemotherapy: A randomized controlled trial. *Journal of Pain and Symptom Management, 31,* 148–161.

Renfroe, K. L. (1988). Effect of progressive relaxation on dyspnea and state anxiety in patients with chronic obstructive pulmonary disease. *Heart and Lung, 17,* 408–413.

Rhodes, V. A., McDaniel, R. W., & Matthews, C. A. (1998). Hospice patients' and nurses' perceptions of self-care deficits based on symptom experience. *Cancer Nursing, 21,* 312–319.

Rhodes, V. A., Watson, P. M., & Johnson, M. H. (1984). Development of reliable and valid measures of nausea and vomiting. *Cancer Nursing, 7,* 33–41.

Rhoten, D. (1982). Fatigue and the post-surgical patient. In C. M. Norris (Ed.), *Concept clarification in nursing* (pp. 277–300). Rockville, MD: Aspen.

Richardson, A. (1995). Fatigue in cancer patients: A review of the literature. *European Journal of Cancer Care, 4,* 20–32.

Richardson, A., & Ream, E. K. (1996). The experience of fatigue and other symptoms in patients receiving chemotherapy. *European Journal of Cancer Care, 5*(Suppl. 2), 24–30.

Richardson, J., Smith, J. E., McCall, G., Richardson, A., Pilkington, K., & Kirsch, I. (2007). Hypnosis for nausea and vomiting in cancer chemotherapy: A systematic review of the research evidence. *European Journal of Cancer Care, 16,* 402–412.

Rosser, R., & Guz, A. (1981). Psychological approaches to breathlessness and its treatment. *Journal of Psychosomatic Research, 25,* 439–447.

Sanzero Eller, L. (1999). Guided imagery interventions for symptom management. *Annual Review of Nursing Research, 17,* 57–84.

Sassi-Dambron, D., Eakin, E., Ries, A. L., & Kaplan, R. M. (1995). Treatment of dyspnea in COPD: A controlled clinical trial of dyspnea management strategies. *Chest, 107,* 724–729.

Schroeder, D., & Hill, G. L. (1991). Postoperative fatigue: A prospective physiological study of patients undergoing major abdominal surgery. *Australian and New Zealand Journal of Surgery, 61,* 774–779.

Schwartz, J. E., Jandorf, L., & Krupp, L. B. (1993). The measurement of fatigue: A new instrument. *Journal of Psychosomatic Research, 37,* 753–762.

Sidani, S. (1991). *Effects of sedative music on the respiratory status of clients with chronic obstructive airway disease.* Unpublished master's thesis, University of Arizona College of Nursing, Tucson.

Smets, E. M., Garssen, B., Bonke, B., & de Haes, J. C. (1995). The multidimensional fatigue inventory: Psychometric qualities of an instrument to assess fatigue. *Journal of Psychosomatic Research, 39,* 315–325.

Smets, E. M. A., Garssen, B., Cull, A., & de Haes, J. C. J. M. (1996). Application of the multidimensional fatigue inventory (MFI-20) in cancer patients receiving radiotherapy. *British Journal of Cancer, 73,* 241–245.

Smets, E. M. A., Garssen, B., Schuster-Uitterhoeve, A. L. J., & de Haes, J. C. J. M. (1993). Fatigue in cancer patients. *British Journal of Cancer, 68,* 220–224.

Smith, C., & Hale, L. (2007). The effects of non-pharmacological interventions on fatigue in four chronic illness conditions: A critical review. *Physical Therapy Reviews, 12,* 324–334.

Smith, M. C., Holcombe, J. K., & Stullenbarger, E. (1994). A meta-analysis of intervention effectiveness for symptom management in oncology nursing research. *Oncology Nursing Forum, 21,* 1201–1210.

Stanton, A. L., & Snider, P. R. (1993). Coping with a breast cancer diagnosis: A prospective study. *Health Psychology, 12*(1), 16–23.

Stoller, J., Ferranti, R., & Feinstein, A. (1986). Further specification and evaluation of a new index for dyspnea. *American Review of Respiratory Disease, 134,* 129–134.

Sutcliffe-Chidgey, J., & Holmes, S. (1996). Developing a symptom distress scale for terminal malignant disease. *International Journal of Palliative Nursing, 2*, 192–198.

Taylor, D. (1999). Effectiveness of professional-peer group treatment: Symptom management for women with PMS. *Research in Nursing and Health, 22*, 496–511.

Thornby, M. A., Haas, F., & Axen, K. (1995). Effect of distractive auditory stimuli on exercise tolerance in patients with COPD. *Chest, 107*, 1213–1217.

Tsay, S-L. (2004). Acupressure and fatigue in patients with end-stage renal disease—a randomized controlled trial. *International Journal of Nursing Studies, 41*, 99–106.

Tucci, R. A., & Bartels, K. L. (1998). Patient use of the symptom reporting tool. *Clinical Journal of Oncology Nursing, 2*(3), 97–99.

University of California, San Francisco, School of Nursing Symptom Management Faculty Group. (1994). A model for symptom management. *Image: Journal of Nursing Scholarship, 26*, 272–275.

van der Molen, B. (1995). Dyspnea: A study of measurement instruments for the assessment of dyspnea and their application for patients with advanced cancer. *Journal of Advanced Nursing, 22*, 948–956.

Van Fleet, S. (2000). Relaxation and imagery for symptom management: Improving patient assessment and individualizing treatment. *Oncology Nursing Forum, 27*, 501–510.

Vasterling, J., Jenkins, R. A., Tope, D. M., & Burish, T. G. (1993). Cognitive distraction and relaxation training for the control of side effects due to cancer chemotherapy. *Journal of Behavioral Medicine, 16*(1), 65–80.

Visowsky, C., & Schneider, S. M. (2003, September 23). Cancer-related fatigue. *Online Journal of Issues in Nursing, 8*(3). Retrieved March 25, 2009, from http://www.nursingworld.org/MainMenuCategories/ANAMarketplace/ANAPeriodicals?OJIN/TableofCo

White, C. L. (1992). Symptom assessment and management of outpatients receiving biotherapy: The application of a symptom report form. *Seminars in Oncology Nursing, 8*(4, Suppl. 1), 23–28.

Whitehead, L. (2009). The measurement of fatigue in chronic illness: A systematic review of uni-dimensional and multidimensional fatigue measures. *Journal of Pain and Symptom Management, 37*, 107–128.

Winningham, M. L. (1995). Fatigue: The missing link to quality of life. *Quality of Life—A Nursing Challenge, 4*(1), 2–7.

Winningham, M. L., Nail, L. M., Burke, M. B., Brophy, L., Cimprich, B., Jones, L. S., et al. (1994). Fatigue and the cancer experience: The state of the knowledge. *Oncology Nursing Forum, 21*, 23–35.

Winstead-Fry, P. (1998). Psychometric assessment of four fatigue scales with a sample of rural cancer patients. *Journal of Nursing Measurement, 6*, 111–122.

Worcester, M., Pesznecker, B., Albert, M., Grupp, K., Horn, B., & O'Connor, K. (1991). Cancer symptom management in the elderly. *Home Health Care Services Quarterly, 12*(2), 53–69.

Wu, H-S., Lin, L-C., Wu, S-C., & Lin, J-G. (2007). The physiologic consequences of chronic dyspnea in chronic pulmonary obstruction disease: The effects of acupressure on depression. *Journal of Alternative and Complementary Medicine, 13*, 253–261.

Yancey, R., Given, B. A., White, N. J., DeVoss, D., & Coyle, B. (1998). Computerized documentation for a rural nursing intervention project. *Computers in Nursing, 16*, 275–284.

Yoshitake, H. (1971). Relations between the symptoms and the feeling of fatigue. *Ergonomics, 14*, 175–186.

Yoshitake, H. (1978). Three characteristic patterns of subjective fatigue symptoms. *Ergonomics, 21*, 231–233.

Youngblut, J. M., & Casper, G. R. (1993). Single-item indicators in nursing research. *Research in Nursing and Health, 16*, 459–465.

Pain as a Symptom Outcome

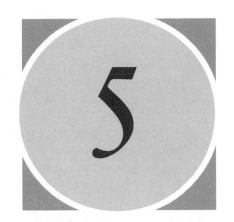

Judy Watt-Watson, RN, PhD
Michael McGillion, RN, PhD

INTRODUCTION

Pain is a symptom that has been documented as an indicator of inadequate pain management for over 35 years, since Marks and Sachar's (1973) seminal work. Patients continue to report inadequate pain relief despite major advances in our understanding of pain mechanisms, treatment approaches, and advocacy efforts by pain societies (Brennan, Carr, & Cousins, 2007; Fishman, 2007; Watt-Watson et al., 2004). To establish determinants of this problem, investigators in the 1980s and early 1990s focused primarily on describing health professionals' pain-related knowledge gaps, and then later on education programs, to solve the problem. However, the intervention's impact on patients' pain was either not measured, or findings were equivocal because of methodological problems. In a meta-analysis examining the effectiveness of nonpharmacological interventions for pain management, the strong heterogeneity between studies resulted in a pooled effect size of only 0.06 (Sindhu, 1996). More recently, the question of whether nursing initiatives actually change pain management practices stimulated an examination of patients' pain as a critical outcome measure. Studies subsequently began to measure pain as a symptom outcome to determine the effect of interventions such as education both for nurses (Bédard, Purden, Sauvé-Larose, Certosini, & Schein, 2006; Dahlman, Dykes, & Elander, 1999; Dalton et al., 1999; Dalton, Keefe, Carlson, & Youngblood, 2004; De Rond, De Wit, Van Dam, & Muller, 2000; De Rond et al., 1999; De Wit & Van Dam, 2001; Francke et al., 1997; Holzheimer, McMillan, & Weitzner, 1999; Neitzel, Miller, Shepherd, & Belgrade,

1999; Seers, Crichton, Carroll, Richards, & Saunders, 2004) and for patients (Ahles et al., 2001; Closs, Briggs, & Everitt, 1999; Clotfelter, 1999; Edwards et al., 2005; LeFort, Gray-Donald, Rowat, & Jeans, 1998; Lorig, Ritter, & Plant, 2005; McDonald, Freeland, Thomas, & Moore, 2001; McGillion et al., 2008; Neitzel et al.; Puntillo & Ley, 2004; Ward, Donovan, Owen, Grosen, & Serlin, 2000; Ward et al., 2008; Watt-Watson et al., 2004). Studies also began to measure pain as a symptom outcome to determine the effect of interventions such as music, cutaneous stimulation, foot reflexology, relaxation, therapeutic touch, or an incision compression garment (Broscious, 1999; Good et al., 2001; Keller & Bzdek, 1986; King et al., 2006; Kubsch, Neveau, & Vandertie, 2000; Kwekkeboom, Kneip, & Pearson 2003; Kwekkeboom, Wanta, & Bumpus, 2008; Meehan, 1993; Phumdoung & Good, 2003; Tanabe, Thomas, Paice, Spiller, & Marcantonio, 2001; Tsay, Chen, Chen, Lin, & Lin, 2008).

This chapter reviews pain as a symptom outcome in evaluating nursing care for adults. The review will include a discussion of (a) the theoretical background for the concept of pain, including a definition and factors influencing pain, (b) issues in the assessment of pain, (c) evidence concerning the relationship between nursing and pain as a symptom outcome, (d) evidence concerning approaches to measurement, and (e) recommendations and directions for future research.

The criteria for selecting studies for this review included (a) a pain-related outcome as the major dependent variable being examined, (b) an experimental or quasi-experimental design, (c) a nursing intervention—either analgesic administration or nonpharmacological, (d) an adequate sample size of at least 10 patients per group, and (e) the use of established measures to evaluate nurse-sensitive patient outcomes. After a review of PsychLIT (1987–2009), Sociological Abstracts (1963–2009), CINAHL (1982–2009), and MEDLINE (1966–2009), 40 studies were selected. Sources were excluded if (a) pain-related outcomes were not measured as a distinct variable, (b) the intervention was nonnursing or was implemented by nonnurses, or (c) the impact of the intervention on actual practices was not evaluated using patient outcomes.

The key words used in the search were *pain*, *interventions*, *education*, *analgesics* (nonnarcotic/opioid), *relaxation* (simple/techniques), *music* (therapy), *imagery* (simple/guided), and *muscle relaxation*. These words were combined with the term nurse to confine the literature to those sources relevant to nursing. The search yielded a total of 371 relevant sources from which 41, all from journal articles, met the criteria.

THEORETICAL BACKGROUND OF THE OUTCOME

Pain continues to be the most common reason people seek help from health professionals. It is also a common cause of disability and diminished quality of life. However, many people with acute and/or chronic pain do not experience the level of adequate pain relief possible through the application of current knowledge about pain and its management. Moreover, unrelieved pain from surgery can precipitate adverse responses, including pulmonary and cardiovascular dysfunction (Benedetti, Bonica, & Belluci, 1984; Dahl et al., 2003; O'Gara, 1988), and may predispose a patient to long-term pain (Katz, 1997; Kehlet, Jensen, & Woolf, 2006; Watt-Watson et al., 2008). Also, chronic noncancer pain is a frequent cause of suffering and disability affecting 29% of Canadians over the age of 18 (Millar, 1996; Moulin, Clark, Speechley, & Morley-Forster, 2002). Therefore, reliable and valid measures to evaluate the effectiveness of pain practices using patient outcomes are critical.

Definition

Pain is a subjective phenomenon that varies with each individual and each painful experience (Melzack & Wall, 1965). The International Association for the Study of Pain (IASP) has defined pain as "an unpleasant sensory and emotional experience associated with actual or potential tissue damage, or described in terms of such damage" (Merskey & Bogduk, 1994, p. 210). The explanatory note with this definition emphasizes the subjectivity of the pain experience, that pain is more than a noxious stimulus, and that patients' self-reports of pain should be accepted even when tissue damage is not clearly evident.

Pain Theory

The most prevalent theory from which this definition was developed is Melzack and Wall's (1965) gate control theory. It has been seminal in stimulating new ideas to explain painful phenomena and to explore new therapies for pain relief. They developed their model of pain mechanisms as an alternative to two main theories, the specificity and pattern theories. They challenged von Frey's (1894, as cited in Melzack & Wall, 1965) prevalent specificity theory that pain intensity is proportional to the degree of tissue damage. Gate control theory emphasizes that pain is not a simple, sensory experience but a complex integration of sensory, affective, and cognitive dimensions. One of Melzack and Wall's major contributions is their suggestion that pain perception involves modulation of noxious input at several levels of the central nervous system. The perception of pain and responsiveness to noxious stimuli are variable and unpredictable because of inhibitory mechanisms that include both endogenous neural activity and individuals' unique cognitive factors.

Modulation of pain perception was only minimally described by Melzack and Wall (1965). More recently, researchers have found that changes occur in the peripheral and central nervous systems in response to painful stimuli, particularly if they are prolonged (Basbaum & Jessell, 2000; Benarroch, 2008; Woolf & Salter, 2000). Peripheral sensitization related to chemicals released from damaged tissues after injury, surgery, or inflammation can decrease the activation threshold of nociceptors. Consequently, nociceptors may discharge spontaneously with a decreased threshold for both noxious and nonnoxious stimuli. Prolonged severe and persistent injury, such as with trauma or surgery, stimulates spinal cord neurons in the dorsal horn to respond to all inputs, painful or not, resulting in a phenomenon called central sensitization. This sensitization can result in abnormal interpretation of normal stimuli and chronic pain that lasts long after the original noxious stimulus. Increasing evidence suggests that preventing or minimizing acute pain may reduce the incidence of long-term pain (Katz, 1997; Kehlet et al., 2006; Woolf & Salter). Therefore, pain relief after interventions such as opioid analgesia, the cornerstone of acute pain management (Agency for Health Care Policy and Research [AHCPR], 1992; Gordon et al., 2004), is a very important outcome to measure. Also, additional outcomes that are helpful in understanding the broader impact of interventions include improvement in activity and other pain-related quality-of-life issues.

Melzack and Dennis (1978) developed this conceptualization further by emphasizing that noxious stimuli enter an already active nervous system that is a substrate of past experience, culture, anticipation, and emotions. A person's cognitive processes act selectively on sensory input and motivation to influence pain transmission via the descending tracts to the dorsal horn. As a result, the amount, quality, and impact of pain are determined by individual factors such as previous pain experiences and one's concept of the cause of pain and its consequences. Therefore, pain is a highly personal experience and more than a noxious stimulus. Consequently, researchers are now looking at outcomes besides pain sensation to understand the impact of pain on mood and usual activities, such as sleeping and walking. They are now delineating pain and its direct impact from the more global experience of suffering. The terms *pain* and *suffering* have tended to be used interchangeably in the literature (Khan & Steeves, 1996). The distinction between the two—that pain is a perception of a sensation related to trauma or disease, whereas suffering takes place at the level of the person's lived experience—has not always been made clear. Spross (1996) defined suffering as being more than a perception or sensation, and as an evaluation of the meaning of pain for the person. Similarly, Kahn and Steeves emphasized that suffering is determined by the relationship between the self and the event rather than by the inherent characteristics of the event itself.

In summary, Melzack and Wall (1965) emphasized that pain is a complex subjective phenomenon. Pain perception and responsiveness to a given stimulus are variable and unpredictable because of inhibitory mechanisms that include both endogenous neural activity and cognitive factors that are unique to each person (Fields, 1987; Wall, 1996). Pain mechanisms have a plasticity in that they can change in response to tissue injury such as surgery; pain perceptions can vary because of factors such as the meaning of pain (Wall). Although process outcomes such as pain intensity and pain relief are important to measure, they are unidimensional and focus only on pain sensation. Outcomes, such as changes in usual activities and abilities, reflect broader dimensions beyond the sensory and are increasingly being included as important indicators of whether the intervention has been successful.

Conceptual Definition

Based on the theoretical work in pain, one can conclude that pain is a subjective, multidimensional phenomenon that varies with each individual and each painful experience. The perception of pain and responsiveness to noxious stimuli are variable and unpredictable because of inhibitory mechanisms that include both endogenous neural activity and individuals' unique cognitive factors (Kehlet et al., 2006). Pain sensation and its direct impact are different from the broader concept of suffering.

Factors that Influence Pain

Pain perception is influenced by both internal and external factors. The nervous system has a functional plasticity that allows it to react to changing situations by altering its functions (Basbaum & Jessell, 2000; Benarroch, 2008; Woolf & Salter, 2000). As a result, the nervous system does not respond in a fixed way to a given stimulus, but can alter its response properties dynamically. A person's cognitive processes act selectively on sensory input and motivation to influence pain transmission via the descending tracts to the dorsal horn (Melzack & Wall, 1965). Therefore, the amount and quality of pain are determined by individual factors such as previous pain experiences, mood, and one's concept of the cause of pain and its consequences. Also, cultural values can influence how one feels and responds to pain.

With repeated noxious stimuli, receptive fields can expand from the injured peripheral site to surrounding uninjured tissue. Alterations in perceptions of stimuli can occur, for example, so that a normal stimulus such as touch may be felt as painful. Therefore, pain not only involves the periphery, but also can result from an altered central nervous system that is interpreting normal signals in an abnormal way. Consequently, a treatment implication is that prevention of pain signals from reaching the central nervous system peri- and postoperatively may reduce immediate pain and long-term pain problems (Katz, 1997; Watt-Watson et al., 2008; Woolf & Salter, 2000).

ISSUES IN THE ASSESSMENT AND MEASUREMENT OF PAIN

A broad review of the literature provided considerable evidence that pain assessment and its related management are problematic. Key issues that emerged are the need to (a) use standardized pain measures to guide assessment and related management, (b) control for nurse and patient mediators of effective assessment, and (c) use other outcomes and pain intensity to determine the impact of the pain problem and its management.

Using Standardized Pain Measures to Guide Assessment and Related Management

Standardized measures such as the 11-point numerical rating scale for pain intensity or the Brief Pain Inventory (BPI) have not routinely been a component of nursing assessment practices, and patients have not perceived nurses as resources in assessing and managing their pain (Watt-Watson, Garfinkel, Gallop, Stevens, & Streiner, 2000). Moreover, nurses have underestimated the pain experienced by their patients, although they believed that mild pain or less was ideal.

Although nurses have identified asking the patient as the most frequently used method of determining pain intensity, fewer than 50% actually regarded it as the most influential factor (Ferrell, McCaffery, & Grant, 1991). Instead, patient behaviors, such as movement and verbal expressions like moaning, have been used to assess pain and determine analgesic interventions. These behaviors were ranked as more important than the patient's self-report. This finding is unfortunate because patients frequently do not express pain or their need for help with management; instead, they realize that their pain will be minimal if they do not move or breathe deeply and cough (Watt-Watson, Garfinkel, et al., 2000; Watt-Watson et al., 2004). Nurses have expected patients to communicate their pain and ask for help, but the majority of patients indicated that they would not voluntarily tell nurses and doctors because they expected them to know when they needed help (Watt-Watson, Stevens, Streiner, Garfinkel, & Gallop, 2001). Therefore, patients' perceptions of their nurse as a resource with their pain were not positive (Watt-Watson et al., 2001). It is problematic that less than 50% of prescribed analgesia was given despite patients' reports of moderate to severe pain (Watt-Watson, Garfinkel, et al., 2000; Watt-Watson et al., 2004).

Controlling for Nurse and Patient Mediators of Assessment

For over 30 years, evidence has demonstrated that nurses' experience and personal beliefs can influence their pain assessment. Nurses who experienced their own intense pain were more aware of their patients' pain (Holm, Cohen, Dudas, Medema, & Allen, 1989). In addition, almost three quarters of nurses in Dalton's (1989) study reported that they were more empathic with patients having difficult pain management problems. Also, nurses have inferred greater pain when patients verbalized their discomfort (Baer, Davitz, & Lieb, 1970). Similarly, patients who asked for pain relief were thought to suffer more than other patients (Oberst, 1978). Nurses have held problematic beliefs or misbeliefs about the validity of patients' reports of pain and assumed that patients would tell them when they needed help (Watt-Watson et al., 2001).

Patient characteristics such as diagnosis, age, gender, and culture may influence caregivers' perceptions of patients' pain and need for intervention. For example, female patients have received fewer analgesics after surgery than male patients (Calderone, 1990; Faherty & Grier, 1984; McDonald, 1994), older adult patients have received fewer analgesics than younger adult patients (Duggleby & Lander, 1994; Melzack, Abbott, Zackon, Mulder, & Davis, 1987; Winefield, Katsikitis, Hart, & Rounsefell, 1990), and patients from ethnic minority groups have received less opioid analgesia postoperatively than Caucasian patients (McDonald, 1994). As well, Bernabei et al. (1998) reported similar data in a study of 13,625 cancer patients aged 65 or older and living in a nursing home; predictors of unrelieved pain and minimal or no analgesic administration included being older, from a minority racial group after language adjustment, cognitively less able, and female. Todd, Samaroo, and Hoffman's (1993) research indicated that Hispanics with long-bone fractures were twice as likely as non-Hispanic Whites to receive no pain medication in emergency departments, although other research has found no racial differences in the amount of analgesia given in emergency departments (Choi, Yate, Coats, Kalinda, & Paul, 2000). Cleeland, Baez, Loehrer, and Pandya (1997) suggested that the inadequate analgesia for Hispanic patients found in their research may relate to patients' concerns about addiction and adverse effects, but the latter concerns have been consistently documented for many patients (Ward et al., 1993; Watt-Watson et al., 2001).

Patients' own beliefs about pain may influence their seeking and accepting help (Ward et al., 1993; Watt-Watson et al., 2004); they identified opioid side effects such as constipation and nausea, as well as fears of addiction, as the major reasons for not seeking help with pain or taking analgesics. Several studies have documented that patients do not necessarily tell a caregiver when they are in pain (Bédard et al., 2006; Carr, 1990; Chen, Miaskowski, Dodd, & Pantilat, 2008; Lavies, Hart, Rounsefell, & Runciman, 1992; Owen, McMillan, & Rogowski,

1990; Watt-Watson, Garfinkel et al., 2000; Watt-Watson et al., 2004), yet nurses infer more pain when patients verbalize their discomfort or ask for relief (Baer et al., 1970; Oberst, 1978; Watt-Watson et al., 2001).

Using Other Outcomes and Pain Intensity to Determine the Impact of the Pain Problem

Pain is multidimensional and not directly proportional to tissue damage (Melzack & Wall, 1965). Although sensation is important, other dimensions, such as the quality and impact of pain, also need to be assessed. Only nine trials in this review used measures to determine the impact of pain on everyday relationships and activities or health-related quality of life along with pain intensity (Bédard et al., 2006; Dalton et al., 1999, 2004; De Wit & Van Dam, 2001; Edwards et al., 2005; LeFort et al., 1998; McGillion et al., 2008; Ward et al., 2000; Watt-Watson et al., 2004).

The approach to determining a person's pain commonly involves using quantitative measures of pain intensity and its location, and/or temporal features. Documented reports of the pain symptom have included primarily well-established unidimensional ratings to measure pain intensity, such as visual analogue scales (VASs) or numerical rating scales (NRSs). The internationally recognized McGill Pain Questionnaire, or MPQ (Melzack, 1975), developed from gate control theory, expanded pain assessment to include both qualitative and quantitative dimensions of pain sensation. Further development has included multidimensional measures, such as the BPI (Daut, Cleeland, & Flanery, 1983), which examine not only intensity but also pain-related interference in usual activities.

More recently, the paucity of measures to examine patients' expectations and perceptions of their pain management experience has been recognized. However, most of these measures have been utilized in single studies with major design issues and have only rudimentary reliability and validity; therefore, they will not be discussed here. The Barriers Questionnaire, both long and short forms, has established reliability and validity and asks about concerns patients have that would prevent them from taking analgesics or asking for help with pain (Ward, Carlson-Dakes, Hughes, Kwekkeboom, & Donovan, 1998; Ward et al., 1993). Because concerns are a mediator of pain but not a direct measure of pain sensation or its impact on everyday activities, this measure will not be included in this review. However, data related to this measure are included in the three studies that used concerns as a mediator variable (Ward et al., 2000; Watt-Watson et al., 2001, 2004). Well-established health-related quality-of-life measures such as the MOH-SF36 were used in four studies (de Wit & Van Dam, 2001; Edwards et al., 2005; LeFort et al., 1998; McGillion et al., 2008) and are discussed in the chapter on functional status in this book (Chapter 2).

Therefore, only measures used almost exclusively in the 41 studies selected for this review will be discussed in this chapter. These measures include the VAS or NRS, the MPQ, and the BPI.

EVIDENCE CONCERNING THE RELATIONSHIP BETWEEN NURSING AND PAIN AS A SYMPTOM OUTCOME

The 41 empirical studies that were identified are reviewed in **TABLE 5-1**. In all but two of the studies, pain as a primary outcome was operationalized as intensity and measured by the VAS or the NRS. Fewer researchers used the MPQ or the BPI. In 17 studies, however, additional outcomes along with pain intensity were examined, including pain-related quality-of-life or activity interference issues ($n = 8$), analgesic prescription and administration ($n = 5$), or both ($n = 4$). The nursing contexts included (a) acute care ($n = 24$ including emergency [2] or labor [1]); (b) home (10) or rural care (1); (c) outpatient or oncology practice (5); or (d) university health service/community (2). More recently, nurses have systematically examined the influence of interventions on patient outcomes related to pain management by using randomized controlled trials. In this review, 31 studies were randomized controlled trials, and the remainder had quasi-experimental pre/posttest designs.

The evidence supporting pain as a relevant outcome for measuring nursing interventions is equivocal. The nursing interventions identified in this review include (a) nonpharmacological strategies, including music alone or combined with relaxation or ibuprofen (Broscious, 1999; Good et al., 2001; McCaffrey & Freeman, 2003; Phumdoung & Good, 2003; Tanabe et al., 2001); therapeutic touch (Keller & Bzdek, 1986; Meehan, 1993); cutaneous stimulation (Kubsch et al., 2000); imagery (Kwekkeboom et al., 2003, 2008; Menzies, Taylor, & Bourguignon, 2006); and physical strategies of foot reflexology (Tsay et al., 2008) or breast compression bandage (King et al., 2006); (b) patient education (Ahles et al., 2001; Closs et al., 1999; Clotfelter, 1999; Dalton et al., 2004; LeFort et al., 1998; Lorig et al., 2005; McDonald et al., 2001; McGillion et al., 2008; Miaskowski et al., 2004; Neitzel et al., 1999; Ward et al., 2000, 2008; Watt-Watson et al., 2004); (c) nurses' education (Bédard et al., 2006; Dahlman et al., 1999; Dalton et al., 1999; de Rond et al., 1999, 2000; de Wit & Van Dam, 2001; Edwards et al., 2005; Francke et al., 1997; Holzheimer et al., 1999; Neitzel et al.; Seers et al., 2004); and (d) nurses' individual feedback related to assessment and pain treatment flowchart (Duncan & Pozehl, 2000). Two studies were also reviewed that reported systematic reviews of the use of relaxation techniques, including imagery, hypnosis, visualization, and cognitive therapy (Seers & Carroll, 1998), and nonpharmacological interventions (Sindhu, 1996).

TABLE 5-1   Studies Investigating the Relationship Between Nursing Interventions and Pain as a Symptom Outcome

Author/date	Design	Sample characteristics/setting	Definition of the outcome concept	Intervention being evaluated	Results	Limitations
Ahles et al. (2001)	Pilot RCT, randomized to usual care group or telephone-based pain intervention; baseline screening for pain and mailed outcome assessment at 3–6 months postenrollment	744 patients from four U.S. rural primary care practices with mild to severe pain in last 4 weeks; RR = 32 randomized to usual care (n = 320) or intervention groups (n = 295, RR = 92%), with or without psychosocial problems; mean age = 48; 55% women	Pain defined as intensity (NRS 0–5), duration, location, and adequacy of treatment; psychosocial functioning (SF-36); Functional Interference Estimate	Telephone-based pain assessment and tailored education strategies by phone and mail	Patients in the intervention group had significantly better scores on SF-36 for pain, physical, emotional, and social subscales and on the total Functional Interference Scale.	Description of methodology unclear; patient response rate low to study (32%) and final questionnaires (53%); follow-up period postintervention varied from 3 to 6 months; despite randomization, significant differences between groups for age, sex, emotional distress, and poor health status
Bédard et al. (2006)	Quasi-experimental design with unequal pretest/posttest comparison; patient pain status, satisfaction and beliefs measured prior to (Phase I) and after (Phase II) program implementation	Convenience sampling from across the surgical divisions for both Phase I: n = 76 patients, mean age = 58.1, 50.0% female, and Phase II: n = 71 patients; RR = 78%, mean age = 64.5, 39.4% female	Overall, worst and average pain measured using NRS from the American Pain Society Patient Outcome Questionnaire	2-year comprehensive evidence-based management program for patients, professionals, and the organization; aimed to increase the number of evidence-based orders for pain management	More patients received evidence-based orders in Phase II than in Phase I; Phase II patients' average pain and worst pain scores were lower than those of Phase I patients, and the evidence-based orders variable was a mediator of these group differences; less interference with sleep, walking, general activities.	Nonrandom sampling; patients who refused participation in Phase II were more likely to be fatigued, in pain, or not feeling well, and this self-selection bias may have led to better results in Phase II; significant differences between groups for age and language.
Broscious (1999)	Experimental single-blind, pretest/posttest three-group design; random assignment using blinded group chip selection for control, white noise, or music prior to chest tube removal (CTR); pain measured at baseline, 5–7 and 20–22 minutes after CTR	156/189 patients having elective open heart surgery in U.S. (4 withdrew, 29 became ineligible because of complications or surgery cancellation). Surgeries included 81% coronary bypass graft, 9% valve, and 9% both; chest tubes were mediastinal (100%) plus one (80%) or two (20%)	Pain intensity measured by a NRS (0–10)	Music vs white noise vs control; experimental groups listened to tape 10 minutes pre-chest tube removal, either to the same white noise or to music chosen from 10 options at preadmission testing; controls had standard care not described.	No significant differences at any time period, and mean score for total group 5–7 minutes after procedure was 5.62 ± 2.79.	Further work needed on dosing, timing, and type of music

Source	Design	Sample	Pain measure	Intervention	Results	Comments/Limitations
		pleural tubes. Mean (*SD*) age = 66 (9.7) years; 38% women				Information intervention did not address toxicity and addiction concerns
Closs et al. (1999)	Pre/posttrial with a control and intervention ward sample over 9 months; interviewed for 15–30 minutes on the morning of second day postsurgery	417 patients from two matched orthopedic wards in four groups in England; convenience sample of elective or trauma patients; excluded if working nights, had terminal disease, confused, or cognitively impaired; RR and demographics not stated	Experience of post-op nighttime pain defined by pain intensity (verbal rating scale, 0–4), analgesics given, pain documentation, and patient-initiated reports	Patient information and structured pain assessment to improve pain after surgery at night	Significant reductions in overnight worst and average pain scores and increase in documented pain assessments; no differences in patients' reporting pain or analgesic administration	
Clotfelter (1999)	Quasi-experimental pretest/posttest design; patients randomly assigned; pain measured at baseline, 2 weeks later twice on same day	36 elderly people (≥ 65 years) with cancer from a U.S. private oncology practice; RR = 88% (17 rated pain as zero at three time periods and were removed); mean age = 77; 64% women	Pain intensity measured by VAS (0–100)	Education video and booklet; experimental group received booklet and saw video, *vs* control, who received only instructions from office staff.	Significantly less pain for experimental group than control group (F34 = 5.8, $p < 0.02$)	Small sample, although differences significant; use of VAS with elderly may have influenced pain ratings; generalizable to this sample only.
Dahlman et al. (1999)	Pretest/posttest design with two different convenience samples; all patients rated pain daily and were asked for a retrospective review before discharge; one group given open-ended questions pre-study day and one group at 3 months post.	75 patients (RR = 94%) with thorax surgery via sternotomy in Sweden; no demographic data reported	Pain intensity using VAS (0–10), satisfaction with pain relief, pain experience, but domains unclear	A study day for nurses on pain; all nurses in thoracic surgery (N > = 75–6 = 69) attended a study day focused on physiology, pharmacology, pain assessment, and treatment strategies.	Patients reported lower pain ratings postintervention; all pain scores were low, but postgroup significantly lower; 95% satisfied with pain relief.	Quasi-experimental with nonequivalent control group; not clear if pain ratings at rest or on movement.

(continues)

BPI = Brief Pain Inventory; IASP = International Association for the Study of Pain; MPQ-SF = McGill Pain Questionnaire-Short Form; NRS = numerical rating scale; PPI = present pain intensity; PRI = pain rating index; RCT = randomized controlled trial; SF-36 = Medical Outcomes Study-Short Form; VAS = visual analogue scale.

TABLE 5-1   Studies Investigating the Relationship Between Nursing Interventions and Pain as a Symptom Outcome (continued)

Author/ date	Design	Sample characteristics/ setting	Definition of the outcome concept	Intervention being evaluated	Results	Limitations
Dalton et al. (1999)	RCT, random selection of 6/14 hospitals having interest in an education intervention, and random assignment to experimental or control; data were collected from convenience patient samples and charts at baseline, end of program, and 6 months later on experimental sites.	Cohorts of 50 patients per site at discharge after abdominal, thoracic, or orthopedic surgery in three community hospitals of 100–500 beds in North Carolina; median age = 49; 69% women; 84.5% Caucasian, 14.8% African American	Pain defined as an unpleasant sensory and emotional experience arising from actual or potential damage or described in terms of such damage (IASP), pain-related interference, and patient satisfaction using American Pain Society questionnaire	A pain education program for nurses, physicians, and pharmacists; teams of 10–15 RNs, 1–2 MDs, and 2 pharmacists designated per site for the program; a Delphi-developed program was given in three 4.5-hour sessions over 8 weeks on pain assessment, pharmacology, and patient role in evaluation of relief.	Outcome data to be reported.	No patient outcome data reported.
Dalton et al. (2004)	Three-arm experimental, repeated measures design; patients randomly assigned; data collected pre- and postintervention and at 1 month and 6 months postintervention.	131 cancer patients who had an elevated score on at least one Biobehavioral Pain Profile Scale from four clinical sites; 121 completed preintervention, 53 completed postintervention, 28 completed the entire study.	Symptom severity measured with Karnofsky Performance Status Scale; pain intensity and interference measured with BPI.	Compared profile-tailored cognitive behavioral therapy (CBT) treatment program with standard CBT or usual care in changing patients' self-reported cognitive-affective, behavioral, and physiologic cancer-related pain outcomes.	Overall pattern (n = 28): The profile-tailored CBT group improved substantially in the short term but decreased at 6 months; standard CBT group changed little until 6 months, when substantial improvement occurred; usual care group showed little change across study; overall slight advantage of profile-tailored CBT.	High rate of attrition for full data collection (71%); statistical analysis limited by attrition rate; description in results section unclear at times; authors modified study protocol many times to enhance patient participation and retention, but this may have affected patient outcomes.
de Rond et al. (1999)	Part of larger study using a quasi-experimental nonequivalent control group design; this study includes the intervention group experiencing daily pain assessments in the hospital.	Patients from one medical and two surgical wards in each of three hospitals in the Netherlands; included if in pain or had an analgesic prescription; diagnoses included acute malignant, chronic malignant, acute noncancer, and chronic noncancer pain; N = 315, RR = 315/369: 24 declined	Feasibility and value of daily pain assessments (NRS, 0–10) as determined by patient opinion; experimental group were asked four open-ended questions about daily pain assessment at second interview.	Nurses' compliance with daily, systematic pain assessment and value for nurses and patients; all nurses working in areas (n = 227) were given 3-hour education about pain assessment, NRS, and pharmacological and nonpharmacological management.	75% of patients were positive about using NRS twice daily; instructions confused some patients.	Quasi-experimental with nonequivalent control group; not clear how sites chosen.

Study	Design	Sample	Measures	Intervention	Results	Notes
		as older and female, and 30 older patients left after first interview; mean (SD) age = 58.6 (17.3); 56.2% women.				
de Rond et al. (2000)	Quasi-experimental with nonequivalent control group; interviewed twice: on admission and either before discharge (control) or postintervention.	480 Dutch patients from two surgical wards and one medical ward from each of three general hospitals; patients stratified for duration of pain (acute/chronic) and type of pain (non-cancer/cancer); RR = 68%; mean (SD) age = 59.5(16.8); 58.5% female.	Prescribed analgesics by MDs, administered analgesics by RNs, and the discrepancy between the two	3-hour pain education for nurses and implementation of two daily pain assessments (NRS 0–10)	The Pain Monitoring Program improved nurses' administration of analgesics ($p <$ 0.05), particularly with moderate-severe pain; discrepancy between orders and administration did not change; PRNs excluded from this.	Quasi-experimental with nonequivalent control group; excluded PRN analgesia from total administration calculations; some postintervention interviews completed after discharge at home.
de Wit & Van Dam (2001)	Randomized, longitudinal study with pretest/posttest experimental design; stratified by sex, age, metastatic site; interviewed at baseline and 2, 4, and 8 weeks postdischarge	104 cancer patients with chronic pain at home; at 8 weeks attrition, 20% control vs 41% intervention group due to deaths; 68.6% women; mean (SD) age = 58.1 (12.4).	Pain intensity (NRS 0–10) and experience (location, time since onset, analgesic use); Quality of Life (EORTC QLQ-C30)	Pain education program tailored for individual patients	No significant differences between groups for pain	Despite randomization, groups differed on analgesics administered, physical and cognitive functioning at baseline; 41% vs 20% intervention group died postdischarge.
Duncan & Pozehl (2000)	Quasi-experimental pretest/posttest design with data collected from two convenience samples of patients over 17 weeks; pre-nurse feedback and postintervention follow up over 15 months, along with retrospective chart data	240 patients had a total knee arthroplasty (pre = 121, post = 119) on a unit where PCA morphine was standard in first 24–28 hours postop in U.S.; 243 patient records were audited postop and 3 excluded due to complications; mean age = 70; 62% women.	Pain intensity (NRS 0–10); analgesic use from chart data: morphine equivalents given during 4-day postop stay; postanalgesic effectiveness (NRS, 0–10).	Intervention involves performance feedback to nurses on patients' postoperative pain outcomes; 30 nurses (23 RNs, 7 LPNs) working on the unit for minimum of 6 months received individual feedback and a pain treatment flowchart related to their q4h assessment, postanalgesic assessments, follow-up, and documentation of patients' acceptable pain level.	Significant changes from pre- to posttest included a decline in mean pain ratings from 3.59 to 3.16, increase in analgesic use from 12.70 mg to 14.54 mg morphine equivalents, decrease in postanalgesic ratings from 3.07 to 2.68, and decrease in unacceptable levels of pain after analgesia from 1.12 to 0.84.	Quasi-experimental with nonequivalent control group; patient pain outcomes were taken from documented ratings.

BPI = Brief Pain Inventory; IASP = International Association for the Study of Pain; MPQ-SF = McGill Pain Questionnaire-Short Form; NRS = numerical rating scale; PPI = present pain intensity; PRI = pain rating index; RCT = randomized controlled trial; SF-36 = Medical Outcomes Study-Short Form; VAS = visual analogue scale.

(continues)

TABLE 5-1   Studies Investigating the Relationship Between Nursing Interventions and Pain as a Symptom Outcome (continued)

Author/date	Design	Sample characteristics/setting	Definition of the outcome concept	Intervention being evaluated	Results	Limitations
Edwards et al. (2005)	Sequential RCT; random assignment of patients to intervention or control group; data collected at pretest and 12 weeks after study admission.	56 patients with chronic venous leg ulcers from regional treatment centers; generally ≥ 60 years of age; 46.4% female.	Rand Medical Outcomes Study Pain Measures used to assess pain frequency and duration.	10 community nurses were trained to provide the intervention, which involved patients visiting a weekly club meeting where they received comprehensive health assessment, ulcer treatment, peer support, social interaction, and goal-setting and preventative care advice.	At 12 weeks, the intervention group reported reductions in the amount of pain experienced ($p < .001$), the degree to which pain affected mood ($p < .01$), sleep ($p < .01$), and normal work ($p < .05$); group also experienced significantly improved ulcer healing. No improvements in pain for the control group.	Number of novel components of intervention makes it difficult to identify which were related to decreased pain; data analysis partially ignores group comparisons in favor of within-group analyses.
Francke et al. (1997)	Pretest/posttest control group design; in each of five hospitals, one ward randomly allocated to CE Program for nurses or control (no program); data collected for 3 months before and 3–6 months after the program; interviewed the day before about 4:00 a.m. and at 2 and 4 days after surgery.	152 surgical patients with curative resection of colon or breast cancer in five Dutch hospitals in four groups per hospital: pre/post groups on intervention ward and pre/post control groups on control ward; nurse recruiters reported less than 10% refusals; mean (*SD*) age = 68.6 (13.6, colon) and 61.2 (25.5, breast); women = 55.5% for colon and 100% for breast	Pain intensity NRS (0–10), pain duration during day, and sleep disruption because of pain (two items from McGill Pain Quality of Life Questionnaire)	Continuing pain education program for nurses on surgical cancer units; all qualified nurses on ward team given 8 weekly 3-hour sessions on pain assessment and management and one follow-up session 4 months after the program.	Pain intensity Day 2 was less for treatment group, but not Day 4 ($p < 0.02$); no differences in pain duration and number of sleepless hours from pain.	Not clear which changes in intervention program related to decreased patient pain
Good et al. (2001)	Secondary analysis of RCT; random assignment to one of four groups (relaxation, music, combined, and control); baseline and Days 1 and 2 postsurgery.	468 abdominal surgery patients in five U.S. hospitals; RR = 76%; mean (SD) age = 45 (11); 84% women	Pain: Used IASP definition, pain intensity (NRS 0–100), distress (NRS 0–100); jaw relaxation as lowering jaw slightly, let tongue rest quietly, allow lips to get soft, breathe slowly, and stop thinking; music types: synthesizer, harp, piano	Relaxation and/or music to reduce postoperative pain	Treatment groups had less pain and distress across days, but interventions were not statistically different in effect.	

			orchestra, or slow modern jazz			
Holzheimer et al. (1999)	Pretest/posttest design using secondary analysis of two studies, one before a nurse intervention and one about 2 years later; measures taken twice for pretest group within 48 hours of admission to hospice care and at Week 4, and once for posttest group over a wide range of time periods > 48 hours.	Pretest (*n* = 47) and posttest (*n* = 255) home care hospice patients with cancer in the U.S.; mean (*SD*) age for both groups = 71 (10.2–12.1); women = 48–52%	Pain intensity defined as worst pain in the past week (NRS 0–10); pain relief (NRS 0–10) rated from *none* to *complete relief* in past week.	Nurse-focused hospicewide four-part intervention consisting of education, policies and procedures, documentation, and performance evaluation	Adjusted mean scores improved from 1995 to 1997 for worst pain (X = 6.7–6.1) and pain relief (X = 6.0–8.4)	Nonequivalent control group; timing of data collection differed; different pain scales were used for each group
Keller & Bzdek (1986)	RCT, two-group design with convenience samples; measures taken prior to, 5 minutes after, and 4 hours after intervention.	60 volunteers from a U.S. university with tension headache who were not taking medication 4 hours before the intervention; mean age = 30; women = 75%	Pain defined as tension headache with no prodrome, neurological deficit, infectious process, or recent head trauma; pain intensity measured using MPQ–Pain Rating Index, number words chosen, PPI	Therapeutic touch (TT) vs placebo; treatment group given a standardized 5-minute therapeutic touch procedure; other group given a mimicked TT (MTT) using counting rather than a meditative state; both groups told to use deep breathing during the postintervention 5-minute interval.	TT group had greater relief than MTT group at first posttest time, MPQ reduction X = 70% (TT) vs 37% (MTT) *p* < 0.002, but no significant differences at 4 hours posttest.	Small sample size; overall results presented as positive, although no significant differences at 4 hours postintervention; minimized the contribution effect of deep breathing in a 5-minute quiet break.
King et al. (2006)	RCT to examine the efficacy of early use of compression undergarment to reduce pain and discomfort over 12 weeks post–median sternotomy after first cardiac surgery; in four sites	385,481 women completed WREST Trial; 23/241 from the intervention group and 29/240 from the usual care group participated; mean age = 65.66 (11.327)	Pain and discomfort related to their sternal incision and breasts was measured using 11-point numeric scales (0–10).	Intervention group used a compression undergarment over the sternotomy versus the usual care group wearing their own bra.	The intervention group were less likely to experience breast pain and discomfort but not sternal pain or discomfort.	Analgesic protocols varied by site, and these data were not collected; minimal discussion of findings at 12 weeks.

BPI = Brief Pain Inventory; IASP = International Association for the Study of Pain; MPQ-SF = McGill Pain Questionnaire-Short Form; NRS = numerical rating scale; PPI = present pain intensity; PRI = pain rating index; RCT = randomized controlled trial; SF-36 = Medical Outcomes Study-Short Form; VAS = visual analogue scale.

(continues)

TABLE 5-1   Studies Investigating the Relationship Between Nursing Interventions and Pain as a Symptom Outcome (continued)

Author/date	Design	Sample characteristics/setting	Definition of the outcome concept	Intervention being evaluated	Results	Limitations
Kubsch et al. (2000)	One group pretest/posttest design with convenience sample having cutaneous stimulation.	50 people entering a U.S. emergency department over a 6-month period who were experiencing pain due to nonemergent/non-life-threatening conditions and who had not self-medicated for pain in the previous 4 hours. 12 < 18 years; women = 64%.	Pain intensity (NRS 0–10) and VAS, blood pressure, and heart rate.	Cutaneous stimulation; certified emergency nurse was trained and implemented the intervention.	Significant reductions in pain scores ($t = 7.09$, $p < 0.0001$), heart rate ($t = 2.79$, $p < 0.008$), and BP ($t = 3.42$, $p < 0.0013$) after cutaneous stimulation using circular pressure/massage to a localized site (over, contra-lateral, or proximal to pain site).	Small sample size; one group pre/posttest design
Kwekkeboom et al. (2003)	Pilot one group, pretest/posttest design	69 inpatients with a wide range of cancers currently experiencing cancer-related pain rated as ≥ 3 on a 0–10 scale; mean age = 55.6 (14.92); 65% female; 97% Caucasian; 10.1% attrition	Pain intensity and pain-related distress (both 0–10 NRS); affect measured using the Positive and Negative Affect Scale; perceived control over pain measured using the control subscale of the Survey of Pain Attitudes	One session listening to a 12-minute audio recording in analgesic imagery with verbal instruction and no background music	Pain intensity decreased from pretest to posttest ($p < .01$); patients' imaging ability was a predictor for mean pain intensity ($\beta = -.26$, p < .01), positive affect ($\beta = .29$, p < .05), and perceived control over pain ($\beta = .31$, p < .05).	Small sample and high number of outcome variables; lack of control group; t-test data only reported for one of three dependent variables; high rate of patients declined study (48.5%) and possibly did so because of negative opinions of guided imagery.
Kwekkeboom et al. (2008)	Pilot study with crossover design; participants received one control trial and two trials of progressive muscle relaxation (PMR) or analgesic imagery over a 2-day period; pain intensity and distress measured before and after each trial; perceived control over pain measured after each trial	40 patients with cancer-related pain from academic hospital; blocked by average pain severity (2–4 vs 5–8) and randomized to one of two orders of interventions; data lost for 8–9 patients for each treatment condition; mean age = 49 (16); 55% female	Current pain intensity measured using 0–10 scale; percent change calculated from pre-to posttrial ratings; pain-related distress using a 0–10 scale; perceived control over pain assessed using control subscale from the Survey of Pain Attitudes	Control recording described members of the healthcare team, explained patients' rights (time = 14:09); PMR recording guided patients though instructions to tense and relax muscles in a series of muscle groups from head to feet (time = 13:36); analgesic imagery recording described a glove anesthesia technique (time = 14:29).	Greater change in pain intensity ($p < .05$); pain-related distress ($p < .01$); and greater perceived control over pain ($p < .05$) for PMR versus control and analgesic imagery versus control; 13/32 PMR patients and 16/31 analgesic imagery patients had a meaningful improvement in pain (≥ 30% reduction in pain intensity).	Small sample size; more intervention trials than control trials on each day; experimenter not blinded when providing each recording to the patient; unequal number of persons randomized to each order; effects from the interventions were short lived (less than 1 hour); timing of control trial (always first) may introduce bias.

LeFort et al. (1998)	RCT, consenting adults randomly allocated to one of two conditions; measures at pretreatment and posttreatment 3 months later; 11 programs with 6–10 participants each	110 people in Newfoundland (treatment = 57, control = 53) with idiopathic chronic noncancer pain longer than 3 months; 5 from treatment and 3 from control groups did not complete the study; patients self-referred or from pain specialists; women = 75%; mean age = 40; attrition = 7%.	Pain sensation (MPQ-SF, VAS [0–100]); disability: subscale of Survey of Pain Attitudes (SOPA-D) and severity (VAS 0–100); health-related quality of life: SF-36	A community-based chronic pain self-management psychoeducation program included six 2-hour sessions given by the principal investigator.	Significant improvement in treatment group, who reported reduced severity of pain problem, less disability (SOPA-D), and greater improvement for bodily pain, physical role functioning, and vitality (SF-36)	Examined effect to 3 months only; only one facilitator used
Lorig et al. (2005)	Blinded randomized two-group comparison study; sample randomly assigned to Arthritis Self-Management Program (ASMP) or Chronic Disease Self-Management Program (CDSMP) and measured at 4 months and 1 year	355 participants with arthritis as their primary concern; 239 randomized to ASMP and 116 to CDSMP; mean age = 65.2; 91.3% female; 85% completed 4-month follow-up and 86.2% completed the 1-year follow-up	Visual Numeric Pain scale included among 12 self-report instruments	ASMP is a 6-week program attended by 10–15 individuals with arthritis; CDSMP is a 6-week program designed for individuals with symptomatic chronic conditions (not arthritis specific).	4 months and 1 year: ASMP group's pain decreased ($p < .05$); CDSMP group's pain did not change from baseline; no difference between the groups for change in pain at 4 months; trend ($p = .088$) suggests ASMP group had improved pain vs CDSMP group at 1 year. For all measures, ASMP better at 4 months, with effect diminishing at 1 year	Unequal patient distribution to conditions; predominantly female, highly educated population with high incidence of diseases other than arthritis; limits generalizability
McCaffrey & Freeman (2003)	RCT, convenience sample randomly assigned to experimental group or control group; data measured on Day 1, Day 7, and Day 14 of the study	66 community-dwelling elders (> 65 years) with chronic osteoarthritis pain; pain rating of at least 3 on 1–10 scale for 15 days per month; 22 women and 11 men per group; mean age = 76.1	SF-MPQ: Pain descriptor scale measured evaluative aspects of pain, and the VAS (100 mm in length) measured pain intensity. Used Rogers's Science of Unitary Human Beings as a framing.	Experimental group listened to music for 20 minutes daily in the morning; the control group sat quietly for the same period of time; elders completed SF-MPQ immediately before (pretest) and after (posttest) the 20 minute bouts.	Experimental group's pre-to-post change was greater than the control group for the PRI and VAS on all 3 days ($p < .001$); repeated-measures ANOVA showed that the experimental group had continued pain decrease over the study duration ($p < .001$); control group the same across study.	Convenience sample, though effective randomization techniques were employed; elders completed study at home, so adherence to study protocol may be questioned; use of pre-to-post change scores for some analyses; study lacked control for nonnarcotic analgesic therapies.

BPI = Brief Pain Inventory; IASP = International Association for the Study of Pain; MPQ-SF = McGill Pain Questionnaire-Short Form; NRS = numerical rating scale; PPI = present pain intensity; PRI = pain rating index; RCT = randomized controlled trial; SF-36 = Medical Outcomes Study-Short Form; VAS = visual analogue scale.

(continues)

TABLE 5-1   Studies Investigating the Relationship Between Nursing Interventions and Pain as a Symptom Outcome (continued)

Author/date	Design	Sample characteristics/setting	Definition of the outcome concept	Intervention being evaluated	Results	Limitations
McDonald et al. (2001)	Two-group, double-blind RCT; data collected prospectively over three points (presurgery, and postsurgery on Days 1 and 2).	31 people ≥ 65 years old having elective single total hip or knee replacement; mean age (SD) = 74 (6); 74% women; attrition = 23%.	Pain as measured by MPQ-SF	A PowerPoint slide show to teach basic pain management, communication skills, and two intensity rating scales	Patients receiving the intervention reported less postoperative pain over the course of their hospital stay	Small sample size; asked for first rating the evening of surgery, which may have influenced communication abilities; usual care included pain scales
McGillion et al. (2008)	Blinded pilot RCT, sample randomized to 6-week intervention group or 3-month wait-list control group; study outcomes assessed 3 months from baseline.	131 community-dwelling patients with chronic stable angina recruited from three teaching hospitals; mean age = 68; 80% male; attrition = 10%	Health-related quality of life measured using the SF-36 and measured specifically for angina using the Seattle Angina Questionnaire	A low-cost 6-week angina psychoeducation program aimed to encourage individual experimentation with self-management techniques and to facilitate mutual support; delivered weekly by a RN using a group format (8–15 patients)	At 3 months, patients' angina pain frequency ($p < .02$) and stability ($p < .001$) improved more for treatment vs control group; improved physical functioning ($p < .01$) and general health ($p < .01$) for the treatment vs control group.	Change score analyses though ANCOVA supported their use; short-term study requires longitudinal data to confirm findings.
Meehan (1993)	A single-blind three-group design with convenience samples over a 7-month period; measures taken prior to and 1 hour after intervention during the evening.	108 U.S. patients scheduled for major elective abdominal or pelvic surgery and requesting opioid analgesia during the evening of data collection; age range of 23–79 years; women = 70%.	Pain intensity (VAS 0–100) and verbal descriptor scale of no pain, mild pain, moderate pain, severe pain, and pain as bad as it could be.	Therapeutic touch vs opioid analgesia vs placebo; experimental group given a standardized 5-minute TT procedure, and the other groups, the standard opioid care or a mimicked TT using counting rather than a meditative state	Pain intensity reduced only in the group receiving opioid analgesics; 56% of all patients requested opioids.	Control of placebo effect
Menzies et al. (2006)	Prospective, longitudinal two-group RCT; randomized to usual care plus guided imagery or usual care alone groups	48 patients community living from MD offices with a Fibromyalgia Impact Questionnaire score > 20; mean age = 49.6, 47 of 48 female	Pain assessed using SF-MPQ: Sensory and affective pain, total pain, and pain on a VAS	Examined effectiveness of guided imagery in improving self-report of pain, and functional status; three guided imagery audiotapes used during 6-week treatment and 4-week follow-up	No clinically significant differences in pain between the usual care plus guided imagery and usual care alone groups	Small sample; potentially only generalizable to this particular sample due to patients' high levels of education and income

Miaskowski et al. (2004)	Two-group double-blinded RCT; patients randomized to standard care or the PRO-SELF Pain Control Program	212 oncology outpatients with pain from bone metastasis recruited from seven locations; 174 completed the study; illness and death reported as reasons for attrition; mean age PRO-SELF = 60 (11.6) and standard = 58.8 (12.9).	Pain intensity scores: least, average, and worst over the 6 weeks of the study using numeric scale from 0 to 10; secondary outcomes were increase in opioid analgesic intake and increase in percentage of patients with appropriate analgesic prescriptions	Standard care: Three home visits in Weeks 1, 3 and 6 and telephone interviews in Weeks 2, 4, and 5; PRO-SELF group: Tailored sessions to patient's individual learning needs, same number of home visits and telephone interviews as the standard group	Over the 6 weeks, the PRO-SELF group experienced reductions in average pain ($p < .001$), worst pain ($p < .001$), and least pain ($p < .001$); PRO-SELF group had reduced pain vs the standard group on average pain ($p = .026$), and worst pain ($p = .033$), but not least pain ($p = .117$).	Difficult to isolate if reductions in pain for PRO-SELF group are due to changes in analgesic prescriptions, changes in intake, or changes in patients' pain perceptions; short-term study period, therefore, longitudinal effects need to be studied.
Neitzel et al. (1999)	Pretest/posttest design with convenience samples of patients prior to patient and health professional pain education interventions, and 8 months later with a different sample.	118 patients (57 preintervention and 61 after having total knee or hip replacement surgery) in the U.S.; 3 pretest patients excluded with incomplete medical record data; age range 30–89.	Patient pain experience defined as pain intensity (VAS 0–10 for current and average), function (VAS 0–10 for walking, sleeping, and relating to others), opioid side effects, and satisfaction.	Education program for health professionals (program, revised orders, and documentation) and patients (information); all nurses on an orthopedic unit ($n = 28$) attended 8 hours of pain education; also, all patients given pain education material either before or after surgery.	No decrease in pain and no significant differences in pain, function, side effects, or satisfaction.	Pretest/posttest non-equivalent control group; intervention time variable.
Phumdoung & Good (2003)	RCT; convenience sample randomized to intervention or control group; randomization stratified and controlled for several extraneous variables; pain measured at start of study and every hour for the 3 study hours.	110 primiparous women in the active phase of labor; 23% did not complete the 3 posttests; no differences between those who withdrew and those who remained in the study; mean age = 24 (3).	Sensory and affective pain separately measured on a horizontal 100-mm VAS	Patients listened to their choice of soft music for first 3 hours of active labor.	Groups were equivalent at baseline, but the control group reported more severe sensations and distress of pain at the three posttests ($p < .05$) and had greater gains than the music group.	As pain increased with labor time, reliability of VAS scales was reduced; may have a ceiling effect on the VAS on the latter posttests.

(continues)

BPI = Brief Pain Inventory; IASP = International Association for the Study of Pain; MPQ-SF = McGill Pain Questionnaire-Short Form; NRS = numerical rating scale; PPI = present pain intensity; PRI = pain rating index; RCT = randomized controlled trial; SF-36 = Medical Outcomes Study-Short Form; VAS = visual analogue scale.

TABLE 5-1 Studies Investigating the Relationship Between Nursing Interventions and Pain as a Symptom Outcome (continued)

Author/date	Design	Sample characteristics/setting	Definition of the outcome concept	Intervention being evaluated	Results	Limitations
Puntillo & Ley (2004)	Randomized double-blind quasi-experimental trial; pain measured before, during, and 20-minutes after chest tube removal.	Convenience sample of 74 patients who had a chest tube inserted during cardiac surgery; mean age = 65.9 (11.4); 74.3% male; tubes removed 26 (12) hours after surgery	Pain intensity and pain distress measured using 0–10 NRS; pain quality measured using MPQ-SF; level of sedation measured using Observer's Assessment of Alertness/Sedation Scale	Four interventions: (1) 4 mg intravenous morphine + procedure information; (2) 30 mg intravenous ketorolac + procedure information; (3) 4 mg intravenous morphine + procedure information + sensory information related to procedure; and (4) 30 mg intravenous ketorolac + procedure information + sensory information related to procedure	Pain intensity ($F = 0.82$; $p = 0.49$), pain distress ($F = 2.48$; $P = .07$), and levels of sedation ($F = 0.47$; $P = .71$) did not differ significantly across time among the four treatment groups; pain quality also did not differ between groups.	Lack of a control group; small sample size; generalizability is quite limited.
Seers & Carroll (1998)	Systematic review of published studies of relaxation techniques	Seven RCTs involving 362 patients, of whom 150 received relaxation; 33/40 studies excluded: 11 not RCTs, 22 RCTs for small sample size less than 10/group, combination interventions, and/or no pain outcomes; six settings were after surgery and one during femoral angiography	Pain (VAS 0–10, MPQ), analgesic data, and length of stay from chart	Relaxation techniques including imagery, hypnosis, visualization, and cognitive therapy	Three studies reported less pain and/or distress if used muscle relaxation with or without imagery, but methodology and validity problems; no difference for 4 remaining vigorously-designed studies.	Heterogeneity amongst studies
Seers et al. (2004)	RCT; convenience sample randomly assigned to intervention and control groups; patient records audited at 3 months for both groups; intervention then implemented on control wards and outcomes reassessed after 3 months	120 patients (>18 years) from four surgical wards; healthcare professionals on two wards received intervention; extensive demographic data reported for various stages on each ward	Pain intensity using a 0–10 scale	Interactive sessions with healthcare professionals describing the need for the study, choice of drugs, principles of evidence-based health care, and a facilitation and change workshop	No significant difference between intervention and control groups at 3 months; control group changed from baseline to 3 months, suggesting an external bias unknown to the researchers.	At baseline, the control group had significantly more pain at rest; one control ward was female only; performance bias possible on control wards; authors reported difficulties standardizing the intervention; control ward changed during intervention period.

			Nonpharmacological methods		Heterogeneity among studies; pooled effect size 0.06
Sindhu (1996)	Meta-analysis of RCTs assessing the effectiveness of nonpharmacological interventions for pain management	49 RCTs (14 unpublished) of nonpharmacological therapies in acute pain management with 3,357 patients		Strong heterogeneity between studies making pooled effect size of 0.06 (range −2.25 to 1.78) difficult to interpret; subgroup analysis also showed considerable heterogeneity, although some evidence that patient teaching and relaxation reduced pain scores	Heterogeneity among studies; pooled effect size 0.06
Tanabe et al. (2001)	Three-group RCT; prospective data collection at baseline and 30 and 60 minutes postintervention	76 patients in an emergency department of a suburban U.S. hospital, with pain rating ≥ 4 (0–10) from minor extremity trauma distal to and including the knee or elbow; mean (SD) age = 41 (18)	Pain intensity (NRS 0–10) and two questions for satisfaction related to total treatment (Likert scale 1–6) and binary yes/no response to immediate attention in triage	Use of ibuprofen or music along with standard care of ice, elevation, and immobilization	Standard care alone, or with ibuprofen or music, did not decrease moderate pain with musculoskeletal trauma.	Small sample size and nonrandom assignment
Tsay et al. (2008)	Two-group RCT with outcomes assessed at baseline (T1) and Day 5 (MPQ-SF), and daily to Day 5 (VAS)	62 postoperative gastric and liver cancer patients from four wards—1 lost from control group (n = 30); mean (SD) age = 59.8 (14.70); 52.46% female	Pain intensity measured by the MPQ-SF (T1 & Day 5) and a VAS (0–100, T1 & daily to Day 5)	Intervention group received 20-min foot reflexology Days 2, 3, and 4 after surgery, plus usual analgesic care received by controls.	Less pain and as-needed opioid analgesic use were demonstrated for the intervention group.	Usual care not clear; PCA opioid analgesic given for 4 days to both groups was not analyzed; no discussion of effect of attention to intervention group; not "double-blinded" as stated.
Ward et al. (2000)	Randomized two-group pilot over an 18-month period; consenting adults randomly allocated to care-as-usual (n = 22) or informational intervention group (n = 21); measures at baseline, 1-, and 2-month follow-up after education intervention.	43 women with metastatic gynecological cancers in a U.S. outpatient comprehensive care cancer center; attrition by third interview = 41%; reason given was too ill. No difference in dropout between groups; mean (SD) age = 58(12); RR = 56%	Pain intensity: Now, worst pain, and least pain in last week (BPI-NRS 0–10); congruence between severity of pain and medication used (Pain Management Index); interference in activities (BPI); Concerns by Barriers Questionnaire.	Pain information vs usual care; individually tailored information about concerns (barriers) and side effect management discussed related to a booklet previously developed; two highest rated concerns then clarified; booster telephone calls given at 1 week postintervention and post time two measures.	No differential improvement in outcome evident for any group; both groups reported decrease in barriers and pain interference.	Small sample size and attrition = 41%, may be floor effect due to selection bias as refusal related to severe pain; short follow-up; intervention did not explore basis for individual barriers.

(continues)

BPI = Brief Pain Inventory; IASP = International Association for the Study of Pain; MPQ-SF = McGill Pain Questionnaire-Short Form; NRS = numerical rating scale; PPI = present pain intensity; PRI = pain rating index; RCT = randomized controlled trial; SF-36 = Medical Outcomes Study-Short Form; VAS = visual analogue scale.

TABLE 5-1   Studies Investigating the Relationship Between Nursing Interventions and Pain as a Symptom Outcome (continued)

Author/date	Design	Sample characteristics/setting	Definition of the outcome concept	Intervention being evaluated	Results	Limitations
Ward et al. (2008)	Two-group RCT with outcome and mediating variables assessed at baseline (T1), 1 month (T2) later, and 2 months (T3) later	176 patients with pain related to metastatic cancer from outpatient oncology clinics; subjects were stratified by level of pain before being randomized; no difference in dropout between groups; mean age = 55.11; attrition rate = 14.8%	Pain intensity: Now, worst pain, and least pain in last week (BPI-NRS 0–10); congruence between severity of pain and medication used (Pain Management Index); interference in activities (BPI); Concerns by Barriers Questionnaire.	RIDcancer educational intervention: Patient describes beliefs about pain, pain-related misbeliefs are discussed, misbeliefs are addressed and replaced, benefits of adopting information is discussed; session lasts 20–60 minutes for each patient, and a telephone call follow-up takes place 2–3 days later.	No difference in pain intensity from T1 to T2; treatment group had reduced usual severity of pain between T1 and T3 vs the control group ($p < .01$); no group differences for pain interference or well-being; regression showed that change in patients' barrier scores mediated change in usual severity of pain from T1 to T3.	Dropouts had higher baseline pain severity and pain interference than those completing the study; difference between T2 and T3 not addressed; change scores used for analyses; some selection bias for patients with low pain ratings at baseline; authors' limitations oriented to explain why an effect was not discovered, showing some bias.
Watt-Watson, Stevens et al. (2000)	RCT pilot, consenting adults randomly allocated to control (standard care) or two treatment conditions (standard + booklet or standard + booklet and interview) measures at preadmission clinic and Days 3 and 5 after surgery.	Of 50 consenting patients, 45 responded at all three periods; 2 from Group 2 too ill at Day 3; 3 too ill to complete any measures after surgery; patients were having their first elective coronary artery bypass graft surgery in Toronto; mean (SD) age = 60.46 (9.49), 5 women.	Pain intensity and quality (NRS 0–10 [rest on movement, present, & past 24 hours]; analgesic data from chart; interference in activities (interference subscale of BPI); concerns measured by short form of Barriers Questionnaire.	Pain education; eight-page pain-focused booklet given to patients prior to surgery	No significant differences using ANOVA among three groups for pain, including worst 24h NRS Day 3: $X = 6.63 \pm 2.46$; Day 5: $X = 6.0 \pm 2.91$; PPI Day 3: $X = 2.43 \pm 1.07$; Day 5: $X = 2.29 \pm 1.06$. No differences for interference because of pain or analgesia; intervention groups had significantly fewer concerns ($F2$, $42 = 4.17, p < 0.02$) and were more satisfied with treatment ($F2,40 = 2.96$, $p < 0.06$).	

| Watt-Watson et al. (2004) | RCT, consenting adults randomly allocated to standard care + booklet or standard care only; pain measured at baseline and on Days 3 and 5 postsurgery | 406 elective patients undergoing their first coronary artery bypass graft surgery; loss to follow-up or patient being too ill led to 183 in treatment and 177 in control groups; mean age = 61.8; 14.7% female | Pain-related interference in activities in the previous 24 h using interference subscale of the BPI (BPI-I); pain measured by the MPQ-SF; analgesics prescribed and administered | Eight-page booklet, *Pain Relief After Surgery*, developed from previous research given to patients prior to surgery, discussed with individual patients and families for ~20 minutes | No significant differences using RM ANOVA among groups for pain-related interference ($p = 0.49$) or NRS scores ($p = 0.3$); at Day 5, control group reported more pain-related interference ($p < .01$); women had significantly more interference due to pain than men ($p < .05$). | Gender data based on small sample of female patients; health-care professionals' lack of understanding of pain management problematic. |

BPI = Brief Pain Inventory; IASP = International Association for the Study of Pain; MPQ-SF = McGill Pain Questionnaire-Short Form; NRS = numerical rating scale; PPI = present pain intensity; PRI = pain rating index; RCT = randomized controlled trial; SF-36 = Medical Outcomes Study-Short Form; VAS = visual analogue scale.

Nonpharmacologic Strategies

Broscious (1999) demonstrated no significant differences in NRS scores for pain intensity with the music intervention group during chest-tube removal for elective open heart surgical patients. Tanabe et al. (2001) also reported no clinically significant pain relief for patients with moderate pain from minor musculoskeletal pain in the emergency department, using standard care (ice, elevation, immobilization) alone or with ibuprofen or music. However, positive results were demonstrated in three trials. Good et al. (2001) found that music alone or with relaxation, or relaxation alone, did reduce pain at rest and on ambulation for patients following abdominal surgery. McCaffrey and Freeman (2003) also found that music for 20 minutes a day for 14 days reduced chronic osteoarthritic pain for community-living people older than 66 years of age. Phumdoung and Good's (2003) music intervention for primiparous women in early labor provided significant pain relief. However, in a systematic review of 51 studies involving 3,663 patients to evaluate the effect of music on acute, chronic, or cancer pain intensity, pain relief, and analgesic requirements, Cepeda, Carr, Lau, and Alvarez (2006) concluded that music should not be considered a first-line treatment for pain relief because the magnitude of positive effects, and therefore, the clinical relevance in clinical practice, remains unclear.

A Cochrane review to evaluate the effectiveness of touch therapies (including healing touch, therapeutic touch, and reiki) on relieving both acute and chronic pain concluded that the studies had methodological limitations and only a modest effect. Nursing studies have included therapeutic touch; Keller and Bzdek (1986) reported greater pain relief for this group on the MPQ at the first posttest time, which did not last to the 4-hour time for university volunteers with tension headaches. In contrast, Meehan (1993) found that therapeutic touch did not make any difference in pain intensity on a VAS for elective abdominal or pelvic surgical patients. Kubsch et al. (2000) reported significant reductions in pain intensity and interference scores using a VAS for patients receiving cutaneous stimulation in an emergency setting. Women in King et al.'s (2006) breast compression undergarment group after sternotomy had less breast pain but not sternotomy pain and distress compared with the usual care group. Although positive outcomes were demonstrated for foot reflexology (Tsay et al., 2008), major methodological issues were evident in this study.

Two nursing systematic reviews that examined the benefits of nonpharmacological nursing interventions also pointed to equivocal findings. Sindhu (1996) found some evidence that relaxation reduces pain scores, although heterogeneity in design and methods between studies made findings of this meta-analysis difficult to interpret. Similarly, Seers and Carroll (1998) found that three studies with methodological problems did report reduced pain with muscle relaxation with or without imagery; however, four other more rigorously designed studies reported no differences.

Patient Education

Patient education interventions have increasingly attended to individual learning needs, working with standardized information and face-to-face and/or telephone methods. Ahles et al. (2001) reported that patients from four rural primary care practices who received a telephone-based nurse educator pain intervention scored significantly better than controls on pain; physical, emotional, and social SF-36 subscales; and functional interference scores. Also, Closs et al. (1999) demonstrated significant reductions in overnight pain intensity on a 1–5 verbal descriptor scale for orthopedic patients receiving a pain education booklet, although analgesic administration did not differ between groups. Clotfelter (1999) also found that older cancer patients who received a booklet and saw a video reported less pain on a VAS than the control group. Similarly, McDonald et al.'s (2001) sample of elderly patients receiving pain education related to communication, management, and intensity scales reported less pain after total hip or knee replacement surgery. Ward et al. (2000) reported that all women with metastatic gynecological cancer in a trial of individually tailored information about concerns and side effect management experienced less pain interference (BPI-interference) at 1 month regardless of their randomized group. In contrast, Neitzel et al. (1999) demonstrated no decrease in pain on a VAS for an orthopedic group who received a pain booklet. Watt-Watson, Stevens, Costello, Katz, and Reid (2000) also found no significant differences in pain on the MPQ-SF or in analgesic administration for coronary bypass surgical patients receiving a randomized controlled trial (RCT) pilot pain education booklet.

Four more recent studies that were designed to offer patients individualized education as compared with usual care also reported mixed results. Dalton et al.'s (2004) cognitive- behavioral therapy-focused 50-minute sessions were tailored to individual patients and reduced worst cancer pain scores, interference with sleep, and confusion up to a month. Watt-Watson et al.'s (2004) booklet addressing consequences of unrelieved acute pain, ways to communicate pain, common misbeliefs and concerns about pain management and management strategies, along with a discussion of questions and concerns, did not demonstrate differences with the usual care group for pain ratings or analgesic use up to 5 days after coronary artery bypass graft surgery; however, the intervention group had significantly lower scores for interference with usual activities and concerns, including concerns about addiction, at Day 5. Miaskowski et al.'s (2004) PRO-SELF Pain Control Program with individualized tailored sessions involving home visits and telephone interviews for oncology outpatients did result in reductions in most pain ratings. Ward et al.'s (2008) positive RIDcancer educational intervention addressed cancer patients' beliefs and misbeliefs in the initial 20- to 60-minute session and included telephone follow-up; usual pain severity scores were reduced between baseline and 3 months, mediated by changes in patients' beliefs about pain.

Three RCTs with rigorous methodology demonstrated positive outcomes using a version of Lorig's Arthritis Self-Management Program. All these psychoeducation programs included 2-hour sessions weekly for 6 weeks that were standardized but allowed for individual choice of priority management strategies and pacing. Two programs were delivered by an experienced health professional (LeFort et al., 1998; McGillion et al., 2008) and the third by an experienced peer (Lorig et al., 2005). LeFort et al. found that a community patient sample with chronic noncancer pain reported reduced pain severity on the MPQ and a VAS at 3 months following her Chronic Pain Self-Management Program. Similarly, McGillion et al.'s (2008) Chronic Angina Self-Management Program resulted in improved anginal pain symptoms using the SF-36 and the Seattle Angina Questionnaire, and an improved ability to manage pain at 3 months. Lorig et al. followed patients for the longest period, up to 1 year, in comparing the specific Arthritis Self-Management Program (ASMP) with the more general Chronic Disease Self-Management Program for arthritis patients; pain scores (NRS, 0–10) improved in both but significantly more so in the specific ASMP. These results support the adapted versions for specific populations demonstrated by LeFort et al. and McGillion et al.

Nurses' Education

Educational pain-focused programs for nurses have resulted in reduced pain scores for patients having thoracic (Dahlman et al., 1999), colon, or breast surgery (Francke et al., 1977) and for those in a home care hospice program (Holzheimer et al., 1999). De Rond and colleagues (1999, 2000) concluded from their findings that using a simple numerical rating scale along with pain education for nurses improved the analgesic administration for medical and surgical patients in three Dutch hospitals. De Wit and Van Dam (2001) found that district nurses who received additional information about the pain of patients being discharged to them better estimated patients' pain intensity and were more satisfied with patients' pain management, but were no different from the control group on assessing patients' relief. However, Neitzel et al. (1999) demonstrated no statistically significant decrease in pain ratings for an orthopedic patient sample despite their being given educational material either before admission or postoperatively. Outcome data are yet to be reported for an 8-week program for nurses working with surgical patients (Dalton et al., 1999). Across studies, variability was evident in the length of programs (3–13.5 hours) and duration of teaching (1 day to 8 weeks).

More recent studies have continued to focus on nurse and/or health team education as a way to improve patient education and pain management outcomes (Bédard et al., 2006; Edwards et al., 2005; Seers et al., 2004). Bédard et al.'s intervention involved a new evidence-based guideline including preprinted orders, posters, and a 2-day course on pain management for clinicians. Patients were given pain management materials along with a discussion about their beliefs and ways to manage their pain. Positive outcomes included more patient evidence-based orders, lower pain scores, less interference with usual activities, and reduction in some concerns about asking for help. Edwards et al. educated 10 community nurses through seminars and treatment guidelines about wound care; these nurses then cared for patients in the home versus a weekly club setting, offering an informal drop-in environment for socialization and support as well as information. At 12 weeks, the group attending the club had significantly reduced pain levels and related interference with mood, sleep, and usual work as compared with the group receiving nursing care at home. Seers et al. (2004) also used an evidence-based intervention with clinicians from two surgical wards; the four interactive sessions focused on baseline audits, analgesic algorithms, critical appraisal principles, and change approaches. There were no significant differences in pain levels or use of drugs between the intervention and control wards, probably because changes in practice occurred in the control wards as well.

Individual Nurse Feedback

Duncan and Pozehl (2000) demonstrated a statistically significant decline in mean pain ratings and an increase in analgesic use for orthopedic patients when nurses received performance feedback about their pain management practices. Nurses were evaluated on four practices that included pain assessments every 4 hours, assessments after analgesic administration, action for unacceptable pain ratings, and documentation of the patient's acceptable pain level. Each nurse received a copy of the feedback and a pain treatment flow chart. Although Holzheimer et al. (1999) included performance improvement monitors as a part of their nurse intervention, this component's effectiveness was not reported.

In summary, a significant improvement in pain following nursing intervention was reported in some of the studies reviewed. However, responses to these pain interventions are equivocal, which may relate more to issues such as the individuality of the pain experience, complexity of the pain management context, and/or methodology issues like uncontrolled designs than to the measures themselves. When the evidence from the most rigorous clinical trials is examined, nursing interventions such as patients' and nurses' education improved patients' pain outcomes. However, the interventions vary considerably in both design and implementation. Nevertheless, based on the evidence from the clinical trials, there is reason to suggest that pain is an outcome that is relevant and sensitive to nursing practice.

EVIDENCE CONCERNING APPROACHES TO MEASUREMENT

This review included only those measures used to examine the relationship between nursing interventions and patient outcomes related to pain. Three measures of pain sensation and/or pain-related impact on usual activities were identified in this review of the empirical nursing literature. The following characteristics of these measures are summarized in **TABLE 5-2**: (a) target population; (b) domains of measurement, number of items, and response format; (c) method of administration; (d) reliability; (e) validity; and (f) sensitivity to nursing intervention.

The approach to assessing pain in all studies was to use the instrument as a self-report measure or interview guide. Therefore, the inclusion criteria for all studies included the ability to speak, read, and understand the primary language of the country (i.e., Dutch, English); patients were excluded if they were cognitively impaired. All patients in this review were adults; because pain is a subjective phenomenon, this approach was appropriate.

The most frequently used approach to examine outcomes has focused on pain intensity, along with its location and/or temporal features. Unidimensional measures to document pain intensity have included visual analogue scales or numerical rating scales, the latter having clinical utility and established reliability and validity. In 20 studies in this review, additional measures were used to examine pain, mainly the short forms of the MPQ and/or components of the BPI. To assess both the qualitative and quantitative aspects of pain sensation, Melzack (1975) developed the MPQ to include not only a VAS for pain intensity but also adjectives that patients could use to describe the sensory, affective, and evaluative components of pain sensation. From the MPQ, Daut et al. (1983) developed the BPI, a multidimensional measure that examines the impact of pain on mood and usual activities, and the person's response to treatment. The use of the longer or shorter versions of the MPQ and BPI depends on the nursing context, that is, shorter forms for more acute care settings.

The three measures that were used almost exclusively in the 41 studies selected for this review include the (a) VASs and/or the NRS version, (b) MPQ, and (c) Brief Pain Inventory (BPI).

Visual Analogue Scale/Numerical Rating Scale

The VASs have been used primarily to measure patients' perceived pain intensity or pain relief. The NRS is an alternative format that asks patients to verbally choose a number between 0 (*no pain*) and 10 (*worst pain ever*) instead of marking their intensity on a line. Scott and Huskisson (1976) established that retest reliability of the VAS was higher (0.94) with literate patients than with nonliterate ones (0.71), whereas the NRS did not differ significantly because of literacy

(0.96 and 0.95, respectively). Responses have been defined as *mild* (1–3), *moderate* (4–6), or *severe* (7–10) (Cleeland & Syrjala, 1992).

The sensitivity to change in pain over time was evident in several nursing trials in this review for both VAS (Clotfelter, 1999; Dahlman et al., 1999; Kubsch et al., 2000; McCaffrey & Freeman, 2003; Meehan, 1993; Phumdoung & Good, 2003; Seers & Carroll, 1998; Sindhu, 1996) and NRS (Ahles et al., 2001; Bédard et al., 2006; Dalton et al., 1999; De Rond et al., 1999, 2000; Duncan & Pozehl, 2000; Francke et al., 1997; Good et al., 2001; Holzheimer et al., 1999; King et al., 2006; Kubsch et al.; Kwekkeboom et al., 2003, 2008; Lorig et al., 2005; Miaskowski et al., 2004; Tsay et al., 2008; Ward et al., 2008). Although both kinds of measures were used in the studies reviewed, the NRS was used in the majority of studies, perhaps because of its greater clinical utility. NRSs are easier to administer and score, require no costs for measures, and have a high rate of correct response regardless of literacy (Ferraz, Quaresma, & Aquino, 1990; Guyutt, Townsend, & Berman, 1987).

McGill Pain Questionnaire

The long form of the MPQ includes (a) a diagram for pain location; (b) a global pain rating scale (Present Pain Intensity [PPI]); (c) sensory, affective, and evaluative adjectives (Pain Rating Index [PRI]); and (d) adjectives to describe the pattern in relation to duration and frequency of pain. The short form of the MPQ includes a VAS for pain intensity, a global pain rating scale (PPI), and sensory, affective, and evaluative adjectives (PRI). Both forms of the MPQ are easy to score. However, difficulties may arise with interpreting some of the adjectives, particularly if English is not the participant's first language. No manual is available for administration instructions or scoring procedures, which must be gleaned from Melzack's (1975) original paper (Wilkie, Savedra, Holzemer, Tesler, & Paul, 1990). The time required to complete the MPQ-LF has been found to be greater than the 10–15 minutes reported by Melzack (1975). McGuire (1984) observed that hospitalized cancer patients required an average of 24 minutes to complete the MPQ. Moreover, Cohen and Tate (1989) described the MPQ as too long for their postoperative sample and recommended using a shorter version. The MPQ-SF requires at least 5 minutes to complete and has been used with acutely ill patients, such as those undergoing surgery (Watt-Watson, Garfinkel et al., 2000; Watt-Watson et al., 2004), chest-tube removal (Puntillo & Ley, 2004), or those living in the community with chronic arthritic pain (McCaffrey & Freeman, 2003) or fibromyalgia (Menzies et al., 2006). The VAS of the MPQ-SF can be replaced with NRSs for clinical utility.

Of the 10 studies using one or more components of the MPQ, sensitivity to change was evident over time for a continuing education trial of nurses working in acute care (Francke et al., 1997), for a chronic pain self-management trial (LeFort

TABLE 5-2   Instruments Measuring Pain

Instrument (author)	Target population	Domains (number of items and response format)	Method of administration	Reliability	Validity	Sensitivity to nursing care
Brief Pain Inventory (Cleeland & Syrjala, 1992)	Adults	20 items; pain history, etiology, intensity, location, quality, and interference with activities	Self-administered	Internal consistency of pain intensity range from 0.80 to 0.86 (McDowell & Newell, 1996); reliability for the interference subscale range from 0.86 to 0.91 (McDowell & Newell).	Discriminant validity (Cleeland, 1991); construct validity (McDowell & Newell)	Sensitivity to change in 5-day postoperative period in a nursing study (Watt-Watson, Stevens et al., 2000; Watt-Watson et al., 2004), but not sustainable at 2 months (Ward et al., 2000) or 6 months (Dalton et al., 2004)
McGill Pain Questionnaire (Melzack, 1975, 1987)	Adults	Domains: (1) body outline for pain location; (2) present pain intensity (6 items); (3) a pain rating index (78 adjectives); and (4) pain pattern (9 items)	Self-report or by interview	Good test-retest reliability (Wilkie et al., 1990)	Construct (Lowe, Walker, & McCallum, 1991) and concurrent validity (Dudgeon, Raubertas, & Rosenthal, 1993)	Sensitivity to change in a nursing evaluation of a pain self-management trial (LeFort et al., 1998); an education trial for nurses in acute care (Francke et al., 1997); a surgical patient education trial (McDonald et al., 2001); and a music intervention for people with osteoarthritic persistent pain (McCaffrey & Freeman, 2003)

Visual analogue scale (VAS) and numeric rating scales (NRSs): numerous author-generated versions (McDowell & Newell, 1996)	Adolescent and cognitively intact adults	One item measuring, measured with 11-point scale; perceived pain intensity or relief	Self-administered	High test-retest reliability (Scott & Huskisson, 1976; Grossman, Sheidler, Swedeen, Mucenski, & Piantadosi, 1991)	Concurrent, construct validity (Grossman et al.; Jenson, Karoly, & Braver, 1986; Jenson, Karoly, O'Riordan, Bland, & Burns, 1989; Price, Bush, Long, & Harkins, 1994)	Evidence of sensitivity to change in nursing trials for the VAS (Clotfelter, 1999; Dahlman et al., 1999; Kubsch et al., 2000; McCaffrey & Freeman, 2003; Meehan, 1993; Phumdoung & Good, 2003; Seers & Carroll, 1998) and for the NRS (Ahles et al., 2001; Bédard et al., 2006; De Rond at al., 1999, 2000; Duncan & Pozehl, 2000; Francke et al., 1997; Good et al., 2001; Holzheimer et al., 1999; King et al., 2006; Kubsch et al., 2000; Kwekkeboom et al., 2003, 2008; Lorig et al., 2005 Miaskowski et al., 2004; Tsay et al., 2008; Ward et al., 2008).

et al., 1998), for a surgical patient education trial (McDonald et al., 2001), and for a music intervention for people with persistent osteoarthritic pain (McCaffrey & Freeman, 2003). In contrast, no change in MPQ scores over time was demonstrated in Keller and Bzdek's (1986) trial of therapeutic touch; in Menzies et al.'s (2006) trial of imagery with fibromyalgia patients; in Watt-Watson, Stevens et al.'s (2000) pilot and later trial (Watt-Watson et al., 2004) of a pain booklet for surgical patients; in Puntillo and Ley's (2004) trial about chest tube removal with cardiac surgical patients; or in Tsay et al.'s (2008) trial of foot reflexology. Those studies, including a VAS or NRS, were also discussed in the previous section, Visual Analogue Scale/Numerical Rating Scale.

Brief Pain Inventory

The BPI is a multidimensional pain measure that addresses pain history, etiology, intensity, location, quality, and interference with activities. A subscale can be used to measure how much pain interferes with everyday function in the seven categories of mood, walking, other physical activities, work, social activity, relations with others, and sleep (BPI-I). The standard measure takes 10–15 minutes to complete, and results are comparable for the self- and interviewer-administered versions. The BPI-short form has even more clinical utility because it is short, easy to read, self-administered, and easy to score. The BPI has been recommended as a comprehensive tool in the Cancer Pain Management Clinical Practice Guidelines (AHCPR, 1994). The BPI-SF is incorporated in the American Pain Society Patient Outcome Questionnaire to be used for quality improvement initiatives (American Pain Society Quality of Care Committee, 1995). However, only four studies (Dalton et al., 2004; Ward et al., 2000; Watt-Watson et al., 2004; Watt-Watson, Stevens et al., 2000) used any form of the BPI in the studies reviewed.

The BPI-I was sensitive to changes over the 5-day postoperative period (Watt-Watson et al., 2004; Watt-Watson, Stevens et al., 2000). However, as Ward et al. (2000) reported, it demonstrated decreased interference for both control and intervention groups of gynecological cancer patients 2 months after the intervention; the time period may have been too long to detect any immediate change resulting from the information given. Dalton et al. (2004) also found that the demonstrated initial improvement from a cognitive behavioral therapy intervention decreased by 6 months. In summary, all measures reviewed have well-established reliability and validity in nursing studies that examined pain and/or its impact with patients in a variety of clinical settings. In addition, these measures have been translated into several languages and are useful for nurses working with multicultural patients. The shorter versions of the MPQ and BPI measures have greater clinical utility than the other forms. However, the NRS, although unidimensional, has demonstrated the most clinical utility of all measures, particularly with people who have less education. The BPI is unique in that it examines broader issues of the impact of pain that would be important to assess, particularly for people with persistent pain. Also, the BPI can be used as a long, short, or interference subscale version, all with established reliability and validity. This review affords considerable evidence that VASs and NRSS are sensitive to changes in outcomes. In addition, the MPQ and the BPI are both sensitive measures that include important outcomes other than pain intensity. It is noteworthy that the short form of the BPI has been used in acute pain settings and with cancer patients in the studies in this review.

RECOMMENDATIONS AND DIRECTIONS FOR FUTURE RESEARCH

Intervention studies have not always measured patient outcomes, particularly in evaluating the effectiveness of nurses' pain education programs. What nurses say they know and believe about pain may not be reflected in their practices (Watt-Watson, Garfinkel et al., 2000; Watt-Watson et al., 2004), and changes in knowledge and beliefs in a posttest may not be retained over time (Howell, Butler, Vincent, Watt-Watson, & Stearns, 2000). Therefore, patient outcomes that are responsive to a variety of interventions are critical to changing practices.

In this review, the most frequently chosen pain outcomes were pain intensity and analgesic administration, which reflect nursing pain management practices, particularly with acute pain problems. The measures chosen, mainly VAS/ NRS and MPQ, were sensitive to these outcomes: Change was demonstrated in response to nursing interventions. Where change did not occur, outcomes may have been influenced by the complexity of the pain management context or methodological issues; results may not be related to the measure. Several studies used a pretest/posttest design with two different groups and did not discuss intervening variables that could have confounded the study results.

In the future, multidimensional measures must be used to determine the degree to which interventions affect an outcome, reflecting not only the sensory experience of pain but also its effect on change in usual activities. Pain intensity and function or disability are not necessarily correlated, given that tissue damage is not directly proportional to pain (Melzack & Wall, 1965). Therefore, data about other outcomes, such as the degree to which pain-related interference continues despite intervention, would provide a clearer picture of the efficacy and utility of the intervention. Only four studies in this review used interference related to pain as an outcome measure. Pain measures such as the VAS and MPQ are responsive to changes in pain intensity. However, measures such as the BPI allow a multi-dimensional assessment of pain that would give more direction to nursing interventions and form a better basis for evaluating the effectiveness of nursing care.

Nurse and patient factors can influence pain assessment. Interventions in the future need to be focused to a greater degree on both nurses' and patients' beliefs and concerns about pain management, and the impact of any intervention needs to be evaluated by using patient-related outcomes. Further work is needed to examine relationships between outcomes such as pain and analgesic use, and those reflecting pain-related activities and beliefs. Although pain outcomes after an intervention did not change in two studies, concerns about taking analgesics were significantly reduced (Ward et al., 2000; Watt-Watson, Stevens et al., 2000; Watt-Watson et al., 2004). Therefore, we need to include different kinds of outcomes for assessing the effectiveness of nursing interventions within this domain of practice. Pain is one such outcome, but others are relevant, including patients' concerns about following effective treatments.

REFERENCES

Agency for Health Care Policy and Research. (1994). *Management of cancer pain: Clinical practice guidelines* (No. 94–0692). Rockville, MD: U.S. Department of Health and Human Services.

Agency for Health Care Policy and Research. (1992). *Acute pain management: Operative or medical procedures and trauma* (No. 92–0032). Rockville, MD: U.S. Department of Health and Human Services.

Ahles, T., Seville, J., Wasson, J., Johnson, D., Callahan, E., & Stukel, T. (2001). Panel-based pain management in primary care: A pilot study. *Journal of Pain and Symptom Management, 22,* 584–590.

American Pain Society Quality of Care Committee. (1995). Quality improvement guidelines for the treatment of acute and cancer pain. *Journal of the American Medical Association, 274,* 1874–1880.

Baer, E., Davitz, L., & Lieb, R. (1970). Inferences of physical pain: In relation to verbal and nonverbal communication. *Nursing Research, 19,* 388–392.

Basbaum, A., & Jessell, T. (2000). The perception of pain. In E. Kandel, J. Schwartz, & T. Jessell (Eds.), *Principles of neural science* (pp. 472–491). New York: McGraw-Hill.

Bédard, D., Purden, M. A., Sauvé-Larose, N., Certosini, C., & Schein C. (2006). The pain experience of post surgical patients following the implementation of an evidence-based approach. *Pain Management Nursing, 7*(3), 80–92.

Benarroch, E. (2008). Descending monoaminergic pain modulation. *Neurology, 71,* 217–221.

Benedetti, C., Bonica, J., & Belluci, G. (1984). Pathophysiology and therapy of postoperative pain: A review. In C. Benedetti, C. R. Chapman, & G. Moricca (Eds.), *Recent advances in the management of pain* (pp. 373–407). New York: Raven Press.

Bernabei, R., Gambassi, G., Lapane, K., Landi, F., Gatsonis, C., Dunlop, R., et al. (1998). Management of pain in elderly patients with cancer. *Journal of the American Medical Association, 279,* 1877–1882.

Brennan, F., Carr D., & Cousins, M. (2007). Pain management: A fundamental human right. *Anesthesia Analgesia, 105,* 205–221.

Broscious, S. K. (1999). Music: An intervention for pain during chest tube removal after open heart surgery. *American Journal of Critical Care, 8,* 410–415.

Calderone, K. (1990). The influence of gender on the frequency of pain and sedative medication administered to postoperative patients. *Sex Roles, 23*, 713–725.

Carr, E. (1990). Postoperative pain: Patients' expectations and experiences. *Journal of Advanced Nursing, 15*, 89–100.

Cepeda, M. S., Carr, D. B., Lau, J., & Alvarez, H. (2006). Music for pain relief. *Cochrane Database of Systematic Reviews Issue 1* (No. CD004843). doi:10.1002/14651858.CD004843.pub2

Chen, L. M., Miaskowski, C., Dodd, M., & Pantilat, S. (2008). Concepts within the Chinese culture that influence the cancer pain experience. *Cancer Nursing, 31*(2), 103–108.

Choi, D. M., Yate, P., Coats, T., Kalinda, P., & Paul, E. (2000). Ethnicity and prescription of analgesia in an accident and emergency department: Cross sectional study. *British Medical Journal, 320*, 980–981.

Cleeland, C. (1991). Pain assessment in cancer: In D. Osoba (Ed.), *Effect of cancer on quality of life* (pp. 293–305). Florida: CRC Press.

Cleeland, C., Baez, L., Loehrer, P., & Pandya, K. (1997). Pain and treatment in minority patients with cancer. *Annals of Internal Medicine, 127*, 813–816.

Cleeland, C., & Syrjala, K. (1992). How to assess cancer pain. In D. Turk & R. Melzack (Eds.), *Handbook of pain assessment* (pp. 362–387). New York: Guilford Press.

Closs, S. J., Briggs, M., & Everitt, V. E. (1999). Implementation of research findings to reduce postoperative pain at night. *International Journal of Nursing Studies, 36*, 21–31.

Clotfelter, C. (1999). The effect of an educational intervention on decreasing pain intensity in elderly people with cancer. *Oncology Nursing Forum, 26*, 27–33.

Cohen, M., & Tate, R. (1989). Using the McGill Pain Questionnaire to study common postoperative complications. *Pain, 39*, 275–279.

Dahl, J., Gordon, D., Ward, S., Skemp, M., Wochos, S., & Schurr, M. (2003). Institutionalizing pain management: The Post-Operative Pain Management Quality Improvement Project. *Journal of Pain, 4*, 361–371.

Dahlman, G., Dykes, A., & Elander, G. (1999). Patients' evaluation of pain and nurses' management of analgesics after surgery: The effect of a study day on the subject of pain for nurses working at the thorax surgery department. *Journal of Advanced Nursing, 30*, 866–874.

Dalton, J. (1989). Nurses' perceptions of their pain assessment skills, pain management practices, and attitudes toward pain. *Oncology Nursing Forum, 16*, 225–231.

Dalton, J., Blau, W., Lindley, C., Carlson, J., Youngblood, R., & Greer, S. M. (1999). Changing acute pain management to improve patient outcomes: An educational approach. *Journal of Pain and Symptom Management, 17*, 277–287.

Dalton, J. A., Keefe, F. J., Carlson, J., & Youngblood, R. (2004). Tailoring cognitive-behavioral treatment for cancer pain. *Pain Management Nursing, 5*(1), 3–18.

Daut, R., Cleeland, C., & Flanery, R. (1983). Development of the Wisconsin Brief Pain Questionnaire to assess pain in cancer and other diseases. *Pain, 17*, 197–210.

de Rond, M., de Wit, R., van Dam, F., & Muller, M. (2000). A pain monitoring program for nurses: Effect on the administration of analgesics. *Pain, 89*, 25–38.

de Rond, M., de Wit, R., van Dam, F., van Campen, B., den Hartog, Y., Klievink, R., et al. (1999). Daily pain assessment: Value for nurses and patients. *Journal of Advanced Nursing, 29*, 436–444.

de Wit, R., & Van Dam, F. (2001). From hospital to home care: A randomized controlled trial of a pain education program for cancer patients with chronic pain. *Journal of Advanced Nursing, 36*, 742–754.

Dudgeon, D., Raubertas, R., & Rosenthal, S. (1993). The short-form of the McGill Pain Questionnaire in chronic cancer pain. *Journal of Pain and Symptom Management, 8*, 191–195.

Duggleby, W., & Lander, J. (1994). Cognitive status and postoperative pain: Older adults. *Journal of Pain and Symptom Management, 9*, 19–27.

Duncan, K., & Pozehl, B. (2000). Effects of performance feedback on patient pain outcomes. *Clinical Nursing Research, 9*, 379–401.

Edwards, H., Courtney, M., Finlayson, K., Lindsay, E., Lewis, C., Shuter, P., et al. (2005). Chronic venous leg ulcers: Effect of a community nursing intervention on pain and healing. *Nursing Standard, 19*(52), 47–54.

Faherty, B., & Grier, M. (1984). Analgesic medication for elderly people post-surgery. *Nursing Research, 33*, 369–372.

Ferraz, M., Quaresma, M., & Aquino, L. (1990). Reliability of pain scales in the assessment of literate and illiterate patients with rheumatoid arthritis. *Journal of Rheumatology, 17*, 1022–1024.

Ferrell, B., McCaffery, M., & Grant, M. (1991). Clinical decision making and pain. *Cancer Nursing, 14*, 289–297.

Fields, H. (1987). *Pain*. New York: McGraw-Hill.

Fishman, S. (2007). Recognizing pain management as a human right: A first step. *Anesthesia Analgesia, 105*, 8–9.

Francke, A. L., Garssen, B., Luiken, J. B., de Schepper, A. M. E., Grypdonck, M., & Abu-Saad, H. H. (1997). Effects of a nursing pain programme on patient outcomes. *Psycho-Oncology, 6*, 302–310.

Good, M., Stanton-Hicks, M., Grass, J., Anderson, G., Lai, H., Roykulcharoen, V., et al. (2001). Relaxation and music to reduce post surgical pain. *Journal of Advanced Nursing, 33*, 208–215.

Gordon, D., Dahl, J., Phillips, P., Frandsen, J., Cowley, C., Foster, R., et al. (2004). The use of "as-needed" range orders for opioid analgesics in management of acute pain: Consensus statement of the American Society for Pain Management Nursing and the American Pain Society. *Pain Management Nursing, 5*(2), 53–58.

Grossman, S., Sheidler, V., Swedeen, K., Mucenski, J., & Piantadosi, S. (1991). Correlation of patient and caregiver ratings of cancer pain. *Journal of Pain and Symptom Management, 6*, 53–57.

Guyutt, G., Townsend, M., & Berman, L. (1987). A comparison of Likert and visual analogue scales for measuring change in function. *Journal of Chronic Diseases, 40*, 1129–1133.

Holm, K., Cohen, F., Dudas, S., Medema, P., & Allen, B. (1989). Effect of personal pain experience on pain assessment. *Image, 21*, 72–75.

Holzheimer, A., McMillan, S. C., & Weitzner, M. (1999). Improving pain outcomes of hospice patients with cancer. *Oncology Nursing Forum, 26*, 1499–1504.

Howell, D., Butler, L., Vincent, L., Watt-Watson, J., & Stearns, N. (2000). Influencing nurses' knowledge, attitudes, and practice in cancer pain management. *Cancer Nursing, 23*, 55–63.

Jenson, M., Karoly, P., & Braver, S. (1986). The measurement of clinical pain intensity: A comparison of six methods. *Pain, 27*, 117–126.

Jenson, M., Karoly, P., O'Riordan, E., Bland, E., & Burns, R. (1989). The subjective experience of acute pain: An assessment of the utility of 10 indices. *Clinical Journal of Pain, 5*, 153–159.

Katz, J. (1997). Perioperative predictors of long-term pain following surgery. In T. Jensen, J. Turner, & Z. Wiesenfeld-Hallin (Eds.), *Proceedings of the 8th World Congress on Pain: Vol. 8. Progress in pain research and management* (pp. 231–240). Seattle: IASP Press.

Kehlet, H., Jensen, T. S., & Woolf, C. J. (2006). Persistent postsurgical pain: Risk factors and prevention. *Lancet, 367*, 1618–1625.

Keller, E., & Bzdek, V. M. (1986). Effects of therapeutic touch on tension headache pain. *Nursing Research, 35,* 101–106.

Khan, D., & Steeves, R. (1996). An understanding of suffering grounded in clinical practice and research. In B. Ferrell, *Suffering* (pp. 3–27). Sudbury, MA: Jones and Bartlett.

King, K. M., Tsuyuki, R , Faris, P., Currie, G., Maitland, A.,&. Collins-Nalai, R. (2006). A randomized controlled trial of women's early use of a novel undergarment following sternotomy: The Women's Recovery from Sternotomy Trial (WREST). *American Heart Journal, 152,* 1187–1193.

Kubsch, S. M., Neveau, T., & Vandertie, K. (2000). Effect of cutaneous stimulation on pain reduction in emergency department patients. *Complementary Therapies in Nursing and Midwifery, 6,* 25–32.

Kwekkeboom, K. L., Kneip, J., & Pearson L. (2003). A pilot study to predict success with guided imagery for cancer pain. *Pain Management Nursing, 4*(3), 112–123.

Kwekkeboom, K. L., Wanta, B., & Bumpus, M. (2008). Individual difference variables and the effects of progressive muscle relaxation and analgesic imagery interventions on cancer pain. *Journal of Pain and Symptom Management, 36,* 604–615.

Lavies, N., Hart, L., Rounsefell, B., & Runciman, W. (1992). Identification of patient, medical and nursing attitudes to postoperative opioid analgesia: Stage 1 of a longitudinal study of postoperative analgesia. *Pain, 48,* 313–319.

LeFort, S. M., Gray-Donald, K., Rowat, K. M., & Jeans, M. (1998). Randomized controlled trial of a community-based psychoeducation program for the self-management of chronic pain. *Pain, 74,* 297–306.

Lorig, K., Ritter, P. L., & Plant, K. (2005). A disease-specific self-help program compared with a generalized chronic disease self-help program for arthritis patients. *Arthritis and Rheumatism, 53,* 950–957.

Lowe, N., Walker, S., & McCallum, R. (1991). Confirming the theoretical structure of the McGill Pain Questionnaire in acute clinical pain. *Pain, 46,* 53–60.

Marks, R., & Sachar, E. (1973). Undertreatment of medical inpatients with narcotic analgesics. *Annals of Internal Medicine, 78,* 173–181.

McCaffrey, R., & Freeman, E. (2003). Effect of music on chronic osteoarthritis pain in older people. *Journal of Advanced Nursing, 44,* 517–524.

McDonald, D. (1994). Gender and ethnic stereotyping and narcotic analgesic administration. *Research in Nursing and Health, 17,* 45–49.

McDonald, D., Freeland, M., Thomas, G., & Moore, J. (2001). Testing a preoperative pain management intervention for elders. *Research in Nursing and Health, 24,* 402–409.

McDowell, I., & Newell, C. (1996). *Measuring health: A guide to rating scales and questionnaires.* New York: Oxford University Press.

McGillion, M. H., Watt-Watson, J., Stevens, B., LeFort, S. M., Coyte, P., & Graham, A. (2008). Randomized controlled trial of a psychoeducation program for the self-management of chronic cardiac pain. *Journal of Pain and Symptom Management, 36,* 126–140.

McGuire, D. (1984). The measurement of clinical pain. *Nursing Research, 33,* 152–156.

Meehan, T. C. (1993). Therapeutic touch and postoperative pain: A Rogerian research study. *Nursing Science Quarterly, 6,* 69–78.

Melzack, R. (1975). The McGill Pain Questionnaire: Major properties and scoring methods. *Pain, 1,* 277–299.

Melzack, R. (1987). The short-form McGill Pain Questionnaire. *Pain, 30,* 191–197.

Melzack, R., Abbott, F., Zackon, W., Mulder, D., & Davis, M. (1987). Pain on a surgical ward: A survey of the duration and intensity of pain and the effectiveness of medication. *Pain, 29,* 67–72.

Melzack, R., & Dennis, S. (1978). Neurophysiological foundations of pain. In R. Steinbach (Ed.), *The psychology of pain* (pp. 1–26). New York: Raven Press.

Melzack, R., & Wall, P. (1965). Pain mechanisms: A new theory. *Science, 150,* 971–979.

Menzies, V., Taylor, A. G., & Bourguignon, C. (2006). Effects of guided imagery on outcomes of pain, functional status, and self-efficacy in persons diagnosed with fibromyalgia. *Journal of Alternative and Complementary Medicine, 12*(1), 23–30.

Merskey, H., & Bogduk, N. (1994). *Classification of chronic pain: Descriptions of chronic pain syndromes and definitions of pain terms* (2nd ed.). Seattle, WA: IASP Press.

Miaskowski, C., Dodd, M., West, C., Schumacher, K., Paul, S. M., Tripathy, D., et al. (2004). Randomized clinical trial of the effectiveness of a self-care intervention to improve cancer pain management. *Journal of Clinical Oncology, 22,* 1713–1720.

Millar, W. (1996). Chronic pain. *Health Reports, 7,* 47–53.

Moulin, D., Clark, A. J., Speechley, M., & Morley-Forster, P. (2002). Chronic pain in Canada: Prevalence, treatment, impact and the role of opioid analgesia. *Pain Research and Management, 7,* 179–184.

Neitzel, J. J., Miller, E. H., Shepherd, M. F., & Belgrade, M. (1999). Improving pain management after total joint replacement surgery. *Orthopaedic Nursing, 18,* 37–64.

Oberst, M. (1978). Nurses' inferences of suffering: The effects of nurse-patient similarity, and verbalizations of distress. In M. J. Nelson (Ed.), *Clinical perspectives in nursing research* (pp. 38–60). New York: Teachers College Press.

O'Gara, P. (1988). The hemodynamic consequences of pain and its management. *Journal of Intensive Care Medicine, 3,* 3–5.

Owen, H., McMillan, V., & Rogowski, D. (1990). Postoperative pain therapy: A survey of patients' expectations and their experiences. *Pain, 41,* 303–307.

Phumdoung, S., & Good, M. (2003). Music reduces sensation and distress of labor pain. *Pain Management Nursing, 4*(2), 54–61.

Price, D., Bush, F., Long, S., & Harkins, S. (1994). A comparison of pain measurement characteristics of mechanical visual analogue and simple numerical rating scales. *Pain, 56,* 217–226.

Puntillo, K., & Ley, S. J. (2004). Appropriately timed analgesics control pain due to chest tube removal. *American Journal of Critical Care, 13,* 292–301.

Scott, J., & Huskisson, E. (1976). Graphic representation of pain. *Pain, 2,* 175–184.

Seers, K., & Carroll, D. (1998). Relaxation techniques for acute pain management: A systematic review. *Journal of Advanced Nursing, 27,* 466–475.

Seers, K., Crichton, N., Carroll, D., Richards, S., & Saunders, T. (2004). Evidence-based postoperative pain management in nursing: Is a randomized-controlled trial the most appropriate design? *Journal of Nursing Management, 12,* 183–193.

Sindhu, F. (1996). Are non-pharmacological nursing interventions for the management of pain effective?: A meta-analysis. *Journal of Advanced Nursing, 24,* 1152–1159.

Spross, J. (1996). Coaching and suffering: The role of the nurse in helping people face illness. In B. Ferrell (Ed.), *Suffering* (pp. 173–207). Sudbury, MA: Jones and Bartlett.

Tanabe, P., Thomas, R., Paice, J., Spiller, M., & Marcantonio, R. (2001). The effect of standard care, ibuprofen, and music on pain relief and patient satisfaction in adults with musculoskeletal trauma. *Journal of Emergency Nursing, 27,* 124–131.

Todd, K. H., Samaroo, N., & Hoffman, J. R. (1993). Ethnicity as a risk factor for inadequate emergency department analgesia. *Journal of the American Medical Association, 269*, 1537–1539.

Tsay, S. L., Chen, H. L., Chen, S. U., Lin, H. R., & Lin, K. C. (2008). Effects of reflexology on acute postoperative pain and anxiety among patients with digestive cancer. *Cancer Nursing, 31*, 109–115.

Wall, P. (1996). Comments after 30 years of the gate control theory. *Pain Forum, 5*(1), 12–22.

Ward, S., Carlson-Dakes, K., Hughes, S., Kwekkeboom, K., & Donovan, H. (1998). The impact of patient-related barriers to pain management on quality of life. *Research in Nursing and Health, 21*, 405–413.

Ward, S., Donovan, H., Owen, B., Grosen, E., & Serlin, R. (2000). An individualized intervention to overcome patient-related barriers to pain management in women with gynecologic cancers. *Research in Nursing and Health, 23*, 393–405.

Ward, S., Goldberg, N., Miller-McCauley, B., Mueller, C., Nolan, A., Pawlik-Plank, D., et al. (1993). Patient-related barriers to management of cancer pain. *Pain, 52*, 319–324.

Ward, S., Gunnarsdottir, S., Shapiro, G. S., Donovan, H., Serlin, R. C., & Hughes, S. (2008). A randomized trial of representational intervention to decrease cancer pain (RIDcancerPain). *Health Psychology, 27*, 59–67.

Watt-Watson, J., Choiniere, M., Carrier, M., Cogan, J., Bussieres, J., Costello, J., et al. (2008). Risk factors in the transition of acute to chronic pain after cardiac surgery. *Canadian Cardiovascular Congress, Abstract 0386*, 151.

Watt-Watson, J., Garfinkel, P., Gallop, R., Stevens, B., & Streiner, D. (2000). The impact of nurses' empathic responses on patients' pain management in acute care. *Nursing Research, 49*, 1–10.

Watt-Watson, J., Stevens, B., Costello, J., Katz, J., & Reid, G. (2000). Impact of preoperative education on pain management outcomes after coronary artery bypass graft surgery: A pilot. *Canadian Journal of Nursing Research, 31*, 41–56.

Watt-Watson, J., Stevens, B., Katz, J., Costello, J., Reid, G. J., & David, T. (2004). Impact of preoperative education on pain outcomes after coronary artery bypass graft surgery. *Pain, 109*, 73–85.

Watt-Watson, J., Stevens, B., Streiner, D., Garfinkel, P., & Gallop, R. (2001). Relationship between nurses' pain knowledge and pain management outcomes for their postoperative cardiac patients. *Journal of Advanced Nursing, 36*, 535–545.

Wilkie, D., Savedra, M., Holzemer, W., Tesler, M., & Paul, S. (1990). Use of the McGill Pain Questionnaire to measure pain: A meta-analysis. *Nursing Research, 39*, 36–41.

Winefield, H., Katsikitis, M., Hart, L., & Rounsefell, B. (1990). Postoperative pain experiences: Relevant patient and staff attitudes. *Journal of Psychosomatic Research, 34*, 543–552.

Woolf, C. J., & Salter M. W. (2000). Neuronal plasticity: Increasing the gain in pain. *Science, 288*, 1765–1768.

Adverse Patient Outcomes

Peggy White, RN, MN
Linda McGillis Hall, RN, PhD, FAAN
Michelle Lalonde, RN, MN

INTRODUCTION

Patient safety is a rising concern in health care today. People enter the healthcare system trusting that the system will not harm them. However, increasing evidence suggests that this may not always be true. Although serious problems in the quality of health care are infrequent compared with the amount of care provided, when they do occur, they can have devastating consequences for patients and their families (Kohn, Corrigan, & Donaldson, 2000). Reports on errors and adverse events in the United States, the United Kingdom, and Canada depict a system that is fragmented and prone to errors. These documents have heightened awareness of patient safety (Baker et al., 2004; Kohn et al.; National Health Service [NHS], 2000) and led to an increased focus on the prevention of adverse events in health care.

DEFINITION OF THE CONCEPT OF ADVERSE PATIENT OUTCOMES

Patient safety has been defined as freedom from accidental injury (Kohn et al., 2000). Much of the literature has operationalized patient safety in relation to adverse occurrences, which can be defined as "unintended injuries or complications that are caused by health care management, rather than by the patient's underlying disease, and that lead to death, disability at the time of discharge or prolonged hospital stays" (Baker et al., 2004, p. 1678). Adverse events include falls, pressure ulcers, medication errors, nosocomial infections, treatment errors, and mortality (American Nurses Association [ANA], 1995; Pierce, 1997).

In the United States, the Institute of Medicine (IOM) (Kohn et al., 2000) examined two studies of adverse events among large samples of hospitalized patients and estimated that healthcare error may have accounted for close to 100,000 patient deaths (Kohn et al.). In U.K. hospitals, adverse events were found to occur in around 10% of admissions, or at a rate in excess of 850,000 a year (NHS, 2000). In a study examining the health records of over 30,100 patients admitted to 51 acute care hospitals in New York State, adverse events occurred in 3.7% of admissions (Brennan et al., 1991). Wilson et al. (1995) reported adverse events in 16.6% of admissions to Australian hospitals, of which 13.7% resulted in permanent disability and 4.9% in death. A New Zealand study reported adverse events in 12.9% of admissions to public hospitals (Davis et al., 2001). Baker et al. (2004) conducted a chart review of 3,745 charts across 20 randomly selected Canadian adult hospitals located in five provinces (British Columbia, Quebec, Alberta, Ontario, and Nova Scotia) in 2000 to examine the incidence of adverse events in Canadian hospitals. The authors found that the rate of adverse events was 7.5 per 100 hospital admissions. Thirty-six percent of the adverse events were judged to be preventable, and 20.8% resulted in death. Based on their results, the authors estimated that of the 2.5 million similar hospital admissions in Canada in 2000, 141,250 to 232,250 admissions were associated with an adverse event. Of the patients whose adverse events resulted in death, 9,250 to 23,750 were preventable. All these reports emphasize that the majority of health services are of a very high standard and that serious failures are uncommon.

Although the reports on adverse events examined errors and the system issues that contribute to them, they did not explore nursing's role in patient safety. As a profession, nursing is accountable for enhancing health and promoting quality outcomes. Patient safety outcomes are an essential component of quality. Buerhaus and Norman (2001) maintained that efforts to improve quality will continue to shape healthcare delivery and that nurses need to be knowledgeable in the "theories, methods and practices of quality improvement." To achieve this goal, nurses will require good data on the measures of quality. Research on the relationship between nursing and patient safety outcomes can provide nurses with the evidence to advocate for safe patient care.

This chapter includes a discussion of adverse occurrences as patient safety outcomes that are sensitive to nursing. An analysis of the current nursing research on medication errors, nosocomial infections, patient falls, and pressure ulcers will be conducted to explore the association between these outcomes and nursing. Factors that influence adverse events, including perceptions about error and system issues, and a review of the empirical research on the relationship between nursing structural variables and adverse events are presented. This chapter also addresses issues with the state of the science in relationship to nursing and adverse patient outcomes and makes recommendations for future directions in this area. The review examines literature relating to the current state of thinking in the area of adverse patient outcomes—specifically, adverse events in relationship to nurse staffing from 1985 to the present.

LINKING ADVERSE PATIENT OUTCOMES TO NURSING

Medication errors, nosocomial infections, patient falls, and pressure ulcers are adverse events that consistently appear in the nursing literature as being theoretically linked to aspects of nursing practice (ANA, 1995, 1996a, 1996b, 1997, 2000; Blegen, Goode, & Reed, 1998; Cho, Ketefian, Barkauskas, & Smith, 2003; Dunton, Gajewski, Taunton, & Moore, 2004; Hugonnet, Chevrolet, & Pittet, 2007; Kovner & Gergen, 1998; Krauss et al., 2005; Lichtig, Knauf, & Milholland, 1999; McCloskey & Diers, 2005; McGillis Hall et al., 2001; McGillis Hall, Doran, & Pink, 2004; Needleman, Buerhaus, Mattke, Stewart, & Zelevinsky, 2002a, 2002b; Potter, Barr, McSweeney, & Sledge, 2003; Sovie & Jawad, 2001; Stegenga, Bell, & Matlow, 2002; Taunton, Kleinbeck, Stafford, Woods, & Bott, 1994).

Medication Errors

A medication error can occur at any of three stages: when the drug is prescribed, when it is dispensed, and when it is administered. A prescribing error is the result of a physician ordering the incorrect drug or dosage, a dispensing error is a mistake made by pharmacy staff when distributing medication to nursing units, and an administration error occurs when a nurse administers the drug incorrectly (ANA, 1995). Leape et al. (2000) found that 39% of medication errors occurred in the prescribing stage, 12% during pharmacy dispensing, and 38% in the nurse administration stage.

In acute care hospitals and long-term care facilities, the administration of medications is primarily a nursing role; therefore, the administration error rate may be associated with the availability and quality of nursing staff (ANA, 1995). Given that approximately one-third of these errors were attributed to nursing, it is important for nurse researchers to understand the factors that contribute to these and to develop strategies to manage them.

Medication administration errors can occur in many forms, including omitting doses; giving extra doses; administering a wrong dose; administering a drug not ordered; or administering a drug at the wrong time, through the wrong route, or at an incorrect rate (Chang & Mark, 2009; Mark & Burleson, 1995). Nurses are responsible for administering the correct dosage of the prescribed drug through the appropriate route to the right patient at the right time. In an American Nurses Association survey (1995), nurses reported that short staffing, particularly to the extent that it leads to increased workload and frequent interruptions, can result in medication administration errors. Other factors, such as inexperienced staff and limited knowledge or skills, may also increase the risk of a nurse making a medication administration error (ANA, 1995).

When exploring linkages between nursing and medication errors, it is important to consider the source and definition of the medication error. The research on medication errors is hampered by a lack of reliable data on the number and type of errors. Investigations have shown that the vast majority of medication errors are not recorded on the patients' charts. D. S. Wakefield et al. (1999a, 1999b) surveyed nurses in two Iowa hospitals to determine their perceptions of why medication errors occur, why they are not reported, and what percentage of medication errors are reported. According to the results, nurses perceived that approximately 60% of medication errors are reported. The rationale for underreporting included fear, administrative response, disagreement over error, and reporting effort (D. S. Wakefield et al., 1999b). Needleman and Buerhaus (2000) suggested that in some organizations, medication errors are only documented if something happens to the patient that requires medical attention. Iezzoni et al. (1994) found that even medication errors that are recorded internally on the patient's chart are often not recorded on the discharge abstract of the patient's chart. The lack of reliable data has been noted in nursing, although studies have demonstrated that data on medication error could be collected consistently (Mark & Burleson, 1995).

The literature on the relationship between medication errors and the quality of nursing care reveals varied results. According to Fuqua and Stevens (1988), stress, nursing shortages, and distractions while administering medication contribute to error. The authors also reported on a study in Pennsylvania that found that medication errors decrease as nursing experience increases. Prescott, Dennis, Creasia, and Bowen (1985) found that when fewer nurses were available for patient care, monitoring of patients decreased, treatment omissions and delays occurred, and medication errors increased. In more recent research, McGillis Hall et al. (2001, 2004) found that units with a higher proportion of regulated professional nursing staff had fewer medication errors. Taylor (2007) found a positive relationship between nursing hours and medication errors, where each increase of 1 hour of nursing per patient day was associated with an 8% increase in the odds of medication errors. The author suggested that perhaps the increase in nursing hours provides nurses with more time to recognize and report medication errors. Other studies did not find a direct correlation between the adequacy of nurse staffing or nurse workload and the incidence of medication errors (Potter et al., 2003; Taunton et al., 1994). Chang and Mark (2009) argued that medication errors that lead to severe physical injury or death may not have the same underlying causal factors as those medication errors that are nonsevere or that do not result in injury or death. These authors contended that research that combines these two potentially different types of medication errors may generate inaccurate results. The authors examined the relationships between nursing unit characteristics and the antecedents of severe and nonsevere medication errors in 286 nursing units over 6 months. They found that severe and nonsevere medication errors had different predictors. Nursing expertise, as rated by the nursing team, and units with more experienced registered nurses (RNs) were negatively associated with non-severe medication errors. A nursing unit with more Bachelor of Science in Nursing-(BScN) educated nurses had fewer severe medication errors, but only up to 54%, after which any further increase in the percentage of BScN nurses did not further decrease severe medication errors.

The literature on medication administration errors suggests that medication errors may be linked to some aspects of nursing, although a direct causal link has not been established (ANA, 1995; Blegen et al., 1998). It has been suggested that each error may be influenced by a unique set of factors and that more research is needed to understand these factors and how they influence medication administration errors (ANA, 1995; Institute of Medicine [IOM], 2000; 2007).

Nosocomial Infections

Nosocomial infections are infections originating in a healthcare organization (Centers for Disease Control [CDC], 2000). The most common types of hospital-acquired infections are urinary tract infections, surgical wound infections, bloodstream infections, and pneumonia (Weinstein, 1998). Nosocomial infections are considered a quality indicator, yet methodological issues, such as the need for complex risk adjustment and differences in the intensity of surveillance in different settings, have limited the use of nosocomial infection rates as a quality indicator in the past (Flood & Diers, 1988; Larson, Oram, & Hedrick, 1988). Mark and Burleson (1995), in a study to determine consistency in the collection of patient outcome data, reported challenges with consistently collecting data on nosocomial infections.

According to Weinstein (1998), one-third of nosocomial infections are preventable. Certain patient care practices, such as proper aseptic and antiseptic techniques in hand washing, skin preparation, wound dressing, and prudent monitoring of invasive medical devices, are under the scope of nursing practice. Nurses minimize the risk of spreading infection in their daily practice by using aseptic techniques when changing dressings to prevent wound infections, and in the care and maintenance of tubing such as catheters and chest tubes. Hand washing is considered the most effective preventative practice with respect to nosocomial infections (Larson et al., 1988). RNs also perform a role in the assessment and monitoring of risk factors for infection, such as age, nutritional status, and medical treatment (ANA, 1995). Given nursing's pivotal role in infection control practices, the incidence of nosocomial infections can be expected to reflect the availability and quality of nursing care (ANA, 1995).

Flood and Diers (1988) found that units with inadequate staffing had higher levels of complications such as general infections and urinary tract infections. Although Taunton et al. (1994) found no relationship between urinary tract infections and nursing workload, they did find evidence that nosocomial infection rates were related to registered nursing staff absenteeism. The authors surmised that staff absenteeism may interrupt continuity of care.

A study conducted by Fridkin, Pear, Williamson, Galgiani, and Jarvis (1996) found that a higher nurse-to-patient ratio was an indicator of a bloodstream infection in patients with a central venous line. The authors hypothesized that an increase in the nurse-to-patient ratio, as well as an increase in the number of central lines, may have placed time constraints on the nursing staff, preventing them from taking proper care of the catheters. American Nurses Association-funded studies piloting quality indicators eliminated the nosocomial infection indicator (central/peripheral line infection) because it occurred so infrequently (Grobe et al., 1998; Langemo, Anderson, & Volden, 2002).

Stegenga et al. (2002) reported that the incidence of nosocomial gastrointestinal infections on a pediatric unit was positively associated with the patient-to-nurse ratio. They also found that patients were three times more at risk of developing a nosocomial gastrointestinal infection within 3 days following an understaffed day, which the authors defined as a day when patients receive less than 10.5 nursing hours per patient. More recently, Hugonnet et al. (2007) found that higher nurse staffing was associated with reduced risk of acquiring a nosocomial infection while in the intensive care unit and that the daily proportion of infected patients was associated with the nurse-to-patient ratios of the previous 2–4 days. Mark, Harless, McCue, and Xu's (2004) findings suggest that RN and licensed practical nurse (LPN) staffing might interact to affect pneumonia, such that increasing RN staffing decreases incidences of pneumonia more when coupled with increased LPN staffing. McGillis Hall et al.'s (2004) study of 19 teaching hospitals in Ontario, Canada, reported that units employing a lower proportion of professional nurses (RNs and registered practical nurses) were associated with greater wound infections. Kane, Shamliyan, Mueller, Duval, and Wilt's (2007a) systematic review of RN staffing and patient outcomes found that each additional patient to a registered nurse's assignment was associated with a 7% relative increase in developing pneumonia. An increase of one RN full-time equivalent per patient day was associated with a 30% decrease of pneumonia in intensive care unit patients and a 31% decrease of nosocomial bloodstream infections in surgical patients. Also, greater overtime hours and the proportion of float nurses were positively associated with nosocomial infections.

Recent studies have examined nosocomial infections (urinary tract infections, pneumonia) and found a relationship between nurse staffing and these nosocomial infections (ANA, 2000; Cho et al., 2003; Kovner & Gergen, 1998; Lichtig et al.,

1999; McCloskey & Diers, 2005; McGillis Hall et al., 2001, 2004; Needleman et al., 2002a, 2002b; Sovie & Jawad, 2001). Further research is needed to understand how these nursing-related variables influence the incidence of nosocomial infections.

Patient Falls

A fall is defined as unintentionally coming to rest on the floor or other lower level, but not as a result of syncope or overwhelming external force (Agostini, Baker, & Bogardus, 2001). In Canada, falls are the sixth leading cause of death among older adults and cost the Canadian healthcare system approximately $2.8 billion annually (SMARTRISK, 1998). A previous fall is one of the strongest predictors of falls (Agostini et al.). Rawsky (1998) contended that the effect of patient falls extends beyond physical injury and cost because older people who fall fear a subsequent fall and may reduce their activities to prevent further falls, which leads to a reduction of independence and further functional decline.

Morse (1993) suggested that most falls in institutions are not random events, but the result of a pattern, and that the opportunity therefore exists to reduce their incidence. In the acute care, long-term care, and home care setting, nurses are responsible for identifying patients who are at risk for falls and developing and implementing a plan of care to minimize risk and reduce the number of falls.

The American Nurses Association feasibility studies addressed whether patients were assessed for risk of fall on admission, whether patients who had previous falls were identified as "at risk," and whether fall protocols were in place prior to falls (Grobe et al., 1998; Langemo et al., 2002). Grobe et al. argued for the use of standardized fall-risk scales and severity scales to add validity to the data. This study also highlights the variation in data on the number and types of injuries associated with falls, the lack of data on the level of patient activity prior to the fall, and whether restraints were in use at the time of the fall. The authors suggested that this information is required to ensure reliable reporting and to allow comparison of rates of falls within units and across organizations.

In an effort to reduce the number of falls, many hospitals, long-term care facilities, and communities have implemented fall prevention programs as part of quality improvement efforts. However, there are limited studies exploring the effect of fall prevention programs and the assessment of risk for falls on the number of falls within organizations (Rawsky, 1998). According to Hernandez and Millar (1986), many older patients fall in institutions when getting up to use the bathroom. A study by Bakarich, McMillan, and Prosser (1997) found that significantly fewer falls occurred in an at-risk group assessed for confusion and mobility status and toileted on a regular basis, as compared with an at-risk group assessed but not toileted. Whedon and Shedd (1989) found that patient acuity, the use of supplemental staffing or inexperienced nursing staff, and a discrepancy between recommended and actual hours of staffing contributed to an increased number of falls. Some studies found no relationship between nursing staffing variables and patient falls (Donaldson et al., 2005; Morse, Tylko, & Dixon, 1987; Taunton et al., 1994; Tutuarima, De Haan, & Limburg,1993), whereas others found that units with a higher proportion of RNs (Blegen & Vaughn, 1998; Dunton et al., 2004; Sovie & Jawad, 2001), higher nurse-to-patient ratios (Krauss et al., 2005), and greater hours of nursing care per patient day (Dunton et al.; Potter et al., 2003; Taylor, 2007) had lower fall rates. One study found that lower inpatient fall rates were associated with higher nurse staffing up to 15 hours per patient day on step-down, medical, and medical-surgical units and when total hours exceeded 15 hours on surgical units (Dunton et al.). Kane et al.'s (2007a) systematic review found that an increase in nursing turnover was associated with a 0.2% increase in patient fall rates.

Many factors, such as patient characteristics, the onset of acute illness, medical treatments, new medications, or an alteration of medication regimen increase the risk for falls (Agostini et al., 2001). Current methods for collecting data on falls are inadequate. Further research is required to better understand the relationship among nurse staffing, nursing interventions, and patient falls. This research needs to be grounded with consistent definitions that capture the level of activity, whether the patient was assessed about "risk for falls" and whether restraints were in place.

Pressure Ulcers

Pressure ulcers are localized areas of tissue damage or necrosis that develop as a result of pressure over a bony prominence (Agostini et al., 2001). Pressure ulcers have been linked to a 50% increase in nursing care time, increased length of stay, higher hospital costs, increased comorbidity, sepsis, and a fourfold increase in mortality in cases developing bacteremia (ANA, 1995). Current clinical practice guidelines for the management of pressure ulcers include systematic skin inspection at least once per day, routine skin cleansing, reduction of pressure by positioning, and minimizing skin exposure to moisture. Even with these practices in place, patients may still develop skin breakdown because of underlying pathologic conditions (National Pressure Ulcer Advisory Panel [NPUAP], 1992). Nursing plays a significant role in assessing the skin condition, implementing treatment plans aimed at reducing pressure, and minimizing exposure to moisture.

The National Pressure Ulcer Advisory Panel has developed clear definitions for staging pressure ulcers that are reflected in current clinical practice guidelines. There is corroboration for capturing the incidence and prevalence of stage 2–4 pressure ulcers (NPUAP, 1992; Registered Nurses Association of Ontario [RNAO], 2002). Frantz, Gardner, Specht, and McIntire (2001) cited a National

Pressure Ulcer Advisory Panel recommendation to exclude stage 1 pressure ulcers because the reliability of the identification of stage 1 ulcers has not been substantiated. However, the feasibility study conducted by the Texas Nurses' Association (Grobe et al., 1998) contended that valuable data were lost by excluding stage 1 pressure ulcers. Although identifying stage 1 ulcers presents a challenge, it may be beneficial to include them in future studies.

Most studies of pressure ulcers have examined the impact of different interventions, rather than the influence of nurse staffing, in relation to assessment (Bostrum et al., 1996; Frantz, Berquist, & Specht, 1995; Hopkins et al., 2000; Lyder, 2002). However, some studies (ANA, 2000; Blegen et al., 1998; Dellefield, 2006; Lichtig et al., 1999; McCloskey & Diers, 2005) found that nursing staff mix was related to lower pressure ulcer rates. Kane et al.'s (2007a) systematic review found that an increase of 1 total nurse hour per patient day was associated with a 2.26% decrease in pressure ulcer rates. Additionally, Mark et al. (2004) found that a decrease in nursing full-time equivalents and nursing hours was related to an increase in the incidence of pressure ulcers. By contrast, Cho et al. (2003) found that all productive hours by all nursing personnel were related to higher pressure ulcer rates. They suggested that perhaps nursing units that have greater nursing hours provide care to higher acuity patients who have higher rates of pressure ulcers and that this greater staffing allows nurses to detect more pressure ulcers because they have more time to assess skin integrity. Many organizations have implemented quality improvement initiatives, such as practice guidelines, aimed at preventing the incidence of skin breakdown. The translation of these clinical practice guidelines into routine practice has been problematic because studies have limited the scope of evaluation to short-term effects of the quality improvement initiatives rather than evaluating whether these strategies are sustained within organizations (Frantz et al., 2001). Researchers who evaluated the integration of a research-based pressure ulcer treatment protocol 5 years after its implementation at a veterans hospital found consistency in the way the protocol had been maintained. Unique factors in this organization included higher staff salaries and benefits, higher total hours of nursing care, above-average levels of nursing personnel, and less staff turnover compared with national averages (Frantz et al., 2001). The organization was also known for promoting autonomy and accountability in individual nurses and involving them in decision-making about patient care.

Although the current evidence on the impact of nurse staffing on pressure ulcers is limited, nursing is responsible for assessing patients and implementing protocols to prevent and treat pressure ulcers (Mark & Burleson, 1995). Changes in the staff mix and/or the number and type of nurses may affect the nurses' capacity to assess patients and implement treatment plans (ANA, 1995; Cho et al., 2003).

To understand the relationship between nursing and the incidence of pressure ulcers, accurate data are required. Grobe et al. (1998) argued for standardization of data collection and risk assessment using a recognized scale. This information would facilitate future research to inform decisions about the nursing inputs required to prevent and/or reduce pressure ulcers. Lake and Cheung (2006) contended that the most accurate method for measuring the prevalence of pressure ulcers is through observational studies, in which the researcher conducts regular assessments of all patients for the presence of pressure ulcers. However, because this method is time- and resource intensive, Lake and Cheung suggested that a second appropriate method for measuring the prevalence of pressure ulcers is through the use of administrative data that clearly indicate if a pressure ulcer developed during a hospital admission.

FACTORS THAT INFLUENCE ADVERSE PATIENT OUTCOMES

According to the literature, a number of factors influence adverse patient outcomes, including perceptions about error and systems issues in the healthcare environment.

Perceptions about Error

Recent reports provide evidence that some errors can be prevented (Kohn et al., 2000; NHS, 2000). Leape et al. (1991) maintained that more than two-thirds of adverse events are preventable, which means that they are caused by an error. Baker et al. (2004) found that in a Canadian sample of acute care hospitals, 36% of adverse events were judged to be preventable. These adverse occurrences do not happen intentionally. In their daily practice, healthcare workers do not plan to commit errors. These errors are the result of the complicated interface between providers and technology, providers and the system, and the complex interaction among the many different healthcare providers (Leape et al., 2000). Furthermore, adverse events do not necessarily signal poor-quality care. For example, Brennan et al. (1991) pointed out that although a drug reaction in a patient who has been appropriately prescribed a specific drug for the first time is, by definition, an adverse event, this type of error is not preventable.

Organizational culture significantly affects the number and type of errors reported. Researchers acknowledge that because of underdetection and underreporting by healthcare professionals, only a fraction of the true incidence of errors is known (Fuqua & Stevens, 1988). Although the current focus is on creating cultures of safety, healthcare organizations have typically handled errors by taking disciplinary action against the individual involved (Keepnews, 2000). This "culture of blame" has discouraged individuals from reporting errors, which leads to underreporting and, ultimately, a failure to identify or correct systems problems that cause or contribute to errors. Meurier (2000) examined the clinical errors for

20 RNs and found that nurses are reluctant to report and discuss errors because of fear of disciplinary action.

Organizations that promote a "culture of safety" acknowledge the high-risk and error-prone nature of health care and encourage individuals to report errors. Within these organizations, executives and clinicians work together to change practice, develop systems to monitor quality, and commit resources to support these changes (M. K. Wakefield & Maddox, 2000). Organizations that encourage open reporting and balanced analysis, both in principle and in practice, are able to have a positive and quantifiable impact on quality outcomes (NHS, 2000).

System Issues

In a systems approach to errors, humans are viewed as fallible, and errors can occur even in good organizations (Reason, 2000). Researchers have learned that the reason people make errors is often largely due to the way that work is designed (Nolan, 2000). From this perspective, if a person makes a mistake, the question should not be who committed the error, but rather why it happened and whether there is a way to redesign the work so that it will not happen again (Reason). Moreover, there is evidence that even when processes are well designed, there will be situations in which mistakes occur (Nolan). Cognitive psychologists and human factors engineers confirm that people make mistakes when they are rushed, under pressure, overworked, emotionally distraught, or working in a difficult environment (Buerhaus, 1999). The current environment, in which nurses are caring for patients with complex needs and are being pressured to work overtime and extra shifts because of inadequate staffing, has the potential to impact adverse patient outcomes (Foley, 1999).

A major role of RNs involves coping with the complexity of patient care and, in particular, the gaps that complexity generates. Cook, Render, and Woods (2000) defined these gaps as "discontinuities in care" that appear in diverse ways, such as loss of information or interruptions in delivery of care. In daily practice, these gaps rarely lead to an adverse event because expert clinicians are able to anticipate, recognize, and bridge these gaps. The authors characterize some bridges to manage these gaps as robust and reliable, whereas others are frail and brittle. It is easier to manage these gaps in a stable milieu than in a complex environment characterized by numerous admissions and discharges, complex patients, increased nurse-to-patient ratios, frequent interruptions, and staffing patterns that may involve inexperienced staff or relief staff (Cook et al., 2000). Expert nurses are able to manage gaps better than are novice nurses (Cook et al.). Nurses report that as they gain more experience, they develop better ways of managing errors and learning from their mistakes (Meurier, Vincent, & Parmar, 1997). With the introduction of unregulated workers, nurses have had to change how they structure their work. In addition to having more patients to manage, they also have to supervise the work of these unregulated workers (Sovie & Jawad, 2001). This further increases the potential for gaps in patient care.

Decision-making by senior management may create conditions that contribute to adverse occurrences. For example, inadequate systems to support communication, lack of orientation and/or ongoing training, and the failure to supply and maintain equipment required to deliver care may lead to conditions that jeopardize patient safety (Meurier, 2000). In the past, healthcare organizations have failed to address systems problems such as written orders that are illegible, medications that have a similar name or that are packaged in a similar way, and potentially dangerous medications that are part of floor stock (Keepnews, 2000). Decreased operating budgets has led to a reduction in nurse managers, educators, and clinical nurse specialists—roles that ensure the structure and expertise to support patient safety and quality (Foley, 1999).

The quality of working environments and quality of interactions with other professionals distinguish hospitals with lower mortality and complications from those with higher adverse events (Aiken, Smith, & Lake, 1994; Knaus, Draper, Wagner, & Zimmerman, 1986; Mitchell & Shortell, 1997; Sovie & Jawad, 2001). In terms of working environments, RNs are dissatisfied with their working conditions. They report that they are spending less time taking care of patients with more complex needs (Aiken, Clarke, & Sloane, 2001), and they believe that the safety and quality of care are deteriorating. Taylor (2007) found that higher levels of nurses' stress recognition were associated with 1.5 to 3 times the odds of patient falls, medication errors, and decubitus ulcers. Additionally, nurses' safety climate was negatively associated with the odds of patients developing a decubitus ulcer. In terms of the quality of interactions with other professionals, communication among the diverse disciplines managing patient care has been shown to affect patient outcomes (Shortell et al., 1994; Sovie & Jawad).

RELATIONSHIPS BETWEEN NURSING STRUCTURAL VARIABLES AND ADVERSE PATIENT OUTCOMES

Nightingale was one of the first nurse researchers to recognize the importance of data collection and the impact that measurement has on patient outcomes. Nightingale logged infection rates and implemented interventions based on her findings (Reed, Blegen, & Goode, 1998). Over the years, there has been an increase in research examining the relationships between nursing structural variables and their impact on adverse patient outcomes.

As rapid changes have occurred within health care, many organizations have reengineered or redesigned work to maximize the expertise and productivity of RNs as a means of controlling costs. Many studies have examined different models of care delivery and their effects on staff and organizational outcomes.

Although these studies have demonstrated that care delivery changes affect organizational outcomes such as cost, their impact on patient outcomes is inconclusive (Barter, McLaughlin, & Thomas, 1997; Blegen et al., 1998; Grillo-Peck & Risner, 1995; Krapohl & Larson, 1996; Lengacher & Mabe, 1993; McGillis Hall, 1998; Tourangeau, White, Scott, McAllister, & Giles, 1999). Recent nursing research is beginning to fill the gap in our understanding of how structural indicators influence quality indicators.

A 1996 report by the Institute of Medicine concluded that there was a lack of empirical evidence to draw conclusions about nurse staffing in hospitals and that although the "literature on the effect of RNs on mortality and on factors affecting the retention of nursing staff is available, there is a serious paucity of recent research on the definitive effects of structural measures, such as specific staffing ratios, on the quality of patient care in terms of patient outcomes when controlling for all other likely explanatory or confounding variables" (Wunderlich, Sloan, & Davis, 1996, p. 9). This report argued that rigorous research on the relationship between nursing variables and quality of care would have significant payoffs for administrators, decision makers, and policy makers. Since that report, a number of studies have provided evidence that links nurse staffing variables to quality of care and patient outcomes (ANA, 2000; Blegen et al., 1998; Blegen & Vaughn, 1998; Flood & Diers, 1988; Kovner & Gergen, 1998; Lichtig et al., 1999; McGillis Hall et al., 2001; Needleman et al., 2002a, 2002b; Sovie & Jawad, 2001). See **TABLE 6-1**.

One of the early studies to examine the effect of nurse staffing levels on patient outcomes compared two medical units with similar capacities, patient mix, and staff mix to assess the effect of nurse staffing levels on patient complications, acuity level, length of stay, and cost (Flood & Diers, 1988). The authors found that the unit with adequate staffing had fewer complications, including infections, length of stay, and decreased patient requests for pain medication, than the unit with less than adequate staffing. This study controlled for the case mix of patients and was conducted in a single setting using organizational-specific definitions for understaffing.

Taunton et al. (1994) examined whether adverse occurrences, such as bloodstream and urinary tract infections, patient falls, and medication errors, were correlated with staff nurse absenteeism, staff nurse separation from the work unit by resignation or transfer, and nursing workload. This study, which was conducted in four large acute care urban hospitals, found an association between patient infections and staff nurse absenteeism. The authors hypothesized that absenteeism and the replacement of staff by less-skilled nurses may disrupt continuity of care and affect patient safety. Although data for this study were collected from hospital documents and each hospital participated in defining the study outcomes, the authors maintained that there may have been underreporting, measurement errors, errors related to the operational definitions, and inconsistent adherence to reporting schematics (Taunton et al.).

TABLE 6-1   Studies Investigating the Relationship Between Nursing Structural Variables and Adverse Events

Author date	Design	Sample characteristics/ setting	Independent variables	Outcomes being investigated and approach to measurement	Results	Limitations
ANA (2000)	Correlational	All-payor sample of more than 9.1 million pts in almost 1,000 hospitals. Medicare sample of more than 3.8 million pts in over 1,500 hospitals across 9 U.S. states.	RN hrs/NIW adjusted day; licensed hrs/NIW adjusted day; % RN licensed hrs.	Mix of RNs, LPNs, and UAPs = % of RN care hours as a total of all nursing care hrs (acute care units); total nursing care hrs provided per patient day = total number of productive hrs worked by nursing staff with direct pt care responsibilities per patient (pts) day. Pressure ulcers = # of pts with NPUAP-AHCPR Stage I, II, III or IV ulcers/# of pts in a prevalence study. Patient falls = the rate per 1,000 pt days at which pts experience an unplanned descent to the floor during the course of the day (total # of pt falls × 1,000/total # of pt days). Patient satisfaction with pain management; nosocomial infections = # of laboratory-confirmed bacteremia associated with sites of central lines/1,000 pt days per unit.	Secondary bacterial pneumonia, postoperative infection, pressure ulcer, and UTI infection rates were lower in hospitals with higher RN skill mixes and in some instances with greater staffing levels.	Poor quality of nurse staffing data: (1) FTEs rather than paid & worked hrs; (2) does not report where nurses work in site; (3) may include psychiatry and rehab units in some sites.
Blegen et al. (1998)	Correlational	42 inpatient units (21,783 discharges); one large 880-bed university hospital (U.S.).	Hrs of care per pt day from all nursing personnel = RN/LPN/NA hrs direct/unit PD for month. Hours of care provided by RNs = RN hrs direct pt care/unit PD for month. RN proportions = RN	Decubiti = incidences of skin breakdown secondary to pressure or exposure to urine/feces. Infections = nosocomial infections not present or incubating at the time of admission (only UTIs and respiratory infections were included). Patient falls = suddenly and involuntarily leaving a position and coming to rest on the floor or some object. Medication errors = wrong dose, duplication, omission, transcrip	RN proportion was inversely related to rates of medication errors, decubiti, and pt complaints. As RN proportions increased, rates of adverse outcomes decreased up to a staff mix of 87.5%.	Concern re: the rigor of incident reports for the reporting of medication errors and pt falls on pt care units; acuity measure may not have been sensitive to higher levels of acuity for pts in critical care and intensive care units.

					Results are less generalizable as single-site study.
			tion, wrong route/pt/solution/ time (per 10, 000 doses).		Data abstracted retrospectively from hospital records may lead to underreporting, measurement errors at initial data point, measurement error in relation to operational definitions of variables.
			Patient complaints = both pt and family complaints about the aspects of the pt's care such as nursing care, medical care, food, and housekeeping (standardized as rate per 1000 pt days).		
			Mortality rates per 1,000 pt days.	Units with higher proportion of RNs had lower rates of pt falls.	Patient outcomes data collected from chart reviews.
Blegen & Vaughn (1998)	Correlational	39 hospital units in 11 hospitals (U.S.).	Hours of care = all hours of care (RN/LPN/ NA) per pt day. RN proportion = proportion of those hours of care delivered by RNs.	Nurse staffing was not related to cardiac arrest.	Dose-based denominators for medication errors were not available for capturing ratios.
			hours PD/all hours PD.		
			Data from comparative occurrence reporting system (CORS)—medication administration errors (MAE); pt falls and cardiac arrest.		
			MAEs = both oral and intravenous medications and includes: omissions, wrong method, wrong pt, wrong dose, inappropriate continuation, wrong drug, administrations to pts with allergies, and adverse drug reactions (MAE = # of errors on the unit in the quarter per 1,000 pt days, and # of errors on the unit in the quarter per 10, 000 doses).		
			Patient falls = # of pt falls on the unit during the quarter per 1,000 pt days.		
			Cardiac arrests = # of cardiac arrests on the unit during the quarter per 1,000 pt days of care (did not include pt with DNR orders).		

BSIs = bloodstream infections; CMI = case mix index; DRG = diagnosis-related group; DVT = deep venous thrombosis; FTE = full time equivalent; GI = gastrointestinal; HCUP = Health Care Utilization Project; hrs = hours; LOS = length of stay; NAP or UAP = unlicensed assistive personnel; NIW = nursing intensity weight; NPU = nosocomial pressure ulcer; PD = patient day; PR = pulmonary embolism; pt = patient; UTI = urinary tract infection.

(continues)

TABLE 6-1 Studies Investigating the Relationship Between Nursing Structural Variables and Adverse Events (continued)

Author date	Design	Sample characteristics/setting	Independent variables	Outcomes being investigated and approach to measurement	Results	Limitations
Chang & Mark (2009)	Longitudinal	$N = 286$ units from a random sample of 146 U.S. hospitals.	Work dynamics: Level of which the nursing unit experiences many interruptions or unexpected events. RN hrs: Percentage of nursing care delivered by RNs. Nursing expertise: RNs rated their nursing teams' level of expertise in recognizing critical patient concerns. Education level. Experience.	Medication errors are errors in the administration of medication, such as wrong dose, wrong patient, wrong time, wrong medication, wrong route, and did not administer a prescribed drug. Measured via incident reports. Errors at different levels of severity: (1) Severe medication errors are those that result in increased nursing care/observation or technical monitoring, diagnostic testing, medical interventions, or transfer to a different nursing unit. (2) Nonsevere medication errors encompass everything else.	None of the independent variables predicted both levels of medication errors. Nursing expertise was negatively associated with nonsevere medication errors ($p < .01$). A unit with more BScN-educated nurses had fewer severe medication errors, but only up to 54%, after which any further increase in the percentage of BScN nurses did not further decrease severe medication errors ($p < .01$). Nursing units with more experienced RNs had more nonsevere medication errors ($p < .01$).	Use of voluntary incident reports; underreporting may underestimate the number of nonsevere medication errors. Did not account for patient health risk/health characteristics.
Cho et al. (2003)	Correlational	California Acute Care Hospitals ($N = 232$); 124,204 pts in 20 surgical DRGs.	Nurse staffing measured in three ways: (1) All hrs: Total productive hrs worked by all nursing personnel per pt day. (2) RN hrs: Total hrs per RN per pt day.	Seven outcomes based on ICD-9-CM codes: (1) fall/injury; (2) pressure ulcer; (3) adverse drug event; (4) pneumonia; (5) UTI; (6) wound infection; and (7) sepsis. LOS used to indirectly measure the impact of adverse events on morbidity. Individual pt costs were estimated by multiplying charges and the hospital-specific cost-to-charge ratio.	All hrs were positively associated with pressure ulcers ($p < .05$). RN hrs ($p < .01$) and RN proportion ($p < .05$) had an inverse relationship with pneumonia. A 1 RN hr increase was associated with an 8.9% decrease in the odds of developing pneumonia.	Nurses' characteristics not included (i.e., education, experience). Nurse staffing data aggregated over the year without accounting for daily fluctuations in pt census and nurse staffing.

			(3) RN proportion: Skill mix of nursing hrs.		All seven adverse events were associated with greater LOS and increased cost. Sepsis, pneumonia, and wound infection positively associated with increased mortality.
Dellefield (2006).	Correlational	California nursing homes (N= 897).	Centralization: Proportion of RN hrs to LVN hrs per census. Proportion of LVN hrs to CNA hrs per census. Specialization: Total RN hrs and LVN hrs per resident. Total CNA hrs per resident. Total nursing staff hrs (including contract, FT, and PT).	Prevalence and risk adjusted prevalence of PU. Deficiency citation.	Greater proportion of RN to LVN associated with a lower risk-adjusted pressure ulcer (PU) prevalence ($p < .001$). Organizations with lower total nursing staff hrs per pt day were more likely to receive a deficiency citation ($p < .001$). Facilities with greater skill mix (RN, LVN, and CNA) were more likely to receive a deficiency citation ($p < .001$). 507 organizations were excluded from the original sample because of missing data or because electronic data were not available.

BSIs = bloodstream infections; CMI = case mix index; DRG = diagnosis-related group; DVT = deep venous thrombosis; FTE = full time equivalent; GI = gastrointestinal; HCUP = Health Care Utilization Project; hrs = hours; LOS = length of stay; NAP or UAP = unlicensed assistive personnel; NIW = nursing intensity weight; NPU = nosocomial pressure ulcer; PD = patient day; PR = pulmonary embolism; pt= patient; UTI = urinary tract infection.

(continues)

TABLE 6-1 Studies Investigating the Relationship Between Nursing Structural Variables and Adverse Events (continued)

Author date	Design	Sample characteristics/ setting	Independent variables	Outcomes being investigated and approach to measurement	Results	Limitations
Donaldson et al. (2005)	Comparison of nurse staffing on pt outcomes prior to and after implementation of mandated ratios	$N = 268$ units in 68 CalNOC hospitals representing $N = 196,000$ pt days. Prevalence of PU and restraint use: $N = 162$ units in 38 CalNOC hospitals.	Nursing care hrs: Productive hrs worked by RN, LVN, non-RN, and non-LVN caregiver staff. RN nursing care hrs. LVN nursing care hrs. Non-RN/LVN caregiver hrs. Contracted hrs. Skill mix.	Total pt days. Pt fall incidence: rate of falls per 1,000 pt days. Hospital-acquired PU prevalence: Total number of pts within facility that have a PU on the day of the prevalence study. Restraint use prevalence.	No statistically significant changes in PU, falls, and restraint use after the implementation of ratios.	Only the California Nursing Outcomes Coalition (CalNOC) hospitals that had at least 2 months of available data during the first 6 months prior to premandated ratios in 2002 and 6 months after the postmandated ratios in 2004. Not all hospitals in California participate in CalNOC; unknown if participant and nonparticipant hospitals differ. Authors used a p of .0042 as significance level for interpreting the relationships among skill mix, staffing, and falls.
Dunton et al. (2004)	Cross-sectional	2,351 nursing units (step-down, medical, surgical, med-surg, and critical care) from 282 acute care hospitals in 45 states.	Nursing hrs per patient day. Skill mix (RN, LPN/LVN, and unlicensed assistive personnel). Percent contract.	Patient fall rate (total number of falls/total number of pt days $\times 1,000$). Fall injury level (total number of falls resulting in an injury/total number of pt days $\times 1,000$). Five injury levels: (1) no injury, (2) mild injury, (3) moderate injury requiring sutures or fractures, (4) major injury requiring surgery or casting, and (5) death.	On step-down, medical, and combined med-surg units, lower fall rates were associated with higher staffing up to 15 hrs per pt day. On surgical units, lower fall rates were associated with greater staffing when the total hrs per pt day exceeded 15 hrs.	Nurses' characteristics not included (i.e. education, experience). Only controlled for hospital size. Did not account for pt DRGs/co morbidities.

Study	Design	Sample/Setting	Measures	Findings	Limitations
Flood & Diers (1988)	Descriptive	482-bed university teaching hospital (northeast U.S.). 2 medical units. Unit B with adequate staffing and Unit A with less than adequate staffing as defined by the hospital; N = 497 pts; 199 male; 298 female.	Staffing workload index = number of required nursing personnel and number of available nursing personnel per shift/per unit as defined by the hospital. Patient complications listed on the Uniform Hospital Discharge Data Summary (infections, heart conditions, and GI disorders). Acuity levels range from 1 (*requiring minimal care*) to 4 (*requiring intensive nursing care*) (San Joaquin PCS); LOS; Cost (room and board charges plus nursing) for pts < or < geographic mean LOS.	For step-down and medical units, lower fall rates were associated with higher RN skill mix. On combined med-surg units, there was a positive association between falls and the percent of contract nursing hrs. On medical units, lower injury falls were associated with higher staffing up to 9 hrs per pt day. Unit A: The frequency and mean number of complications per pt were higher; generalized infections (N = 88) & UTI (N = 62) most common complications. Unit A had a slightly greater LOS than Unit B when controlled for DRG; Unit A had higher % PD at acuity level = 3 (Unit A = 75%; Unit B=57%). Unit A projected to have a greater loss in net revenues.	Only allowed for 1 time point, 15 hrs in model. Did not examine possibility of multiple knots. Study did not measure the amount of care received by pts on both units. It only examined pt complications. It may be that the pts on Unit A had DRGs that were more complex and required more nursing care.
Hugonnet et al. (2007)	Prospective cohort study	N = 1,883 pts Medical ICU in Geneva, Switzerland.	Workload as measured by the RN: pt ratio. (Total number of RNs during a 24-hr period/# pts that day) Occurrence of ICU-acquired infection, which utilized the CDC's definition and criteria for nosocomial infections, including pneumonia.	The daily proportion of infected patients was associated with the RN: pt ratio of 2, 3, and 4 days prior ($p < .05$). Higher nurse staffing was associated with lower risk of infection.	Pts were not followed after discharge from the ICU; infections acquired close to discharge may not be captured. Specific ICU pt population limits generalizability of results. Only a pt's first acquired infection was included in the analysis.

(continues)

BSIs = bloodstream infections; CMI = case mix index; DRG = diagnosis-related group; DVT = deep venous thrombosis; FTE = full time equivalent; GI = gastrointestinal; HCUP = Health Care Utilization Project; hrs = hours; LOS = length of stay; NAP or UAP = unlicensed assistive personnel; NIW = nursing intensity weight; NPU = nosocomial pressure ulcer; PD = patient day; PR = pulmonary embolism; pt= patient; UTI = urinary tract infection.

TABLE 6-1   Studies Investigating the Relationship Between Nursing Structural Variables and Adverse Events (continued)

Author date	Design	Sample characteristics/ setting	Independent variables	Outcomes being investigated and approach to measurement	Results	Limitations
Kane et al. (2007a)	Systematic review	94 primary studies conducted in acute care hospitals in the U.S. and Canada.	Ratio of FTE of RNs per pt day. # of pts assigned to 1 RN per shift.	Hospital-related mortality, failure to rescue, cardiac arrest, shock, unplanned extubation, respiratory failure, thrombosis (DVT and pulmonary embolus), upper GI bleeding, surgical bleeding, falls, NPU, nosocomial infections, UTI, hospital acquired pneumonia, and nosocomial pneumonia.	Each ↑ of one pt per RN shift was associated with a 7% ↑ in the relative risk of pneumonia, 45% ↑ in unplanned extubation, and 53% ↑ in pulmonary failure. An ↑of one RN FTE per pt day was associated with a 30% ↓ in pneumonia in ICU pts and 31% ↓ in nosocomial BSIs in surgical pts. Greater overtime hrs and the proportion of float RNs were positively associated with nosocomial infections. ↑ in nursing turnover was associated with a 0.2 % ↑in pt falls. An ↑ of one total RN hr per pt day was associated with a 2.26% ↓ in NPU rates.	Secondary data analyses excluded.
Kane et al. (2007b)	Systematic review (part of a larger study; Kane et al., 2007a)	28 primary studies conducted in acute care hospitals in the U.S. and Canada that reported adjusted odds ratios of pt outcomes.	Ratio of FTE of RNs per pt day. # of pts assigned to 1 RN per shift in the unit.	Hospital-related mortality, failure to rescue, cardiac arrest, shock, unplanned extubation, respiratory failure, DVT, upper GI bleeding, surgical bleeding, falls, NPU, nosocomial infections, UTI, hospital-acquired pneumonia, and nosocomial pneumonia.	↑ RN staffing was associated with 19% lower odds of developing hospital-acquired pneumonia for all pts and 30% for ICU pts. 1 RN FTE ↑ per pt day was associated with a 36% reduction in the odds of nosocomial blood infections in surgical pts, 60% lower odds of respiratory failure, and 51% lower odds of unplanned extubation in ICU pts.	Only included studies that reported adjusted odds ratios. Excluded secondary data analyses.

| Koyner & Gergen (1998) | Correlational | 589 acute care community hospitals in 10 U.S. states. | # of FTE RNs working in the hospital and outpatient departments per adjusted pt day. | Nine postsurgical outcomes based on ICD-9-CM codes Nurse-sensitive indicators: Venous thrombosis, or pulmonary embolism after major surgery and after invasive vascular procedure, excluding from the population at risk discharged pts with venous thrombosis as principal diagnosis; UTIs after major surgery, excluding from the population at risk discharged pts in MDC 11 (renal), MDC 12 (male genital), or MDC 13 (female genital): pneumonia after major surgery excluding from the population at risk discharged pts in MDC 4 (respiratory), with cancer, or with AIDS; pneumonia after invasive vascular procedure, excluding from the population at risk discharged pts in MDC 4 (respiratory), with cancer, or with AIDS. Non-nurse-sensitive indicators: Pulmonary compromise after surgery (pulmonary congestion, lung edema, or respiratory insufficiency or failure); acute myocardial infarction after major surgery; GI hemorrhage or ulceration after major surgery; mechanical complications due to device, implant, or graft. | A positive association between the number of pts per RN shift and pt outcomes, such as failure to rescue, pulmonary failure, unplanned extubation, and cardiopulmonary resuscitation. Significant inverse relationships between FTE RNs per adjusted inpt day (RNAPD) & UTIs after major surgery ($p < 0.0001$); pneumonia after major surgery ($p < 0.001$); thrombosis after major surgery ($p < 0.01$); pulmonary compromise after major surgery ($p < 0.05$); ↑ nurse staffing related to ↓ UTIs, pneumonia, thrombosis, & pulmonary compromise after surgery. | Coding inconsistencies may have occurred in the nine indicators and/or discharge abstracts. Selection process eliminated pts with multiple diagnoses who may have responded differently to nurse staffing. |

(continues)

BSIs = bloodstream infections; CMI = case mix index; DRG = diagnosis-related group; DVT = deep venous thrombosis; FTE = full time equivalent; GI = gastrointestinal; HCUP = Health Care Utilization Project; hrs = hours; LOS = length of stay; NAP or UAP = unlicensed assistive personnel; NIW = nursing intensity weight; NPU = nosocomial pressure ulcer; PD = patient day; PR = pulmonary embolism; pt= patient; UTI = urinary tract infection.

TABLE 6-1 Studies Investigating the Relationship Between Nursing Structural Variables and Adverse Events (continued)

Author date	Design	Sample characteristics/ setting	Independent variables	Outcomes being investigated and approach to measurement	Results	Limitations
Kovner et al. (2002)	Descriptive Cross-sectional	13 U.S. states; HCUP data.	# RNs FTEs/PD adjustment.	Venous thrombosis or pulmonary embolism after major surgery: Discharges with venous thrombosis or pulmonary embolism in any secondary diagnosis/all nonmaternal/nonneonatal discharges aged 18 or older with major surgery procedure on Day 1 or 2 of admission.	# RN hrs/PD adjusted significantly inversely related to pneumonia.	Data do not distinguish between RN direct care providers and indirect or management roles.
			# LPN FTEs/PD adjustment.	Pulmonary compromise after major surgery: Discharges with pulmonary congestion, lung edema, or respiratory insufficiency or failure in any secondary diagnosis/all nonmaternal/nonneonatal discharges aged 18 or older with major surgery procedure on Day 1 or 2 of admission.		Data reflect paid hours and may overestimate productive hours.
						Data exclude UAPs.
				UTIs after major surgery: Discharges with UTIs in any secondary diagnosis/all nonmaternal/nonneonatal discharges aged 18 or older with major surgery procedure on Day 1 or 2 of admission.		
				Pneumonia after major surgery: Discharges with pneumonia in any secondary diagnosis/all nonmaternal/nonneonatal discharges aged 18 or older with major surgery procedure on Day 1 or 2 of admission.		
Krauss et al. (2005)	Case control	N = 106 inpatient falls.	Pt-to-RN ratio at time of fall.	Inpatient falls.	Increased pt-to-nurse ratio associated with a greater risk of falls.	Inpatient falls were reported voluntarily, which may underestimate the incidence of falls.
		N = 318 case control subjects randomly selected and matched on approximate LOS.	History of falls, fall risk level, medications taken within		Patients whose nurses had a ratio greater than 5:1 were 2.6 times more likely to have a fall	

Study	Design	Sample	Measures	Outcomes / Data Collection	Findings	Comments
			the last 24 hrs, side rail and bed position, medical diagnosis at time of fall, activity level, footwear.		than those with fewer than 5 pts.	Interviews regarding pts' risk of falls were conducted with nurses for the participant group, and pts/family for the control group. Recall bias.
Lichtig et al. (1999)	Correlational	Hospitals: California ($N = 462$) and New York ($N = 229$). Patient: California–3.5 million discharges; New York–2.5 million discharges.	RN hours as a percentage of total nursing hours; Total nursing hours per NIW-adjusted pt day.	Collected from Discharge Data Abstract using ICD-9-CM codes that appeared as a secondary diagnosis: pressure ulcers; pneumonia; UTIs; postoperative infections; LOS; rates calculated by DRG for each hospital & for each state - < or < statewide average outcome rates.	Nursing skill mix related to lower pressure ulcer rates. Higher mix of RNs associated with lower levels of pneumonia. In California only, higher % RNs associated with lower postoperative infections. Nursing skill mix related to UTI rates.	Quality of data was inconsistent, especially reported nursing hrs; in some instances, nonreporting of nurse staffing data. Possible under-reporting and inaccurate coding of secondary diagnoses.
Mark et al. (2004)	Retrospective longitudinal with panel data	$N = 422$ hospitals in 11 U.S. states.	RN staffing: RN FTEs/1,000 inpatient days. LPN staffing: LPN FTEs/1000 inpatient days. Non-RN staffing: Non-RN FTEs/1000 inpatient days.	Mortality. Decubitus ulcers. Pneumonia. UTIs. All calculated by: Risk-adjusted observed/expected	A small nonlinear relationship between RN staffing and pt mortality ($r = -.087$, $p < .001$). Suggest that RN and LPN staffing may interact to affect pneumonia, where increasing RN staffing decreases pneumonia more with increased LPN staffing ($r = -.047$, $p < .05$).	Observations were excluded if fewer than 15 adverse events were expected between two time periods. The HCUP data set from which the outcomes were retrieved do not specify whether a diagnosis was present on admission or occurred while in hospital.

(continues)

BSIs = bloodstream infections; CMI = case mix index; DRG = diagnosis-related group; DVT = deep venous thrombosis; GI = gastrointestinal; HCUP = Health Care Utilization Project; hrs = hours; LOS = length of stay; NAP or UAP = unlicensed assistive personnel; NIW = nursing intensity weight; NPU = nosocomial pressure ulcer; PD = patient day; PR = pulmonary embolism; pt= patient; UTI = urinary tract infection.

TABLE 6-1 Studies Investigating the Relationship Between Nursing Structural Variables and Adverse Events (continued)

Author date	Design	Sample characteristics/ setting	Independent variables	Outcomes being investigated and approach to measurement	Results	Limitations
McCloskey & Diers (2005)	Retrospective longitudinal time series	N = 3.3 million medical and surgical inpatient discharges from 1989 to 2000. N = 65,221 nurses (RNs and LPNs) from 1993 to 2000. Acute care hospitals in New Zealand.	Number of nursing FTE. Number of nursing hrs worked. Skill mix (percentage of total RN FTEs).	An adverse outcome was considered for any discharges with an adverse outcome ICD code in the three secondary discharge diagnoses. For all pts: CNS complications, decubitus ulcers, DVT and PE, pneumonia, sepsis, shock and cardiac arrest, upper GI bleed, and UTI. LOS and mortality. For surgical pts only: Pulmonary failure, physiologic and metabolic derangement, and surgical wound infections.	Suggest that the decrease in nursing FTEs and nursing hrs and an increase in skill mix that occurred during New Zealand's hospital restructuring in the early to mid-1990s were associated with higher rates of adverse outcomes, such as CNS complications, decubitus ulcers, and sepsis for medical pts, and CNS complications, decubitus ulcers, DVT/PE, sepsis, UTI, pulmonary failures, and physiologic and metabolic derangement in surgical pts.	Nursing data from the Nursing Workforce data set did not differentiate between inpatient and outpatient nurses. The nursing data set had missing data. Between 1993 and 2000, the nursing data set measured number of hrs worked differently; some years were aggregated by 5 hrs worked, and some years were reported as percentages. The National Minimum Dataset does not account for any diagnoses that may be present on admission.
McGillis Hall et al. (2001)	Descriptive repeated measure	19 Canadian teaching hospitals, 77 units; 2,046 pts.	Proportion of regulated staff (RNs & RPNs) = # RNs & RPNs on Unit × 100/# Total Nursing Personnel on Unit.	Data on medication errors, wound infections, UTIs, and pt falls collected from chart review. Other outcomes collected by survey. Functional status; perceptions of pain; patient satisfaction with nursing care; medication errors; wound infections; UTIs; patient falls.	Higher proportion of RNs/RPNs in the staff mix associated with better functional health and pt satisfaction outcomes at discharge and with lower unit rates of medication errors and wound infections.	Missing data within the health records for secondary data.

McGillis Hall et al. (2004)	Descriptive correlational	N = 19 acute care teaching hospitals in Ontario (N = 77 adult medical, surgical, and obstetrics units).	Proportion of RNs = # RNs on Unit × 100/# Total Nursing Personnel on Unit. RN/RPN staff mix. All RN staff mix. Proportion of regulated to unregulated staff (URW). RN/RPN/URW staff mix. Nursing resource use. Patient complexity.	Falls, medication errors, wound infections, and UTIs.	Units with a lower proportion of RNs/RPNs had higher medication errors (p < .05) and wound infections (p < .01).	The availability and quality of nurse staffing data. Missing data within the health records for secondary data.
Needleman et al. (2002a, 2002b)	Correlational	799 hospitals from 11 states. 5,075,969 medical pts & 1,1104,659 surgical pts.	# of hours per pt for (RNs, LPNs, aides), individual & totaled. Proportion (%) of total RN hours & LPN hours. # hrs/day by licensed nurses; RN hrs as a proportion of licensed nurse hours.	All pts administrative data: UTIs; pressure ulcers; hospital-acquired pneumonia; deep vein thrombosis/pulmonary embolism; upper GI bleed: central nervous system complications; sepsis; shock/cardiac arrest; mortality; failure to rescue. Additional outcomes for surgical pts only: Surgical wound infection, pulmonary failure, metabolic derangement.	Medical patients: Consistent relationships between nurse staffing variables and five pt outcomes (UTIs, pneumonia, LOS, upper GI bleed, and shock). Surgical patients: Relationship between failure to rescue and nurse staffing was strong and consistent (weaker evidence was found for UTIs and pneumonia). Stronger evidence of an association between pt outcomes and levels of RN staffing compared with the evidence linking pt outcomes to mix of LPN.	Concerns about the quality of discharge abstract data, that is, missing data or data recorded incorrectly; staffing data collected from diverse data sets; data not consistently available.

BSIs = bloodstream infections; CMI = case mix index; DRG = diagnosis-related group; DVT = deep venous thrombosis; FTE = full time equivalent; GI = gastrointestinal; HCUP = Health Care Utilization Project; hrs = hours; LOS = length of stay; NAP or UAP = unlicensed assistive personnel; NIW = nursing intensity weight; NPU = nosocomial pressure ulcer; PD = patient day; PR = pulmonary embolism; pt= patient; UTI = urinary tract infection.

(continues)

TABLE 6-1 Studies Investigating the Relationship Between Nursing Structural Variables and Adverse Events (continued)

Author date	Design	Sample characteristics/ setting	Independent variables	Outcomes being investigated and approach to measurement	Results	Limitations
Potter et al. (2003)	Prospective correlational	N = 3,418 patients from 32 units.	Total hrs of nursing care per pt day. Percentage of direct nursing care provided by RNs.	Fall index: Number of falls on unit/number of patient days × 1,000. Medication error index: Number of medication errors on unit/number of patient days × 1,000. Inpatient self-report of self-care, health status, and symptom management (pain, distress, anxiety, and quality of the previous night's sleep). Patient satisfaction from hospital's postdischarge satisfaction measure.	Percentage of direct nursing care provided by RNs was negatively associated with pts' perception of pain and self-care ability and positively associated with pts' satisfaction and health status. Total hrs of nursing care per pt day was negatively associated with patient distress, self-care ability, symptom management, and fall index.	Reliance on voluntary report of falls and medication errors. Recall bias of patient self-report measures.
Sovie & Jawad (2001)	Correlational	29 U.S. teaching hospitals with more that 300 beds. 1 medical unit & 1 surgical unit per site.	FTEs for each type of nursing staff. Skill mix. Hours worked per pt day for all staff and for selected categories of staff (i.e., RNs, UAPs, and a category that included other roles, i.e., LPNs, clerks and managers); LPNs were included in the other category because of the small number of LPNs in these	Patient falls: Any fall or slip in which a pt came to rest unintentionally on the floor, whether it resulted in injury or was witnessed. Multiple falls by the same pt were considered separate events. (# of falls in a unit × 1,000/# of pt days). NPUs: Lesions caused by unrelieved pressure, thus resulting in damage to underlying tissue, had to involve broken skin (# of pts with NPUs in the unit or hospital/total # of pts evaluated in the area (unit or hospital) and expressed as an annual rate). UTIs: Nosocomial if there was no evidence that the infections were present or incubating at the time of admission to the hospital or within 72 hours after admission, and if the infection met the criteria for symptomatic bacteri-	Fall rate declined as # RNs/PD ↑ NPU rates declined on surgical unit, remained constant on medical units, not related to nurse staffing. UTI rates ↑ on both units, not related to nurse staffing.	CMI used for adjustment at hospital level; no risk adjustment at unit level.

Stegenga et al. (2002)	Retrospective descriptive	N = 2,929 admissions to a 44-bed general pediatric unit in Canada.	Labor costs per discharge.	bacteriuria established by the Centers for Disease Control National Nosocomial Infection Surveillance System (# of infections × 100/# of pts discharged).		
			Day patient-to-RN ratios.	Nosocomial viral GI infections (NVGIs).	Monthly NVGIs were positively associated with both day (r = .50, p < .05) and night patient-to-RN ratios (r = .56, p < .05).	Nursing hrs included educational time, which might have overestimated actual time spent on patient care.
			Night patient-to-RN ratios.			Did not account for patient acuity.
			Nursing hrs per patient day.		The risk of NVGIs was almost three times greater during the 72-hr period after an understaffed day (less than 10.5 nursing hrs per patient day).	Patient-to-nurse ratios were used as a surrogate measure of nurse workload.

(continues)

BSIs = bloodstream infections; CMI = case mix index; DRG = diagnosis-related group; DVT = deep venous thrombosis; FTE = full time equivalent; GI = gastrointestinal; HCUP = Health Care Utilization Project; hrs = hours; LOS = length of stay; NAP or UAP = unlicensed assistive personnel; NIW = nursing intensity weight; NPU = nosocomial pressure ulcer; PD = patient day; PR = pulmonary embolism; pt= patient;   UTI = urinary tract infection.

TABLE 6-1 Studies Investigating the Relationship Between Nursing Structural Variables and Adverse Events (continued)

Author date	Design	Sample characteristics/ setting	Independent variables	Outcomes being investigated and approach to measurement	Results	Limitations
Taunton et al. (1994)	Correlational	Four large acute care hospitals (Midwest U.S.). One teaching hospital. 65 pt care units.	Absenteeism: Individual staff RN variable averaged for work unit = Total days absent per quarter/Total days scheduled per quarter × 100. Unit separation (Resignation or transfer) = # staff RNs leaving work unit per quarter/# staff RNs on unit at beginning of quarter × 100. Workload = required pt care hours/actual pt care hours.	UTI: Monthly average for UTIs per quarter/Monthly average for pt days per quarter × 1000. BSIs = monthly average for BSIs per quarter/Monthly average for pt days per quarter × 1,000. Falls: Total pt falls per quarter/Total pt days per quarter × 1,000. Medication errors: Total medication errors per quarter/Total nursing care hours per quarter × 10,000.	An association between UTIs & staff RN absenteeism and between BSIs & RN absenteeism; no meaningful relationships among falls, medication errors, and any of the organizational variables that were examined.	Data abstracted retrospectively from hospital records may lead to underreporting; measurement errors at initial data point, measurement error in relation to operational definitions of variables. Patient outcomes data collected from chart reviews; dose-based denominators for medication errors were not available for capturing ratios.

Taylor (2007)	Retrospective cross-sectional doctoral dissertation	N = 28,876 inpatients from 29 units in one acute care hospital for falls and medication errors. N = 28,260 discharges from 29 units in 1 acute care hospital for PE/DVTs and decubitus ulcers.	Turnover. Nursing hrs per pt day. Safety attitude questionnaire (includes nurses' stress, safety and morale).	PE/DVT extracted from the discharge data by applying the Patient Safety Indicators. Falls extracted from Patient Safety Net. Decubitus ulcers extracted from the discharge data by applying the Patient Safety Indicators. Medication errors extracted from Patient Safety Net.	Increasing RN stress recognition was associated with a 1.5 to 3 times the odds of patient falls, medication errors, and decubitus ulcers. RNs safety climate was negatively associated with the odds of patients developing a decubitus ulcer. Nursing hrs per pt day had a negative relationship with pt falls and a positive relationship with medication errors. Each increase of 1 hour of productive nursing per pt was related to a 10% decrease in the odds of pt falls and an 8% increase in the odds of medication errors.	Skill mix not included. Influence of nursing characteristics not included. Did not account for patient health risks/characteristics.

BSIs = bloodstream infections; CMI = case mix index; DRG = diagnosis-related group; deep venous thrombosis = DVT; FTE = full time equivalent; GI = gastrointestinal; HCUP = Health Care Utilization Project; hrs = hours; LOS = length of stay; NAP or UAP = unlicensed assistive personnel; NIW = nursing intensity weight; NPU = nosocomial pressure ulcer; PD = patient day; PR = pulmonary embolism; pt= patient; UTI = urinary tract infection.

Kovner and Gergen (1998) examined the relationship between nurse staffing and the adverse events of patient mortality, medication error rate, and nosocomial infections for 589 acute care hospitals. Controlling for case mix, the researchers collected information on hospital-level variables such as teaching status, ownership, bed size, hospital resources, and region. The researchers examined outcomes that could theoretically be linked to nursing, as well as outcomes that did not have a theoretical link to nursing. They found a strong relationship between full-time-equivalent RNs per adjusted day and urinary tract infections and pneumonia after surgery, and a less robust relationship between full-time-equivalent RNs per adjusted day and thrombosis after surgery. The researchers found no relationship between nurse staffing and pneumonia or venous thrombosis. The authors cautioned that coding inconsistencies and inaccuracies in discharge abstracts may have influenced the results of the study. Also, the selection process eliminated patients with multiple diagnoses, who may have responded differently to nurse staffing.

Blegen et al. (1998) examined the role of nurse staffing on patient outcomes. Data were collected from hospital records on 42 inpatient units on the following outcomes: patient falls, medication errors, pressure ulcers, patient complaints, respiratory and urinary tract infections, and mortality. The researchers controlled for patient severity by using nursing acuity system data. They found that units with higher than average patient acuity had lower rates of medication errors and patient falls. They also found that these same units had higher rates of other adverse occurrences such as skin breakdown, patient and family complaints, infections, and deaths. When they controlled for average patient acuity, the proportion of hours of care delivered by RNs was inversely related to the unit rates of medication errors, decubiti, and patient complaints. Total hours of care from all nursing personnel were associated directly with the rates of decubiti, complaints, and mortality. This study also reported an unexpected finding: The relationship between registered nursing staff proportion of care was curvilinear. As the RN proportion increased, rates of adverse outcomes decreased up to 87.5%. At that level, as RN proportion increased, adverse occurrences also increased. The authors theorized that their indicator for acuity might not have been sensitive enough to control for the sharply higher acuity levels in critical care units and intermediate care units.

Blegen and Vaughn (1998) conducted a multisite study to describe the relationship between nurse staffing and the outcomes of medication errors, patient falls, and cardiopulmonary arrests. They collected unit-level data and controlled for patient acuity and reported that units with a higher proportion of RNs had lower rates of patient falls. In addition, there was a "nonlinear" relationship between the proportion of RNs in the staff mix and medication administration errors. Medication errors declined as the proportion of RNs increased up to 85%; however, any further increase in the proportion of RNs resulted in increased medication administration errors. The authors indicated that further research is required to provide a fuller explanation of these findings.

Lichtig et al. (1999) examined the impact of nurse staffing on adverse events for hospitals in California and New York. Using statewide data collected in the Uniform Hospital Discharge Data Set, they collected information on the following outcomes: pressure ulcers, pneumonia, urinary tract infections, postoperative infections, and length of stay. They found that the higher the percentage of registered nursing staff and, to a lesser degree, the more nursing hours per acuity-adjusted day, the better the patient outcomes for pressure ulcers, pneumonia, postoperative infections, and urinary tract infections.

In 1994, the American Nurses Association initiated the Patient Safety and Quality Initiative, a multifaceted approach to examining the impact of staffing changes on the quality of patient care. It included a focus on research using large databases to identify indicators that have a strong relationship to patient outcomes. The indicators selected for the Patient Safety and Quality Initiative were specific to nursing, could be tracked over time, and had a strong link to nursing quality. After an extensive literature review, expert consultations, and focus groups, the initiative identified 21 nursing quality care indicators for potential use in a report card for nursing. The American Nurses Association experienced difficulties in measuring and tracking these indicators and, in a pilot study conducted in 48 hospitals in California and New York, collected information on only seven indicators: total nursing care hours per nursing intensity weight; RN hours as a percentage of all nursing hours; length of stay; pressure ulcers; pneumonia; urinary tract infections; and postoperative infections. According to the findings, a higher proportion of RNs was significantly associated with lower length of stay and lower rates of pressure ulcers, pneumonia, postoperative infection, and urinary tract infections (ANA, 1997).

One component of the American Nurses Association initiative is the development, testing, storage, and evaluation of nursing-sensitive indicators by the University of Kansas School of Nursing and Medical Center Research Institute (Midwest Research Institute [MRI], 1999). To support a National Database of Nursing Quality Indicators, which is housed at the University of Kansas, the American Nurses Association conducted six pilot projects with State Nursing Associations in Arizona, California, Virginia, Minnesota, North Dakota, and Texas and collected data on the following indicators: nursing hours per patient day, nursing skill mix, pressure ulcers, falls, nosocomial infections, patient satisfaction with pain management, patient satisfaction with educational information, patient satisfaction with nursing care, patient satisfaction with overall care, and nurse job satisfaction. More than 256 hospitals across 37 states were participating in this initiative by 2000 (Rowell, 2001). Currently, more than 1,400 U.S. hospitals are participating in this initiative (ANA, 2009).

A second American Nurses Association study examined the relationship between nurse staffing and five outcome measures: length of stay, pneumonia, postoperative infections, pressure sores, and urinary tract infections (ANA, 2000). Nursing intensity weights (NIWs) were used to identify the differences in patients' acuity or need for nursing care. This study found that secondary bacterial pneumonia, postoperative infections, pressure ulcers, and urinary tract infections were lower in hospitals with higher RN skill mixes and, in some instances, greater staffing levels. In examining adverse occurrences, the American Nurses Association also considered two other factors that influence healthcare practice: hospital teaching status (primary medical school affiliate, other teaching, or nonteaching) and setting (defined as large urban, urban, or rural). The American Nurses Association report highlights the difficulty of obtaining data that measure the amounts and type of nursing care provided. Researchers found that nurse staffing data are not collected universally on a comprehensive basis.

McGillis Hall et al. (2001) assessed the composition and mix of nursing care staff in 19 teaching hospitals on patient, nurse, and system outcomes. More than 2,046 patients, 1,116 nurses, 63 unit managers, and 50 senior executives participated in the study. The authors controlled for other possible determinants of health outcomes, such as case mix, baseline health status, patient age, gender, and complexity of illness. Unit-level data were collected from the discharge abstract database of patient health records on patient falls, medication errors, urinary tract infections, and wound infections, using consistent definitions. Nursing staff mix was found to be a significant predictor of four patient health outcomes (functional independence, pain, social functioning, and satisfaction with obstetrical care) and two quality outcomes (medication errors and wound infections). This study is significant because it measured outcomes at the individual patient level rather than at the inpatient unit or hospital level. The authors of this study also expressed concern about the availability and quality of nurse staffing data. Given that the secondary data for patient falls, pressure ulcers, and nosocomial infections were collected from the health records, it is impossible to know if data were missing or recorded incorrectly.

Needleman et al. (2002a, 2002b) conducted an analysis of the discharge records of more than 6 million patients, of whom 5 million were admitted to the hospital because of a medical diagnosis and 1 million for a surgical problem. This study examined whether there was a correlation between the levels of RNs and patient outcomes. In hospitals with higher RN staffing, patients' stays were 3–5% shorter, and patient complication rates 2–9% lower, than in hospitals with lower staffing. Researchers found that a higher proportion of hours of care by RNs was associated with lower rates of pneumonia, shock and cardiac arrest, upper gastrointestinal bleeding, sepsis, and deep venous thrombosis. For surgical patients, the higher the proportion of care provided by RNs, the lower the rate of urinary tract infections, and the greater the number of hours of care per day provided by a RN, the lower the rate of "failure to rescue." No association was found between increased levels of staffing by RNs and the rate of in-hospital death, or between increased staffing by LPNs or nurses' aides and the rate of adverse events. The study underscored the weaknesses of currently available data. Nurse staffing data are inconsistent in data sets. When using secondary diagnosis, it is not always possible to ascertain whether the conditions were present on admission. Discharge abstract data are vulnerable to missing data or data that are recorded incorrectly.

Sovie and Jawad (2001) collected data from 29 teaching hospitals to evaluate the impact of hospital restructuring initiatives on outcomes. Data were collected on rate of patient falls, nosocomial pressure ulcers, urinary tract infections, and patient satisfaction. The data were collected from incident reports (patient falls), prevalence studies (nosocomial pressure ulcers), and hospital infectious disease reports or quarterly retrospective chart audits (urinary tract infections). Researchers found that increased RN hours worked per patient day were associated with lower fall rates. They also reported a strong relationship between RN staffing and urinary tract infections. In this study, the prevalence of pressure ulcers decreased, and the authors surmised that this was the result of monthly prevalence surveys, which resulted in increased assessment and planning by nurses. Although case mix index was available at the hospital level, the authors argued that for risk adjustment purposes, this information is required at the unit level.

Kovner, Jones, Zhan, Gergen, and Basu (2002) examined the impact of nurse staffing on four postsurgical events: venous thrombosis/pulmonary embolism, pulmonary compromise after surgery, urinary tract infection, and pneumonia. To limit variation in severity in this study, the authors eliminated data for patients admitted from nursing homes, other hospitals, and elsewhere. They reported a significant inverse relationship between RN hours per adjusted patient day and pneumonia. The authors pointed to the limitations of available staffing data. Databases do not differentiate between direct care providers and indirect care providers. Also, only paid hours are captured. This may diminish the relationship between nurse staffing and adverse events. Stegenga et al. (2002) examined the relationship between nurse staffing and the development of nosocomial gastrointestinal infections in a Canadian pediatric population admitted on one nursing unit. The authors found that monthly infection rate was associated with the nurse-to-patient ratios on both day and night shifts. They also found that the risk of acquiring a nosocomial gastrointestinal infection was three times greater during the 72-hour period after an understaffed day. The authors defined understaffing as less than 10.5 nursing hours per patient day. Similar to Kovner et al. (2002), the authors reported limitations of the available nurse staffing data. Nurses' educational time is included in the nursing hours per patient day. This may overestimate the actual time nurses spent on patient care in this study.

Dellefield (2006) examined the impact of nurse staffing on risk-adjusted pressure ulcer prevalence and deficiency citation in California nursing homes. Using the Online Survey Certification and Reporting system and the Office of Statewide Health Planning and Development data sources for California nursing homes, the author collected information on RN, LPN, and certified nursing assistant staffing, the prevalence of pressure ulcers and nursing homes' deficiency citations, and nursing home size, ownership, and proportion of Medicaid residents. Residents' clinical risk factors were accounted for by calculating the risk-adjusted pressure ulcer prevalence. Findings indicate that a greater proportion of RNs to LPNs was related to lower risk-adjusted prevalence of pressure ulcers and that lower total nursing personnel hours per patient day and greater skill mix were associated with a greater number of deficiency citations. The author cautioned that the data sources used had inherent limitations, such as missing data, data at the facility level instead of the resident level, and misreported staffing data.

Mark et al. (2004) conducted an analysis of data from the American Hospital Association, the Centers for Medicare and Medicaid Services, InterStudy and Area Resource Files, and the Healthcare Cost and Utilization Project to examine the relationship between changes in nurse staffing and adverse events, such as decubitus ulcers, pneumonia, urinary tract infections, and mortality. Longitudinal data for 422 American hospitals were examined. The authors included case mix, payer mix, number of hospital beds, and whether hospital was public or private in their analysis. Findings suggest that RN and LPN staffing may interact to affect patient pneumonia rates, such that increasing RN staffing decreases pneumonia more when LPN staffing is higher. Caution on the weaknesses of the available adverse events data was highlighted. The Healthcare Cost and Utilization Project data set does not specify whether a diagnosis was present on admission or occurred while in the hospital.

McCloskey and Diers (2005) examined medical and surgical patient discharges from New Zealand's public hospitals and survey data from the nursing workforce to determine the effects of hospital reengineering on nurse staffing and patient adverse events. The authors found that the decrease in nursing hours and full-time equivalents and an increase in skill mix that took place during New Zealand's public hospitals reengineering were associated with greater rates of adverse events, such as decubitus ulcers and sepsis for medical patients, and decubitus ulcers, deep venous thrombosis/ pulmonary embolism, wound infections, sepsis, and urinary tract infections for surgical patients. The authors highlighted several limitations of working with administrative data sets. The Nursing Workforce data set did not differentiate between inpatient and outpatient nurses and had missing data, and the variable *number of nursing hours worked* was measured differently at different points in time. Also, the National Minimum Dataset did not differentiate between diagnoses present on admission versus those acquired during hospitalization.

More recently, Lake and Cheung (2006) conducted a critical analysis of studies examining the relationships between nurse staffing, and falls and pressure ulcers in acute care hospitals. The inclusion criteria for this analysis were: articles were published in peer-reviewed journals; studies were conducted in acute care sites; falls or pressure ulcers were the outcomes examined; and the authors used multivariate analysis of nurse staffing. Eleven articles met these inclusion criteria. The authors reported that their analysis could not provide conclusive evidence for the relationships between nurse staffing, and falls and pressure ulcers. They suggested that the varied research methodologies used across these studies may partially account for the equivocal findings.

Kane et al. (2007a) conducted a systematic review ($N = 94$ studies) for the Agency for Healthcare Research and Quality to examine the associations between nurse staffing in hospitals and patient outcomes. The analysis was adjusted for patient acuity at both the individual and hospital levels. The authors also created two standardized nurse staffing rates: the number of patients per nurse/shift and RN full-time equivalent per patient day. Although the results of this systematic review support the contention that nurse staffing is associated with patients' outcomes, the authors were unable to assert the causality of this relationship. This study resulted in a publication of the subfindings of the systematic review (Kane et al., 2007b).

ISSUES WITH NURSING RESEARCH ON ADVERSE PATIENT OUTCOMES

This critical review of the current literature exploring the relationship between nursing and adverse patient outcomes has highlighted a number of important concerns. Most of the challenges relate to methodological concerns with the collection and the quality of the data. The studies on adverse occurrences are based on chart reviews of the antecedents of these occurrences and whether an error occurred that led to the event (Hayward & Hofer, 2001). Much of the literature on medical errors is hampered by a lack of workable operational definitions, imprecision in measurement, and conceptual overlap of the terms used to discuss adverse events (Hofer, Kerr, & Hayward, 2000).

One of the limitations with the work to date has been the limited use of conceptual frameworks to guide the field of patient safety research. A number of conceptual models exist that could serve as a framework. For example, Irvine, Sidani, and McGillis Hall (1998) developed the Nursing Role Effectiveness model that conceptualizes nurses' contribution to health care in terms of the roles they assume in health care and relates those roles to patient outcome achievement. Patient safety can be a result of the quality of nurses' independent roles (e.g., precision in patient assessment), medical care-related roles (e.g., nurses' clinical judgment and implementation of a medical order), or interdependent roles (e.g., accurate and timely communication among members of the healthcare team).

Affonso and Doran (2002) developed a theoretical framework that conceptualizes patient safety in terms of four cornerstones: (a) building technological tools to create safer ways for dealing with drugs and devices (Kohn et al., 2000); (b) applying human-factors designs to create healthy work environments; (c) reforming the organizational culture to foster critical thinking for decision-making and teamwork; and (d) delivering processes to optimize safe care via precision in assessments, monitoring and tracking patient responses, and performing ongoing evaluations of processes to prevent errors from occurring. Mitchell, Ferketich, and Jennings (1998) extended Donabedian's 1966 (Donabedian, 1966) structure, process, and outcomes framework to develop a dynamic and reciprocal Quality Health Outcomes model that would be more sensitive to nursing inputs. This model has four components: (1) system characteristics, which includes individuals, organizations, and/ or groups, allowing for multiple levels of analysis; (2) interventions; (3) clients' characteristics; and (4) outcomes that reflect the effects of nursing interventions on clients' health. This model proposes that interventions are not directly linked to outcomes, but instead that outcomes reflect a more dynamic process with interactions among system characteristics, client characteristics, and interventions.

Comparisons of adverse occurrences are limited by variations in patient characteristics. Of particular concern are characteristics, such as comorbidities, that can affect the probability of an adverse outcome. Mitchell, Heindrich, Moritz, and Hinshaw (1997) argued for the inclusion of risk adjustment when examining adverse occurrences. Without adjusting for variations in these characteristics, it is impossible to determine whether a seemingly bad outcome (e.g., a high number of pressure ulcers) reflects a substandard quality of care or whether it results from the treatment of a disproportionate number of patients with high-risk characteristics. Lake and Cheung (2006) also argued that future nurse staffing and patient adverse events research must include patient-specific risk or characteristics. Blegen et al. (1998) reported that many studies examining nurse-sensitive outcomes use adjustments for severity at the hospital level (i.e., case-mix adjustments), but these cannot reflect severity of patients' conditions on separate units (i.e., an obstetrical unit versus an acute medical unit). Because the impact of nurse staffing is at the unit level, future research on adverse occurrences should adjust for acuity at this level. Lake and Cheung contended that studies conducted only at the hospital level do not account for the clustering of patients at the unit level or, by contrast, that units are clustered within hospitals. They argued that future research must use multilevel modeling to appropriately address the multilevel nature of nurse staffing and patient adverse events.

Nursing research continues to be limited by the variables captured in existing databases. There is a lack of reliability in how the data are reported within and among sites. In the early work on testing the American Nurses Association indicators, challenges were encountered with diverse definitions within organizations, lack of agreed-on instrumentation for measuring outcomes, and difficulty capturing data at the unit level (Mowinski Jennings, Loan, DePaul, Brosch, & Hildreth, 2001). Many early empirical studies on outcomes were conducted in single settings, which affects researchers' ability to compare the role of nursing on various patient outcomes across settings. Researchers are beginning to conduct large-scale examinations of patient outcomes. Multi-site research needs to be grounded in consistent and comparable definitions of outcomes that are of interest to nursing and that incorporate standardized, sensitive acuity measures (Blegen et al., 1998; Mark & Burleson, 1995). Rowell (2001) emphasized the need for cost-effective databases and data retrieval systems to capture nursing indicator data.

To provide variables that will assist researchers in understanding how different numbers and types of nurses affect patient safety outcomes, the quality of the nursing structural variables in databases must be improved. Currently, the nursing variables in administrative databases are inconsistent. The variables include all nurses in the organization rather than only the nurses who provide direct care (Blegen el al., 1998). This limits researchers' ability to understand the relationships between nurse staffing and patient safety outcomes. To understand the relationship between nurse staffing and adverse patient occurrences, researchers need to know the direct nurse staffing hours by skill level and cost center. Additionally, to ensure consistent interpretation of findings, there must be uniformity in how researchers conceptualize and measure staffing hours and skill mix (Lake & Cheung, 2006).

Pierce (1997) warned that studying outcomes alone will be insufficient if they are analyzed in isolation. Donabedian's (1982) framework for measuring the quality of care through structure, process, and outcomes indicators continues to underlie how we view nursing's role in adverse occurrences. Within healthcare organizations, the relationship between the structure of nursing and outcomes of care is not clearly understood. In addition, nursing practice is situated within an increasingly complex environment. A working group on the relationship between nurse staffing and healthcare-associated infections suggested that the inconsistencies in nursing research may be reflective of a systems layer that has not yet been identified (Jackson, Chiarello, Gaynes, & Gerberding, 2002). This should not preclude us from moving forward with the collection of data on adverse patient outcomes. Further research requires consistent reliable data to explore the links between nursing inputs, processes of care, and outcomes of care. Also, future research must collect data on organizational variables that shape nursing environments.

To date, much of the nursing research on adverse patient outcomes has occurred in acute care settings. This reflects the availability of staffing data in this sector. However, health care occurs across a continuum of community care, acute care, and long-term care settings. As the population ages, its need for health care changes, and many people move through these different sectors. Because nursing plays a role in health care across the continuum of care, future research should examine the relationship between nursing and adverse patient outcomes in all healthcare sectors. This will require administrators, policy makers, researchers, and funders to identify the staffing and nursing-sensitive outcome variables required to support research.

EMERGING THEMES IN ADVERSE PATIENT OUTCOMES RESEARCH

Researchers have started looking at novel ways to gain a greater understanding of the process through which nurse staffing affects patient care, as well as new ways of defining and examining adverse patient outcomes. Schubert et al. (2008) examined the impact of nurses' decisions to ration care to gain a greater understanding of the process of how nurse understaffing affects patient care. Rationing of nursing care occurs when nurses perceive that there is a lack of time to perform essential nursing tasks for various reasons, such as low staffing levels or skill mix, and must subsequently decide which tasks cannot be carried out or withheld altogether. They found that higher levels of rationing of care were associated with higher levels of nurse-reported nosocomial infections, patient falls, pressure ulcers, and medication errors, even after controlling for nurse-to-patient ratios. The authors suggest that the process of rationing nursing care may partially explain how lower staffing may influence patient outcomes. Chang and Mark's (2009) study examining the antecedents of medication errors distinguished between errors at different levels of severity, specifically severe and nonsevere errors. The authors contended that severe and nonsevere medication errors may not have the same underlying causal factors and that studies combining these potentially different types of errors may generate inaccurate results. This study found that these two types of medication errors did have different predictors; nursing expertise and experience were negatively associated with nonsevere medication errors, and BScN-prepared nurses were associated with fewer severe medication errors.

CONCLUSION

As the only healthcare providers who are with patients 24 hours a day, 7 days a week, nurses play a role in preventing adverse patient outcomes. The literature examined in this review suggests that nurses may be important in the prevention of patient falls, pressure ulcers, nosocomial infections, and medication errors. Researchers have begun examining the process through which nurse staffing affects patient care in unique ways. Continued research is required to further the system's understanding of the relationship between nursing and adverse events and to help inform the decisions that administrators and policy makers make regarding nurse staffing. This review also highlights the challenges in conducting rigorous adverse patient outcomes research, such as those relating to the methodological concerns with the collection, the consistency, and the quality of the data. Efforts need to be directed toward improving the quality and consistency of the data collected. There is also a need to examine the relationships between nurses and adverse patient outcomes in settings other than acute care, such as home care and long-term care settings. The role of nurses in the provision of quality patient care in these settings is as important as in acute care. Structuring nursing to create an optimum practice environment to promote patient safety is, and will continue to be, of concern to administrators, decision makers, policy makers, and the public.

REFERENCES

Affonso, D., & Doran, D. (2002). Cultivating discoveries in patient safety research: A framework. *Journal of International Nursing Perspectives, 2*(1), 33–47.

Agostini, J. V., Baker, D. I., & Bogardus, S. T. (2001, July). *Making health care safer: A Critical analysis of patient safety practices* (Evidence Report/Technology Assessment No. 43; AHRQ Publication No. 01-E058). Retrieved June 6, 2002 from http://www.ahrq.gov/clinic/ptsafety/index.html

Aiken, L. H., Smith, H. L., & Lake, E. T. (1994). Lower Medicare mortality among a set of hospitals known for good nursing care. *Medical Care, 32*(8), 171–187.

Aiken, L. H., Clarke, S. P., & Sloane, D. M. (2001). Hospital restructuring: Does it adversely affect care and outcomes? *Journal of Health and Human Services Administration, 23,* 416–442.

American Nurses Association. (1995). *Nursing report card for acute care.* Washington, DC: American Nurses Publishing.

American Nurses Association. (1996a). *Nursing quality indicators.* Washington, DC: American Nurses Publishing.

American Nurses Association. (1996b). *Nursing quality indicators: Guide for implementation.* Washington, DC: American Nurses Publishing.

American Nurses Association. (1997). *Implementing nursing's report card.* Washington, DC: American Nurses Publishing.

American Nurses Association. (2000). *Nurse staffing and patient outcomes in the inpatient hospital setting.* Washington, DC: American Nurses Publishing.

American Nurses Association. (2009). *NDNQI: Transforming data into quality care.* Retrieved July 1, 2009, from http://www.nursingworld.org/MainMenuCategories/ThePracticeofProfessionalNursing/PatientSafetyQuality/Research-Measurement/The-National-Database/NDNQIBrochure.aspx

Bakarich, A., McMillan, V., & Prosser, R. (1997). The effect of a nursing intervention on the incidence of older patient falls. *Australian Journal of Advanced Nursing, 15*(1), 26–31.

Baker, R. G., Norton, P. G., Flintoft, V., Blais, R., Brown, A., Cox, J., et al. (2004). The Canadian adverse events study: The incidence of adverse events among hospital patients in Canada. *Canadian Medical Association Journal, 170,* 1678–1686.

Barter, M., McLaughlin, F. E., & Thomas, S. A. (1997). Registered nurse role changes and satisfaction with unlicensed assistive personnel. *Journal of Nursing Administration, 27*(1), 29–38.

Blegen, M. A., Goode, C. J., & Reed, L. (1998). Nurse staffing and patient outcomes. *Nursing Research, 47*(1), 43–50.

Blegen, M. A., & Vaughn, T. (1998). A multisite study of nurse staffing and patient occurrences. *Nursing Economic$, 16*, 196–203.

Bostrum, J., Mechanic, J., Lazar, N., Michelson, S., Grant, L., & Nomura, L. (1996). Preventing skin breakdown: Nursing practice, costs, and outcomes. *Applied Nursing Research, 9*, 184–188.

Brennan, T. A., Leape, L. L., Laird, N. M., Herbert, L., Localio, R., Lawthers, A. G., et al. (1991). Incidence of adverse events and negligence in hospitalized patients. *New England Journal of Medicine, 324*, 370–376.

Buerhaus, P. I. (1999). Lucian Leape on the causes and prevention of errors and adverse events in health care. *Image: Journal of Nursing Scholarship, 31*, 281–286.

Buerhaus, P. I., & Norman, L. (2001). It's time to require theory and methods of quality improvement in basic and graduate nursing education. *Nursing Outlook, 49*(2), 67–69.

Centers for Disease Control. (2000, March 3) *Monitoring hospital-acquired infections to promote patient safety—United States, 1990–1999.* Retrieved July 25, 2002, from http://www.cdc.gov/mmwr/preview/mmwrhtml/mm4908a1.htm

Chang, Y-K., & Mark, B. A. (2009). Antecedents of severe and nonsevere medication errors. *Journal of Nursing Scholarship, 41*, 70–78.

Cho, S. H., Ketefian, S., Barkauskas, V. H., & Smith, D. G. (2003). The effects of nurse staffing on adverse events, morbidity, mortality, and medical costs. *Nursing Research, 52*(2), 71–79.

Cook, R. I., Render, M., & Woods, D. D. (2000). Gaps in the continuity of care and progress on patient safety. *British Journal of Medicine, 320*, 791–794.

Davis, P., Lay-Yee, R., Briant, R., Schug, S., Johnson, S., & Bingley, W. (2001). *Adverse events in New Zealand public hospitals: Principal findings from a national survey.* Wellington, New Zealand: Ministry of Health. Retrieved from http://www.moh.govt.nz/moh.nsf/49ba80c00757b8804c256673001d47d0/d255c2525480c8a1cc256b120006cf25

Dellefield, M. A. (2006). Organizational correlates of the risk-adjusted pressure ulcer prevalence and subsequent survey deficiency citation in California nursing homes. *Research in Nursing and Health, 29*, 345–358.

Donabedian, A. (1966). Evaluating the quality of medical care. *Milbank Memorial Fund Quarterly, 44*, 166–206.

Donabedian, A. (1982). Quality, cost, and health: An integrative model. *Medical Care, 20*, 975–992.

Donaldson, N., Burnes Bolton, L., Aydin, C., Brown, D., Elashoff, J. D., & Sandhu, M. (2005). Impact of California's licensed nurse-patient ratios on unit-level nurse staffing and patient outcomes. *Policy, Politics, and Nursing Practice, 6*, 198–210.

Dunton, N., Gajewski, B., Taunton, R. L., & Moore, J. (2004). Nurse staffing and patient falls on acute care hospital units. *Nursing Outlook, 52*(1), 53–59.

Flood, S. D., & Diers, D. (1988). Nurse staffing, patient outcome and cost. *Nursing Management, 19*(5), 35–43.

Foley, M. (1999). *Written testimony of the American Nurses Association before the Senate Committee on health education, labor, and pensions on medical errors.* Retrieved April 30, 2000, from http://www.nursingworld.org/gova/federal/legis/testimon/2000/mf0126.htm

Frantz, R. A., Berquist, S., & Specht, J. (1995). The cost of treating pressure ulcers following implementation of a research-based skin care protocol in a long term care facility. *Advanced Wound Care, 8*(1), 36–45.

Frantz, R. A., Gardner, S., Specht, J. K., & McIntire, G. (2001). Integration of pressure ulcer treatment protocol into practice: Clinical outcomes and care environment attributes. *Outcomes Management for Nursing Practice, 5*, 112–120.

Fridkin, S. K., Pear, S. M., Williamson, T. H., Galgiani, J. N., & Jarvis, W. R. (1996). The role of understaffing in central venous catheter-associated bloodstream infections. *Infection Control and Hospital Epidemiology, 17*, 150–158.

Fuqua, R. A., & Stevens, K. R. (1988). What we know about medication errors. A literature review. *Journal of Nursing Quality Assurance, 3*(1), 1–17.

Grillo-Peck, A. M., & Risner, P. B. (1995). The effect of a partnership model on quality and length of stay. *Nursing Economic$, 13*, 367–372, 374.

Grobe, S. J., Becker, H., Calvin, A., Biering, P., Jordan, C., & Tabone, S. (1998). Clinical data for use in assessing quality: Lessons learned from the Texas Nurses' Association report card. *Seminars for Nurse Managers, 6*, 126–138.

Hayward, R. A., & Hofer, T. P. (2001). Estimating hospital deaths due to medical errors. *Journal of the American Medical Association, 286*(4). Retrieved July 25, 2001, from http://www.ncbi.nlm.nih.gov/pubmed/11466119

Hernandez, M., & Millar, J. (1986). How to reduce patient falls. *Geriatric Nursing, 7*(2), 97–102.

Hofer, T. P., Kerr, E. A., & Hayward, R. A. (2000). What is an error? *American College of Physicians Online.* Retrieved June 19, 2002, from http://www.acponline.org/journals/ecp/novdec00/hofer.htm

Hopkins, B., Hanlon, M., Yauk, S., Sykes, S., Rose, T., & Cleary, A. (2000). Reducing nosocomial pressure ulcers in an acute care facility. *Journal of Nursing Care Quality, 14*(3), 28–36.

Hugonnet, S., Chevrolet, J-C., Pittet, D. (2007). The effect of workload on infection risk in critically ill patients. *Critical Care Medicine, 35*(1), 76–81.

Iezzoni, L. I., Daley, J., Heeren, T., Foley, S. M., Hughes, J. S., Fisher, E. S., et al. (1994). Using administrative data to screen hospitals for high complication rates. *Inquiry, 31*, 40–55.

Institute of Medicine. (2000). *To err is human: Building a safer health system.* Washington, DC: National Academy Press. Retrieved from http://www.nap.edu/openbook.php?isbn=0309068371

Institute of Medicine. (2007). *Preventing medication errors.* Washington, DC: National Academy Press. Retrieved July 1, 2009, from http://www.iom.edu/?id=35961

Irvine, D. M., Sidani, S., & McGillis Hall, L. (1998). Linking outcomes to nurses' roles in health care. *Nursing Economic$, 16*, 58–64, 87.

Jackson, M., Chiarello, L., Gaynes, R. P., & Gerberding, J. L. (2002). Nurse staffing and healthcare-associated infections: Proceedings from a working group meeting. *Journal of Nursing Administration, 32*(6), 314–322.

Kane, R. L., Shamliyan, T. A., Mueller, C., Duval, S., & Wilt, T. J. (2007a). *Nursing staffing and quality of patient care* (Evidence Report/Technology Assessment No. 151; AHRQ Publication No. 07-E005). Retrieved July 1, 2009, from http://www.ahrq.gov/downloads/pub/evidence/pdf/nursestaff/nursestaff.pdf

Kane, R. L., Shamliyan, T. A., Mueller, C., Duval, S., & Wilt, T. J. (2007b). The association of registered nurse staffing levels and patient outcomes. *Medical Care, 45*, 1195–1204.

Keepnews, D. (2000). A systems approach to health care errors: Experts say we'll need a "culture of safety" to reduce errors. *American Journal of Nursing, 100*(6), 77–78.

Knaus, W. A., Draper, E. A., Wagner, D. P., & Zimmerman, J. E. (1986). An evaluation of outcomes from intensive care in major medical centers. *Annals of Internal Medicine, 104*, 410–418.

Kohn, L. T., Corrigan, J. M., & Donaldson, M. S. (2000). *To err is human: Building a safer health system.* Washington, DC: National Academy Press.

Kovner, C., & Gergen, P. (1998). Nurse staffing levels and adverse events following surgery in U.S. hospitals. *Image: Journal of Nursing Scholarship, 30*, 315–321.

Kovner, C., Jones, J., Zhan, C., Gergen, P. J., & Basu, J. (2002). Nurse staffing and postsurgical adverse events: An analysis of administrative data from a sample of U.S. hospitals, 1990–1996. *HSR: Health Services Research, 37*, 611–629.

Krapohl, G. L., & Larson, E. (1996). The impact of unlicensed assistive personnel on nursing care delivery. *Nursing Economic$, 14*, 99–109.

Krauss, M. J., Evanoff, B., Hitcho, E., Ngugi, K. E., Dunagan, W. C., Fisher, I., et al. (2005). A case-control study of patient, medication, and care-related risk factors for inpatient falls. *Journal of General Internal Medicine, 20*, 116–122.

Lake, E. T., & Cheung, R. B. (2006). Are patient falls and pressure ulcers sensitive to nurse staffing? *Western Journal of Nursing Research, 28*, 654–677.

Langemo, D. K., Anderson, J., & Volden, C. M. (2002). Nursing quality outcome indicators. The North Dakota study. *Journal of Nursing Administration, 32*(2), 98–105.

Larson, E., Oram, L. F., & Hedrick, E. (1988). Nosocomial infection rates as an indicator of quality. *Medical Care, 26*, 676–684.

Leape, L. L., Brennan, T. A., Laaird, N., Lawthers, A. G., Logalio, A. R., Barnes, B. A., et al. (1991). The nature of adverse events in hospitalized patients. *New England Journal of Medicine, 324*, 377–384.

Leape, L. L., Kabcenell, A. I., Gandhi, T. K., Carver, P., Nolan, T. W., & Berwick, D. M. (2000). Reducing adverse drug events: Lessons from a breakthrough series collaborative. *Joint Commission Journal on Quality Improvement, 26*, 321–331.

Lengacher, C. A., & Mabe, P. R. (1993). Nurse extenders. *Journal of Nursing Administration, 23*(3), 16–19.

Lichtig, L. K., Knauf, R. A., & Milholland, D. K. (1999). Some impacts of nursing on acute care hospital outcomes. *Journal of Nursing Administration, 29*(2), 25–33.

Lyder, C. H. (2002). Pressure ulcer prevention and management. *Annual Review of Nursing Research, 20*, 35–61.

Mark, B. A., & Burleson, D. L. (1995). Measurement of patient outcomes. Data availability and consistency across hospitals. *Journal of Nursing Administration, 25*(4), 52–59.

Mark, B. A., Harless, D. W., McCue, M., & Xu, Y. (2004). A longitudinal examination of hospital registered nurse staffing and quality of care. *Health Services Research, 39*, 279–300.

McCloskey, B. A., & Diers, D. K. (2005). Effects of New Zealand's reengineering on nursing and patient outcomes. *Medical Care, 43*, 1140–1146.

McGillis Hall, L. (1998). The use of unregulated workers in Toronto hospitals. *Canadian Journal of Nursing Administration, 11*(1), 9–31.

McGillis Hall, L., Doran, D., & Pink, G. H. (2004). Nurse staffing models, nursing hours, and patient safety outcomes. *Journal of Nursing Administration, 34*(1), 41–45.

McGillis Hall, L., Irvine, D., Baker, G. R., Pink, G., Sidani, S., O'Brien Pallas, L., et al. (2001). *A study of the impact of nursing staff mix models and organizational change strategies on patient, system and nurse outcomes.* Toronto: Faculty of Nursing, University of Toronto and Canadian Health Services Research Foundation/Ontario Council of Teaching Hospitals.

Meurier, C. E. (2000). Understanding the nature of errors in nursing: Using a model to analyse critical incident reports of errors which had resulted in an adverse or potentially adverse event. *Journal of Advanced Nursing, 32,* 202–207.

Meurier, C. E., Vincent, C. A., & Parmar, D. G. (1997). Learning from errors in nursing practice. *Journal of Advanced Nursing, 26,* 111–119.

Midwest Research Institute. (1999). *National Database for Nursing Quality Indicators.* Retrieved July 1, 2002, from http://www.medscape.com/viewarticle/569395

Mitchell, P. H., Ferketich, S., & Jennings, B. M. (1998). Quality health outcomes model. *Image: Journal of Nursing Scholarship, 30,* 43–46.

Mitchell, P. H., Heindrich, J., Moritz, P., & Hinshaw, A. S. (1997). Outcome measures and care delivery systems. *Medical Care Supplement, 35*(11, Suppl.), NS19–NS32.

Mitchell, P. H., & Shortell, S. M. (1997). Adverse outcomes and variations in organization and delivery of care. *Medical Care, 35*(11, Suppl.), NS19–NS32.

Morse, J. M. (1993). Nursing research on patient falls in health care institutions. *Annual Review of Nursing Research, 11,* 299–316.

Morse, J. M., Tylko, S. J., & Dixon, H. A. (1987). Characteristics of the fall prone patient. *The Gerontologist, 27,* 516–522.

Mowinski Jennings, B., Loan, L. A., DePaul, D., Brosch, L. R., & Hildreth, P. (2001). Lessons learned while collecting ANA indicator data. *Journal of Nursing Administration, 31*(3), 121–131.

National Health Service. (2000). *An organisation with memory: Report of an expert group on learning from adverse events in the NHS.* Retrieved April 19, 2010, from http://www.dh.gov.uk/prod_consum_dh/groups/dh_digitalassets/@dh/@en/documents/digitalasset/dh_4065086.pdf

National Pressure Ulcer Advisory Panel. (1992). *Statement on pressure ulcer prevention.* Retrieved June 5, 2000, from http://www.npuap.org

Needleman, J., & Buerhaus, P. I. (2000). *Nurse staffing and quantity of care in inpatient units in acute care hospitals: Phase one report* (Contract No. 230–99–0021). Health Resources Services Administration.

Needleman, J., Buerhaus, P., Mattke, S., Stewart, M., & Zelevinsky, K. (2002a). Nurse-staffing levels and the quality of care in hospitals. *New England Journal of Medicine, 346,* 1715–1722.

Needleman, J., Buerhaus, P., Mattke, S., Stewart, M., & Zelevinsky, K. (2002b). *Nurse staffing and patient outcomes in hospitals* (Final report). Boston: Harvard School of Public Health.

Nolan, T. W. (2000). System changes to improve patient safety. *British Medical Journal, 320,* 771–773.

Pierce, S. F. (1997). Nurse-sensitive health care outcomes in acute care settings: An integrative analysis of the literature. *Journal of Nursing Quality, 11*(4), 60–72.

Potter, P., Barr, N., McSweeney, M., & Sledge, J. (2003). Identifying nurse staffing and patient outcome relationships: A guide for change in care delivery. *Nursing Economic$, 21,* 158–166.

Prescott, P., Dennis, K. E., Creasia, J., & Bowen, S. (1985). Nursing shortage in transition. *Image: Journal of Nursing Scholarship, 18,* 127–133.

Rawsky, E. (1998). Review of the literature on falls among the elderly. *Image: Journal of Nursing Scholarship, 38,* 47–52.

Reason, J. (2000). Human error: Models and management. *British Medical Journal, 320,* 768–770.

Reed, L., Blegen, M., & Goode, C. S. (1998). Adverse patient occurrences as a measure of nursing quality. *Journal of Nursing Administration, 28*(5), 62–69.

Registered Nurses Association of Ontario. (2002). *Risk assessment and prevention of pressure ulcers.* Toronto, Ontario, Canada: Registered Nurses Association of Ontario.

Rowell, P. (2001). Lessons learned while collecting ANA indicator data: The American Nurses Association responds. *Journal of Nursing Administration, 31*(3), 130–131.

Schubert, M., Glass, T. R., Clarke, S. P., Aiken, L. H., Schaffert- Witvliet, B., Sloane, D. M., et al. (2008). Rationing of nursing care and its relationship to patient outcomes: The Swiss extension of the International Hospital Outcomes Study. *International Journal of Quality in Health Care, 20,* 227–237.

Shortell, S. M., Zimmerman, J. E., Rousseau, D. M., Gillies, R. R., Wagner, D. P., Draper, E. A., et al. (1994). The performance of intensive care units: Does good management make a difference? *Medical Care, 32,* 508–525.

SMARTRISK. (1998). *The economic burden of unintentional injury in Canada.* Retrieved July 15, 2002, from http://www.smartrisk.ca/researchers/economic_burden_studies/canada.html

Sovie, M. D., & Jawad, A. F. (2001). Hospital restructuring and its impact on outcomes. *Journal of Nursing Administration, 31,* 588–600.

Stegenga, J., Bell, E., & Matlow, A. (2002). The role of nurse understaffing in nosocomial viral gastrointestinal infections on a general pediatrics ward. *Infection Control and Hospital Epidemiology, 23,* 133–136.

Taunton, R. L., Kleinbeck, S. V., Stafford, R., Woods, C. Q., & Bott, M. J. (1994). Patient outcomes: Are they linked to registered nurse absenteeism, separation, or workload? *Journal of Nursing Administration, 24*(4S), 48–55.

Taylor, J. A. (2007). *Utility of patient safety case finding methods and associations among organizational safety climate, nurse injuries, and errors.* Unpublished doctoral dissertation, John Hopkins University, Baltimore, Maryland.

Tourangeau, A. E., White, P., Scott, J., McAllister, M., & Giles, L. (1999). Evaluation of a partnership model of care delivery involving registered nurses and unlicensed assistive personnel. *Canadian Journal of Nursing Leadership, 12*(2), 4–20.

Tutuarima, J. A., de Haan, R. J., & Limburg, M. (1993). Number of nursing staff and falls: A case-control study on falls by stroke patients in acute-care settings. *Journal of Advanced Nursing, 18,* 1101–1105.

Wakefield, D. S., Wakefield, B. J., Borders, T., Uden-Holman, T., Blegen, M., & Vaughn, T. (1999a). Understanding and comparing differences in reported medication administration error rates. *American Journal of Medical Quality, 14*(2), 73–80.

Wakefield, D. S., Wakefield, B. J., Uden-Holman, T., Borders, T., Blegen, M., & Vaughn, T. (1999b). Understanding why medication administration errors may not be reported. *American Journal of Medical Quality, 14*(2), 81–88.

Wakefield, M. K., & Maddox, P. J. (2000). Patient quality and safety problems in the U.S. heath care system: Challenges for nursing. *Nursing Economic$, 18,* 58–62.

Weinstein, R. A. (1998). *Nosocomial infection update: Emerging infectious diseases.* Retrieved April 19, 2010, from http://www.cdc.gov/ncidod/eid/vol4no3/weinstein.htm

Whedon, M., & Shedd, P. (1989). Prediction and prevention of patient falls. *Image: Journal of Nursing Scholarship, 21,* 108–114.

Wilson, R. M., Runciman, W. B., Gibberd, R. W., Harrison, B.T., Newby, L., & Hamilton, J. D. (1995). The Quality of Australian Health Care Study. *Medical Journal of Australia, 163,* 458–476.

Wunderlich, G. S., Sloan, F. S., & Davis, C. K. (Eds.). (1996). *Nursing staff in hospitals and nursing homes: Is it adequate?* Washington, DC: National Academy Press.

Psychological Distress as a Nurse-Sensitive Outcome

Doris Howell

INTRODUCTION

Psychological distress monitoring and evidence-based psychosocial care is emerging as an integral component of routine clinical practice and a transformed person-centered healthcare system attentive to the needs of the whole person (Institute of Medicine [IOM], 2001, 2008). Evaluating and monitoring psychological distress in all medically ill populations, especially those with chronic disease, is important given the prevalence of chronic illness and its replacement of acute illness as the predominant disease pattern in developed countries (Petrie & Revenson, 2005). Recently, psychological distress ("distress") was endorsed as the "sixth" vital sign (Bultz & Carlson, 2005) with processes for assessment of distress established as an expectation of clinical practice in cancer (Howell, Currie et al., 2009; Jacobsen et al., 2005). Monitoring for distress is also a standard for quality performance in cancer organizations (Accreditation Canada, 2009) and primary care systems (Dietrich et al., 2004). Routine screening of psychological distress followed by effective assessment and management is urgent because it is a significant risk factor for mental health disorders, including major (clinical) depression and anxiety disorders (Andrews & Slade, 2001; Harvey & Ismail, 2008). Mental health problems are projected to become a major contributor to disease burden (Mathers & Loncar, 2006) and health costs in the future (Stephens & Joubert, 2001).

Psychological distress as an outcome sensitive to psychosocial nursing interventions has gained increasing attention in the nursing literature (Fulcher, Badger, Gunter, Marrs, & Reese, 2008; Given & Sherwood, 2005). Psychological distress has figured prominently in nursing practice as part of therapeutic care and inter-personal communication with patients facing illness stressors (Arnold, 1999). Psychological distress and related terms such as *adjustment* and *coping* feature heavily in nursing classification systems (McCloskey & Bulechek, 1996) and theories to guide nursing practice, such as Gordon's (1994) functional health patterns and Roy's Adaptation Model (Roy & Andrews, 1999). These examples support the recognition of the important role for nursing in facilitating psychological adjustment to illness and minimizing its adverse effects on patient/family experience of illness and health-related quality of life.

The purpose of this chapter is to review the empirical evidence to determine if psychological distress is sensitive to psychosocial nursing interventions. This chapter reviews the available conceptual and empirical literature on psychological distress and theoretical knowledge regarding psychological adjustment in chronic illness. The first section describes the methods and search strategies used to identify relevant literature. The second section presents an overview of how psychological distress is conceptualized and operationally defined in concept analysis research and in empirical literature. The third section reviews evidence for psychosocial nursing interventions on reducing psychological distress to evaluate its sensitivity to psychosocial nursing practice variables as an outcome. Finally, issues in the assessment and measurement of psychological distress are discussed and the measures used in the studies reviewed for their psychometric properties and their sensitivity to change in response to nursing interventions.

BACKGROUND ON PSYCHOLOGICAL DISTRESS

Psychological distress is a normal reaction to systemic physical illness, particularly with illnesses that require adjustment in aspirations, relationships, employment, and social activities (Turner & Kelly, 2000). Psychological distress usually resolves quickly once the stressor is removed but can be prolonged depending on the characteristics of illness (Balderson & Towell, 2003; Sharpe & Curran, 2006), including its severity, the extent of disruption it causes in daily living, and its life-threatening nature (Kissane et al., 2004; Pincus, Griffith, Pearce & Isenberg, 1996; Westlake, Dracup, Fonarow, & Hamilton, 2005). Chronic illness that is long term or permanent and severe enough to interfere with a person's ordinary physical, psychological, or social functioning (Hymovich & Hagopian, 1992) is associated with the highest risk of developing psychological distress (Currie & Wang, 2004). Chronic illnesses can overwhelm an individual's coping resources and support systems because of the numerous threats posed, including loss of dignity, diminished self-esteem, stigma, pain, physical impairment, changes to future goals, lifestyle disruptions, and life threat (Bisschop, Kriegsman, Beekman, & Deeg, 2000; Devins & Binik, 1996). Highly prevalent chronic diseases such as arthritis, cancer, diabetes, epilepsy, heart disease, respiratory illness, stroke, neurological disorders, and HIV/AIDS can lead to significant psychological distress because they require adaptation in multiple life domains and demand ongoing psychological adjustment (Stanton, Revenson, & Tennen, 2007).

Variation in the prevalence of psychological distress is reported across studies because of differing definitions and data sources. However, it is estimated that up to 50% of chronically ill patients with heart disease, diabetes, arthritis, asthma, and hypertension are at high risk of psychological distress, depression, and/or depressive symptoms (Anderson, Freedland, Clouse, & Lustman, 2001; McVeigh, Mostashari, & Thorpe, 2004; Shih, Hootman, Strine, Chapman, & Brady, 2006). Prevalence in cancer is reported as ranging from 20 to 40% (Howland & Rowland, 1998), with higher rates of up to 65% documented for advanced cancer populations (Hotopf, Chidgey, Addington-Hall, & Ly, 2002). Persons with multiple interacting comorbid chronic conditions (multimorbidity) are particularly vulnerable, with an estimated five times higher odds of developing psychological distress compared with those with only one chronic illness (Fortin et al., 2006). In a study of over 8,000 older adults in a population based survey, Polsky and colleagues (2005) reported an increased risk of depressive symptoms in the first 2 years following a diagnosis of cancer, heart disease, arthritis, diabetes, and chronic lung disease that persisted years postdiagnosis. Cancer survivors show higher rates of psychological distress compared with population norms that can be prolonged for as long as 6 years post–cancer treatment in a small proportion of the population (Hoffman, 2009).

Strong empirical evidence shows that psychological variables such as depression are associated with disease outcomes in a number of chronic illnesses such as congestive heart disease, cancer, HIV/AIDS (Schneiderman, 2004), and diabetes (Katon, Rutter, Simon, & 2005). Psychological distress intensifies the effect of physical illness by increasing pain, functional limitations, and disability (Ciechanowski, Katon, & Russo, 2000; Fortin et al., 2006; Strine et al., 2004; Wells & Sherbourne, 1999) and weakening motivation for self-care and adherence to medical regimes (Dimatteo, Lepper, & Croghan, 2000). Psychological distress also alters the clinical course of illness, leading to an increased rate of complications (Stanton et al., 2007) and lower overall health (Moussavi et al., 2007; Shih & Simon, 2008). Moreover, psychological distress negatively impacts quality of life (Michael, Berkman, Colditz, Holmes, & Kawachi, 2002).

Psychological distress is also linked to lower disease-free survival in cancer (Bottomley, 1998; Garssen & Goodkin, 1999; Speigel & Kato, 1996) and recurrent infarction in cardiac disease (Bush et al., 2001). Critically ill cardiac patients experiencing the physiological effects associated with anxiety are at higher risk for a number of cardiac complications, such as recurrent ischemia and arrhythmias (Moser et al., 2003; Moser & Dracup, 1996; Moser, McKinley, Reigel, Doering, & Garvin, 2002). Higher mortality has been associated with even minimal depressive symptoms following myocardial infarction (Bush et al.) and doubling the risk of recurrent cardiac events following cardiac bypass surgery (Blumenthal et al., 2003). Higher mortality in populations with diabetes (Katon et al., 2005), cancer (Greer, 1991; Hamer, Chida, & Malloy, 2009), and heart disease (Covinsky et al., 1999) is associated with psychological distress. Increased healthcare costs are also associated with psychological distress because of greater utilization of healthcare services, prolonged hospitalization, and support-seeking healthcare behavior (Koopmans & Lamers, 2007; Stern, Pascale, & Ackerman, 1977).

CONCEPTUALIZATION AND DEFINITIONS OF PSYCHOLOGICAL DISTRESS

Literature Review Method

A review of the literature was conducted to identify empirical evidence of a relationship between psychological distress and nursing interventions (**TABLE 7-1**). The databases searched included CINAHL, MEDLINE, PsycINFO, and Sociological Abstracts (SCA). The search terms were adapted according to requirements of the database searched. Primary search terms used included *nursing, intervention, randomized trials*, and *quasi-experimental*. A total of 559 citations were retrieved, and studies were included if they met the following inclusion criteria: (a) psychological distress, anxiety, or depression as a primary outcome; (b) an experimental design (either randomized controlled trial [RCT] or quasi-experiment); (c) non-pharmacological nursing intervention; (d) an adequate sample size (> 10 per group); (e) use of an established measure(s) of psychological distress; (f) covering the years 1999–2009; and (g) adult population (over age 18) with systemic illness. Articles were excluded based on the following criteria: (a) non-English-speaking; (b) pediatric population; and (c) focus on caregiver/family distress. Studies of nursing interventions in pain were also excluded because pain is the subject of a specific chapter in this review (Chapter 5). After reviewing the abstract of each article, 53 articles that met the inclusion and exclusion criteria were included for further examination.

Conceptual Search: In addition to the search strategy described above, a search for conceptual articles was conducted to identify papers that provided a conceptual overview of psychological distress or, more specifically, depression, anxiety, or the process of psychological adjustment. This search strategy was conducted in MEDLINE, CINAHL, and PsycInfo, and included MeSH terms (adaptation, psychological/; stress, psychological/; exp emotions/; depression/anxiety) or key words (*psychological distress, psychosocial function*, and *psychosocial support*) combined with terms to identify reviews or concept papers (concept formation/; "review literature as topic"/; (concept adj2 analysis).mp.; state adj2 science.mp.). This search strategy resulted in 496 articles, of which 15 were included for further review, meeting the criteria of a concept analysis or theory paper. Opinion papers were excluded.

Conceptual Definitions

Psychological distress is defined as the emotional condition that one feels in response to having to cope with situations that are unsettling, frustrating, or perceived as harmful or threatening (Lazarus & Folkman, 1984). Psychological distress has also been conceptualized as encompassing emotional states, including lack of enthusiasm, problems with sleep, feeling downhearted or blue, feeling hopeless about the future, feeling emotional (i.e. crying easily or feeling like crying), feeling bored or a passing interest in things, and thoughts of suicide (Burnette & Mui, 1994). The term *emotional distress* is often used interchangeably with the term *psychological distress* or the nonspecific term *distress* because these are considered to be more acceptable and less stigmatizing to patients and denotes psychological distress as a normal response (Jacobsen et al., 2005; Trask et al., 2002). However, psychological distress can signal a maladaptive response when it is prolonged and accompanied by other risk factors or defining characteristics such as those of major (clinical) depression or other types of adjustment or anxiety disorders (Stanton et al., 2007). Consequently, psychological distress is also defined as an outcome of poor adjustment (Stanton et al.) or maladaptive psychological functioning (Abelhoff, Armitage, Lichter, & Neiderhuber, 2000).

In a concept analysis to clarify terms, Ridner (2003) noted that psychological distress is seldom defined as a unique concept but is embedded within the context of strain, stress, and distress. She recommended that the term *strain* not be used because it is unlikely to contribute to psychological distress, whereas terms such as *stress* and *distress* are nonspecific responses to a demand or stressor that can be either harmful (distress) or not harmful (stress) to the individual. *Distress* is the term recommended for use in current cancer guidelines and is defined as "unpleasant emotions of a psychological (cognitive, behavioral, emotional), social, and/or spiritual nature extending along a continuum, ranging from common normal feelings of vulnerability, sadness, and fear to problems that can become disabling, leading to psychological states such as depression, anxiety, panic, social isolation, and existential and spiritual crisis" (National Comprehensive Cancer Network [NCCN], 2008). Ridner suggested that the term *psychological distress* is more accurate than the nonspecific term *distress* for describing the individual's response to illness for which nurses intervene. Psychological distress was subsequently defined "as the unique, discomforting emotional state experienced by an individual in response to a specific stressor or demand that results in harm, either temporary or permanent, to the person" (p. 539).

Psychological distress is also defined as an unpleasant mood or an affective state that can be measured as positive or negative affect usually assessed as subjective symptoms of depression and/or anxiety because these constructs can be easily measured with standardized instruments in clinical practice (Portenoy & Bruera, 2003). Further diagnostic assessment is necessary for the population that scores high on subjective self-report measures for the presence of symptoms of anxiety and depression for a definitive clinical diagnosis and/or designation of major (clinical) depression or an adjustment or anxiety disorder. A clinical diagnosis of depression or anxiety disorder must be preceded by a structured diagnostic interview (SCID). The current gold standard instruments for structured diagnostic interviews include the Composite International Diagnostic Interview (CIDI) (Witchen, 1994) and the Structured Diagnostic Interview for Depression (SCID) (Ekselius, Lindstrom, von Knorring, Bodlund, & Kullgren, 1994). Depression and anxiety are further defined based on concept analysis studies identified in this review and according to psychiatric classification diagnostic criteria as specified by the American Psychiatric Association (APA) (2000).

Anxiety: Anxiety is defined as feelings of stress or tension from known or unknown stimuli (Lehmand & Rabins, 1999). Anxiety is considered a natural response and necessary warning of the need for adaptation to a perceived threat to homeostasis, or impending change of a physical, social, or psychological nature (Bay & Algese, 1999). Anxiety is "a heightened sense of uneasiness to a potential non-specific threat that is inconsistent with the expected event and results when there is a mismatch between the next likely event and the actual event" (Bay & Algese, p. 105). Anxiety is characterized by a number of typical physical signs and symptoms, particularly those associated with autonomic overactivity such as sweating, palpitations, tachycardia, and tremor (Stark et al., 2002). Physical symptoms of anxiety can also include loss of appetite, abdominal distress, headaches, and perception of dyspnea or shortness of breath. Psychological symptoms of anxiety have also been described for illnesses such as cancer, including recurrent thoughts about diagnosis and treatment, concerns about changes in functioning, fears and worries about the future and death, hypervigilance, and difficulty concentrating (Sheldon, Swanson, Dolce, Marsh, & Summers, 2008).

Two distinct types of anxiety are described in the literature: state anxiety and trait anxiety (Spielberger, Gorsuch, Lushene, Vagg, & Jacobs, 1983). State anxiety is considered a transitory emotional response to a stressor, whereas trait anxiety reflects a more long-standing quality or stable predisposition to anxiety, as determined by personality pattern (Spielberger et al., 1983). Anxiety is considered a pathologic disorder when it is excessive and uncontrollable, requires no specific external stimulus, and manifests with a wide range of physical and affective symptoms and changes in behavior and cognition. Abnormality is defined as symptoms that are out of proportion to the threat, with persistence and deterioration in emotional or other functioning. As outlined in the *Diagnostic and Statistical Manual of Mental Disorders* (DSM IV-TR), anxiety disorders include generalized anxiety disorder (GAD), social anxiety disorder (also known as social phobia), specific phobia, panic disorder with and without agoraphobia, obsessive-compulsive disorder (OCD), posttraumatic stress disorder (PTSD), anxiety secondary to medical condition, acute stress disorder (ASD), and substance-induced anxiety disorder. Anxiety is highly correlated with depression (Portenoy & Bruera, 2003).

Depression: The term *depression* has been used to denote the full range of depressive symptoms, including normal sadness in response to loss, as well as chronic depressed emotional affect and clinical depression meeting specific criteria for psychiatric disorder (Barsevick, Sweeney, Haney, & Chung, 2002). The term *clinical depression* is often used interchangeably with the term *major depression* (Ballenger et al., 2001). Clinical depression as a psychiatric disorder is defined as a syndrome characterized by physical and psychological symptoms including depressed mood, loss of interest or pleasure, feelings of guilt or low self-worth, disturbed sleep and/or appetite, low energy, changes in movement (agitation or slowed movements), poor concentration, and thoughts of death or suicide (Ballenger et al.). The symptoms must persist for most of the day, nearly every day, for at least 2 consecutive weeks. The episode must be accompanied by clinically significant distress or impairment in social, occupational, or other important areas of functioning (APA, 2000).

Essential Attributes of Psychological Distress

Even when patients do not meet the criteria for a clinical diagnosis of depression or anxiety, they can have some form of psychological distress, which could be regarded as a sign of poor adjustment (Polonsky, 2000). Psychological distress is described as evolving along a continuum, progressing from initial emotional responses such as sadness, grief, or loss to more serious affective states such as anxiety and depression (NCCN, 2008). A number of essential attributes of psychological distress were identified by Ridner (2003), including perceived inability to cope effectively; change in emotional status; discomfort; communication of discomfort; and harm. Critical attributes identified for anxiety by Bay and Algese (1999) include a subjective state of uneasiness; rising apprehension; and transformation of these subjective states into behaviors focused on obtaining relief, such as restlessness or agitation.

Antecedent of Psychological Distress

The antecedents of psychological distress were identified as: unique to human beings; presence of a stressor either a symptom or an event; perception of the stressor as a personal threat, thus triggering a stress response; loss of control; and ineffective coping (Ridner, 2003). Antecedents of anxiety were identified as a perceived threat to homeostasis and presence of an impending change, such as employment or career, physical function, or a source of loss (Bay & Algese, 1999). Antecedents of psychological distress can also be biological in nature, related either to the specific release of catecholamines (epinephrine and norepinephrine, cortisol) as part of the "fight or flight" response to the stressor (Selye, 1978), or to the release of proinflammatory substrates (cytokines) triggered by illness

TABLE 7-1   Studies Investigating the Relationship Between Nursing Interventions and Psychological Distress as a Nurse-Sensitive Outcome

Author/ Date	Design of study (method of participant assignment, number of measurement occasions)	Setting/subjects (characteristics of the sample and response rate, and the setting: acute care, community, long-term care)	Definition of the primary outcome concept and measure(s) used, including reliability coefficient	Nurse intervention variables investigated	Major results	Limitations
Allard (2007)	RCT; random allocation of participants; repeated-measures design—T1 (pretest), T2, and T3 (1 week following the first and second intervention sessions, respectively). Sample stratification.	N = 117; RR = 64%; mean age = 53.6 years old; women newly diagnosed with breast cancer and scheduled to undergo first surgery; 40% had stage 1 and 25% had stage 2 breast cancer; acute care setting.	Primary outcome: Emotional distress, defined as a person's inability to regulate his or her response when facing a stressful health experience, namely surgery for breast cancer. Profile of Mood States-SF (POMS); contains 37 items; used the translated French-Canadian version; α = .75–.94.	Psychoeducational intervention sessions completed over the telephone by nurses to help women redirect their focus of attention on the symptom experience (cognitive), decisions made to alleviate physical symptoms, and attainment of physical and emotional well-being/emotional regulation (therapeutic listening).	A significant difference was detected in the POMS-SF pretest and posttest at T2 scores between the control and intervention (lower distress) groups. Faster decrease in emotional distress after surgery in the intervention group as compared with the control group (trend).	Small sample size but was justified for a moderate effect.
Ambler et al. (1999)	Quasi-experimental design; time sequential design; three measurements: T1 (before surgery), T2 (2 week follow-up), and T3 (6-month follow-up).	N = 103 females with breast cancer whose treatment involved surgery for malignant or benign lumps (conventional care N = 46; intervention N = 21); diagnosis of malignancy was made in 65% and 35% had a benign lump; mean age = 50 years old; RR = 64%; acute care.	Primary outcomes: Psychological well-being, anxiety, depression. HADS; 14 items, 7 relating to anxiety and 7 to depression; α = .41–.76 (anxiety) and .3–.6 (depression); cut-off scores for "casesness" = 11. Rotterdam Symptom Checklist (RSCL); 34 items creating two subscales: psychological (α = .88–.94) and physical (α = .71–.88).	Special breast cancer nurses trained by a psychologist to deliver an advocacy intervention to reduce psychological stress by providing support prior to the diagnostic consultation appointments. Emotional support and counseling; Eliciting concerns, developing a list of questions for the surgeons, and accompanying the patient to the appointment.	Anxiety significantly lower 2 weeks postsurgery; lower in intervention group vs conventional care group. Level of "caseness" (cut-off of > 11) for anxiety and depression lower 2 weeks postsurgery in intervention group. No difference in psychological scales between groups on the RSCL.	Potential contamination of intervention to control group (one nurse). Potential selection bias and group differences due to treatment at 6-month measure. Small sample in intervention group.

			Primary outcomes:			
Arving et al. (2007)	RCT; four measurements: T1 (pretest), T2 (1 month after intervention), T3 (3 months after intervention), and T4 (6 months after intervention).	N = 172 primary breast cancer patients about to start adjuvant therapy; RR = 62%; mean age = 55; acute care.	Primary outcomes: Quality of life, anxiety, depression. HADS, State-Trait Anxiety Inventory (STAI); European Organisation of Research and Treatment of Cancer Quality of Life Questionnaire (EORTC-QLQ-C30). Reliability not reported.	Psychosocial support provided by trained nurses (INS), psychologists (IPS), or standard care (SC). INS during a 4-month period. CBT techniques included relaxation, distraction, activity scheduling, and ways to improve communication. Patients received at least one session and decided whether future sessions were needed.	Significant differences between intervention and control groups on emotional functioning subscale and impact of events scale and on quality of life measure (EORTC), but not for HADS or STAI. Significant differences in anxiety when IPS and INS compared with standard care.	Significant missing data. Improvement in all groups over time. Possible ceiling or floor effects.
Badger et al. (2005)	Experimental, repeated-measures design; three assessment points: T1 (pretest), T2 (after 6-week intervention), and T3 (1 month after completion of intervention).	N = 48; women with breast cancer with stage 1–3 receiving adjuvant treatment; mean age 54 (usual care) and 53 (intervention group); acute care and community. Usual care group received phone calls for patient and partner but only received resources and no counseling (9 min).	Primary outcomes: Depression, positive and negative affect, fatigue, and stress. CES-D; cut-off scores ≥ 16 indicate depression, in present study α > .90. PANAS in present study α ≥ .88. ICS in present study α > .96.	Clinical nurse specialists in mental health nursing and oncology (32 hours of training on interpersonal psychotherapy techniques and supervised counseling). Telephone interpersonal counseling (TIP-C). Participants received six weekly telephone calls: cancer education, interpersonal role disputes, social support, awareness, management of depressive symptoms, and role transitions; partners received three TIP-C sessions. (32.9 min.)	Depression declined over time, but no significant differences between groups. Positive affect increased over time significantly in both groups but no decline in negative effect. Significant reduction in stress over time in both groups but no differences between groups.	Small sample size. No justification for sample size.

α = Cronbach's alpha coefficients; BAI = Beck's Anxiety Inventory; CES-D = Center for Epidemiological Studies–Depression; GDS = Geriatric Depression Scale; GDS-SF = Geriatric Depression Scale-Short Form; HADS = Hospital Anxiety and Depression Scale; HARS = Hamilton Anxiety and Depression Scale; HDRS = Hamilton Depression Rating Scale; HRQOL = health-related quality of life; IBS = irritable bowel syndrome; ICS = Index of Clinical Stress; IES = Impact of Events Scale; IRR = interrater reliability; MOS-SF-36 = Medical Outcomes Study-Short Form-36; MSAS = Memorial Symptom Assessment Scale; MUIS = Mishel's Uncertainty in Illness Scale; N = sample size; NRS = numeric rating scale; PAIS-SR = Psychosocial Adjustment to Illness Scale-Self-Report; PANAS = Positive and Negative Affect Scale; POMS = Profile of Mood States; RCT= randomized controlled trial; STAI = State-Trait Anxiety Inventory; VAAS = visual analogue for anxiety scale; VAS = visual analogue scale; ZSDS = Zung Self-Rating Depression Scale.

(continues)

TABLE 7-1   Studies Investigating the Relationship Between Nursing Interventions and Psychological Distress as a Nurse-Sensitive Outcome (continued)

Author/ Date	Design of study (method of participant assignment, number of measurement occasions)	Setting/subjects (characteristics of the sample and response rate, and the setting: acute care, community, long-term care)	Definition of the primary outcome concept and measure(s) used, including reliability coefficient	Nurse intervention variables investigated	Major results	Limitations
Chaboyer et al. (2007)	Quasi-experimental, time-series design: four blocks (4 months in duration) with a wash-out period in between of 1 month.	N = 100 patients and families: Transfer of patient from an ICU (≥ 3 days) to a ward was occurring; 58% male patients; mean age = 59 (control), 57 (intervention); RR = 60%; acute care.	Primary outcomes: Transfer anxiety—anxiety experienced by the individual when he/she moves from a familiar, somewhat secure environment to unfamiliar place. Similar to state anxiety. STAI- Form Y-1 State; 20 items that measure "state"; reported α = .91 and α .59–.62 for study.	Education/ assessment of patient/family for transfer to the ward, coordination of ICU patient transfer and nurse liaison role: Communicating with staff, assessing skill mix and resources, preparing both the ICU and ward staff for patient transfer, and assessing bed status; provided practical and emotional support and education to patients and families pre- and postdischarge.	No effect on patient or family pretransfer anxiety.	Anxiety measured only once, just after planned transfer notification. Low reliability of STAI in ICU population. Sample size low: Post hoc analysis suggested N = 300 needed to show effect.
Cheung et al. (2002)	RCT; three measurement time points post-operatively: T1 (1 week), T2 (5 weeks), and T3 (10 weeks).	N = 59 colorectal cancer patients after stoma surgery; mean age = 56, and 60 for control and study groups, respectively; 67% and 69% male (control and study groups, respectively); RR = 89%; acute care.	Primary outcome: Anxiety. The Chinese version of the STAI (C-STAI) used to assess anxiety; 40 items; α = .76–.90: quality of life assessed by several scales, Quality of Life Index for Colostomy (23 items, each with a 10-cm linear VAS, α = .71–.90); and Hong Kong Chinese version of the WHO QOL Measure-Abbreviated Version (WHOQOL-BREF-HK) (28 items, α = .92–.93).	Progressive muscle relaxation training (PMRT) for a 20-min period (two sessions); required subjects to tense and relax different muscle groups in combination with deep breathing during post-operative period. At home, patients practiced using an audio-tape at least two to three times per week for 1 week. Follow-up calls every 2 weeks were conducted by study research nurse.	Significant decrease in state anxiety and improved generic quality of life in the domains of physical, psychological, social health.	

Study	Design	Sample	Measures	Intervention	Results	Limitations
Cole et al. (2006)	Nonexperimental design; population-based cohort.	N = 35 patients with depression and congestive heart failure (CHF); 35 of 101 CHF patients referred had a major depressive or adjustment disorder; of these, 24 received follow-up evaluations; acute-care and community.	Primary outcome: Depression (no definition provided). An interactive voice response version of HADS and Patient Health Questionnaire were used; questionnaire data not reported.	Nurse practitioner trained in coaching and depression management. A 13-month telephonic nurse double-disease management program (DDMP): changes in delivery system design, decision support (education for primary care providers), patient self-management/emotional support, clinical information management support, organizational support, and community linkages.	82% of patients with major depression and 75% of patients with "other depression" (PHQ score < 10) responded. Mean change in PHQ scores for the sample as a whole improved significantly over the 24 weeks of the program, and for those with major depression and other depression.	Small sample size.
Cote & Pepler (2002)	RCT; two measurement points: T1 (preintervention) and T2 (postintervention).	N = 90 hospitalized HIV-infected males; mean age = 40; RR = 78%.	Primary outcomes: Mood, psychological distress, anxiety. Mood was assessed with the PANAS; contains 20 descriptors; Cronbach's α ranging from 0.86 to 0.90 for PA and from 0.84 to 0.87 for NA; in current study, α = 0.76 for PA, and 0.87 for NA; IES measured subjective distress; 15 items; Cronbach's α = .78–.86 in previous and present studies: VAS measured anxiety.	Psychoeducation interventions by the first author and a nurse experienced in AIDS care: 20% of interventions were analyzed by an independent observer to assess consistency within groups. Three groups: cognitive coping skills (CCSs), expression of emotions (EE), or control; 3 days in 20–30 minute sessions: strengthen cognitive coping skills/regulating emotional responses. Empathy a fundamental component of interaction.	Beneficial effect on negative affect following first daily session. No change in positive affect. Significant decrease in distress for cognitive skills training group and anxiety presession and immediately after session.	Sample size and no justification of sample size. Potential for selection bias randomization method not clear.

α = Cronbach's alpha coefficients; BAI = Beck's Anxiety Inventory; CES-D = Center for Epidemiological Studies–Depression; GDS = Geriatric Depression Scale; GDS-SF = Geriatric Depression Scale–Short Form; HADS = Hospital Anxiety and Depression Scale; HARS = Hamilton Anxiety and Depression Scale; HDRS = Hamilton Depression Rating Scale; HRQOL = health-related quality of life; IBS = irritable bowel syndrome; ICS = Index of Clinical Stress; IES = Impact of Events Scale; IRR = interrater reliability; MOS-SF-36 = Medical Outcomes Study–Short Form-36; MSAS = Memorial Symptom Assessment Scale; MUIS = Mishel's Uncertainty in Illness Scale; N = sample size; NRS = numeric rating scale; PAIS-SR = Psychosocial Adjustment to Illness Scale-Self-Report; PANAS = Positive and Negative Affect Scale; POMS = Profile of Mood States; RCT = randomized controlled trial; STAI = State-Trait Anxiety Inventory; VAAS = visual analogue for anxiety scale; VAS = visual analogue scale; ZSDS = Zung Self-Rating Depression Scale.

(continues)

TABLE 7-1 Studies Investigating the Relationship Between Nursing Interventions and Psychological Distress as a Nurse-Sensitive Outcome (continued)

Author/ Date	Design of study (method of participant assignment, number of measurement occasions)	Setting/subjects (characteristics of the sample and response rate, and the setting: acute care, community, long-term care)	Definition of the primary outcome concept and measure(s) used, including reliability coefficient	Nurse intervention variables investigated	Major results	Limitations
Crogan et al. (2008)	RCT; repeated measures, pretest/posttest.	$N = 10$ completed the pretest and 7 completed posttest; acute care.	Primary outcomes: Mood, stress, coping. ICS measured subjective stress with 25 items; $\alpha = .96$. Cantril's Ladder: 4-item subjective measure of global quality of life; test-retest reliability; $r = 1.0$. Brief Depression Rating Scale: 8 items; based on clinical observation; IRR, $r = .91–.94$.	Nurse-led (training of 8 hours) story-telling group intervention. Participants assigned to twelve 1.5-hour sessions of story-telling: searching for a personal narrative, caring, equalizing power of participants, building community by guiding, respect, and listening, community-building practices, and helping meaning to emerge.	Decreased stress in story-telling group despite disease progression. No differences on other variables.	Small sample size but justified for moderate effects. Randomization procedure not specified.
P. Davidson et al. (2008)	Quasi-experimental design, two measurement time points: T1 (preintervention) and T2 (postintervention).	$N = 54$ women with heart disease; mean age = 60; acute care.	Anxiety, depression, and stress not defined. Depression, Anxiety, Stress Scales (DASS) used to measure psychological variables; 21 items with three self-report subscales; $\alpha = 0.81$ (depression), .73 (anxiety), and .81 (stress).	Cardiac nurse/ researcher facilitated sessions. Heart Awareness for Women: 6-week program, each session lasting 2 hours with 5–10 women in each session; mutual aid and discussions around heart disease, coping with changing roles, activity, depression/anxiety, challenges, stress, effective communication.	No significant changes in depression, anxiety, stress, cardiac control, role integration, or perceived social support.	
Deshler et al. (2006)	RCT; four-arm (three study and one control); two measurement time points: T1 (preintervention) and T2 (3 weeks post).	$N = 52$ newly registered cancer patients and their support people; 30% lung cancer patients; 63% male; acute care.	Primary outcome: State and trait anxiety assessed with POMS anxiety subscale; coefficients not reported; trait anxiety measured with STAI; $\alpha = .90$	Orientation video/ booklet delivered in class, during drop-in sessions, or by mail. Control group received a resource booklet as part of routine care.	No effect on anxiety.	

Dirksen & Epstein (2008)	RCT; two measurement points: T1 (pretreatment) and T2 (posttreatment).	N = 72, women diagnosed with stage 1–3 breast cancer at least 3 months postcompletion of primary treatment without current evidence of disease; mean age = 57 (intervention), and 59 (control); RR = 23%; acute care.	Primary outcomes: Fatigue and mood (anxiety, depression), and quality of life. Anxiety assessed with STAI; 40 items; α = .91–.97 (state) and .88–.94 (trait) for both groups in present study. Depression assessed with CES-D; 20 items; a score ≥ 16 indicates depression; α = . 86 and .92 for both groups in present study.	Master's nurses conducted the four weekly classes and two phone call sessions (manualized). Intervention group received a 1-week (2 weeks pretreatment, 6 weeks treatment, and 2 weeks posttreatment) CBT program; stimulus control instructions, sleep restriction therapy, and sleep education and hygiene. The component control group received sleep education and hygiene only. The treatment phase comprised four in-class sessions and two telephone sessions.	Significant improvements in fatigue, trait anxiety, depression, and quality of life.
Dougherty et al. (2004)	RCT; three measurement points: T1 (discharge from hospital), T2 (1 month after ICD [implantable cardioverter defibrillator] therapy), and T3 (3 months after ICD therapy).	N = 168; mean age = 63 (intervention) and 65 (control); 79% male; sudden cardiac arrest survivors receiving ICD; RR = 69%; acute care. Control group received usual care.	Primary outcomes: Physical function and psychological adjustment. Definitions were not provided. STAI: Used the state scale of the inventory only; α = 0.84. CES-D for depressive symptomatology; α = 0.87. Physical function assessed with the Patient Concerns Assessment (PCA) and SF-12 Short Form Health Survey.	Expert cardiovascular nurses trained to deliver 8-week intervention: (1) structured information provided in a mailed booklet, and (2) telephone support to teach specific knowledge and behavioral skills needed to manage ICD recovery, enhance self-confidence (self-efficacy) in one's ability to deal with illness demands, and reduce emotional arousal and anxiety.	Significant reduction in the intervention group on PCA symptoms at 1 month and reduced anxiety and enhanced knowledge at 3 months.

α = Cronbach's alpha coefficients; BAI = Beck's Anxiety Inventory; CES-D = Center for Epidemiological Studies–Depression; GDS = Geriatric Depression Scale; GDS-SF = Geriatric Depression Scale–Short Form; HADS = Hospital Anxiety and Depression Scale; HARS = Hamilton Anxiety Rating Scale; HDRS = Hamilton Depression Rating Scale; HRQOL = health-related quality of life; IBS = irritable bowel syndrome; ICS = Index of Clinical Stress; IES = Impact of Events Scale; IRR = interrater reliability; MOS-SF-36 = Medical Outcomes Study-Short Form-36; MSAS = Memorial Symptom Assessment Scale; MUIS = Mishel's Uncertainty in Illness Scale; N = sample size; NRS = numeric rating scale; PAIS-SR = Psychosocial Adjustment to Illness Scale-Self-Report; PANAS = Positive and Negative Affect Scale; POMS = Profile of Mood States; RCT= randomized controlled trial; STAI = State-Trait Anxiety Inventory; VAAS = visual analogue for anxiety scale; VAS = visual analogue scale; ZSDS = Zung Self-Rating Depression Scale.

(continues)

TABLE 7-1 Studies Investigating the Relationship Between Nursing Interventions and Psychological Distress as a Nurse-Sensitive Outcome (continued)

Author/Date	Design of study (method of participant assignment, number of measurement occasions)	Setting/subjects (characteristics of the sample and response rate, and the setting: acute care, community, long-term care)	Definition of the primary outcome concept and measure(s) used, including reliability coefficient	Nurse intervention variables investigated	Major results	Limitations
Duffy et al. (2006)	RCT; 2 measurement points: T1 (baseline) and T2 (6 months postintervention).	N = 184 neck and head cancer patients with at least one of smoking, alcoholic, or depression issues; mean age = 58 (usual care) and 56 (intervention); over 61% of the sample had stage 3/4 cancers: RR =42%: acute care. Control group received "enhanced" usual care.	Primary outcomes: Depression, smoking, and alcohol problems. No definitions provided. GDS-SF; used cut-off score of ≥ 4 to indicate probable depression; reliability coefficients not provided.	Primary nurse trained on CBT and trained other nurses; supervision from a psychiatrist: 45 min nursing assessment of smoking, alcohol problems, or depression. CBT intervention: Workbook, 9–11 telephone sessions of CBT counseling, and pharmacologic management: Goal setting, self-monitoring, analyzing behavioral antecedents, coping skills, and social skills training.	Significant differences in 6 months in smoking cessation and depression rates, but no significant differences between groups.	
Erci et al. (2009)	RCT; four measurement time points: T1 (baseline), T2 (preoperative), T3 (postoperative), and T4 (prior to discharge from hospital).	N = 120 patients attending a surgery clinical and scheduled for surgery; 60% and 46.7% female, study and control groups respectively; acute care.	Primary outcome: Pre-/postoperative anxiety; anxiety defined as an energy source inextricably related to human development from infancy to death; is required for biological and emotional growth. Anxiety was measured using the Beck Anxiety Inventory (BAI); 21 items; in the current study, α = .87, and previous studies reported α = .93.	1-week intervention based on Peplau's therapeutic relationship: Orientation (define and identify patient health problem), identification (issues with anxiety and fear around surgery explored and discussed; self-care management options discussed), exploitation (continued development of therapeutic relationship), and resolution.	Levels of anxiety in the intervention group decreased significantly between intervention and control group.	

Study	Design	Sample	Outcomes/Measures	Intervention	Results	Limitations
Fillion et al. (2008)	RCT; three measurement points: T1 (baseline), T2 (postintervention), and T3 (3-month follow-up).	N = 87 French-speaking Canadian females who had completed treatment for nonmetastatic breast cancer; mean age = 52; RR = 19%; acute care.	Primary outcomes: Emotional distress (anxiety and depression). Secondary outcomes: Fatigue, quality of life, energy levels, and fitness. Emotional distress measured using the POMS; 14 items; translated French version of the original POMS; α = .92 (original study).	Nurses trained in CBT over 6 hours. Lazarus and Folkman stress-coping theoretic framework and Salmon's theory of physical activity, combining stress management psychoeducation and physical activity. The intervention comprised four weekly group meetings, 2.5 hours each, and 1 brief (15 min) booster telephone session. For each session, 1 hour was devoted to walking training and 1.5 hours to psychoeducative stress.	Greater improvement in fatigue, energy level, and emotional distress at 3-month follow-up compared with control. Overall nonsignificant improvement in emotional distress.	Small sample size.
Fitzsimmons (2001)	RCT; two measurement points: T1 (baseline) and T2 (posttest).	N = 39 residents in long-term care with diagnosis or symptoms of depression; mean age = 80, 72% male; 79% with depression diagnosis; RR = 82%; long-term care.	Primary outcome: Depression, no definition provided. GDS-SF; 15 items; score of 4 or higher indicated presence of depression, and a score of 5 or higher is strongly associated with depression; simple test for those with low reading level; test can be read to the patient and is not affected by visual acuity.	Therapeutic biking completed in groups of 4. Nurses and aides trained by a certified therapeutic recreation specialist. A 2-week trial of wheelchair biking therapy: (1) residents have small-group discussions about bike riding in the past, tapping into long-term memory; (2) each resident gets 15 minutes to ride the bike and tell others about the ride afterward.	Significant improvements in depression scores in intervention group compared with control.	Small sample size. Gender mix: More men limiting generalizability. Cognitive impairment in some study subjects.

(continues)

α = Cronbach's alpha coefficients; BAI = Beck's Anxiety Inventory; CES-D = Center for Epidemiological Studies–Depression; GDS = Geriatric Depression Scale; GDS-SF = Geriatric Depression Scale-Short Form; HADS = Hospital Anxiety and Depression Scale; HARS = Hamilton Anxiety and Depression Scale; HDRS = Hamilton Depression Rating Scale; HRQOL = health-related quality of life; IBS = irritable bowel syndrome; ICS = Index of Clinical Stress; IES = Impact of Events Scale; IRR = interrater reliability; MOS-SF-36 = Medical Outcomes Study-Short Form-36; MSAS = Memorial Symptom Assessment Scale; MUIS = Mishel's Uncertainty in Illness Scale; N = sample size; NRS = numeric rating scale; PAIS-SR = Psychosocial Adjustment to Illness Scale-Self-Report; PANAS = Positive and Negative Affect Scale; POMS = Profile of Mood States; RCT = randomized controlled trial; STAI = State-Trait Anxiety Inventory; VAAS = visual analogue for anxiety scale; VAS = visual analogue scale; ZSDS = Zung Self-Rating Depression Scale.

TABLE 7-1　Studies Investigating the Relationship Between Nursing Interventions and Psychological Distress as a Nurse-Sensitive Outcome (continued)

Author/Date	Design of study (method of participant assignment, number of measurement occasions)	Setting/subjects (characteristics of the sample and response rate, and the setting: acute care, community, long-term care)	Definition of the primary outcome concept and measure(s) used, including reliability coefficient	Nurse intervention variables investigated	Major results	Limitations
Gallagher et al. (2003)	RCT; two measurement time points: T1 (before hospital discharge) and T2 (12 weeks postdischarge). Individually tailored.	$N = 196$ females hospitalized for coronary artery diseases; mean age = 67 (range 34–92); RR = 93%; acute care. Usual care consisted of an education program and referral to cardiac rehabilitation programs.	Primary outcomes: Psychosocial recovery, defined as psychosocial adjustment, anxiety, and depression. PAIS; 46 items; reported α >.65, and in this study, α >.68. HADS anxiety and depression; 14 items; scores > 11=clinical diagnosis: inter-item correlations ranged from .41 to .76.	Intervention delivered by cardiac nurse. Goal-setting for self-management of symptoms, diet, exercise, smoking, medication, and stress response. Initial evaluation during admission followed by telephone counseling at 1, 3, and 6 weeks postdischarge.	No effect on psychosocial adjustment, anxiety, or depression at T2.	
Gümüs & Cam (2008)	Quasi-experimental, single-group design; two measurement time points: preintervention and postintervention.	$N = 30$ women newly diagnosed with breast cancer in the first treatment process; mean age = 44.5; acute care. International: Turkey.	Primary outcome: Psychosocial adjustment, including psychological distress. PAIS-SR was used to assess psychological distress; 46 items; scores < 35 indicate *good psychosocial adjustment*; 35–51 indicate *fair psychosocial adjustment*; and > 51 indicate *poor psychosocial adjustment*; available in Turkish language; previously reported in Turkish population α = .80–.95; α in present sample ranged from .50 to .87.	The general purpose of the emotional support-focused interventions was to get patients to share their feelings, thoughts, and experiences; to facilitate their adjustment to their daily lives; and to improve their ability to cope with their illness. The intervention included semistructured face-to-face intensive individual interview sessions once a week for 1–1.5 hours for a total of seven sessions.	Significant increase in adaptation and decrease in psychological distress.	Relevance to Canadian healthcare system. Significant loss to follow-up from pre to post (91 to 30). Self-selection bias and not clear how many patients approached to participate.

Harkness et al. (2003)	RCT; three measurement time points: T1 (beginning of waiting period), T2 (2 weeks prior to scheduled elective cardiac catheterization [CATH]), and T3 (at the outpatient pre-CATH appointment). Concealed randomization.	N = 228 patients referred for CATH; mean age = 64 years old; 55% male; RR = 68%; acute care.	Primary outcomes: Anxiety and HRQOL (no definition provided) Anxiety measured with STAI and visual analogue rating (VAR). HRQOL measured with SF-36; 36 items; α = .76–.88. Seattle Angina Questionnaire (SAQ) to measure functional status in coronary artery disease.	Psychoeducational intervention: Intervention group received a nurse-delivered detailed information and education session within 2 weeks of being placed on the waiting list for elective CATH. Usual group received the usual care for patients waiting for CATH, which involved no regular contact from any health professional.	Anxiety increased in both groups during the waiting time, measured by STAI, and HRQOL deteriorated. Significant differences between the intervention (lower scores) and control group in self-reported anxiety measured on VAS.	Effect possibly influenced by support because usual care group received no contact. Lower anxiety (state and trait) in intervention group at baseline. Selection differences for nonparticipants.
Hartford et al. (2002)	RCT; four measurement points: T1 (baseline in hospital), T2 (at home, Day 3), T3 (at home, Week 4), and T4 (at home, Week 8).	N = 131 patients who have undergone elective coronary artery bypass graft surgery and their partners; mean age = 62 (intervention) and 63 (control); 84% and 88% male, intervention and control groups, respectively. Control group received usual care, which did not include systematic follow-up.	Primary outcome: Anxiety Anxiety measured using the BAI; 21 items; four discrete anxiety categories: (1) *minimal* (1–7), (2) *mild* (8–15), (3) *moderate* (16–25), and (4) *severe* (26–63); α = .92; test-retest at 1 week, r = .75.	Nurse intervention: 20–60 minutes of information and support for patients and partners. Topics included exercise, pain, psychosocial problems, medication, diet, constipation, smoking cessation, cardiac disease, cardiovascular risk factors, diagnostic tests, and sleep. First session of intervention was on day of discharge, followed by six telephone sessions. Partners and patients were spoken to separately.	Anxiety moderate to severe on discharge. Significantly lower in the intervention group than in control group at Day 2 at home. Partners anxiety low pre and post.	Low female participation.

(continues)

α = Cronbach's alpha coefficients; BAI = Beck's Anxiety Inventory; CES-D = Center for Epidemiological Studies–Depression; GDS = Geriatric Depression Scale; GDS-SF = Geriatric Depression Scale-Short Form; HADS = Hospital Anxiety and Depression Scale; HARS = Hamilton Anxiety Rating Scale; HDRS = Hamilton Depression Rating Scale; HRQOL = health-related quality of life; IBS = irritable bowel syndrome; ICS = Index of Clinical Stress; IES = Impact of Events Scale; IRR = interrater reliability; MOS-SF-36 = Medical Outcomes Study-Short Form-36; MSAS = Memorial Symptom Assessment Scale; MUIS = Mishel's Uncertainty in Illness Scale; N = sample size; NRS = numeric rating scale; PAIS-SR = Psychosocial Adjustment to Illness Scale-Self-Report; PANAS = Positive and Negative Affect Scale; POMS = Profile of Mood States; RCT = randomized controlled trial; STAI = State-Trait Anxiety Inventory; VAAS = visual analogue for anxiety scale; VAS = visual analogue scale; ZSDS = Zung Self-Rating Depression Scale.

TABLE 7-1   Studies Investigating the Relationship Between Nursing Interventions and Psychological Distress as a Nurse-Sensitive Outcome (continued)

Author/ Date	Design of study (method of participant assignment, number of measurement occasions)	Setting/subjects (characteristics of the sample and response rate, and the setting: acute care, community, long-term care)	Definition of the primary outcome concept and measure(s) used, including reliability coefficient	Nurse intervention variables investigated	Major results	Limitations
Hayes et al. (2003)	RCT; two measurement points: T1 (baseline, prior to intervention) and T2 (postintervention).	N = 198 patients scheduled for gastrointestinal procedures; mean age = 61 (range 29–84); 97% male; acute care.	Primary: Anxiety—emotional state consisting of feelings of tension, apprehension, nervousness, and worry with activation or arousal of the autonomic nervous system. State anxiety: Transitory emotional state. Trait anxiety is the stable individual difference in being prone to anxiety visible in behaviors. Anxiety measured with STAI; 40 items; α reported at .90 and .93; time to complete in study population = 3 min.	Intervention consisted of 15 minutes of self-selected music (classical, jazz, rock, country, western, or easy listening). Control group received 15 minutes of usual care.	Significantly lower anxiety in the intervention group compared with controls.	Dose of the intervention. External validity beyond VA population.
Heitkemper et al. (2004)	Three-arm RCT; three measurement points: T1 (immediately after the intervention or control group), T2 (6 months postintervention), and T3 (12 months postintervention).	N = 132 women with irritable bowl syndrome who had reported current symptoms during the previous month; mean age = 33; community.	Primary outcomes: Psychological distress, quality of life, and daily GI symptoms. Psychological distress measured using the Symptom Checklist-90R; 90-item checklist; α = .97; published norm = .26 (sample of 480 women).	Intervention delivered by psychiatric NP. Three groups received: (1) 8-week multicomponent, 1 hour individualized: baseline review, physiological arousal and breathing, diet and automatic thoughts, cognitive restructuring and relaxation, problem-solving, goals, plans, coping, strategies; (2) brief condensed: one 90-min session; and (3) usual care as per recommendations from healthcare provider.	Lower psychological distress in the comprehensive group, intervention arm only.	

Hoff & Haaga (2005)	Cohort study with random assignment; two time points: preintervention and postintervention.	Primary outcome: State anxiety. Secondary outcomes: General distress, knowledge, satisfaction with programs. State anxiety assessed with STAI–Form Y; 20 items; α = .95–.95. General distress assessed with POMS-SF; 30 items; α = .86–.92.	Orientation tour; informing patients of support services available to them; self-advocacy and asking for support for needs; and providing them with written information to refer to throughout the course of treatment. Additional information regarding the services available at the clinic and radiation oncologists' emergency contact information.	No difference in anxiety or distress.	Potential contamination between intervention and control.
	$N = 100$ (55 patients and 45 caregivers) new patients with all types of cancers who were undergoing first radiation treatment; age ranged from 27 to 82 ($M = 66$); most common cancers were breast cancer (32%) and prostate cancer (18%); acute care.				
Kim et al. (1999)	Quasi-experimental, two-group design (nonequivalent control and intervention); two measurement points: T1 (baseline) and T2 (postintervention).	Primary outcome: Anxiety related to mechanical ventilation was the primary outcome. Secondary outcomes: Negative mood. Anxiety: STAI; 40 items; α range from .86 to .95; for study, instrument was translated into Korean; α ranged from .74 to .94; α for present study ranged from .88 to 91. Negative mood: Negative affect subscale of the PANAS; α range .85–.89.	Experimental group received both the usual care and intervention. Intervention included providing patients with concrete objective information about the mechanical ventilation during a 30-minute session with the investigators and with a booklet with specific information and communication during mechanical ventilation.	Significantly less anxiety and negative mood during mechanical ventilation than the control group.	Applicability to Canadian healthcare population as Korean cardiac population. Convenience sample, nonrandom assignment. Small sample size.
	$N = 43$ patients scheduled electively to undergo first cardiac surgery and those receiving mechanical ventilation; mean age = 40 (control), 39 (intervention); 59% (control) and 67% (intervention) female; acute care. Usual care: Information about surgery, hospital stay, complications, and anesthesia.				

α = Cronbach's alpha coefficients; BAI = Beck's Anxiety Inventory; CES-D = Center for Epidemiological Studies–Depression; GDS = Geriatric Depression Scale; GDS-SF = Geriatric Depression Scale-Short Form; HADS = Hospital Anxiety and Depression Scale; HARS = Hamilton Anxiety and Depression Scale; HDRS = Hamilton Depression Rating Scale; HRQOL = health-related quality of life; IBS = irritable bowel syndrome; ICS = Index of Clinical Stress; IES = Impact of Events Scale; IRR = interrater reliability; MOS-SF-36 = Medical Outcomes Study-Short Form-36; MSAS = Memorial Symptom Assessment Scale; MUIS = Mishel's Uncertainty in Illness Scale; N = sample size; NRS = numeric rating scale; PAIS-SR = Psychosocial Adjustment to Illness Scale-Self-Report; PANAS = Positive and Negative Affect Scale; POMS = Profile of Mood States; RCT = randomized controlled trial; STAI = State-Trait Anxiety Inventory; VAAS = visual analogue for anxiety scale; VAS = visual analogue scale; ZSDS = Zung Self-Rating Depression Scale.

(continues)

TABLE 7-1 Studies Investigating the Relationship Between Nursing Interventions and Psychological Distress as a Nurse-Sensitive Outcome (continued)

Author/Date	Design of study (method of participant assignment, number of measurement occasions)	Setting/subjects (characteristics of the sample and response rate, and the setting: acute care, community, long-term care)	Definition of the primary outcome concept and measure(s) used, including reliability coefficient	Nurse intervention variables investigated	Major results	Limitations
Lin & Wang (2005)	RCT; four measurement time points: T1 (preintervention), T2 (30 min after posttest), T3 (4 hours after surgery), and T4 (24 hours after surgery). Permuted block randomization.	N = 62 patients undergoing abdominal surgery; mean age = 58 (intervention) and 55 (control); 56% of sample was male; acute care.	Primary outcomes: Preoperative anxiety and pain. Anxiety was measured with the visual analogue scale for anxiety (VASA), consisting of a 10-cm horizontal line with the descriptors *no anxiety on the left and the highest possible anxiety on the right.*	Intervention (20–30 minutes presurgery): (1) explaining the causes of pain and uncomfortable feelings; (2) influence of postoperative pain, importance of pain management and early out-of-bed activities; (3) how to decrease pain with nonmedicinal methods; (4) encouraging requests for analgesics after surgery; and (5) setting a pain control goal, encouraging expression of feelings and concerns, and selecting a favorite nonmedical pain relief method.	Significant decrease in preoperative anxiety and preoperative pain attitude.	Random distribution by selecting from an envelope.
Markle-Reid et al. (2006)	RCT; two-armed, single-blind; two measurement points: T1 (preintervention) and T2 (6 month). Blinding of interviewers to purpose of study, treatment assignment, and obtained assessments.	N = 142 older people (age ≥ 75) eligible for personal support services through community care access center; 76% female; 69% 75–85 years old and 30% > 86 years old; RR = 49.9%; community. Usual care: regular home care support.	Primary outcomes: Cognitive status, mental health (presence of depression), functional quality of life, perceived social support, and coping styles. Depression: CESD; 20 items; no reliability reported.	Intervention to bolster the participant's personal resources and environmental supports to reduce the level of vulnerability, enhance health and quality of life, and reduce on-demand use of expensive healthcare resources. Community nurse visited the home or contacted participants by phone over a 6-month period.	Significantly improved mental health, reduction in depression, and enhanced social support.	Higher functioning group of older people compared with dropouts. Urban setting.

Martensson et al. (2005)	Cluster RCT with primary group practices as unit of randomization. RCT; three measurement points, T1 (preintervention), T2 (3-month follow-up), and T3 (12-month follow-up).	N = 153 patients; 54% males, mean age = 79, 59% in New York Heart Association class III–IV; RR = 68%; primary healthcare team practices in Sweden.	Primary outcomes: HRQOL and depression. Depression: ZSDS; 20 items; cut-off scores available; translated into Swedish for present study. Internal consistency of instrument not assessed in the study.	Primary team trained in a 3-hour session (heart failure nurse and cardiologist) to increase their competence in providing heart failure care (29 nurses and 10 physicians). Intervention: One 2-hour session in the home (spouses included) at the beginning of the study, involving education and counseling followed by telephone support for a 12-month period. The session aimed at enhancing the patient's understanding of heart failure and improving self-management.	Significant difference in depression. Greater depression control over time in the intervention group.	Sample power and not accounting for intraclass correlation.
McCusker et al. (2001)	RCT; three measurement points. Research assistants (blinded to participant assignment) at 1 and 4 months after ED visit.	N = 388 older patients (age ≥ 65) admitted to ER and scored 2–6 on the Identification of Seniors at Risk (ISAR) Tool; 55% and 65% female in intervention and control respectively RR = 91.1%; acute care.	Primary outcomes: Functional dependence and depression. Depressive symptoms were assessed with the GDS-SF; 15 items; validated in both French and English; cut-off point of 5 or more had a sensitivity of 91% and specificity of 54%.	Initial screening using the ISAR, followed by a brief nursing evaluation and referral to appropriate medical and community services for high-risk patients. Nurses provided limited follow-up to ensure services provided. Usual care control ED patients eligible for study were not assessed or received further services.	Nonsignificant changes in depressive scores.	

(continues)

α = Cronbach's alpha coefficients; BAI = Beck's Anxiety Inventory; CES-D = Center for Epidemiological Studies–Depression; GDS = Geriatric Depression Scale; GDS-SF = Geriatric Depression Scale-Short Form; HADS = Hospital Anxiety and Depression Scale; HARS = Hamilton Anxiety Rating Scale; HDRS = Hamilton Depression Rating Scale; HRQOL = health-related quality of life; IBS = irritable bowel syndrome; ICS = Index of Clinical Stress; IES = Impact of Events Scale; IRR = interrater reliability; MOS-SF-36 = Medical Outcomes Study-Short Form-36; MSAS = Memorial Symptom Assessment Scale; MUIS = Mishel's Uncertainty in Illness Scale; N = sample size; NRS = numeric rating scale; PAIS-SR = Psychosocial Adjustment to Illness Scale-Self-Report; PANAS = Positive and Negative Affect Scale; POMS = Profile of Mood States; RCT = randomized controlled trial; STAI = State-Trait Anxiety Inventory; VAAS = visual analogue for anxiety scale; VAS = visual analogue scale; ZSDS = Zung Self-Rating Depression Scale.

TABLE 7-1 Studies Investigating the Relationship Between Nursing Interventions and Psychological Distress as a Nurse-Sensitive Outcome (continued)

Author/Date	Design of study (method of participant assignment, number of measurement occasions)	Setting/subjects (characteristics of the sample and response rate, and the setting: acute care, community, long-term care)	Definition of the primary outcome concept and measure(s) used, including reliability coefficient	Nurse intervention variables investigated	Major results	Limitations
Meeks et al. (2008)	RCT; two measurement points: T1 (preintervention) and T2 (postintervention). Tailored intervention.	N = 25 (including 5 for pilot study and 20 for implementation study); mean age = 75.4; individuals had a score >11 on the GDS and a score > 13 on the Mini Mental State examination; long-term care.	Primary outcome: Depression, a result of interaction of individual vulnerabilities, environmental stressors, disruptions of scripted behavior patterns, and emotional responses. **GDS, Hamilton Depression Scale (HDS),** and **Mini-Mental State Examination.**	BE-ACTIV, a 10-week intervention targeting reduced positive affect by systematically increasing positive events and activities. Individual weekly meetings with residents and mental health consultant, involvement of staff, systematic assessment, increase of pleasant events, behavioral problem-solving, and weekly communication.	Significant improvement in depressive symptoms, increased activity participation, and reduced barriers to participation.	Sample size.
Midgaard et al. (2005)	Cohort; two measurement time points: T1 (baseline) and T2 (6 weeks).	N = 91 patients receiving chemotherapy; mean age = 42; 64% female; acute care.	Anxiety and depression was assessed with the HADS; 14 items, 7 related to anxiety and 7 linked to depression; score ≥ 11 = *clinically significant case;* score 8–10 = *borderline or "doubtful" cases;* 7 or less = *"normal" noncases;* α = .73 (depression) and .89 (anxiety). Aerobic capacity of the participants was indirectly estimated by use of a stepwise work capacity on an exercise bicycle.	A physical training component in specially designed workout rooms located at the hospital was carried out in the mornings in groups (support component). After completion of the program, patients were invited to an open training session once a week.	Anxiety and depression were significantly reduced after the intervention. Improvements in fitness were correlated with improvement in depression but not anxiety.	

Mok & Woo (2004)	RCT; three measurement points: T1 (preintervention) and T2/T3 (postintervention and 3 days after intervention). Systolic and diastolic blood pressure and heart rate measured by an independent assessor.	$N = 102$ elderly patients (65 years of age or older) hospitalized for a stroke; 50% male; ages ranged from 65 to 85, with a mean age of 73.2; RR = 90%; acute care.	Primary outcome: Anxiety, defined as a vague feeling of uneasiness or apprehension. Secondary outcomes: Pain, blood pressure, and heart rate. State anxiety: State subscale of the STAI; $\alpha = 0.83–0.92$ for state anxiety scores; Chinese version (C-STAI) used in this study; has been tested in Hong Kong and was found to possess high reliability.	The intervention consisted of 10 minutes of slow-stroke back massage (SSBM) for seven consecutive evenings. Patients in the experimental group were given a massage near the side of their bed, with a curtain screened both to provide privacy and to minimize unnecessary movement. In addition to the massage, the patients in the intervention group received the standard nursing care.	Significant reduction in anxiety. Positive changes in physiological measures for as long as 3 days postmassage.	Chinese population. Random drawing of lots. Self-report bias.
Palese et al. (2005)	Quasi-experimental group control and intervention group design; three time points: T1 (morning of surgery), T2 (return from surgery), and T3 (48 hours following surgery).	$N = 145$ patients undergoing day surgery for varicose veins, hernia, breast biopsy, and hemorrhoids; mean age = 48 (nurse case model) and 55 (traditional nursing); 45% and 42% male in the intervention and control groups, respectively; acute care.	Primary outcomes: Pain, anxiety, anxiety-related factors, and perceived quality of care. Anxiety: NRS, from 0 (*no anxiety/ no pain*) to 10 (*maximum level of anxiety/ of pain*). Uncertainty was evaluated using the Mitchell Uncertainly in Illness Scale (MUIS); four subscales.	Nurse case management (NCM) model: Follows through a patient's diagnostic, clinical, and nursing care; helps the patient to prepare for surgery; is available and on hand at all times to receive information; gives the patient strategies and advice on handling the operation and the immediate postoperative period; organizes the path of treatment ordered; and, together with the surgeon, decides when the operation will take place.	Significant differences in anxiety between intervention and control group, with lower anxiety in the NCM model.	Use of severity (VAS): Report bias. Stratification of the population: Significant heterogeneity in surgery. Group differences: Higher age in usual care ward control.

α = Cronbach's alpha coefficients; BAI = Beck's Anxiety Inventory; CES-D = Center for Epidemiological Studies–Depression; GDS = Geriatric Depression Scale; GDS-SF = Geriatric Depression Scale-Short Form; HADS = Hospital Anxiety and Depression Scale; HARS = Hamilton Anxiety and Depression Scale; HDRS = Hamilton Depression Rating Scale; HRQOL = health-related quality of life; IBS = irritable bowel syndrome; ICS = Index of Clinical Stress; IES = Impact of Events Scale; IRR = interrater reliability; MOS-SF-36 = Medical Outcomes Study-Short Form-36; MSAS = Memorial Symptom Assessment Scale; MUIS = Mishel's Uncertainty in Illness Scale; N = sample size; NRS = numeric rating scale; PAIS-SR = Psychosocial Adjustment to Illness Scale-Self-Report; PANAS = Positive and Negative Affect Scale; POMS = Profile of Mood States; RCT= randomized controlled trial; STAI = State-Trait Anxiety Inventory; VAAS = visual analogue scale for anxiety scale; VAS = visual analogue scale; ZSDS = Zung Self-Rating Depression Scale.

(continues)

TABLE 7-1 Studies Investigating the Relationship Between Nursing Interventions and Psychological Distress as a Nurse-Sensitive Outcome (continued)

Author/ Date	Design of study (method of participant assignment, number of measurement occasions)	Setting/subjects (characteristics of the sample and response rate, and the setting: acute care, community, long-term care)	Definition of the primary outcome concept and measure(s) used, including reliability coefficient	Nurse intervention variables investigated	Major results	Limitations
Quattrin et al. (2006)	RCT; three measure time points: T1 (pre-intervention), T2 (immediately follow-ing the intervention), and T3 (24 hours after the intervention).	N = 30 cancer patients hospitalized for at least 2 days in an oncol-ogy inpatient unit; 63% female; mean age = 54.2.	Primary outcome: Anxiety; nausea/vomiting, and other side effects of chemotherapy. Anxiety was assessed with the STAI; 40 items made of two subscales for state and trait anxiety; α = .83–92	Reflexology foot mas-sage (30 minutes) provided by nurs-ing assistants trained and monitored in the technique.	Significant differ-ences between anxiety in intervention and control.	
Rabins et al. (2000)	Cluster RCT; two measurement time points: T1 (prein-tervention) and T2 (postintervention).	N = 237 residents of long-term care with significant level of psychiatric symptoms using standardized tools; mean age = 75; 84% (intervention group) and 70% (con-trol group) female; RR = 80%; long-term care.	Depression, mood, and psychiatric symp-toms and behavioral disorders. The Brief Psychiatric Rating Scale (BPRS) measure was used to assess psychiatric symptoms and and behavioral disorders. The Montgomery-Asberg Depression Rating Scale (MADRS) was used to detect change in mood and to measure depressive symptoms.	Psychiatrist-guided intervention by nurses in psychogeriatric assessment and treat-ment in a city hous-ing intervention. Education of staff in evidence-based man-agement of mood dis-order, other mental health disorders, and problems with demen-tia. Weekly support by mental health nurse.	Significant differences in the scores for psy-chiatric rating and depression; reduced between intervention and control postinter-vention, and over time.	Higher education and higher income in inter-vention group. Sample size not accounted for in intra-class correlation.
Rawl et al. (2002)	RCT; three measure-ment time points: T1 (base-line), T2 (halfway through intervention), and T3 (1 month postintervention).	N = 109 new diag-nosed breast (55%), colon (25%), or lung (29%) cancer patients receiving che-motherapy; mean age = 55; 84% female; RR = 48%; acute care.	Primary outcomes: Psychosocial func-tioning, anxiety, and depression. Depression: CES-D-20; 20 items; in pres-ent study α = .85–.89.	Computer-based advanced practice nurse nursing: Provide information on symp-tom management, dis-ease, and treatment; coordinate medical resources; and	Intervention group had significantly less depression between baseline and T2, less anxiety and greater improvement in the role, emotional, and	Low participation rate and high withdrawal in the intervention group. Heterogeneity in sample. Diffusion of intervention.

			STAI was used to measure state anxiety; 20-items; in present study α = .90–.92. MOS-SF-36 used to assess psychosocial functioning; in present study α = .76–93	provide emotional support and counseling. Nine contacts: Five in person, four telephone, conducted over an 18-month period.	mental health subscales of the MOS-SF-36.	Table of random numbers.
Scott et al. (2004)	RCT; three measurement points: T1 (preintervention), T2 (3 months), and T3 (6 months). The placebo intervention consisted of health promotion topics.	N = 88 heart failure patients enrolled in an agency care group; 44% male; mean age =75 (range 33–94); RR = 92% community.	Primary outcome variables: Perceived mental health and quality of life. The Mental Health Inventory-5 (MHI-5), a subscale of the MOS-SF-36; five items; the general population norm is 74.74 (range 0–100); reported α = .65–.81; in present study α = .86.	Eight weeks (1hour) in-home. Three groups: Mutual goal setting, supportive-educative, and placebo. The mutual goal-setting group examined values about heart failure mutually explored and strategies developed for goal attainment. The supportive-educative intervention taught the client self-care management and support.	No significant changes between groups. At 6 months, the mutually supportive group's scores on the MHI-5 were significantly higher than the other two groups. Overall, the participants experienced increased MHI scores over time.	
Sloman (2002)	RCT; four-arm study: (1) progressive muscle relaxation (PMR) training, (2) guided imagery (GI) training, (3) both of these treatments, and (4) control group. Two measurement time points: T1 (preintervention) and T2 (3 weeks after initial session).	N = 56 advanced cancer patients experiencing anxiety and depression; 26 females and 30 males; mean age = 54.5; all were receiving palliative care in their home and were on pain medication; community and acute care.	Primary outcomes: Anxiety defined as "A feeling of apprehension, worry, uneasiness, or dread, especially of the future." Depression: "A feeling involving an element of sadness and helplessness with little drive for socialization or communication." Anxiety and depression assessed with the HADS; no reliability data provided.	Taught relaxation using tape-recorded training. The sessions were one of the following: PMR, GI, or a combination of PMR and GI. Each session lasted approximately 30 min. At the end of the session, participants shared their feelings, and a tape recorder was left to allow patients to practice twice daily.	No improvement in anxiety but improvement in depression and quality of life.	

α = Cronbach's alpha coefficients; BAI = Beck's Anxiety Inventory; CES-D = Center for Epidemiological Studies–Depression; GDS = Geriatric Depression Scale; GDS-SF = Geriatric Depression Scale–Short Form; HADS = Hospital Anxiety and Depression Scale; HARS = Hamilton Anxiety Rating Scale; HDRS = Hamilton Depression Rating Scale; HRQOL = health-related quality of life; IBS = irritable bowel syndrome; ICS = Index of Clinical Stress; IES = Impact of Events Scale; IRR = interrater reliability; MOS-SF-36 = Medical Outcomes Study-Short Form-36; MSAS = Memorial Symptom Assessment Scale; MUIS = Mishel's Uncertainty in Illness Scale; N = sample size; NRS = numeric rating scale; PAIS-SR = Psychosocial Adjustment to Illness Scale-Self-Report; PANAS = Positive and Negative Affect Scale; POMS = Profile of Mood States; RCT= randomized controlled trial; STAI = State-Trait Anxiety Inventory; VAAS = visual analogue for anxiety scale; VAS = visual analogue scale; ZSDS = Zung Self-Rating Depression Scale.

(continues)

TABLE 7-1   Studies Investigating the Relationship Between Nursing Interventions and Psychological Distress as a Nurse-Sensitive Outcome (continued)

Author/Date	Design of study (method of participant assignment, number of measurement occasions)	Setting/subjects (characteristics of the sample and response rate, and the setting: acute care, community, long-term care)	Definition of the primary outcome concept and measure(s) used, including reliability coefficient	Nurse intervention variables investigated	Major results	Limitations
G. D. Smith (2006)	Quasi-experimental; two measurement points: T1 (pre-intervention) and T2 (3 months after treatment).	N = 75 IBS patients; acute care.	Primary outcomes: Symptoms, depression, anxiety, and HRQOL. Anxiety and depression were measured using the HADS questionnaire.	Nurse-led gut-directed hypnotherapy (5- to 7.5-hour sessions) over 3 months in addition to education and support. Hypnotherapy was induced by eye fixation, followed by conventional deepening and relaxation techniques. Self-hypnosis taught and audiocassettes given for home use.	Significant reduction in anxiety scores after treatment. Depression remained unchanged.	Research design.
Strong et al. (2008)	RCT; four measurement points: T1 (preintervention) and T2/T3/T4 (3, 6, and 12 months after treatment).	N = 200 patients with a cancer prognosis more than 6 months and a major depressive disorder; mean age = 56; 71% female; acute care; RR = 60%.	Primary outcome: Depression, anxiety. Depression: Symptom Checklist-20 (SCL-20); derived from the SCl-90. Anxiety measured with a SCL-10; 10 items derived from the SCL-90.	Screening/management of depression: 10 one-to-one sessions over 3 months of education about depression and treatment; problem-solving to overcome feelings of helplessness; improving communication.	Significant improvement in the intervention group regarding anxiety and fatigue as compared with the control group.	Nonblinding of treatment allocation.
Targ & Levine (2002)	RCT; two measurement time points: T1 (baseline) and T2 (postintervention).	N = 181 women with breast cancer diagnosed with metastatic cancer within 18 months; mean age = 49 (intervention) and 47 (standard group); acute care.	Primary outcomes: Anxiety, depression, spiritual well-being, and quality of life. Anxiety and depression assessed with POMS; 65 items; reliability coefficients not provided.	A 12-week standard group support or a 12-week complementary and alternative medicine (CAM) support. CAM group taught the use of meditation, affirmation, imagery and ritual. Standard group (led by a psychiatrist) combined CBT with group support.	Significant decrease in depression and anxiety.	

Study	Design	Sample	Primary outcome	Intervention	Results	Notes
Taylor-Piliac & Chair (2002)	RCT, three-group design; three measurement points: T1 (baseline), T2 (post-intervention), and T3 (after procedure).	N = 45 hospitalized patients undergoing cardiac catheterization (CC).	Primary outcome: Anxiety (temporal feelings of fear and worry) and mood states. State-Anxiety Inventory (SAI); 20 items; questionnaire available in Cantonese/Chinese versions; *low anxiety = 20–39, moderate anxiety = 40–59, and high anxiety = 60–80*; α =.93 in Chinese men. POMS measured mood states; 65-item tool; translated into Chinese language among Chinese population, α =.91 and test/retest = .86.	Three groups: (1) music intervention: cassette recorder and headphones with individual volume control; (2) sensation information: subjects listened to a prerecorded audiotape providing the sensation information, describing what a patient will see, hear, smell, taste, and feel during the CC; (3) control group: usual care.	No significant effect on anxiety or mood, or decreased symptoms of anxiety, including heart and respiratory rate.	Socially desirable responses given Chinese culture. Age differences between groups (older control group). Randomized after collection of baseline data.
Twiss et al. (2007)	RCT; measurement pre/post surgery.	N = 86; mean age: 86.4. recruited prior to Coronary Artery By-pass Graft surgery; RR=not specified; acute care.	STAI was used to measure state anxiety; 20 items; in present study α =.90–.92	Music intervention: Self-selected listening of CDs during surgery and while in recovery room.	Significant reduction in the intervention group compared with control.	Random assignment by picking assignment from box. Attrition: 14 dropouts in intervention.
Wengstrom et al. (1999)	RCT; five measurement points: T1 (baseline), T2/T3 (Weeks 3 and 5, completion of treatment), and T4/T5 (follow-up periods, 2 weeks and 3 months).	N = 134 female breast cancer patients receiving curative radiation therapy (RT); mean age= 58; RR = 77%; acute care.	Primary outcomes: Subjective distress (intrusion and avoidance), side effects, and quality of life. Perceived stress reactions were studied using the IES; 15 items; in present study α =.73–.87.	Intervention: Five 30-min sessions once a week during treatment and two follow-up sessions after treatment; oral and written cognitive information about RT, side-effect education; support and guidance in self-care; psychological support and strategies for coping and emotional regulation.	Positive effect in minimizing stress reaction as measured on the IES.	Randomization by sealed envelope. Attrition.

α = Cronbach's alpha coefficients; BAI = Beck's Anxiety Inventory; CES-D = Center for Epidemiological Studies–Depression; GDS = Geriatric Depression Scale; GDS-SF = Geriatric Depression Scale-Short Form; HADS = Hospital Anxiety and Depression Scale; HARS = Hamilton Anxiety Rating Scale; HDRS = Hamilton Depression Rating Scale; HRQOL = health-related quality of life; IBS = irritable bowel syndrome; ICS = Index of Clinical Stress; IES = Impact of Events Scale; IRR = interrater reliability; MOS-SF-36 = Medical Outcomes Study-Short Form-36; MSAS = Memorial Symptom Assessment Scale; MUIS = Mishel's Uncertainty in Illness Scale; N = sample size; NRS = numeric rating scale; PAIS-SR = Psychosocial Adjustment to Illness Scale-Self-Report; PANAS = Positive and Negative Affect Scale; POMS = Profile of Mood States; RCT= randomized controlled trial; STAI = State-Trait Anxiety Inventory; VAAS = visual analogue for anxiety scale; VAS = visual analogue scale; ZSDS = Zung Self-Rating Depression Scale.

(continues)

TABLE 7-1 Studies Investigating the Relationship Between Nursing Interventions and Psychological Distress as a Nurse-Sensitive Outcome (continued)

Author/Date	Design of study (method of participant assignment, number of measurement occasions)	Setting/subjects (characteristics of the sample and response rate, and the setting; acute care, community, long-term care)	Definition of the primary outcome concept and measure(s) used, including reliability coefficient	Nurse intervention variables investigated	Major results	Limitations
Williams & Schreier (2004)	RCT; three measurement time points: T1 (preintervention); T2 (1 month after treatment began), and T3 (3 months after treatment).	$N = 70$ women receiving their first treatment of chemotherapy; mean age = 50 (range 30–74); primarily in stage 2 of the disease; acute care.	State anxiety (transitory anxiety), side-effect severity, and use and efficacy of self-care behaviors. Anxiety assessed with the STAI; reliability coefficients not reported. The self-care diary (SCD) was used to assess the number of side effects experienced, the severity of each of the side effects, the number of self-care behaviors performed for a given side effect, and effectiveness of self-care behaviors; test-retest reliability, $r = .80$.	Patients in both groups received the standard education, including information about how to handle more frequent side effects, such as nausea, hair loss, and mucositis. Patients in the experimental group were mailed audiotapes (20-minute audiotapes providing information about the nutritional management of side effects, and exercise and relaxation techniques to manage fatigue, anxiety, and difficulty sleeping) and a printed SCD. All subjects were interviewed three times by telephone by the same interviewer.	State anxiety diminished over time in both groups, but no difference was detected between groups.	No assessment of other types of support received. Variation in adherence to audiotapes.

α = Cronbach's alpha coefficients; BAI = Beck's Anxiety Inventory; CES-D = Center for Epidemiological Studies–Depression; GDS = Geriatric Depression Scale; GDS-SF = Geriatric Depression Scale-Short Form; HADS = Hospital Anxiety and Depression Scale; HARS = Hamilton Anxiety Rating Scale; HDRS = Hamilton Depression Rating Scale; HRQOL = health-related quality of life; IBS = irritable bowel syndrome; ICS = Index of Clinical Stress; IES = Impact of Events Scale; IRR = interrater reliability; MOS-SF-36 = Medical Outcomes Study-Short Form-36; MSAS = Memorial Symptom Assessment Scale; MUIS = Mishel's Uncertainty in Illness Scale; N = sample size; NRS = numeric rating scale; PAIS-SR = Psychosocial Adjustment to Illness Scale-Self-Report; PANAS = Positive and Negative Affect Scale; POMS = Profile of Mood States; RCT = randomized controlled trial; STAI = State-Trait Anxiety Inventory; VAAS = visual analogue for anxiety scale; VAS = visual analogue scale; ZSDS = Zung Self-Rating Depression Scale.

or treatment modalities that produce "sickness behaviour" (de Ridder, Geenen, Kuijer, & Middendorp, 2008; M. Watson, 2001). Sickness behavior refers to subjective feelings of fatigue, weakness, malaise, and listlessness presenting along with changes in appetite and weight, altered sleep patterns, diminished interest in one's surroundings, and difficulties in concentration. The inflammatory pathophysiological processes that induce sickness behavior promote psychological symptoms in a number of chronic conditions, including acute myocardial infarction, diabetes, cancer, and arthritis (de Ridder et al.). A number of other factors or antecedents, including personality disposition, life stage, life experiences, previous exposure to stressors, age, culture, ethnicity, gender, spirituality, and quality of, support are associated with psychological adjustment and the subsequent development of psychological distress. Other factors associated with the development of psychological distress are further elaborated in later sections of this chapter.

THEORETICAL BACKGROUND

Physical illness can be viewed as a stressor, the demands of which depend on the characteristics and severity of the illness (Sharpe & Curran, 2006). Because chronic illness affects every aspect of being (physical, emotional, social, financial, spiritual), it represents a threat to everything that is important to a person (Hymovich & Hagopian, 1992). Consequently, patients must find effective ways of coping with the threat and new ways to achieve a rebalancing of their changed living circumstances to achieve positive psychological adjustment (de Ridder et al., 2008). Adjustment is defined as a response to a change in the environment that allows a person to become more suitably adapted to a change (de Ridder et al.) and usually refers to a desirable state or end point (Brennan, 2001). Adjustment in chronic illness is considered a lifelong process because continual adjustment to new symptoms, periods of good health, times of remission, and exacerbations are necessary as the illness trajectory unfolds (Sidell, 1997). Signs of successful adjustment to a chronic illness include mastery of disease-related adaptive tasks, preservation of functional status, maintenance of quality of life across domains, emotional balance, the absence of psychological disorders, presence of low negative affect and high positive affect, and retention of meaning and purpose in life (de Ridder et al.; Stanton, Collins, & Sworowski, 2001; Stanton et al., 2007). Life satisfaction and global self-esteem are also considered indicators of adjustment (Schiaffino, Shawaryn, & Blum, 1998).

Perceived personal growth and positive meaning in illness, also labeled as posttraumatic growth and benefit finding, respectively, have more recently emerged as important indicators of adjustment (Folkman & Greer, 2000; Mols, Vingerhoets, Coebergh, & van de Poll-Franse, 2005). Conversely, the development of clinically significant emotional or behavioral symptoms of psychological distress and, more specifically, anxiety and/or depression, are equated with poor adjustment or labeled as adjustment disorder (Cordova, Cunningham, Carlson, & Andrykowski, 2001; Meijer, Sinnema, Bijstra, Mellenbergh, & Wolters, 2002).

Several models have been proposed regarding how patients adjust to illness, the most popular being identified as the theory of stress and coping (Folkman & Lazarus, 1980; Folkman, Lazarus, Dunkel-Schetter, De Longis, & Gruen, 1986) because it constitutes the foundation for understanding disease-related adjustment. This model is based on the theory that how people cope with stress affects their physical, psychological, and social well-being. Coping refers to the cognitions and behaviors that people use to regulate distressing situations (Folkman & Moskowitz, 2000). The appraisal of the stressor is a critical element in the stress and coping model and is postulated to occur in successive stages of primary and secondary appraisal. In primary appraisal, the individual assesses the nature of the stressor, evaluating the degree of loss, threat, or harm perceived to be associated with it. Secondary appraisal then occurs, whereby the person judges what he or she can do to deal with the situation by considering the options available, including his or her personal coping repertoire, environmental constraints, and the availability of social support. Self-efficacy, one's belief in his or her capability or confidence to accomplish tasks associated with an illness (Bandura, 1997), is also identified as an important element of secondary appraisal (Folkman & Greer, 2000).

Appraisal processes trigger the selection of coping strategies according to whether the individual views the stressor as a threat, harm, loss, or challenge. Amelioration of the perceived harm or threat is achieved by both regulating distressing emotions and changing the problem that is causing the discomfort, labeled emotion-focused coping and problem-focused coping, respectively (Lazarus & Folkman, 1984). Coping is regarded as context specific and varies as the adaptive tasks of illness change (Blalock, DeVellis, Holt, & Hahn, 1993) Active coping strategies, including information-seeking, problem-solving, seeking social support, benefit-finding, and creating outlets for emotional expression, are linked to better adjustment and reduced psychological distress (Carver, Scheier, & Weintraub, 1989; P. Davidson et al., 2008). Avoidant coping strategies, on the other hand, are predictive of poor adjustment when used to manage health problems for cancer (Hack & Degner, 2004), heart disease (Dew et al., 1994), and rheumatic disease (Covic, Adamson, Spencer, & Howe, 2003). More recently, meaning-based coping was added to the stress-coping model (Folkman & Greer) based on research that benefit-finding or positive meaning may be derived from cognitive reframing of the illness and redefining of life purpose. Meaning-based coping can include finding order (incorporating life-changing events into preexisting beliefs) and finding purpose (searching for purposeful life goals) within restricted circumstances (Park & Folkman, 1997; Thompson & Janigan, 1988). Consequently, the experience of illness is not always negative, with positive outcomes labeled as posttraumatic growth or benefit-finding (Janoff-Bulman, 1989).

Benefit-finding has been reported for cancer (Antoni et al., 2001; Andrykowski et al., 2005; Bower et al., 2005; Sears, Stanton, & Danoff-Burg, 2003; Tomich & Helgeson, 2004), rheumatoid arthritis (Danoff-Burg & Revenson, 2005), multiple sclerosis (Pakenham, 2005), myocardial infarction (Petrie, Buick, Weinman, & Booth, 1999), and HIV/AIDS (Seigel & Scrimshaw, 2000).

The self-regulatory model (SRM) (Leventhal, Nerenz, & Steele, 1984), also called the common sense model (Ward, 1993), extends stress and coping theory by emphasizing the role of external cues and information processing as critical to explaining individual variation in adjustment to illness. SRM expands coping to include a broader range of coping procedures and health behaviors (e.g., taking a medication, going to the emergency department) that might be used by an individual to manage a health threat and achieve self-regulation of illness (Leventhal & Deifenbach, 1991). SRM asserts that individuals use internal (past history of symptoms or illness in self or significant others) and external (health providers, family, friends, media) information to construct meaning or cognitive representations of an illness that in turn influence selection of coping procedures. Representations contain information about five aspects of the illness: identity (label placed on the illness); cause (ideas about attributions for the illness); consequences (perceived short- and long-term effects); cure or control (ideas about whether the illness can be treated); and timeline (expectations about duration and course of the disease) (Brownlee, Leventhal, & Leventhal, 2000). Emotional representations (fear, anxiety, and sadness) are processed in parallel with cognitive representations of the health threat, potentially contributing to the potential for psychological distress. Representations (emotional and cognitive) drive efforts to reduce the illness threat through specific self-regulatory actions or coping procedures, which are subsequently appraised for their effectiveness and altered accordingly. Studies in chronic illness support the hypothesis that illness representations influence psychological responses (depression, self-esteem, anxiety, life satisfaction); medical outcomes (pain severity, glycemic control); and health behavior (self-care, return to work, rehabilitation attendance, adherence to medications) (Haggar & Orbell, 2003; Scharloo et al., 1998). Representational educational approaches based on the self-regulatory model (SRT) have been recommended for person-centered, psychoeducational nursing interventions (Donovan & Ward, 2005).

FACTORS THAT INFLUENCE ADJUSTMENT AND PSYCHOLOGICAL DISTRESS

Significant heterogeneity has been noted in psychological adjustment to chronic illness across individuals and chronic diseases and subsequently in the development of psychological distress (Petrie & Revenson, 2005; Stanton et al., 2007). Personality attributes, perceptions of control, and socioeconomic and demographic (gender, age) variables are considered important determinants of psychological adjustment. These variables are further described as:

(a) *Personality attributes:* Personality affects adaptation either by influencing risk or by acting as a protective factor (T. W. Smith & Gallo, 2001). Personality traits such as hardiness and optimism are considered important predictors of psychological adjustment because they are considered to provide the internal resources needed to face challenges constructively and purposefully (de Ridder et al., 2008). Dispositional optimism appears to work by bolstering the use of approach-oriented coping strategies (Scheier & Carver, 1985) and is shown across chronic illnesses such as heart disease and cancer to affect adjustment (Carver et al., 2005; Schou, Ekeberg, & Ruland, 2005; Shneck, Irvine, Stewart, & Abbey, 2001). A higher feeling of personal control (Moser & Dracup, 1996) and a view that one has internal control versus external control (control by powerful others) (Rotter, 1990) are associated with better psychosocial adjustment.

(b) *Socioeconomic status:* Socioeconomic status is considered to predict adjustment because it can have a direct effect on influencing health outcomes or an indirect effect through lower access to healthcare resources (de Ridder et al., 2008). Lower income (< $29,999) was found to be a sensitive predictor of higher levels of psychological distress in chronically ill primary care practice patient populations (Fortin et al., 2006). This is consistent with epidemiologic studies in many countries indicating that populations in the lowest socioeconomic positions fare worse across multiple health outcomes (Marmot, 2003).

(c) *Demographic factors:* Younger populations with physical health problems and chronic illness appear to be more vulnerable to psychological distress such as depression than older populations (Currie & Wang, 2004; Patten, Beck, Williams, Barbul, & Metz, 2003). This may be due to problems of adjustment and coping (Patten & Juby, 2008) and the extent of disruption wrought by the illness in critical stages of the life cycle (Veach, Nicholas, & Barton, 2002). Women tend to report more psychological distress when faced with chronic illness as compared with men who face identical stressors; this is possibly explained by the different coping strategies used by women, including greater use of social support, as compared with men in response to distress (Nolen-Hoeksema, Larson, & Grayson, 1999; Ptacek, Smith, & Zanas, 1992; Stokes & Wilson, 1984; Wohlgemuth & Betz, 1991). Traditional gender-role stereotypes of men and women have been used to explain such findings, suggesting that women are socialized to be emotionally expressive and interdependent, whereas men are socialized to be independent (Greenhaus & Parasuraman, 1994).

(d) *Culture and ethnicity:* Little is known about the role of culture and ethnicity in adjustment to illness because few studies have examined psychological adjustment in diverse multicultural populations (Stanton et al., 2007). Elevated psychological symptoms are reported more frequently in some groups with chronic illness (e.g., Latina cervical cancer patients) (Meyerowitz, Formenti, Ell, & Leedham, 2000), but underlying mechanisms such as income differences that could be contributing to these differences have not been examined.

(e) *Social support:* Social support is hypothesized to either buffer the person from the influence of stressful events (buffering effect model) or have a direct effect (main effects model) (Gonzalez, Goeppinger, & Lorig, 1990). A buffering effect is present when psychosocial resources, such as the presence of social support, modify the relationship between the stressor and depression, whereas a direct effect occurs when psychosocial resources have a beneficial effect on depressive symptoms regardless of the stressor (Broadhead et al., 1983; Cobb, 1976). Social support explains depressive symptoms in a number of chronic illnesses such as arthritis (Demange et al., 2004), trajectories of adjustment in cancer (Helgeson, Snyder, & Seltman, 2004), and heart disease (Bennett et al., 2001). Relationship with a partner is considered vital to psychological adjustment to major stressors (Northouse, Mood, Templen, Mellon, & George, 2000; Schulz & Schwarzer, 2004), with a buffering effect demonstrated across illnesses on the negative influence of disease on depressive symptoms (Bisschop et al., 2000).

SENSITIVITY TO NURSING CARE

Psychological distress is considered a nurse-sensitive outcome (Given & Sherwood, 2005), and psychosocial interventions are recommended for adoption in managing psychological distress such as depression and anxiety (Fulcher et al., 2008; Rodgers et al., 2005). Psychosocial interventions are diverse and typically are identified as relaxation training, cognitive and behavioral coping strategies, education/information support, psychoeducational approaches, individual counseling or family-based therapy, and group social support (Rodgers et al.). Psychosocial interventions usually include more than one component bundled together as part of an intervention package and are classified as a complex nursing intervention (Conn, Rantz, Wipke-Tevis, & Maas, 2001). However, the components of psychosocial interventions are inconsistently defined across studies, with significant variation in the types of interventions and in the combination of the components that constitute the intervention (Rodgers et al.).

Psychosocial interventions have proven efficacy in medically ill patients with cancer, cardiovascular disease, and HIV/AIDS in alleviating the psychological distress associated with these illnesses (Fekete, Antoni, & Schneiderman, 2007). Psychosocial interventions are shown to have positive effects on psychological distress (including depression and a number of other outcomes) such as perceived social support and problem-focused coping, and to potentially influence biological variables linked with disease progression and earlier mortality across chronic conditions (Schneiderman, Antoni, Saab, & Ironson, 2001). Reviews involving other chronic conditions such as arthritis (Lorig, Sobel, Ritter, Laurent, & Hobbs, 2001) and diabetes (Peyrot & Rubin, 2007) have demonstrated effectiveness of psychosocial interventions as part of a comprehensive program of self-management and health behavior change to reduce psychological distress. Systematic reviews in cancer and heart disease are most prominent in the literature given the prevalence of these conditions in the population and were the subject of an extensive scoping review (Rodgers et al., 2005). As reported by Rodgers and colleagues, the beneficial effects of psychosocial interventions on psychological distress are as follows:

(a) *Cancer:* Standard mean differences showed a beneficial effect of psycho-educational interventions on depression, with an overall effect size of 0.54 (95% CI: 0.43, 0.65) and specific effect sizes for education alone (4 studies: d50.50); nonbehavioral/cognitive counseling alone (5 studies; d50.66); muscle relaxation with guided imagery (12 studies; d50.40); and combination treatments with educational, behavioral, or nonbehavioral counseling (12 studies: $d = 0.52$) for anxiety (0.56, 95% CI: 0.42, 0.70) and mood (0.45, 95% CI: 0.32, 0.58). In a proportion of studies reviewed, positive effects were also observed for behavioral (65% of studies), counseling (70%), and education (57%) interventions in relieving depression. In addition, beneficial effects of relaxation therapy on depression (ES: 0.45), tension (ES: 0.51), anxiety (ES: 0.45), and mood (ES: 0.44), documented as effect sizes, were noted. Meta-analytic reviews of psychosocial interventions in other reviews in cancer populations reported small effect sizes for depression (0.19) and emotional adjustment (0.24), and moderate effects for anxiety (0.36) (Meyer & Mark, 1995; Sheard, & McGuire, 1999).

(b) *Heart disease:* Beneficial effects on psychological outcomes were shown for education in cardiac disease, but because of significant heterogeneity in studies, effect sizes were not calculated in any of the reviews identified. Existing reviews of broader psychosocial interventions, such as stress management in cardiac disease, showed beneficial effects on psychological outcomes, including a small decrease in standardized mean difference for anxiety (0.07, CI: 0.16, 0.01) and depression scores (0.32, CI: 0.44, 0.01), and a reduction in psychological distress (effect size: 0.30) from patient education, counseling, and behavioral techniques. Significant heterogeneity in populations and interventions and low quality in systematic reviews were noted.

The benefits of psychosocial interventions support the need for their use in clinical practice as part of a biopsychosocial approach to healthcare delivery (Engel, 1977). Psychosocial interventions recommended for application by nurses in managing depression as a nurse-sensitive outcome in cancer were identified as cognitive-behavioral therapy, education and information, counseling and psychotherapy, behavioral therapy, and supportive interventions because these were supported by the highest levels (RCT or meta-analysis) of evidence for effectiveness (Fulcher et al., 2008). Similarly, psychoeducational and/or cognitive-behavioral therapy interventions were recommended for application in reducing anxiety as a nurse-sensitive outcome based on the strong evidence supporting this type of intervention approach (Sheldon et al., 2008).

None of the reviews identified in the literature focused specifically on evaluating the sensitivity of psychological distress as an outcome of psychosocial interventions delivered by nurses. This section of the chapter examines the empirical evidence in nursing to evaluate psychological distress as sensitive to psychosocial nursing interventions. In this review, a total of 45 empirical studies that met inclusion and exclusion criteria were examined for their effectiveness on psychological distress as a primary study outcome. Psychological distress in these studies was measured as general psychological distress or, more specifically, as subjective symptoms of anxiety and/or depression. Psychosocial nursing interventions in studies reviewed included a variety of components and were targeted toward reducing psychological distress in patients with diverse chronic conditions, including cancer, cardiac disease, diabetes, and HIV, and in elderly nursing home residents. The psychosocial interventions were administered by nurses at different points in the illness trajectory, such as prior to or during diagnostic procedures or during treatment, and usually comprised multiple components. Six types of psychosocial nursing interventions were identified in the studies reviewed: (a) education/informational; (b) cognitive-behavioral therapy; (c) psychoeducation; (d) relaxation; (e) structural supportive care interventions/models of care; and (f) exercise.

Education/Information Support

Nurses have traditionally identified education as one of their core responsibilities and an important strategy to reduce psychological distress (Thomas, 2003). Education/informational support refers to receipt of advice, suggestions, and additional knowledge or information about a situation; it may include education about the medical condition, related symptoms, and what patients might experience emotionally, cognitively, or spiritually in relation to the illness or its treatment (Campbell, Phaneuf, & Deanne, 2004; Helgeson, Cohen, Schultz, & Yasko, 2000). Education/information and support interventions focus on increasing knowledge, informed decision-making, and self-care skills to decrease anxiety, fear, and distress (Lambert & Loiselle, 2007). Information is considered an essential component of a supportive care approach in health care (Fitch, Page, & Porter, 2008).

Effectiveness of education/informational support nursing interventions on psychological distress was examined in nine RCTs (Crogan, Evans, & Bendel, 2008; Deshler et al., 2006; Erci, Sezgin, & Kacmaz, 2009; Harkness, Morrow, Smith, Kiczula, & Arthur, 2003; Hartford, Wong, & Zarkaria, 2002; Lin & Wang, 2005; Rawl et al., 2008; Scott, Setter-Kline, & Britton, 2004; Williams & Schreier, 2004), three quasi-experimental studies (Ambler et al., 1999; R. J. Davidson, Jackson, & Kalin, 2000; Kim, Garvin, & Moser, 1999), and a cohort study (Hoff & Haaga, 2005). All the interventions had an educational component but varied in their supportive care component (therapeutic listening vs self-advocacy), mode of delivery (telephone vs face-to-face vs peer group), intervention dose (two to nine sessions), timing, and length. Mixed findings were observed regarding the sensitivity of this type of psychosocial nursing intervention on psychological distress outcomes.

Randomized Controlled Trials

In an intervention focused on providing education and support to enable self-management as part of a therapeutic relationship in general surgical populations, Erci et al. (2009) reported reduced anxiety across three measurement time points, including prior to discharge, in the intervention group. Similarly, Lin and Wang (2005) reported reduced anxiety when education was combined with anticipatory support in managing feelings and emotions prior to major abdominal surgery. However, the measurement time points were short in the Lin and Wang study—pre, immediate post, and 24 hours after surgery—and whether the effect was sustained during the recovery period is not clear. Interventions administered over longer periods of time with a more intense supportive component reduced anxiety in both cardiac and cancer populations. Following an education and telephone support intervention (six sessions) provided to both patients and their partners, Hartford et al. (2002) demonstrated a reduction in anxiety in the intervention group that was observed in the postdischarge period. Education delivered by computer combined with emotional support in nine sessions (face to face and telephone) over an 18-month time frame in mixed cancer populations was also found to reduce both anxiety and depression (Rawl et al., 2002). Reduced anxiety was also shown for cardiac patients in the period preceding cardiac diagnostic procedures, with significant reductions in anxiety in the intervention group when provided with anticipatory education and support (Harkness et al., 2003). Negative findings were reported for anxiety in a randomized trial in which cancer patients and their support partners were provided with information about treatment delivered in a video-plus-booklet format, regardless of whether it was mailed or delivered in a classroom or drop-in format without a clear support component (Deshler et al., 2006). Similarly, a pilot intervention that focused only on peer support using storytelling facilitated by nurses found no effect on psychological distress (Crogan et al., 2008). However, the study was likely underpowered.

Quasi-Experimental Studies

An education/support intervention to prepare patients prior to cardiac surgery was shown to reduce anxiety and negative mood in the intervention group in a pre-post cohort comparison (Kim et al., 1999). A stress reduction and advocacy support intervention reported a reduction in anxiety (Ambler et al., 1999). No significant change was noted for anxiety or depression in a quasi-experimental group educational/support intervention in women with heart disease (P. Davidson et al., 2008) or in a cohort study comprising male and female patients with heart failure (Hoff & Haaga, 2005). Both of the later interventions were primarily focused on education, with a less clear support component.

Sample sizes across studies ranged from 10 to 131; most studies were adequately powered, although sample sizes were not always justified. The findings regarding psychological distress as sensitive to information/education support interventions are equivocal given that a number of studies reported negative findings. Subtle differences in the interventions, particularly in the supportive care component or in the dose, timing, or length of the intervention may have influenced the findings given the significant heterogeneity across studies regarding intervention components. These findings suggest that psychological distress may be sensitive to nursing psychosocial interventions, but the dose and length of the intervention over time is an important consideration in the design of these interventions. Interventions focused on passive dissemination of education without a support component appear to be ineffective.

Cognitive-Behavioral Therapy

Cognitive-behavioral therapy (CBT) is a psychotherapeutic approach that aims to influence dysfunctional emotions, behaviors, and cognitions through a goal-oriented, systematic procedure with a particular focus on stress management and coping skills training (Keller et al., 2000). In the past, CBT was reserved for use as a specialist intervention delivered by psychologists or psychiatrists, but nurses and other health professionals have been trained to successfully administer CBT interventions (Arving et al., 2007). In this review, there were six randomized trials of nurse-delivered CBT interventions (Arving et al.; Dirksen & Epstein, 2008; Dougherty, Lewis, Thompson, Baer, & Kim, 2004; Duffy et al., 2006; Heitkemper et al., 2004; Targ & Levine, 2002). No differences in anxiety or depression were noted for CBT delivered by nurses (INS) to women starting adjuvant breast cancer chemotherapy, as compared with CBT delivered by psychologists (IPS) (Arving et al.). When the effects of both intervention groups were combined (INS and IPS), statistically significant differences in levels of anxiety and depression were found in the intervention group as compared with usual care. Significant differences were also noted for CBT interventions in reducing anxiety and depression in women with breast cancer who received six sessions focused on physical symptom reduction (fatigue and insomnia) and emotional distress spaced throughout the chemotherapy treatment period (Dirksen & Epstein). Similarly, an 8-week intervention in cardiac populations focused on emotional distress as part of a self-management program reported significant reductions in anxiety and depression in the short term in cardiac populations (Dougherty et al.). Significant decreases in anxiety and depression were also reported for women with advanced breast cancer who received a 12-week intervention that combined CBT and relaxation therapy approaches (Targ & Levine). Significantly lower general psychological distress was reported in women with irritable bowel syndrome who received an 8-week CBT intervention (Heitkemper et al.). A CBT intervention used to alter health risks in head and neck cancer patients observed a reduction in psychological distress at 6 months, but no differences were found between experimental and control groups, suggesting that the observed change may have been attributed to response shift (Duffy et al.).

Most of the trials reviewed for CBT interventions were adequately powered, and psychological distress was sensitive to this type of psychosocial nursing intervention. However, diversity across studies in the components of the CBT intervention make it difficult to recommend a specific combination, and it is not clear which component of the intervention was most active in contributing to the effectiveness of the intervention. Across diverse populations, CBT appeared to perform equally well in reducing psychological distress.

Psychoeducational Approaches

Extensive research has supported the evidence base for psychoeducational interventions as an effective approach for managing psychological distress (Fawzy et al., 1990; Fawzy & Fawzy, 1994; Fawzy, Fawzy, Arndt, & Pasnau, 1995; Fawzy et al., 1993; Rodgers et al., 2005). Psychoeducational interventions usually comprise four primary components—health education, stress management, coping skills, and psychological support (Fawzy et al., 1995)—delivered as a group or individualized approach. Interventions bordering between CBT and psychoeducational interventions make it difficult to differentiate between these interventions. However, CBT interventions usually place greater emphasis on cognitive reframing of illness and/or addressing faulty cognitions or beliefs about illness.

Eight RCTs (Allard, 2007; Badger et al., 2005; Cote & Pepler, 2002; Fillion et al., 2008; Gallagher, McKinley, & Dracup, 2003; Rabins et al., 2000; Strong et al., 2008; Wengstrom, Haggmark, Strander, & Forsberg, 1999) and two quasi-experimental studies (Cole et al., 2006; Gümüs & Cam, 2008) were identified as psychoeducational nursing interventions in the studies reviewed. Allard reported a significant reduction in general psychological distress when women were provided with education and active listening to enhance coping with primary breast cancer surgery initiated prior to and followed by telephone support in the initial days following surgery. In an intervention delivered to hospitalized HIV/AIDS population over a 3-day period, Cote and Pepler also reported a decrease in both anxiety and negative affect measured immediately postintervention. Both anxiety and depression were reduced for long-term care residents with mental health problems who received psychogeriatric assessment and weekly visits by a mental health nurse, and support by trained staff between sessions (Rabins et al., 2000). An intensive 3-month (10 session) psychoeducational nursing intervention that targeted a mixed population of cancer patients with major depressive disorder showed a reduction in depression and anxiety measured over a 12-month time frame (Strong et al.). Similarly, women with breast cancer undergoing radiation therapy who received 30-minute sessions based on a psychoeducational approach once a week for 5 weeks during treatment, followed by two sessions posttreatment, showed a reduction in subjective distress measured as a stress reaction (Wengstrom et al.). A 4-week group psychoeducational intervention for women post–breast cancer treatment combined with physical activity showed a reduction in general psychological distress at 3 months in the intervention group compared with the control, but not at earlier measurement time points (Fillion et al.). Significant nonparticipation rates were reported for this study, raising concerns about selection bias, and women may have been exposed to other interventions during this time frame. No significant differences were found between control and intervention groups in anxiety or depression when the intervention was provided as a telephone counseling intervention alone to cancer patients and their partners (Badger et al.), or for cardiac patients post–acute infarction who received telephone counseling over a 6-week period posthospitalization for heart disease (Gallagher et al., 2003). The interventions in both of these studies had a similar duration of 6 weeks, but it was less clear regarding the components of the intervention and if they were indeed psychoeducational or general support interventions delivered by telephone.

A population-based quasi-experimental study also reported a reduction in major depression in a significant proportion of the population with a double diagnosis of diabetes and depression (Cole et al., 2006). General psychological distress was also reduced over time in a quasi-experimental study (pre-post) that focused on intensive emotional support provided on an individual basis and combined with coping skill training for about an hour in seven sessions with women newly diagnosed with breast cancer (Gümüs & Cam, 2008).

Overall, it appears that psychological distress is sensitive to psychoeducational nursing interventions across differing population groups, but diversity in intervention approaches and the components emphasized make it difficult to determine what aspects of the intervention were most important in achieving the effect. Those with the strongest emphasis on all the components of psychoeducation as defined by Fawzy et al. (1995) and with at least six sessions appeared to be most beneficial. Similar to other interventions reviewed in this chapter, comparison of the intervention to a usual care control group may have introduced attention bias, and few researchers tracked patient exposure to other psychosocial resources.

Relaxation Therapy

Seven RCTs and one quasi-experimental study were identified that included various nurse-delivered forms of relaxation interventions as a method of reducing stress related to acute medical procedures or chronic conditions. These interventions were diverse in their components and included progressive muscle relaxation (Cheung, Molassiotis, & Chang, 2002), hypnosis (G. D. Smith, 2006), massage (Mok & Woo, 2004; Quattrin et al., 2006), imagery (Sloman, 2002; Twiss, Seaver, & McCaffrey, 2007), and music therapy (Hayes, Buffum, Lanier, Rodahl, & Sasso, 2003; Taylor-Piliae & Chair, 2002). A reduction in anxiety was observed in patients following a nurse-delivered music intervention given 15 minutes prior to gastrointestinal procedures (Hayes et al.), whereas a significant change in anxiety was not found when either music or sensory information was provided to patients undergoing cardiac procedures (Taylor-Piliae & Chair, 2002). Positive benefits, including reduced anxiety, were reported in elderly stroke patients with nurse-led massage therapy that elicited a relaxation response measured using standard physiological measures (Mok & Woo). Similarly, hospitalized cancer patients reported reduced anxiety when nurses administered reflexology foot massage for 30 minutes (Quattrin et al.). The use of progressive muscle relaxation in colon cancer patients (Cheung et al.) and in mixed-cancer populations with advanced disease, combined with imagery (Sloman), reduced symptoms of anxiety and/or depression. In a quasi-experiment with hypnotherapy combined with progressive muscle relaxation, symptoms of depression, but not anxiety, were reduced for an inflammatory bowel syndrome population (G. D. Smith, 2006). These mixed results suggest that the use of music may be condition specific and that the threat associated with treatment or procedures may preclude effectiveness of this type of relaxation approach in some populations unless the dose is adequate and monitored to ensure adherence to the intervention. Monitoring of the fidelity of the intervention or adherence was rarely reported across most of the intervention studies reviewed.

Structural Supportive Care Interventions/Models of Care

Two RCTs and two quasi-experimental studies were identified that focused on the delivery of psychosocial nursing interventions using a specific model of nursing care, such as nurse case management (Markle-Reid et al., 2006; McCusker et al., 2001; Palese, Comuzzi, & Bresadola, 2005), a liaison nurse (Chaboyer, Thalib, Acorn, & Foster, 2007), and nurse-led heart failure management (Martensson, Stromberg, Dahlstrom, Karlsson, & Fridlund, 2005). The effects of these interventions were found to be equivocal in reducing psychological distress, with results dependent on the type of intervention. In a quasi-experiment (pre-post), Chaboyer et al. found no effect on pretransfer anxiety when nurses coordinated the transfer from the intensive care unit to a medical ward and prepared both patients and families to reduce transfer-related anxiety. In contrast, nurse-led case management appears to be an effective approach to reducing psychological distress. Markle-Reid and colleagues had nurses follow elderly patients into the home based on a theoretical model of social support and vulnerability that included telephone follow-up over a 6-month period. A reduction in depressive symptoms and enhanced perceptions of social support were reported. McCusker and colleagues also reported a reduction in depressive symptoms when elderly patients received coordinated home care following discharge from the emergency department. Significant differences in anxiety between intervention and control were also reported for a nurse-case management model that emphasized psychological preparation of patients prior to general surgery (Palese et al.). Reduction in major depressive disorder was also found in a cluster population-based trial in primary care practices when interventions were targeted toward management of depression by nurses and physicians using interventions such as screening for distress and decision-support systems (Martensson et al.).

Structure of care interventions assumes an empirical link between the outcome and the structure or organization of care, with less attention paid to the underlying processes of care that are critical to achieving an effect. Consequently, given the mixed findings for these interventions on psychological distress and the lack of clarity regarding the processes of psychosocial interventions provided within these models of care, it is difficult to conclude that psychological distress is sensitive to this type of intervention. Further attention needs to be paid to measuring intervention processes in these models of care to determine their effectiveness and to facilitate replication in future studies.

Exercise

Physical activity or exercise interventions have been shown to have beneficial effects on reducing psychological distress such as depression in physical illness (Salmon, 2001). Three RCTs were reviewed that focused on nurse-delivered exercise interventions to reduce psychological distress across chronic conditions (Fitzsimmons, 2001; Meeks, Looney, Van Haitsma, & Teri, 2008; Midtgaard et al., 2005). A reduction in depression scores was reported in elderly nursing home residents trained in wheelchair biking when combined with group support, as compared with a usual care control group (Fitzsimmons et al., 2001). In a cohort comparison study, an intensive aerobic fitness program (9 hours weekly for 6 weeks) for women receiving chemotherapy demonstrated a significant reduction in both anxiety and depression, with improvements in depression most closely correlated with improvements in cardiovascular fitness (Midtgaard et al.). Similarly, a significant reduction in depressive symptoms was reported in a program targeted toward increasing physical activity and participation in positive events in elderly residents with mental health disorders (Meeks et al.). Psychological distress appears to be sensitive to nurse-led exercise intervention programs, but given the few studies identified with a primary outcome of psychological distress, a further review of studies that include distress as a secondary outcome is needed, which is beyond the scope of this review. In summary, this review has shown that psychological distress is sensitive to psychosocial nursing interventions, but diversity in the types of psychosocial interventions and the components comprising the intervention makes it difficult to make recommendations regarding any particular intervention elements. CBT and psychoeducational interventions were found to be most beneficial, which is consistent with systematic reviews in this area. It is less clear if nurse-led models of care or education alone are psychosocial interventions sensitive to reducing psychological distress. Small sample sizes, variable doses, sample selection procedures, randomization procedures, and monitoring of adherence and intervention fidelity need greater attention in future psychosocial nursing intervention research. In addition, advanced practice nurses or specialized nurses delivered many of the interventions in the studies reviewed, and further research is needed to determine the sensitivity of psychological distress to nursing psychosocial practice variables when delivered by nurses as part of routine practice.

ISSUES IN ASSESSMENT AND MEASUREMENT OF PSYCHOLOGICAL DISTRESS

Psychological distress often goes unrecognized in persons with chronic illness, with potentially detrimental consequences for patients and their families (Biji et al., 2003). Moreover, providers and patients frequently underestimate the seriousness of psychological distress comorbid with chronic illness, assuming that it is a natural reaction rather than a potentially serious condition (Passik et al., 1998). Even when patients do not meet criteria for a definitive clinical diagnosis of depression or anxiety disorder, they can experience milder forms of psychological distress, which might signal poor adjustment and the need for clinical intervention (de Ridder et al., 2008). A number of issues in the assessment and measurement of psychological distress are identified in the literature and summarized as follows:

1. Differentiating between transient and normal levels of psychological distress and affective states of depression and anxiety is critical to effective treatment. The threshold of symptoms required for a diagnosis of major depression in terms of psychiatric classification is arbitrary (Kendlar & Gardner, 1998; Sloan & Kring, 2007).

2. Psychological distress measured only as affective states of anxiety and depression is problematic because patients' definitions of distress may be qualitatively different from symptoms of anxiety and depression, interfering with assessment of milder forms of distress (Trask et al., 2002).

3. Measurement of only negative affective states such as depression and anxiety ignores the importance of positive affective states as measures of psychological adjustment to illness, such as feeling happy, cheerful, interested in life, and life satisfaction (Stewart, Ware, Sherbourne, & Willis, 1992; Ware & Sherbourne, 1992), or benefit finding, now shown to be an important indicator of adjustment in a number of chronic illnesses (Folkman & Greer, 2000; Mols et al., 2005).

4. Depression as an emotional state is not a neatly defined entity, with considerable overlap between depression and anxiety; individuals presenting with one of these problems usually also have the other as an associated condition (Goldberg & Huxley, 1992).

5. Symptoms of depression and/or anxiety, such as fatigue or changes in appetite, might be confused with illness and/or treatment symptoms. For instance, many of the symptoms of "sickness behavior" are similar to those of depression. Somatic symptoms may be assumed to be diagnostic of affective states of depression or anxiety and may not be taken into account in a number of standardized questionnaires (Hotopf et al., 2002; M. Watson, 2001).

6. Sensitivity and specificity of measures are variable, and the standard cut-off scores for identifying "cases" of serious psychological distress may overestimate rates of depression (Hotopf et al., 2002) and is a continuing area of disagreement (M. Watson, 2001). Rarely are clinically meaningful change scores established for measures of anxiety and depression or correlated with the extent of disruption in physical function or interruption in life activities (Given et al., 2008)

7. Gold standard measures for establishing a clinical diagnosis of depression and/or anxiety such as the Structured Clinical Interview for DSM (SCID) can be time consuming to complete and usually depend on resources such as psychologists or psychiatrists, who may not be accessible in some healthcare regions (e.g., rural or remote areas).

8. Identification of psychological distress is highly dependent on self-report, which can be subject to bias given that patients may be reluctant to report for fear of being stigmatized as mentally ill (Moussavi et al., 2007). Moreover, as noted by Moussavi and colleagues, the reporting of symptoms could vary because of cultural differences such as varying interpretations and translated meanings of words such as *distress* in different languages.

9. Screening and assessment for psychological distress are considered distinct processes (Zabora, 1998), with screening identified as a rapid method using brief self-report measures by the clinical team, and assessment involving in-depth clinical interviews by mental health professionals (APA, 2000).

INSTRUMENTS MEASURING PSYCHOLOGICAL DISTRESS

A number of systematic reviews have been conducted to identify instruments and their psychometric properties for the measurement of psychological distress. As many as 45 tools/instruments have been identified that are commonly used to measure psychological distress, with the most common being the Brief Symptom Inventory and the Hospital Anxiety and Depression Scale (Zigmond & Snaith, 1983). In a scoping review to identify outcome measures for measuring psychological distress outcomes in cancer, 15 measures commonly used in cancer patients were identified that were the most content valid, based on conceptual definitions of psychological distress, and psychometrically sound (Howell, Fitch, Bakker, Green, & Doran, 2009). Although a number of instruments exist for the measurement of psychological distress, their sensitivity to nursing care requires evaluation in nursing intervention studies. In this chapter, only those instruments that were used to measure psychological distress in the nursing intervention studies reviewed and their psychometric properties and sensitivity to nursing practice variables are discussed.

Fifteen instruments for the measurement of psychological distress were reviewed, and their characteristics and psychometric properties are summarized in **TABLE 7-2**. All but two of the studies included in this review used a structured, self-report instrument, and most researchers measured psychological distress as subjective symptoms of anxiety and/or depression. Two authors used only a visual analogue scale (VAS) (Cote & Pepler, 2002) and a numeric rating scale (NRS) (Palese et al., 2005) for measuring depression and anxiety. Measures of positive and negative affect or general psychological distress were used less frequently, and a number of researchers used more than one measure. Psychological adjustment was rarely measured, and none of the nursing intervention studies reviewed measured coping as a potential mediating variable of psychological distress. The sensitivity of psychological distress measures are described only for those measures most common in the reviewed studies as follows.

Anxiety

The most frequently used measure of anxiety in the nursing intervention studies reviewed was the STAI-S (state scale) of the State-Trait Anxiety Inventory (STAI) (Spielberger et al., 1983). The STAI is considered the gold standard for measuring anxiety in medical illness, and its reliability and validity are well documented. The items in this scale are consistent with conceptual definitions of anxiety described by Bay and Algese (1999). This scale was used in 12 of the nursing psychosocial intervention studies reviewed (Chaboyer et al., 2007; Cheung et al., 2002; Harkness et al., 2003; Hayes et al., 2003; Hoffman, 2009; Kim et al., 1999;

TABLE 7-2 Instruments Measuring a Psychosocial Outcome

Instrument (Author)	Target population/ practice setting	Domains (# of items and response format)	Method of administration	Reliability (internal consistency, test-retest, interrater)	Content validity	Construct and criterion validity	Evidence of sensitivity to nursing variables
COMBINATION ANXIETY AND DEPRESSION SCALES							
Hospital Anxiety and Depression Scale (Zigmond & Snaith, 1983) (Bjelland, Dahl, Haug, & Neckelmann, 2002; Johnston, Pollard, & Hennessey, 2000; Morrey, Greer, & Watson, 1991, as cited in McDowell, 2006; Morse, Kendell, & Barton, 2005; Skarstein, Aass, & Fossa, 2000, as cited in McDowell, 2006)	Screening instrument for anxiety and depression in hospital, psychiatric, and research settings. Used in various populations	Severity of anxiety and depression (14 items, two subscales; one subscale assesses anxiety, and one assesses depression; 4-point Likert-type scale from 0 to 3)	Self-administered	Internal consistency (coefficient α): Cronbach's α = .82–97 (HADS-A) and .79–90 (HADS-D) in cancer patients Test-retest: $r > .75$ (various time intervals)	HADS was developed based on the conceptual definitions of anxiety and depression.	Construct validity: Many studies reporting a two-factor model. Criterion validity: HADS correlated with clinician ratings ($r = .70$, HADS-D, and .74, HADS-A); with BDI ($r = .61$–.83 HADS-A; $r = .62$–.73 for HADS-D); with State-Trait Anxiety Inventory ($r = .64$–.81 HADS-A; $r = .52$–.65 HADS-D). Ratings distinguished between individuals classified with depression and those with anxiety.	Overall, nursing intervention studies show mixed results on sensitivity of the HADS to a detect change in nursing variables anxiety and depression. Several studies have detected changes in anxiety and depression, whereas others have indicated that changes in depression, as compared with anxiety, are not as consistent. Measurement points ranged from 2 weeks to 12 months.
Profile of Mood States (POMS) (Shacham, 1983) (Baker, Denniston, Zabora, Polland, & Dudley, 2002; Cella et al., 1987; Guadagnoli, & Mor, 1989; McDowell, 2006; McNair, Lorr, & Droppleman, 1971)	Used primarily with ill adult patients in clinical or research settings	Affective, cognitive, behavioral, or somatic (65-item adjective-rating instruments comprising 6 subscales: tension/anxiety; depression/dejection, anger/hostility, vigor-activity, fatigue-inertia, and confusion-bewilderment; items are rated on a 5-point Likert-type scale from 0 to 4)	Self-administered	Internal consistency (coefficient α): Cronbach's α = .84–95 (psychiatric patients) Test-retest: R = .65–.74 (approximately 20 days apart)	Developed based on a series of factor analytic studies, the scale represents the refinement of a total of 100 different adjective scales by means of repeated factor analyses.	Construct validity: Factor analysis has replicated the six-factor model across various samples of patients. Criterion validity: POMS correlated with the Hopkins Symptom Distress Scales, CES-D, Revised Symptom Checklist-90, and HADS ($r > .60$).	Overall, nursing intervention studies have shown that the POMS is sensitive to change in nursing variables such as emotional distress, general distress, and negative affective state (depression/dejection and anxiety/tension) at 1, 3, and 6 months. Several studies did not show a change in POMS scores, including short-term music interventions and center orientation programs.

(continues)

TABLE 7-2   Instruments Measuring a Psychosocial Outcome (continued)

Instrument (Author)	Target population/ practice setting	Domains (# of items and response format)	Method of administration	Reliability (internal consistency, test-retest, interrater)	Content validity	Construct and criterion validity	Evidence of sensitivity to nursing variables
Profile of Mood States-SF (Shacham, 1983) (Baker et al., 2002; Cella et al., 1987; Guadagnoli & Mor, 1989; McDowell, 2006; McNair et al., 1971)	POMS-SF developed and further validated in cancer patients with various tumor sites and across all phases	37 items rated on a 5-point Likert-type scale and the same 6 subscales as the full version (see previous)	Self-administered	Internal consistency (coefficient α): Cronbach's α = .78–.91	N/A	Construct validity: POMS-SF had a similar six-factor model as POMS. Criterion validity: POMS-SF correlated with POMS ($r = .95$) and the POMS Total Mood and Disturbance Scale ($r = .54–.88$); with the Bradburn positive and negative affect scales ($r = .48–.73$); and with the CES-D ($r = .63$); POMS-SF fatigue and vigor subscales correlated with the MOS-SF-20 ($r = -.42$ and .42, respectively) and Karnofsky Performance Score (KPS) score ($r = -.40$ and .39, respectively). POMS-SF scores discriminated between patients with CES-D scores < 16 and those with scores ≥ 16.	Overall, nursing intervention studies have shown that the POMS-SF is sensitive to change in nursing variables such as emotional distress at time points ranging from 1 week to 6 months.

ANXIETY SCALES

Beck Anxiety Inventory (Beck, Epstein, Brown, & Steer, 1988; Beck et al., 1997, as cited in McDowell, 2006) (Fydrich, Dowdall, & Chambless, 1992; Kabacoff, Segal, Hersen, & Van Hasselt, 1997; Osman et al., 1993, as cited in McDowell, 2006; Steer, Ranieri, Beck, & Clark, 1993)	Developed in healthy population but has been used across various chronically ill populations	Subjective, somatic, and behavioral symptoms of anxiety (21 items, two subscales; items are rated on a 4-point Likert-type scale from 0 to 3)	Self-administered or interviewer administered	Internal consistency (coefficient α): Cronbach's α = .70–.92 (for subscales) and .86–.94 (entire scale) Test-retest: *r* = .62–.83 (11 days to 7 weeks)	Content validity: BAI covers most of the DSM-III-R symptoms and 11 of 13 DSM symptoms of panic disorder. However, BAI does not include avoidant behaviors (one of the DSM criteria for social anxiety and phobias).	Construct validity: Several studies including various populations have replicated the original two-factor model. However, studies have also indicated three-, four-, and five-factor models. Criterion validity: BAI has correlated with STAI (*r* = .44–.68); with Hamilton Rating Scale for Anxiety (*r* = .47–.67); with Symptom Checklist-90 (*r* = .75–.81); and with Brief Symptom Inventory (*r* = .69–.78). Studies have indicated that BAI can discriminate among patients with mood, anxiety, and other types of psychiatric disorders.	Limited information is available. Several studies have shown that BAI is sensitive to change in anxiety in nursing interventions.

(continues)

TABLE 7-2 Instruments Measuring a Psychosocial Outcome (continued)

Instrument (Author)	Target population/ practice setting	Domains (# of items and response format)	Method of administration	Reliability (internal consistency, test-retest, interrater)	Content validity	Construct and criterion validity	Evidence of sensitivity to nursing variables
State-Trait Anxiety Inventory (Spielberger et al., 1983) (Okun et al., 1996, as cited in McDowell, 2006; van Knippenberg et al., 1990, as cited in McDowell, 2006)	Various populations (healthy, ill, and chronically ill)	State anxiety (temporary condition for specific situations; STAI-S) and trait anxiety (a tendency to perceive certain situations in a specific way; STAI-T) (20-item measure comprising the STAI-S and STAI-T subscales; items are rated on a 4-point scale from 1 to 4)	Self-administered	Internal consistency (coefficient α): Cronbach's α = .83–.95 (STAI-S) and α = .67–.92 (STAI-T) Test-retest: Several studies have noted a higher stability of the STAI-T (r = .73–.86) as compared with STAI-S (r = .16–.76).	Content validity: According to the DSM-IV, the STAI covers five of the eight domains for generalized anxiety disorder.	Construct validity: Several factor models have been detected, from two to four factors. The correlation between the two subscales appears to be high (r = .70–.80). Criterion validity: STAI correlated with BAI (r = .44–.68); with an anxiety diary (r = .34–.53); and with Depression Anxiety Stress Scale (r = .34–.55). STAI scores discriminated between individuals under stress (expected to have higher anxiety) and those under less stress or not in stressful situations, and between patients with phobias and those with general anxiety disorders.	Most nursing interventions assess state anxiety as compared with trait. Nursing intervention studies show that the STAI's ability to detect change in nursing variables is inconclusive. Several studies indicate that no changes were detected as a result of interventions (measurement point raged from 1 to 6 months). It appears that STAI is able to detect change in anxiety within shorter time frames (1 day to 3 months).
Zung Self-Rating Anxiety Scale (Zung, 1971, 1974, 1980) (McDowell, 2006)	Healthy and ill populations	Affective and physiological symptoms of anxiety (20 items; items are rated on a 4-point scale from 1 to 4)	Clinician and self-administered version available	Internal consistency (coefficient α): Cronbach's α = .61–.85 Split-half reliability = .71	ZSAS based on the conceptual definition of anxiety, with attention paid to distinguishing anxiety from depression.	Criterion validity: Correlation between self-rated version and the clinician ratings was moderate to high, r = .66–.74	Few nursing intervention studies currently use the ZSAS to evaluate anxiety. Results suggest that the ZSAS is not sensitive to change in anxiety scores.

Instrument	Purpose	Description	Administration	Reliability	Content validity	Construct/Criterion validity	Comments	Clinical utility
Hamilton Anxiety Rating Scale (Hamilton, 1960) (Bech, Kastrup, & Rafaelson, 1986; Bech, Stanley, & Zebb, 1999; Beck & Steer, 1991; Beneke, 1987; Clark & Donovan, 1994; Maier et al., 1988, as cited in McDowell, 2006)	Designed for use with patients already diagnosed with an anxiety neurosis	Presence and severity of psychic and somatic anxiety symptoms (13 categories of anxiety and rating of patient's behavior at the interview by clinician; 5-point Likert-type rating scale, 0–4)	Clinician administered	Internal consistency (coefficient α): Cronbach's α = .85–.92 Test-retest: r = .64 (stability after 1 year) to .96 (shorter periods of time) Interrater: r = .74–.93 (ratings between clinicians)	Content selected on the basis of clinician experience.	Construct validity: Factor analysis across several studies has supported a two-factor structure. Criterion validity: Hamilton anxiety (HARS) and depression scales correlated highly (r = .68–.92); HARS correlated with BAI (r = .53); with a global clinician rating of anxiety (r = .75); and with STAI (r = .23–.58). Responsiveness to change was found to be higher for the psychic items as compared with the somatic items.	SAS correlations with the Taylor Manifest Anxiety Scale ranged from .30 to .62, and with the HADS, r = .56–.81. Unable to discriminate between depression and anxiety. However, individual items have been shown to discriminate between individuals with a clinical diagnosis of anxiety and those without.	Few nursing intervention studies currently use the HARS to evaluate anxiety. Limited studies indicate that the HARS was able to detect changes in anxiety as a result of nursing interventions. Measurement time points assessed ranged from 6 to 12 months postintervention.

(continues)

TABLE 7-2   Instruments Measuring a Psychosocial Outcome (continued)

Instrument (Author)	Target population/ practice setting	Domains (# of items and response format)	Method of admin- istration	Reliability (internal consistency, test- retest, interrater)	Content validity	Construct and criterion validity	Evidence of sensitivity to nursing variables
DEPRESSION SCALES							
Beck Depression Inventory (Beck & Beck, 1972; Beck, Steer, et al., 1988; Beck, Ward, Mendelson, Mock, & Erbaugh, 1961) (Allen, Newman, & Souhami, 1997; Berard, Boermeester, & Viljoen, 1998; Dzois, Dobson, & Ahnberg, 1998; Edwards et al., 1984, as cited in McDowell, 2006; Yin & Fan, 2000)	Developed, validated, and used in various populations including healthy individuals, chronically ill patients, and psychiatric patients Often used as a community screening tool and for clinical research	Behavioral, somatic, and cognitive domains of depression (21 items; items are rated on a 4-point Likert-type scale from 0 to 3)	Self-administered or interviewer administered	Internal consistency (coefficient α): Cronbach's α = .76–95 (psychiatric populations) and α = .73–.92 (nonpsychiatric populations) Test-retest: r = .48–.86 (psychiatric patients); r = .60–.83 (nonpsychiatric populations) (various time intervals) for BDI	Content validity: BDI contains six of the nine DSM-III criteria for depression.	Construct validity: Several studies have identified a single factor structure. Criterion validity: The most current version, BDI-II, correlated with the BDI-I (r = .93 and kappa agreement = .70). BDI correlated with clinician ratings, r = .55–.96 (psychiatric patients) and r = .55–.73 (nonpsychiatric patients); with the Hamilton Rating Scale Depression, r = .61–.86; with the ZSDS, r = .71–.76; and with the Geriatric Depression Scale, r = .78–.85. Discriminated between groups with contrasted levels of depression.	Sensitivity to change

				Internal consistency (coefficient α)	Content/Construct validity	Criterion validity	
Beck Depression Inventory-SF (Beck & Beck, 1972; Beck, Epstein, et al., 1988; Beck et al., 1961) (Allen et al., 1997; Berard et al., 1998; Dzois et al., 1998; Edwards et al., 1984, as cited in McDowell, 2006; Yin & Fan, 2000)	Developed, validated, and used in various populations, including healthy individuals, chronically ill patients, and psychiatric patients; often used as a community screening tool and for clinical research	Behavioral, somatic, and cognitive domains of depression (13 items; items are rated on a 4-point Likert-type scale from 0 to 3)	Self-administered or interviewer administered	Internal consistency (coefficient α): Cronbach's $\alpha = .59–.84$	Based on the full version of BDI.	Criterion validity: BDI-SF correlated highly with the long form ($r = .89–.97$) and moderately with clinician ratings ($r = .55–.67$).	N/A
Center for Epidemiologic Studies Depression Scale (Radloff, 1977) (Carpenter et al., 1998; Devins et al., 1988; Hann, Winter, & Jacobsen, 1999; Okun et al., 1996, as cited in McDowell, 2006; Schrovers et al., 1996, as cited in McDowell, 2006; Stommel et al., 1993)	Developed to identify depression in the general population; has been used extensively across various settings and various age and sociodemographic groups	Frequency of depressive symptoms, including negative affect/mood; positive mood/well-being; somatic; and interpersonal (20 items, four subscales; items are rated on a 4-point Likert-type scale from 0 to 3)	Self-administered	Internal consistency (coefficient α): Cronbach's $\alpha > .85$ for various samples of patients. Test-retest: In cancer patients, $r > .50$ (2.5 weeks apart) Interrater: $r = .76$ between versions administered by a nurse and a research assistant	Content validity: CES-D covers seven of the nine DSM-IV criteria for depression.	Construct validity: Four-factor model has been replicated across several populations. Criterion validity: CES-D correlated with clinician rating of depression, $r = .56$; the Hamilton Rating Scale for Depression ($r = .44–.69$); with the depression categorization of the DSM-III ($r = .77$); with the STAI-S ($r = .77$); with the SF-36 mental health subscale ($r = -.65$); with Bradburn's Affect Balance Scale ($r = .61–.77$); and with Symptom Checklist-90 ($r = .72–.87$). In various populations, CES-D discriminated between populations with and without depression.	Overall, the findings indicate that the CES-D is able to detect changes in depression scores as a result of nursing interventions. Measurement time frame ranged from 1 to 6 months.

(continues)

TABLE 7-2   Instruments Measuring a Psychosocial Outcome (continued)

Instrument (Author)	Target population/ practice setting	Domains (# of items and response format)	Method of administration	Reliability (internal consistency, test-retest, interrater)	Content validity	Construct and criterion validity	Evidence of sensitivity to nursing variables
Center for Epidemiologic Studies-Depression Scale–SF (Radloff, 1977) (Carpenter et al., 1998; Devins et al., 1988; Hann et al., 1999; Okun et al., 1996, as cited in McDowell, 2006; Schrovers et al., 1996, as cited in McDowell, 2006; Strommel et al., 1993)	Developed to identify depression in the general population, the elderly, and clinical populations	Frequency of depressive symptoms, including negative affect/ mood; positive mood/well-being; somatic; and interpersonal (15-item and 11-item version available; items are rated on a 4-point Likert-type scale from 0 to 3)	Self-administered	Internal consistency (coefficient α): Cronbach's α > .83 (15 items) and > .68 (11 items)	Based on the CES-D.	Construct validity: CES-D-SF (13 items) has also replicated the four-factor model. Criterion validity: The short form correlates highly with the long form (r = .88–.93).	Limited information is available on the sensitivity of the CES-D-SF because it is rarely used in nursing intervention studies to evaluate depression.
Zung Self-Rating Depression Scale (Zung, 1965) (Biggs, Wylie, & Ziegler, 1978; Dugan et al., 1998; Hwang, Chang, & Kasimis, 2003; McDowell, 2006; Hwang et al., 2003; Lambert et al., 1986, as cited in McDowell, 2006; McKegney et al., 1988, as cited in McDowell, 2006; Moran et al., 1983, as cited in McDowell, 2006; Passik et al., 2000, 2001; Schotte et al., 1996, as cited in McDowell, 2006)	Often used in clinical studies to monitor changes following treatment, a screening instrument on family practice, and cross-cultural studies	Frequency of symptoms of depression, including self-judgment, decreased vital sense, anhedonia, diurnal variation of mood, neurovegetative features, and duration of symptoms (20 items; items are rated on a 4-point Likert-type scale from 1 to 4)	Self-administered	Internal consistency (coefficient α): Cronbach's α .47–.85 Test-retest: R = .61 (1 year apart in elderly populations)	Review of instruments indicated that SDS covers five of the DSM-III criteria well, covers four partially, and overlooks one variable.	Construct validity: A 3-factor model has been identified in most studies. Criterion validity: ZSDS correlated with clinician (r = .38–.80) and psychiatrist (r = .20–.69) ratings of depression; with BDI (r = .60–.83); and with the several other depression scales (r = .55–.70). ZSDS correlated weakly with ECOG scores (r = .17–.30).	Limited information is available on the sensitivity of the ZSDS to nursing variables. Few nursing intervention studies currently use this scale to evaluate depression. One study reported a significant change in depression scores after an education nursing intervention at 3 and 12 months postintervention.

Brief Zung Self-Rating Depression Scale (Zung, 1965) (Biggs et al., 1978; Dugan et al., 1998; Hwang et al., 2003; Lambert et al., 1986, as cited in McDowell, 2006; McKegney et al., 1988, as cited in McDowell, 2006; Moran et al., 1983, as cited in McDowell, 2006; Passik et al., 2000, 2001; Schotte et al., 1996, as cited in McDowell, 2006)	Frequency of symptoms of depression (omits nine items concerning somatic symptoms; 11 items; items are rated on a 4-point Likert-type scale from 1 to 4)	Self-administered	Internal consistency (coefficient α): Cronbach's $\alpha = .84$	Based on the full version of the ZSDS.	Earlier studies suggested that ZSDS can discriminate among patients with depression, anxiety, psychiatric conditions, and controls. Recent meta-analysis argues that it can discriminate well. Criterion validity: Brief ZSDS significantly correlated with the ZSDS ($r = .88$–$.92$) and the Mini International Neuropsychiatric Interview (MINI; $r = -.57$).	N/A

(continues)

TABLE 7-2　Instruments Measuring a Psychosocial Outcome (continued)

Instrument (Author)	Target population/ practice setting	Domains (# of items and response format)	Method of administration	Reliability (internal consistency, test-retest, interrater)	Content validity	Construct and criterion validity	Evidence of sensitivity to nursing variables
Geriatric Depression Scale (Weiss et al., 1986; Yesavage et al., 1983) (Agrell & Dehlin, 1989; Birk et al., 1982, as cited in McDowell, 2006; Feher, Larrabee, & Crook, 1992; Koening et al., 1988, as cited in McDowell, 2006; Lesher, 1989; Lyons et al., 1989, as cited in McDowell, 2006; Rule, Harvey, & Dobbs, 1986; L. C. Watson, Lewis, Kistler, Amick, & Boustani, 2004; Weiss et al., 1986)	Developed and extensively used as a screening test for depression in the elderly; intended for use in clinical applications and in an office setting	Positive and negative affective domains of depression (30 items, dichotomous yes/no scale)	Self-administered or interviewer administered	Internal consistency (coefficient α): Cronbach's α = .80–.94 Split-half reliability = .94 Test-retest: R = .86 (1 hour), r = .85 (1 week), and r = .98 (10–12 days) Interrater: r = .85 (long-term care facility residents)	Developed from a pool; items specifically directed to detect depression in the elderly. These items were chosen by clinicians and researchers. GDS contains more items characteristic of depression in elderly patients than other scales, but, as with other scales, GDS still does not meet all the DSM-III criteria.	Criterion validity: GDS correlated with the Hamilton Rating Scale for Depression (r = .58–.82); with the BDI (r = .85); with ZSDS (r = .82); and with CES-D (r = .82). Agreement between GDS and structured psychiatric interview (kappa = .62). GDS discriminated significantly between depressed and non-depressed cognitively impaired patients. Various cut-off points suggested, with 10/11 most commonly used (sensitivity = 84–92% and specificity = 67–95%). Scores on GDS unrelated to social desirability.	GDS is a commonly used scale to detect depression in the elderly. Several studies indicate that GDS was able to detect a change in depression scores after various nursing interventions. Because of the population of interest, the GDS-SF is more commonly used in nursing interventions than the full version.

Instrument	Purpose	Description	Administration	Reliability	Content	Validity	Comments
Geriatric Depression Scale-Short-Form (Weiss et al., 1986; Yesavage et al., 1983) (Agrell & Dehlin, 1989; Birk et al., 1982, as cited in McDowell, 2006; Feher et al., 1992; Koeing et al., as cited in McDowell, 2006; Lesher, 1989; Lyons et al., 1989, as cited in McDowell, 2006; Rule et al., 1986; L. C. Watson et al., 2004)	Developed and extensively used as a screening test for depression in the elderly; intended for use in clinical applications and in an office setting	Positive and negative affective domains of depression (15 items, dichotomous yes/no scale)	Self-administered or interviewer administered	N/A	N/A	Criterion validity: GDS-SF correlated highly with the GDS ($r = .66–.89$). Compared with the CES-D, GDS-SF was equally sensitive to identifying major depression and superior in identifying minor depression.	Overall, the studies indicate that the GDS-SF is sensitive to detecting change in depression in the elderly after various nursing interventions. Several studies reported a nonsignificant difference in depression scores after a cognitive-behavioral intervention in the experimental group detected at 6 months follow-up. One study reported a significant difference in depression scores of a behavioral intervention.
Hamilton Rating Scale for Depression (Hamilton, 1960, 1967) (Bech et al., 1986; Hammond, 1998; Hedlund & Vieweg, 1979; McDowell, 2006; Onega & Abraham, 1997; Raskin, 1986, as cited in McDowell, 2006; Reynolds & Kobak, 2004)	Intended to be used as a research tool to quantify severity of depression in patients already diagnosed with depression	Severity of depression in those diagnosed with depression; focus on somatic symptoms (21 items; 3-point and 5-point Likert-type scales)	Clinician administered	Internal consistency (coefficient α): Cronbach's $\alpha = .48–.95$ in various populations. Interrater: $r = .70–.98$. Test-retest: $r = .69$ (5-item version) –.72 (original version)	Includes four of eight melancholia symptoms in DSM-III, omits nonreactivity of mood, reduction of concentration, and anhedonia. Neglects cognitive and affective symptoms with focus on somatic symptoms.	Construct validity: Number of factors ranges from 3 to 7. Criterion validity: HRSD correlated with clinician ratings of severity ($r = .67$); with the Raskin scale for Depression ($r = .65–.81$); with the Montgomery-Asberg Depression Rating scale ($r = .71$); with the BDI ($r .21–.82$); and with the ZSDS ($r = .22–.95$). In several review studies, HRSD provided the largest consistent index of change as compared with BDI and ZSDS.	Limited information is available on the sensitivity of the HRS to nursing variables because few studies currently use it to detect depression. One study showed a significant change in depression scores after an exercise intervention, but the study sample was too small to draw conclusions.

Mok & Woo, 2004; Palese et al., 2005; Rawl et al., 2002; Taylor-Piliae & Chair, 2002; Williams & Schreier, 2004). All but three of these studies found sensitivity to psychosocial nursing interventions in reducing anxiety based on this measure. Based on this evidence, the STAI-S is supported as being sensitive to nursing practice variables.

The Beck Anxiety Inventory was also found to be sensitive to nursing practice variables in two studies (Erci et al., 2009; Hartford et al., 2002), but definitive conclusions about its sensitivity cannot be made given the small number of studies that used this as an outcome measure of psychological distress. Two authors used a unidimensional scale for depression and anxiety, including a VAS (Cote & Pepler, 2002) and a NAS (Palese et al., 2005). Single scales are considered adequate only for screening patients as a red flag indicator of psychological distress that should be followed by a more comprehensive assessment using a valid and reliable instrument (Howell, Currie et al., 2009). Unidimensional scales may be particularly sensitive to social desirability report bias and widespread diversity in interpretation because patients may find it difficult to assign a specific number to psychological symptoms. In addition, clinically meaningful changes scores have not been established for a number of these scales, with the exception of the well-established distress thermometer (Jacobsen et al., 2005) embedded in the NCCN guidelines (2008).

Depression

The CES-D (Radloff, 1977) was the most commonly used measure for assessing the effect of nursing psychosocial interventions on depression as an outcome in three of the nursing intervention studies. The CES-D is considered to be a more sensitive measure of depression in medically ill populations because it excludes somatic symptoms that are similar to those associated with subjective symptoms of depression. Of the studies employing the CES-D, three reported improvement in depression as compared with a control group (Markle-Reid et al., 2006; Rawl et al., 2002; Sherwood et al., 2005), whereas a change in depression scores was not observed in other studies (Badger et al., 2005; Dougherty et al., 2004). Those studies that did not show a change in depression were telephone-counseling interventions in cancer (Badger et al.) and post–acute myocardial infarction (Dougherty et al.), which might be attributed to intervention or study design. Anxiety measured on the STAI was sensitive to change in the Dougherty et al. study, suggesting that sensitivity to change in depression on this outcome measure requires a more targeted and intense intervention approach or should include CBT or psychoeducation.

The Geriatric Depression Scale (Weiss, Nagel, & Aaronson, 1986) was used in four of the intervention studies (Duffy et al., 2006; Fitzsimmons, 2001; McCusker et al., 2001; Meeks et al., 2008), given the focus in these studies on an older population. However, a change in depression was noted in only one (Meeks et al.) of the four studies using this measure. Subsequently, the sensitivity of this measure to psychosocial nursing practice variables is unclear, and further attention might need to be paid to the sensitivity of age-specific outcome measures. Other measures of depression were also used including the Zung Self-Rating Depression Scale (Martensson et al., 2005) and a recently disease-specific measure of psychological distress for diabetes (P. Davidson et al., 2008). However, these were single studies precluding definitive conclusions about their sensitivity to psychosocial nursing practice variables.

Anxiety and Depression

Six of the nursing intervention studies reviewed used the Hospital Anxiety and Depression Scale (Zigmond & Snaith, 1983) to measure psychological distress as subjective symptoms of anxiety and depression (Ambler et al., 1999; Arving et al., 2007; Cole et al., 2006; Midtgaard et al., 2005; Sloman, 2002; J. R. Smith et al., 2005). The Hospital Anxiety and Depression Scale is widely used across medically ill populations because of its brevity, its sensitivity in detecting "caseness" for depression, and its classification of depression as mild, moderate, or severe (Zigmond & Snaith). Of the studies employing HADS, the majority reported a change in anxiety alone (Ambler et al.; J. R. Smith et al., 2005), depression and anxiety (Midtgaard et al., 2005), or depression alone (Cole et al.; Sloman). These findings are similar to negative findings for depression measured with the CES-D suggesting that when patients are still experiencing the stressor, a more intensive and targeted intervention approach may be necessary for a longer intervention period. Moreover, the inflammatory biological processes contributing to the development of psychological distress during active treatment in cancer and cardiac disease may render depression refractory to psychosocial intervention unless a combination of pharmacological and nonpharmacological intervention approaches is applied.

General Psychological Distress

Five studies used a more general measure of affective mood, the Profile of Mood States (POMS) (Shacham, 1983). The POMS is commonly used in medically ill populations and measures affective mood states including anger, depression, and tension/anxiety, as well as feelings of vigor, bewilderment, and confusion. The POMS appeared to be sensitive to psychosocial nursing care interventions in four of the five studies that used this as an outcome measure of general psychological distress (Allard, 2007; Dirksen et al., 2008; Fillion et al., 2008; Targ & Levine, 2002). A change in distress was not detected in a population of Chinese patients who received a music intervention prior to a cardiac procedure (Taylor-Piliae &

Chair, 2002), but this intervention appeared inadequate, and adherence was not monitored. This finding might be explained by cultural differences in the endorsement of psychological symptoms or the weakness of the intervention design. Less common measures of psychological distress, such as the Symptom Checklist (Heitkemper et al., 2004) and the Mental Health Inventory (Strong et al., 2008), were also used. However, given the small numbers of studies using these instruments, confidence in their sensitivity to nursing interventions is low.

The Positive and Negative Affect Scale (PANAS) was another general measure of psychological distress used in four of the nursing intervention studies (Antoni et al., 2006; Badger et al., 2005; Cote & Pepler, 2002; Kim et al., 1999). Positive affect increased over time in a study of telephone interpersonal counseling in both the control and intervention group, suggesting response shift rather than sensitivity of the instrument (Badger et al.). No affect was shown in a study focused on strengthening patients' cognitive coping skills (Cote & Pepler), whereas a reduction in negative affect was shown in a quasi-experimental study of educational support (Kim et al.). Given these results and the small numbers of studies that used the PANAS as a measure of psychological adjustment, it is difficult to conclude that this measure is sensitive to psychosocial nursing practice variables.

Psychological Adjustment

Psychological adjustment was used as a measure of psychological distress in only two of the nursing intervention studies (Gallagher et al., 2003; Gümüs & Cam, 2008). Similar to many of the other studies reviewed, mixed findings were found, with no effect observed in one study (Gallagher et al., 2003), whereas a reduction in psychological distress was seen in the second study (Gümüs & Cam, 2008). A definitive conclusion regarding the sensitivity of psychological adjustment measures to psychosocial nursing practice variables is difficult given the limited number of studies that used this outcome.

In summary, a number of psychometrically sound measures that are in common use across medically ill populations in both clinical practice and research such as the HADS and STAI were supported as sensitive to psychosocial nursing practice variables in this review. The Profile of Mood States was also shown to be sensitive to nursing practice variables and is well validated for use in research. There is a wealth of instruments for measuring psychological distress, but further research is required to establish clinically meaningful change scores for these as outcome measures and to determine if statistically significant reductions are associated with improvements in health and other aspects of psychological functioning and health. Further research is needed to assess the feasibility of using these measures in routine clinical practice.

CONCLUSIONS AND RECOMMENDATIONS FOR FUTURE PRACTICE AND RESEARCH

Psychological distress is a normal response when individuals are faced with systemic physical illness, especially if the illness is chronic in nature and disrupts multiple dimensions of daily living such as employment, future goals, and aspirations. However, if individuals are unable to negotiate the multiple tasks associated with chronic illness as part of psychological adjustment, they may develop concomitant psychological distress. Psychological distress is a serious comorbid condition of chronic illness that is often underrecognized and undertreated. It has potentially devastating consequences for patients and families in terms of the clinical course of illness, survival outcomes, and overall health related quality of life. The nursing studies reviewed in this chapter support emerging consensus that psychological distress is a nurse-sensitive outcome, particularly when nursing interventions are sufficiently targeted, are comprised of an adequate dose and intensity, and include approaches with known efficacy. The main points that emerged from this review that examined the sensitivity of psychological distress to psychosocial nursing interventions are as follows:

1. Psychological distress is a common response to physical illness, especially chronic illnesses that demand ongoing adjustment in multiple life domains, requiring early and sustained psychosocial intervention approaches to minimize the development of major depression and other adjustment or anxiety disorders.

2. Psychological distress has detrimental consequences for patients in terms of a more difficult clinical course marked with higher complications, recurrent disease, and exacerbations, possibly contributing to higher mortality and health costs.

3. Screening for psychological distress is becoming an expected part of routine clinical practice and a standard for quality performance in a number of healthcare organizations given its prevalence in populations with systemic and chronic illness.

4. Empirical evidence reviewed for nurse-delivered psychosocial nursing interventions provides support for psychosocial distress as a nurse-sensitive outcome when interventions are appropriately targeted and include support combined with education, or when intervention components include CBT or psychoeducational approaches.

5. Structure of care interventions such as nurse-led case management models show some effect on psychological distress, but further attention to psychosocial care processes is necessary given that an empirical link between structure and outcome cannot be assumed.

6. A wealth of psychological distress outcome measures are available to nurses that can reliably and validly measure this construct, and a number of these appear to be sensitive to psychosocial nursing interventions and feasible for use in clinical practice.

7. Education interventions alone appear to be ineffective unless combined with a supportive component of an adequate dose and intensity, but these findings might be explained by significant heterogeneity in study design and intervention processes.

8. Greater attention needs to be focused on study rigor, including better reporting of study design, characteristics of the intervention, monitoring for intervention fidelity, potential effects of confounders such as use of other services, randomization procedures and their quality as well as sample recruitment and justification of sample size.

9. A theoretical framework supporting how the intervention should work and justification for intervention dose was lacking across a number of studies, and, if present, the causal relationship between constructs in the model and the intervention target was not clear.

10. Psychological adjustment, and the subsequent development of distress, is influenced by a number of variables; some can be altered or should be taken into account as covariates in sample selection procedures.

11. Further research is needed to establish clinically meaningful significant difference for psychological distress measures, and feasibility testing of these measures for use in routine clinical practice is needed.

In conclusion, much of the responsibility for the assessment and management of psychological distress across care settings and disease populations will fall to frontline clinical staff, particularly nurses. Nurses have an important role to play in the assessment of psychological distress by being attentive to visual and verbal cues of psychological distress, using valid and reliable measures to screen for distress, and engaging patients using interpersonal communication skills to open a dialogue with patients (and their families) to assess contributing factors, explore patient and family concerns, and understand their experience of living with and adjusting to illness. Nurses can incorporate screening for distress, followed by a more comprehensive assessment of distress, in routine clinical practice using the many valid and reliable outcome measures available and appropriately target psychosocial interventions relevant to patients' concerns and needs (Howell, Currie et al., 2009). Nurses play a significant role as advocates for routine screening and assessment of psychological distress in healthcare organizations and in ensuring that scores on distress measures inform interdisciplinary care planning. Nurses also have a potential role in minimizing the adverse effects of psychological distress by intervening early in the illness trajectory and applying evidence-based psychosocial interventions known to be sensitive in reducing distress as an integral component of clinical nursing practice. Further, nurse administrators must ensure that nurses are adequately prepared in the assessment of psychological distress and in applying evidence-based psychosocial interventions as part of routine supportive care. Psychosocial care is an essential component of nursing practice, and psychological distress is considered a nurse-sensitive outcome. Finally, further refinement of psychosocial nursing interventions to manage psychological distress is critical to clinical practice and future nursing research.

REFERENCES

Abelhoff, M. D., Armitage, J. O., Lichter, A. S. & Neiderhuber, J. E. (2000). *Clinical oncology* (2nd ed.). New York: Churchill Livingstone.

Accreditation Canada. (2009). *Qmentum Program 2009 standards: Cancer care and oncology services 2008* (Version 2). Ottawa, Ontario, Canada: Canadian Health Services Accreditation.

Agrell, B., & Dehlin, O. (1989). Comparison of six depression rating scales in geriatric stroke patients. *Stroke, 20,* 1190–1194.

Allard, N. C. (2007). Day surgery for breast cancer: Effects of a psychoeducational telephone intervention on functional status and emotional distress. *Oncology Nursing Forum, 34,* 133–141.

Allen, R., Newman, S. P., & Souhami, R. L. (1997). Anxiety and depression in adolescent cancer: Findings in patients and parents at the time of diagnosis. *European Journal of Cancer Care, 33,* 1250–1255.

Ambler, N., Rumsey, N., Harcourt, D., Khan, F., Cawthorn, S., & Barker, J. (1999). Specialist nurse counsellor interventions at the time of diagnosis of breast cancer: Comparing "advocacy" with a conventional approach. *Journal of Advanced Nursing, 29,* 445–453.

American Psychiatric Association. (2000). *Diagnostic and statistical manual of mental disorders* (4th ed., text revision). Washington, DC: Author.

Anderson, R. J., Freedland, K. E., Clouse, R. E., & Lustman, P. J. (2001). The prevalence of comorbid depression in adults with diabetes: A meta-analysis. *Diabetes Care, 24,* 169–1078.

Andrews, G., & Slade, T. (2001). Interpreting scores on the Kessler Psychological Distress Scale (K10). *Australian and New Zealand Journal of Public Health, 25,* 494–497.

Andrykowski, M. A. A., Bishop, M. M., Hahn, E. A., Cella, D. E., Beaumont, J. L., Brady, M. J., et al. (2005). Long-term health-related quality of life, growth, and spiritual well-being after hematopoietic stem-cell transplantation. *Journal of Clinical Oncology, 23,* 599–568.

Antoni, M. H., Lehman, J. M., Kilbourn, K. M., Boyers, A. E., Culver, J. L., Alferi, S. M., et al. (2001). Cognitive-behavioral stress management intervention decreases the prevalence of depression and enhances benefit finding among young women under treatment for early-stage breast cancer. *Health Psychology 20*(6), 2–32.

Antoni, M. H., Wimberly, S. R., Lechner, S. C., Kazi, A., Sifre, T., Urcuyo, K. R., et al. (2006). Reduction of cancer-specific thought intrusions and anxiety symptoms with a stress management intervention among women undergoing treatment for breast cancer. *American Journal of Psychiatry, 163,* 1791–1797.

Arnold, E. (1999). Communicating with clients in stressful situations. In E. Arnold & K. U. Boggs (Eds.), *Interpersonal relationships: Professional communication skills by nurses* (pp. 445–475). Toronto, Ontario, Canada: W. B. Saunders.

Arving, C., Sjoden, P. O., Bergh, J., Hellbom, M., Johansson, B., Glimelius, B., et al. (2007). Individual psychosocial support for breast cancer patients: A randomized study of nurse versus psychologist interventions and standard care. *Cancer Nursing, 30,* E10–E19.

Badger, T., Segrin, C., Meek, P., Lopez, A. M., Bonham, E., & Sieger, A. (2005). Telephone interpersonal counseling with women with breast cancer: Symptom management and quality of life. *Oncology Nursing Forum, 32,* 273–279.

Baker, F., Denniston, M., Zabora, J., Polland, A., & Dudley, W. N. (2002). A POMS short form for cancer patients: Psychometric and structural evaluation. *Psycho-Oncology, 11*, 273–281.

Balderson, N., & Towell, T. (2003). The prevalence and predictors of psychological distress in men with prostate cancer who are seeking support. *British Journal of Health Psychology, 8*, 125–134.

Ballenger, J. C., Davidson, J. R. T., Lecrubier, Y., Nutt, D. J., Jones, R. D., & Berard, R. M. (2001). Consensus statement on depression, anxiety, and oncology. *Journal of Clinical Psychiatry, 62*(Suppl. 8), 64–67.

Bandura A. (1997). *Self-efficacy: The exercise of control.* New York: Freeman.

Barsevick, A. M., Sweeney, C., Haney, E., & Chung, E. (2002). A systematic qualitative analysis of psycho-educational interventions for depression in patients with cancer. *Oncology Nursing Forum, 29*, 73–84.

Bay, E. J., & Algese, D. L. (1999). Fear and anxiety: A simultaneous concept analysis. *Nursing Diagnosis, 10*(3), 103–111.

Bech, P., Kastrup, M., & Rafaelson, O. J. (1986). Mini-compendium of rating scales for states of anxiety, depression, mania, schizophrenia with corresponding DSM-III syndromes. *Acta Psychiatrica Scandinavica, 73* (Suppl. 326), 1–37.

Bech, J. G., Stanley, M. A., & Zebb, B. J. (1999). Effectiveness of the Hamilton Anxiety Rating Scale with older generalized anxiety patients. *Journal of Clinical Geropsychology, 5*, 281–290.

Beck, A. T., & Beck, R. W. (1972). Screening depressed patients in family practice: A rapid technique. *Postgraduate Medicine, 52*, 81–85.

Beck, A. T., Epstein, N., Brown, G., & Steer, R. A. (1988). An inventory for measuring clinical anxiety: Psychometric properties. *Journal of Consulting and Clinical Psychology, 56*, 893–897.

Beck, A. T., & Steer, R. A. (1991). Relationship between the Beck Anxiety Inventory and the Hamilton Anxiety Rating Scale with anxious outpatients. *Journal of Anxiety Disorders, 5*, 213–223.

Beck, A. T., Steer, R. A., & Garbin, M. G. (1988). Psychometric properties of the Beck Depression Inventory: Twenty-five years of evaluation. *Clinical Psychology Review, 8*, 77–100.

Beck, A. T., Ward, C. H., Mendelson, M., Mock, J., & Erbaugh, J. (1961). An inventory for measuring depression. *Archives of General Psychiatry, 4*, 561–571.

Beneke, M. (1987). Methodological investigations of the Hamilton Anxiety Rating Scale. *Pharmacopsychiatry, 20*, 249–255.

Bennett, S. J., Perkins, K. A., Lane, K. A., Deer, M., Brater, D. C., & Murray, M. D. (2001). Social support and health-related quality of life in chronic heart failure patients. *Quality of Life Research, 10*, 671–682.

Berard, R. M. F., Boermeester, F., & Viljoen, G. (1998). Depressive disorders in an out-patient oncology setting: Prevalence, assessment, and management. *Psycho-Oncology, 7*, 117–120.

Biggs, J. T, Wylie, L. T., & Ziegler, V. E. (1978). Validity of the Zung Self-Rating Depression Scale. *British Journal of Psychiatry, 132*, 381–385.

Biji, R. V., de Graaf, R., Hiripi, E., Kessler, R. C., Kohn, R., Offord, D. R., et al. (2003). The prevalence of treated and untreated mental disorders in five countries. *Health Affairs, 22*(3), 122–133.

Bisschop, M. I., Kriegsman, D. M. W., Beekman, A. T. F., & Deeg, D. J. (2000). Chronic diseases and depression: The modifying role of psychosocial resources. *Social Science and Medicine, 59*, 721–733.

Bjelland, I., Dahl, A. A., Haug, T. T., & Neckelmann, D. (2002). The validity of the Anxiety and Depression Scale: An updated literature review. *Journal of Psychosomatic Research, 52*, 69–77.

Blalock, S. J., DeVellis, B. M., Holt, K., & Hahn, P. M. (1993). Coping with rheumatoid arthritis: Is one problem the same as the another? *Health Education Quarterly, 21*, 119–32.

Blumenthal, J. A., Lett, H. S., Babyak, M. A., White, W., Smith, P. K., et al. (2003). Depression as a risk factor for mortality after coronary artery bypass surgery. *Lancet, 362*, 604–609.

Bottomley, A. (1998). Depression in cancer patients: A literature review. *European Journal of Cancer Care, 7*, 181–191.

Bower, J. E., Meyerowitz, B. E., Desmond, K. A., Bernaards, C. A., Rowland, J. H., & Ganz, P. (2005). Perceptions of positive meaning and vulnerability following breast cancer: Predictors and outcomes among long-term breast cancer survivors. *Annals of Behavioral Medicine, 29*, 236–245.

Brennan, J. (2001). Adjustment in cancer-coping or personal transition? *Psycho-Oncology, 10*(1), 1–18.

Broadhead, W. E., Kaplan, B. H., Jones, S. A., Wagner, E. H., Schoenbach, V. J., Grimson, R., et al. (1983). The epidemiological evidence for a relationship between social support and health. *American Journal of Epidemiology, 117*, 521–537.

Brownlee, S., Leventhal, H., & Leventhal, E. (2000). Regulation, self-regulation, and construction of the self in the maintenance of physical health. In M. Boekaerts & P. Pintrich (Eds.), *Handbook of self-regulation* (pp. 369–416). London: Academic.

Bultz, B. D., & Carlson, L. E. (2005). Emotional distress as the sixth vital sign in cancer. *Journal of Clinical Oncology, 23*, 6440–6441.

Burnette, D., & Mui, A. (1994). Determinants of self-reported depressive symptoms by frail elderly persons living alone. *Journal of Gerontological Social Work, 22*(1–2), 3–18.

Bush, B. F., Zeigelstein, R. C., Tayback, M., Richter, D., Stevens, S., Zahalsky, H., et al. (2001). Even minimal symptoms of depression increase mortality risk after acute myocardial infarction. *American Journal of Cardiology, 88*, 337–341.

Campbell, H. S., Phaneuf, M., & Deanne, K. (2004). Cancer peer support programs—do they work? *Patient Education and Counseling, 55*, 3–15.

Carpenter, J. S., Andrykowski, M. A., Wilson, J., Hall, L., Rayens, M. K., Sachs, B., et al. (1998). Psychometrics for two short forms of the Center for Epidemiologic Studies–Depression Scale. *Issues in Mental Health Nursing, 19*, 481–494.

Carver, C. S., Scheier, M. F., & Weintraub, J. K. (1989). Assessing coping strategies: A theoretically based approach. *Journal of Personality and Social Psychology, 56*, 267–283.

Carver, C. S., Smith, R. G., Antoni, M. H., Petronis, V. M., Weiss, S., & Derhagopian, R. P. (2005). Optimistic personality and psychosocial well-being during treatment predict psychosocial well-being among long-term survivors of breast cancer. *Health Psychology, 24*, 508–516.

Cella, D. F., Jacobsen, P. B., Orav, E. J., Holland, J. C., Silberfarb, P. M., & Rafla, S. (1987). A brief POMS measure of distress for cancer patients. *Journal of Chronic Diseases, 40*, 939–942.

Chaboyer, W., Thalib, L., Alcorn, K., & Foster, M. (2007). The effect of an ICU liaison nurse on patients and family's anxiety prior to transfer to the ward: An intervention study. *Intensive and Critical Care Nursing, 23*, 362–369.

Cheung, Y. L., Molassiotis, A., & Chang, A. M. (2002). The effect of progressive muscle relaxation training on anxiety and quality of life after stoma surgery in colorectal cancer patients. *Psycho-Oncology, 12*, 254–266.

Ciechanowski, P. S., Katon, W. J., & Russo, J. E. (2000). Depression and diabetes: Impact of depressive symptoms on adherence, function, and costs. *Archives of Internal Medicine, 160*, 3278–3285.

Clark, D. B., & Donovan, J. E. (1994). Reliability and validity of the Hamilton Anxiety Rating Scale in an adolescent sample. *Journal of the American Academy of Child and Adolescent Psychiatry, 33*, 354–360.

Cobb, S. (1976). Social support as a moderator of life stress. *Psychosomatic Medicine, 38*, 300–314.

Cole, S. A., Farber, N. C., Weiner, J. S., Sulfaro, M., Katzelnick, D. J., & Blader, J. C. (2006). Double-disease management or one care manager for two chronic conditions: Pilot feasibility study of nurse telephonic disease management for depression and congestive heart failure. *Disease Management, 9*, 266–276.

Conn, V. S., Rantz, M. J., Wipke-Tevis, D. D., & Maas, M. L. (2001). Designing effective nursing interventions. *Research in Nursing and Health, 24*, 433–442.

Cordova, M. J., Cunningham, L. L., Carlson, C. R., & Andrykowski, M. A. (2001). Posttraumatic growth following breast cancer: A controlled comparison study. *Health Psychology, 20*, 176–185.

Cote, J. K., & Pepler, C. (2002). A randomized trial of a cognitive coping intervention for acutely ill HIV-positive men. *Nursing Research, 51*, 237–244.

Covic, T., Adamson, B., Spencer, D., & Howe, G. (2003). A biopsychosocial model of pain and depression in rheumatoid arthritis: A 12-month longitudinal study. *Rheumatology, 42*, 1287–1294.

Covinsky, K. E., Kahana, E., Chin, M. H., Palmer, R. M., Fortinsky, R. H., & Landefield, C. S. (1999). Depressive symptoms and nine-year survival of 1001 male veterans hospitalized with medical illness. *Annals of Internal Medicine, 130*, 563–569.

Crogan, N. L., Evans, B. C., & Bendel, R. (2008). Storytelling intervention for patients with cancer: Part 2—pilot testing. *Oncology Nursing Forum, 35*, 265–272.

Currie, S. R., & Wang, J. (2004). Chronic back pain and major depression in the general Canadian population. *Pain, 107*(1–2), 54–60.

Danoff-Burg, S., & Revenson, T. A. (2005). Benefit-finding among patients with rheumatoid arthritis: Positive effects on interpersonal relationships. *Journal of Behavioral Medicine, 28*, 91–103.

Davidson, P., Digiacomo, M., Zecchin, R., Clarke, M., Paul, G., Lamb, K., et al. (2008). A cardiac rehabilitation program to improve psychosocial outcomes of women with heart disease. *Journal of Women's Health, 17*, 123–136.

Davidson, R. J., Jackson, D. C., & Kalin, N. H. (2000). Emotion, plasticity, context, and regulation: Perspectives from affective neuroscience. *Psychology Bulletin, 126*, 890–909.

Demange, V., Guillemin, F., Bauman, M., Suurmeiher, B. M., Moum, T., Doeglas, D., et al. (2004). Are there more than cross-sectional relationships of social support and social networks with functional limitations and psychological distress in early rheumatoid arthritis? *Arthritis Rheumatology, 51*, 782–791.

de Ridder, D., Geenen, R., Kuijer, R., & Middendorp, H. V. (2008). Psychological adjustment to chronic disease. *Lancet, 372*, 246–255.

Deshler, A. M., Fee-Schroeder, K. C., Dowdy, J. L., Mettler, T. A., Novotny, P., Zhao, X., et al. (2006). A patient orientation program at a comprehensive cancer center. *Oncology Nursing Forum, 33*, 569–578.

Devins, G. M., & Binik, Y. M. (1996). Facilitating coping with chronic physical illness. In M. Zeidner & N. S. Endler (Eds.), *Handbook of coping: Theory, research, and application* (pp. 640–696). New York: Wiley.

Devins, G. M., Orme, C. M., Costello, C. G., Binik, Y. M., Frizzell, B., Stam, H. J., et al. (1988). Measuring depressive symptoms in illness populations: Psychometric properties of the Center for Epidemiologic Studies Depression (CES-D) Scale. *Psychology and Health, 2*, 139–156.

Dew, M. A., Simmons, R. G., Roth, L. H., Schulberg, H. C., Thompson, M. E., Armitage, J. M., et al. (1994). Psychosocial predictors of vulnerability to distress in the year following heart transplantation. *Psychological Medicine, 35*, 1215–1227.

Dietrich, A. J., Oxman, T. E., Williams, J. W. Schulberg, H. C., Bruce, M. I., Lee, P. W., et al. (2004). Re-engineering systems for the treatment of depression in primary care: Cluster randomized trial. *British Medical Journal, 329*(7466), 602–608.

Dimatteo, M. R., Lepper, H. S., & Croghan, T. W. (2000). Depression as a risk factor for non-compliance with medical treatment: Meta-analysis of the effects of anxiety and depression on patient adherence. *Archives of Internal Medicine, 60*, 2101–2107.

Dirksen, S. R., & Epstein, D. R. (2008). Efficacy of an insomnia intervention on fatigue, mood, and quality of life in breast cancer survivors. *Journal of Advanced Nursing, 61*, 664–675.

Donovan H. S., & Ward, S. (2005). Representations of fatigue in women receiving chemotherapy for gynecological cancers. *Oncology Nursing Forum, 32*, 113–116.

Dougherty, C. M., Lewis, F. M., Thompson, E. A., Baer, J. D., & Kim, W. (2004). Short-term efficacy of a telephone intervention by expert nurses after an implantable cardioverter defibrillator. *Pacing and Clinical Electrophysiology, 27*, 1594–1602.

Duffy, S. A., Ronis, D. L., Valenstein, M., Lambert, M. T., Fowler, K. E., Gregory, L., et al. (2006). A tailored smoking, alcohol, and depression intervention in head and neck cancer patients. *Cancer Epidemiology, Biomarkers and Prevention, 15*, 2203–2208.

Dugan, W., McDonald, M. V., Passik, S. D., Rosenfeld, B. D., Theobald, D., & Edgerton, S. (1998). Use of the Zung Self-Rating Depression Scale in cancer patients: Feasibility as a screening tool. *Psycho-Oncology, 7*, 483–493.

Dzois, D. J. A., Dobson, K. S., & Ahnberg, J. L. (1998). A psychometric evaluation of the Beck Depression Inventory-II. *Psychological Assessment, 10*, 83–89.

Ekselius, L., Lindstrom, E., von Knorring, L., Bodlund, O., & Kullgren, G. (1994). SCID II interviews and the SCID Screen questionnaire as diagnostic tools for personality disorders in DSM-III-R. *Acta Psychiatrica Scandinavica, 90*, 120–123.

Engel, G. L. (1977). The need for a new medical model: A challenge for biomedicine. *Science, 196*, 129–136.

Erci, B., Sezgin, S., & Kacmaz, Z. (2009). The impact of therapeutic relationship on preoperative and postoperative patient anxiety. *Australian Journal of Advanced Nursing, 26*, 59–66.

Fawzy, F. I., Cousins, N., Fawzy, N. W., Kemeny, M. E. Elashoff, R., & Morton, D. L. (1990). A structured psychiatric intervention for cancer patients: II. Changes over time in immunological measures. *Archives of General Psychiatry, 47*, 729–735.

Fawzy, F. I., & Fawzy, N.W. (1994). A structured psychoeducational intervention for cancer patients (manual). *General Hospital Psychiatry, 16*, 149–192.

Fawzy, F. I., Fawzy, N. W., Arndt, L., & Pasnau, R. (1995). Critical review of psychosocial interventions in cancer care. *Archives of General Psychiatry, 52*, 100–113.

Fawzy, F. I., Fawzy, N. W., Hyun, C., Elashoff, R., Guthrie, D., Fahey, J. L., et al. (1993). Malignant melanoma: Effects of an early structured psychiatric intervention, coping, and affective state on recurrence and survival. *Archives of General Psychiatry, 47*, 720–725.

Feher, E. P., Larrabee, G. J., & Crook, T. H. (1992). Factors attenuating the validity of the Geriatric Depression Scale in a dementia population. *Journal of the American Geriatric Society, 40*(9), 906–909.

Fekete, E. M., Antoni, M. H., & Schneiderman, N. (2007). Psychosocial and behavioral interventions for chronic medical conditions. *Current Opinion in Psychiatry, 20*, 152–157.

Fillion, L., Gagnon, P., Leblond, F., Gelinas, C., Savard, J., Dupuis, R., et al. (2008). A brief intervention for fatigue management in breast cancer survivors. *Cancer Nursing, 31*, 145–159.

Fitch, M., Page, B., & Porter, H. (Eds.). (2008). *Supportive care in cancer.* Pembroke, Ontario, Canada: Pappin Communications.

Fitzsimmons, S. (2001). Easy rider wheelchair biking. A nursing-recreation therapy clinical trial for the treatment of depression. *Journal of Gerontological Nursing, 27*, 14–23.

Folkman, S., & Greer, S. (2000). Promoting psychological well-being in the face of serious illness: When theory, research and practice inform each other. *Psycho-Oncology, 9*, 11–19.

Folkman, S., & Lazarus, R. S. (1980). An analysis of coping in a middle-aged community sample. *Journal of Health and Social Behavior, 210*, 219–239.

Folkman, S., Lazarus, R. S., Dunkel-Schetter, C., De Longis, A., & Gruen, R. (1986). The dynamics of a stressful encounter: Cognitive-appraisal coping and encounter outcomes. *Journal of Personality and Social Psychology, 50*, 992–1013.

Folkman, S., & Moskowitz, J. T. (2000). Positive affect and the other side of coping. *American Psychologist, 55*, 647–654.

Fortin, M., Bravo, G., Hudon, C., Lapointe, L., Dubois, M-F., & Almiral, J. (2006). Psychological distress and multimorbidity in primary care. *Annals of Family Medicine, 4*, 417–422.

Fulcher, C. D., Badger, T., Gunter, A. K., Marrs, J. A., & Reese, J. M. (2008). Putting evidence into practice: Interventions for depression. *Clinical Journal of Oncology Nursing, 12*, 131–141.

Fydrich, T., Dowdall, D., & Chambless, D. L. (1992). Reliability and validity of the Beck Anxiety Inventory. *Journal of Anxiety Disorders, 6*, 55–61.

Gallagher, E., McKinley, S., & Dracup, K. (2003). Effects of a telephone counseling intervention on psychosocial adjustment in women following a cardiac event. *Heart and Lung, 32*, 79–87.

Garssen, B., & Goodkin, K. (1999). On the role of immunological factors as mediators between psychosocial factors and cancer progression. *Psychiatry Research, 85*, 51–61.

Given, B., Given, C. W., Sikorski, A., Jeon, S., McCorkle, R., Champion, V., et al. (2008). Establishing mild, moderate, and severe scores for cancer-related symptoms: How consistent and clinically meaningful are interference-based severity cut-points? *Journal of Pain and Symptom Management, 35*, 126–135.

Given, B. A., & Sherwood, P. R. (2005). Nurse sensitive patient outcomes: A white paper. *Oncology Nursing Forum, 32*, 773–784.

Goldberg D., & Huxley, P. (1992). *Common mental disorders: A biopsychosocial approach.* London: Routledge.

Gonzalez, V. M., Goeppinger, J., & Lorig, K. (1990). Four psychosocial theories and their application to patient education and clinical practice. *Arthritis Care and Research, 3*, 132–142.

Gordon, M. (1994). *Nursing diagnosis: Process and application.* St. Louis, MO: Mosby.

Greenhaus, J. H., & Parasuraman, S. (1994). Work-family conflict, social support, and well-being. In M. J. Davidson & R. J. Burke (Eds.), *Women in management: Current research issues* (pp. 213–229). London: Paul Chapman.

Greer, S. (1991). Psychological response to cancer and survival. *Psychological Medicine, 21*, 43–49.

Guadagnoli, E., & Mor, V. (1989). Measuring cancer patients' affect: Revision and psychometric properties of the Profile of Mood States. *Journal of Consulting and Clinical Psychology, 84*, 907–915.

Gümüs, A. B., & Cam, A. (2008). Effects of emotional support-focused nursing interventions on the psychosocial adjustment of breast cancer patients. *Asian Pacific Journal of Cancer Prevention, 9*, 691–697.

Hack, T. F., & Degner, L. F. (2004). Coping responses following breast cancer diagnosis predict psychological adjustment three years later. *Psycho-Oncology, 13*, 235–247.

Haggar, M., & Orbell, S. (2003). A meta-analytic review of the common-sense model of illness representations. *Psychology and Health, 18*, 141–184.

Hamer, M., Chida, Y., & Malloy, G. (2009). Psychosocial distress and cancer mortality. *Journal of Psychosomatic Research, 66*, 255–258.

Hamilton, M. A. (1960). A rating scale for depression. *Journal of Neurology, Neurosurgery and Psychiatry, 23*, 56–62.

Hamilton, M. (1967). Development of a rating scale for primary depressive illness. *British Journal of Social and Clinical Psychology, 6,* 278–296.

Hammond, M. F. (1998). Rating depression severity in the elderly physically ill patient: Hamilton and the Montgomery-Asberg depression rating scale. *International Journal of Geriatric Psychiatry, 13,* 257–261.

Hann, D., Winter, K., & Jacobsen, P. (1999). Measurement of depression in cancer patients: Evaluation of the Center for Epidemiological Studies Depression Scale (CES-D). *Journal of Psychosomatic Research, 46,* 437–443.

Harkness, K., Morrow, L., Smith, K., Kiczula, M., & Arthur, H. M. (2003). The effect of early education on patient anxiety while waiting for elective cardiac catheterization. *European Journal of Cardiovascular Nursing, 2,* 113–121.

Hartford, K., Wong, C., & Zakaria, D. (2002). Randomized controlled trial of a telephone intervention by nurses to provide information and support to patients and their partners after elective coronary artery bypass graft surgery: Effects of anxiety. *Heart and Lung, 31,* 199–206.

Harvey, S. B., & Ismail, K. (2008). Psychiatric aspects of chronic physical disease. *Lancet, 372,* 471–474.

Hayes, A., Buffum, M., Lanier, E., Rodahl, E., & Sasso, C. (2003). A music intervention to reduce anxiety prior to gastrointestinal procedures. *Gastroenterology Nursing, 26,* 145–149.

Hedlund, J. L., & Vieweg, B. W. (1979). The Hamilton Rating Scale for Depression: A comprehensive review. *Journal of Operational Psychiatry, 10,* 149–165.

Heitkemper, M. M., Jarrett, M. E., Levy, R. L., Cain, K. C., Burr, R. L., Feld, A., et al. (2004). Self-management for women with irritable bowel syndrome. *Clinical Gastroenterology and Hepatology, 2,* 585–596.

Helgeson, V. S., Cohen, S., Schulz, R., & Yasko, J. (2000). Effects of psychosocial treatment in prolonging cancer: Who benefits from what? *Annals of the New York Academy of Science, 840,* 674–683.

Helgeson, V. S., Snyder, P., & Seltman, H. (2004). Psychological and physical adjustment to breast cancer over 4 years: Identifying distinct trajectories of change. *Health Psychology, 23,* 3–15.

Hoff, A. C., & Haaga, D. A. (2005). Effects of an education program on radiation oncology patients and families. *Journal of Psychosocial Oncology, 23,* 61–75.

Hoffman, K. E. (2009). Cancer survivors at increased risk of psychological distress. *Archives of Internal Medicine, 169,* 1274–1281.

Hotopf, M., Chidgey, J., Addington-Hall, J., & Ly, K. L. (2002). Advanced disease: A systematic review Part 1. Prevalence and case finding. *Palliative Medicine, 16,* 81–97.

Howell, D., Currie, S., Mayo, S., Jones, G., Boyle, M., Hack, T., et al. (2009). *A Pan-Canadian clinical practice guideline: Assessment of psychosocial health care needs of the adult cancer patient.* Toronto, Ontario, Canada: Canadian Partnership Against Cancer (Cancer Journey Action Group) and the Canadian Association of Psychosocial Oncology.

Howell, D., Fitch, M., Bakker, D., Green, E., & Doran, D. (2009). *Patient-centered outcomes in cancer care.* Toronto, Ontario, Canada: Report to Canadian Institute of Health Research.

Howland, J. C., & Rowland, J. H. (1998). *Handbook of psychooncology* (2nd ed.). New York: Oxford University Press.

Hwang, S. S., Chang, V. T., & Kasimis, B. S. (2003). A comparison of three fatigue measures in veterans with cancer. *Cancer Investigation, 21,* 363–373.

Hymovich, D. P., & Hagopian, G. A. (1992). *Chronic illness in children and adults: A psychosocial approach.* Philadelphia: W. B. Saunders.

Institute of Medicine. (2001). *Crossing the quality chasm: A new health care system for the 21st century.* Washington, DC: National Academy Press.

Institute of Medicine. (2008). *Cancer care for the whole patient: Meeting psychosocial health needs* (N. E. Adler & Ann E. K. Page, Eds.). Washington, DC: National Academies Press.

Jacobsen, P. B., Donovan, K. A., Trask, P. C., Fleishman, S. B., Zabora, J., Baker, F., et al. (2005). Screening for psychological distress in ambulatory cancer patients. *Cancer, 103,* 1494–1502.

Janoff-Bulman, R. (1989). Assumptive worlds and the stress of traumatic events: Applications of the schema construct. *Social Cognition, 7*(2), 113–136.

Johnston, M., Pollard, B., & Hennessey, P. (2000). Construct validation of the Hospital Anxiety and Depression Scale with clinical populations. *Journal of Psychosomatic Research, 48,* 579–584.

Kabacoff, R. I., Segal, D. L., Hersen, M., & Van Hasselt, V. B. (1997). Psychometric properties and diagnostic utility of the Beck Anxiety Inventory and the State-Trait Anxiety Inventory with older adult psychiatric outpatients. *Journal of Anxiety Disorders, 11,* 33–47.

Katon, W. A., Rutter, C., & Simon, C. (2005). The association of comorbid depression with mortality in patients with type 2 diabetes. *Diabetes Care, 28,* 2668–2672.

Keller, M. B., McCullough, J. P., Klein, D. N., Arnow, B., Dunner, D. L., Gelenberg, A. J., et al. (2000). A comparison of nefazodone, the cognitive-behavioral analysis system of psychotherapy, and their combination for the treatment of chronic depression. *New England Journal of Medicine, 342*(20), 1462–1470.

Kendlar, K. S., & Gardner, C. O. (1998). Boundaries of major depression: An evaluation of DSM-II criteria. *American Journal of Psychiatry, 55,* 172–177.

Kim, H., Garvin, B. J., & Moser, D. K. (1999). Stress during mechanical ventilation: Benefit of having concrete objective information before cardiac surgery. *American Journal of Critical Care, 8,* 118–126.

Kissane, D. W., Grabsch, B., Love, A., Clarke, D. M., Block, S., & Smith, G. (2004). Psychiatric disorder in women with early stage and advanced breast cancer: A comparative analysis. *Australian and New Zealand Journal of Psychiatry, 38,* 320–326.

Koopmans, G. T., & Lamers, L. M. (2007). Gender and health care utilization: The role of mental distress and help-seeking propensity. *Social Science and Medicine, 64,* 1216–1230.

Lambert, S. D., & Loiselle, C. G. (2007). Health information seeking behavior: A concept analysis. *Qualitative Health Research, 17,* 1006–1019.

Lazarus, R. S., & Folkman, S. (1984). *Stress, appraisal and coping.* New York: Springer.

Lehmand, S. W., & Rabins, P. V. (1999). Clinical geropsychiatry. In J. J. Gallo, J. Busby-Whitehead, P. V. Rabins, R. A. Silliman, & J. B. Murphy (Eds.), *Reichel's care of the elderly: Clinical aspects of aging* (pp. 179–189). Philadelphia: Lippincott Williams and Wilkins.

Lesher, E. L. (1989). Validation of the Geriatric Depression Scale among nursing home residents. *Clinical Gerontology, 9,* 37–43.

Leventhal, H., & Deifenbach, M. (1991). The active side of illness cognition. In J. A. Skeleton & K. Croyle (Eds.), *Mental representation in health and illness* (pp. 247–272). New York: Springer-Verlag.

Leventhal, H., Nerenz, D. R., & Steele D. J. (1984). Illness representations, and coping with health threats. In A. Baum, S. E. Taylor, & J. E. Singer (Eds.), *Handbook of psychology and health: Vol. 4. Social psychological aspects of health* (pp. 219–252). Hillsdale, NJ: Erlbaum.

Lin, L. Y., & Wang, R. H. (2005). Abdominal surgery, pain and anxiety: Preoperative nursing intervention. *Journal of Advanced Nursing, 51,* 252–260.

Lorig, K. R., Sobel, D. S., Ritter, P. L., Laurent, D., & Hobbs, M. (2001). Effect of a self-management program on patients with chronic disease. *Effective Clinical Practice, 4,* 256–262.

Markle-Reid, M., Weir, R., Browne, G., Roberts, J., Gafni, A., & Henderson, S. (2006). Health promotion for frail older home care clients. *Journal of Advanced Nursing, 54*, 381–395.

Marmot, M. (2003). Social resources and health. In F. Kessel, P. L. Rosenfeld, & N. B. Anderson (Eds.), *Expanding the boundaries of health and social science* (pp. 259–285). New York: Oxford University Press.

Martensson, J., Stromberg, A., Dahlstrom, U., Karlsson, J. E., & Fridlund, B. (2005). Patients with heart failure in primary health care: Effects of a nurse-led intervention on health-related quality of life and depression. *European Journal of Heart Failure, 7*, 393–403.

Mathers, C. D., & Loncar, D. (2006). Projections of global mortality and burden of disease from 2002 to 2030. *PLoS Medicine, 3, e442. Retrieved from http://dx.doi.org/10.1371%2Fjournal. pmed.0030442*

McCloskey, J., & Bulechek, G. (1996). *NIC: Nursing Intervention Classification System.* St. Louis, MO: Mosby.

McCusker, J., Verdon, J., Tousignant, P., de Courval, L. P., Dendukuri, N., & Belzile, E. (2001). Rapid emergency department intervention for older people reduces risk of functional decline: Results of a multicenter randomized trial. *Journal of the American Geriatrics Society, 49*, 1272–1281.

McDowell, I. (2006). *Measuring health: A guide to rating scales and questionnaires* (3rd ed.). New York: Oxford University Press.

McNair D. M., Lorr, M., & Droppleman, L. F. (1971). *EITS manual for the Profile of Mood States.* San Diego, CA: Educational and Industrial Testing Service.

McVeigh, K. H., Mostashari, F., & Thorpe, L. E. (2004). Serious psychological distress among persons with diabetes—New York City, 2003. *Morbidity and Mortality Weekly Report, 53*, 1089–1092.

Meeks, S., Looney, S. W., Van Haitsma, K., & Teri, L. (2008). BE-ACTIV: A staff-assisted behavioral intervention for depression in nursing homes. *The Gerontologist, 48*, 105–114.

Meijer, S., Sinnema, G., Bijstra, J., Mellenbergh, G., & Wolters, W. (2002). Coping styles and locus of control as predictors of psychological adjustment for adolescents with a chronic illness. *Social Science and Medicine, 54*, 1453–1461.

Meyer, T. J., & Mark, M. M. (1995). Effects of psychological interventions for cancer patients. *Health Psychology, 14*(2), 101–108.

Meyerowitz, B. F., Formenti, S. C., Ell, K. O., & Leedham, B. (2000). Depression among Latina cervical cancer patients. *Journal of Social Clinical Psychology, 19*, 352–371.

Michael, Y. L., Berkman, L. F., Colditz, G. A., Holmes, M. D., & Kawachi, I. (2002) Social networks and health-related quality of life in breast cancer survivors: A prospective study. *Journal of Psychosomatic Research, 52*, 285–293.

Midtgaard, J., Rorth, M., Stelter, R., Tveteras, A., Andersen, C., Quist, M., et al. (2005). The impact of a multidimensional exercise program on self-reported anxiety and depression in cancer patients undergoing chemotherapy: A phase II study. *Palliative and Supportive Care, 3*, 197–208.

Mok, E., & Woo, C. P. (2004). The effects of slow-stroke back massage on anxiety and shoulder pain in elderly stroke patients. *Complementary Therapies in Nursing and Midwifery, 10*, 209–216.

Mols, F., Vingerhoets, A. J., Coebergh, J. W., & van de Poll-Franse, L. V. (2005). Quality of life among long term breast cancer survivors: A systematic review. *European Journal of Cancer, 41*, 2613–2619.

Morse, R., Kendell, K., & Barton, S. (2005). Screening for depression in people with cancer: The accuracy of the Anxiety and Depression Scale. *Clinical Effectiveness in Nursing, 9*, 188–196.

Moser, D. K., Chung, M. L., McKinley, S., Reigel, B., An, K., Cherrington, C. C., et al. . (2003). Critical care nursing practice regarding patient anxiety assessment and management. *Intensive and Critical Care Nursing, 19*, 276–288.

Moser, D. K., & Dracup, K. (1996). Is anxiety after myocardial infarction associated with subsequent arrhythmic events? *Psychosomatic Medicine, 58*, 395–401.

Moser, D. K., McKinley, S., Reigel, B., Doering, L. V., & Garvin, B. (2002). Perceived control reduces in-hospital complications associated with anxiety in acute myocardial infarction. *Circulation, 106*, II-369.

Moussavi, S., Chatterji, S., Verdes, E., Tandon, A., Patel, V., & Ustun, B. (2007). Depression, chronic diseases, and decrements in health: Results from the World Health Surveys. *Lancet, 370*, 851–858.

National Comprehensive Cancer Network. (2008). *NCCN clinical practice guidelines in oncology: Distress management.* Retrieved May 30, 2009, from http://www.nccn.org/professionals/physician_gls/f_guidelines.asp#supportive

Nolen-Hoeksema, S., Larson, J., & Grayson, J. (1999). Explaining the gender differences in depressive symptoms. *Journal of Personality and Social Psychology, 77*, 1061–1072.

Northouse, L. L., Mood, D., Templen, T., Mellon, S., & George, T. (2000). Couples' patterns of adjustment to colon cancer. *Social Science and Medicine, 50*, 271–284.

Onega, L. L., & Abraham, I. L. (1997). Factor structure of the Hamilton Rating Scale for Depression in a cohort of community-dwelling elderly. *International Journal Geriatric Psychiatry, 12*, 760–764.

Pakenham, K. I. (2005). Benefit finding in multiple sclerosis and associations with positive and negative outcomes. *Health Psychology, 24*, 123–132.

Palese, A., Comuzzi, C., & Bresadola, V. (2005). The "nurse case manager" model applied to day surgery in Italy. *Lippincott's Case Management, 10*, 83–92.

Park, C., & Folkman, C. (1997). Meaning in the context of stress and coping. *Review of General Psychology, 1*, 115–144.

Passik, S. D., Dugan, W., McDonald, M. V., Rosenfeld, B., Theobald, D. E., & Edgerton, S. (1998). Oncologists' recognition of depression in their patients with cancer. *Journal of Clinical Oncology, 164*, 1594–1600.

Passik, S. D., Kirsch, K. L., Donaghy, K. B., Theobald, D. E., Lundberg, J. C., Holtsclaw, E., et al. (2001). An attempt to employ the Zung Self Rating Depression Scale as a "lab test" to trigger follow-up in ambulatory oncology clinics: Criterion validity and detection. *Journal of Pain and Symptom Management, 21*, 273–281.

Passik, S. D., Lundberg, J. C., Rosenfeld, B., Kirsch, K. L., Donaghy, K., Theobald, D., et al. (2000). Factor analysis of the Zung Self-Rating Depression Scale in a large ambulatory oncology sample. *Psychosomatics, 41*, 121–127.

Patten, S. B., Beck, C. A., Williams, J. V. A., Barbul, C., & Metz, L. M. (2003). Major depression in multiple sclerosis: A population-based study. *Neurology, 61*, 1524–1527.

Patten, S., & Juby, H. (2008). *A profile of clinical depression in Canada.* Research Data Centre Network: Research Synthesis Series No. 1. Retrieved April 19, 2010, from http://hdl.handle.net/1880/46327

Petrie, K. J., Buick, D. L., Weinman, J., & Booth, R. J. (1999). Positive effects of illness reported by myocardial infection and breast cancer patients. *Journal of Psychosomatic Research, 47*, 537–543.

Petrie, K. J., & Revenson, T. A. (2005). Editorial: New psychological interventions in chronic illness: Towards examining mechanisms of action and improved targeting. *Journal of Health Psychology, 10*, 179–184.

Peyrot, M., & Rubin, R. R. (2007). Behavioral and psychosocial interventions in diabetes: A conceptual review. *Diabetes Care, 30*, 2433–2439.

Pincus, T., Griffith, J. Pearce, S., & Isenberg, D. (1996). Prevalence of self-reported depression in patients with rheumatoid arthritis. *British Journal of Rheumatology, 35*, 879–883.

Polonsky, W. H. (2000). Understanding and assessing diabetes-specific quality of life. *Diabetes Spectrum, 13,* 36–41.

Polsky, D., Doshi, J. A., Marcus, S., Oslin, D., Rothbard, A., Thomas, N., et al. (2005). Long-term risk for depressive symptoms after a medical diagnosis. *Archives of Internal Medicine, 165,* 1260–1266.

Portenoy, R. K., & Bruera, E. (2003). *Issues in palliative care research.* New York: Oxford University Press.

Ptacek, J. T., Smith, R. E., & Zanas, J. (1992). Gender, appraisal and coping: A longitudinal analysis. *Journal of Personality, 60,* 747–770.

Quattrin, R., Zanini, A., Buchini, S., Turello, D., Annunziata, M. A., Vidotti, C., et al. (2006). Use of reflexology foot massage to reduce anxiety in hospitalized cancer patients in chemotherapy treatment: Methodology and outcomes. *Journal of Nursing Management, 14,* 96–105.

Rabins, P. V., Black, B. S., Roca, R., German, P., McGuire, M., Robbins, B., et al. (2000). Effectiveness of a nurse-based outreach program for identifying and treating psychiatric illness in the elderly. *Journal of the American Medical Association, 283,* 2802–2809.

Radloff, L. S. (1977). The CES-D scale: A self-report depression scale for research in the general population. *Applied Psychological Measurement, 1,* 385–401.

Rawl, S. M., Given, B. A., Given, C. W., Champion, V. L., Kozachik, S. L., Kozachik, S. L., et al. (2002). Intervention to improve psychological functioning for newly diagnosed patients with cancer. *Oncology Nursing Forum, 29,* 967–975.

Reynolds, W. M., & Kobak, K. A. (2004). Reliability and validity of the Hamilton depression inventory: A paper-and-pencil version of the Hamilton Depression Rating Scale clinical interview. *Psychological Assessment, 7,* 472–483.

Ridner, S. H. (2003). Psychological distress: Concept analysis. *Journal of Advanced Nursing, 45,* 536–545.

Rodgers, M., Fayter, D., Richardson, G., Ritchie, G., Lewin, R., & Sowden, A. J. (2005). *The effects of psychosocial interventions in cancer and heart disease: A review of systematic reviews.* York, England: Centre for Reviews and Dissemination, University of York.

Rotter, J. B. (1990). Internal versus external control of reinforcement: A case history of a variable. *American Psychologist, 45,* 489–493.

Roy, C., & Andrews, H. (1999). *The Roy Adaptation Model: The definitive statement.* Norwalk, CT: Appleton and Lange.

Rule, B. G., Harvey, H. Z., & Dobbs, A. R. (1986). Reliability of the Geriatric Depression Scale for younger adults. *Clinical Gerontology, 4,* 21–28.

Salmon, P. (2001). Effects of physical activity on anxiety, depression, and sensitivity to stress: A unifying theory. *Clinical Psychology Review, 21*(1), 33–61.

Scharloo, M., Kapstein, A. A., Weinman, J., Hazes, J. M., Willems, L. N. A., Bergman, W., et al. (1998). Illness perceptions, coping, and functioning in patients with rheumatoid arthritis, chronic obstructive pulmonary disease and psoriasis. *Journal of Psychosomatic Research, 44,* 573–585.

Scheier, M. F., & Carver, C. S. (1985). Optimism, coping, health, personality predispositions: Assessment and implications of generalized outcome expectancies. *Health Psychology, 4,* 219–247.

Schiaffino, K. M., Shawaryn, M. A., & Blum, D. (1998). Examining the impact of illness representations on psychological adjustment to chronic illnesses. *Health Psychology, 17,* 262–268.

Schneiderman, N. (2004). Psychosocial, behavioral, and biological aspects of chronic diseases. *American Psychological Society, 13,* 247–251.

Schneiderman, N., Antoni, M. H., Saab, P. G., & Ironson, G. (2001). Health psychology: Psychosocial and behavioral aspects of chronic disease management. *Annual Review of Psychology, 52,* 555–580.

Schou, I., Ekeberg, O., & Ruland, C. M. (2005). The mediating role of appraisal and coping in the relationship between optimism-pessimism and quality of life. *Psycho-Oncology, 14,* 718–727.

Schulz, U., & Schwarzer, R. (2004). Long-term effects of spousal support on coping with cancer after surgery. *Journal of Sociology Clinical Psychology, 23,* 487–497.

Scott, L. D., Setter-Kline, K., & Britton, A. S. (2004). The effects of nursing interventions to enhance mental health and quality of life among individuals with heart failure. *Applied Nursing Research, 17,* 248–256.

Sears, S. R., Stanton, A. L., & Danoff-Burg, S. (2003). The yellow brick road and the emerald city: Benefit finding, positive re-appraisal coping, and post-traumatic growth in women with early-stage breast cancer. *Health Psychology, 22,* 487–492.

Seigel, K., & Scrimshaw, E.W. (2000). Perceiving benefits in adversity: Stress-related growth in women living with HIV/AIDS. *Social Science and Medicine, 51,* 1543–1554.

Selye, H. (1978). *The stress of life.* Columbus, OH: McGraw-Hill Education.

Shacham, S. (1983). A shortened version of the Profile of Mood States. *Journal of Personality Assessment, 47,* 305–306.

Sharpe, L., & Curran, L. (2006). Understanding the process of adjustment to illness. *Social Science and Medicine, 62,* 1153–1166.

Sheard, T., & McGuire, P. (1999). The effect of psychological interventions on anxiety and depression in cancer patients: Results of two meta-analyses. *British Journal of Cancer, 80,* 1770–1780.

Sheldon, L. K., Swanson, S., Dolce, A., Marsh, K., & Summers, J. (2008). Putting evidence into practice: Evidence-based interventions for anxiety. *Clinical Journal of Oncology Nursing, 12,* 789–797.

Sherwood, P., Given, B. A., Given, C. W., Champion, V. L., Doorenbos, A. Z., Azzouz, F., et al. (2005). A cognitive behavioral intervention for symptom management in patients with advanced cancer. *Oncology Nursing Forum, 32,* 1190–1198.

Shih, M., Hootman, J. M., Strine, T. W., Chapman, D. P., & Brady, T. J. (2006). Serious psychological distress in U.S. adults with arthritis. *Journal of General Internal Medicine, 21,* 1160–1166.

Shih, M., & Simon, P. A. (2008). Health-related quality of life among adults with serious psychological distress and chronic medical conditions. *Quality of Life Research, 17,* 521–528.

Shneck, Z. M., Irvine, J., Stewart, D., & Abbey, S. (2001). Psychological factors and depressive symptoms in ischemic heart disease. *Health Psychology, 20,* 141–145.

Sidell, N. L. (1997). Adult adjustment to chronic illness: A review of the literature. *Health and Social Work, 22,* 5–11.

Sloan, D. M., & Kring, A. M. (2007). Measuring changes in emotion during psychotherapy: Conceptual and methodological issues. *Clinical Psychology: Science and Practice, 14,* 307–322.

Sloman, R. (2002). Relaxation and imagery for anxiety and depression control in community patients with advanced cancer. *Cancer Nursing, 25,* 432–435.

Smith, G. D. (2006). Effect of nurse-led gut-directed hypnotherapy upon health-related quality of life in patients with irritable bowel syndrome. *Journal of Clinical Nursing, 15,* 678–684.

Smith, J. R., Mildenhall, S., Noble, M. J., Shepstone, L., Koutantji, M., Mugford, M., et al. (2005). The coping with asthma study: A randomised controlled trial of a home based, nurse led psychoeducational intervention for adults at risk of adverse asthma outcomes. *Thorax, 60,* 1003–1011.

Smith, T. W., & Gallo, L. C. (2001). Personality traits as risk factors for physical illness. In A. Baum, T. A. Revenson, & J. Singer (Eds.), *Handbook of health psychology* (pp. 139–174). Mahwah, NJ: Erlbaum.

Speigel, D., & Kato, P. M. (1996). Psychosocial influences on cancer incidence and progression. *Harvard Review of Psychiatry, 4,* 10–26.

Spielberger, C., Gorsuch, R., Lushene, R., Vagg, P., & Jacobs, G. (1983). *Manual for the State-Trait Anxiety Inventory*. Palo Alto, CA: Consulting Psychologists Press.

Stanton, A. L., Collins, C.A., & Sworowski, L. A. (2001). Adjustment to chronic illness: Theory and research. In A. Baum, T. A. Revenson, & J. Singer (Eds.), *Handbook of health psychology* (pp. 387–403). Mahwah, NJ: Erlbaum.

Stanton, A. L., Revenson, T. A., & Tennen, H. (2007). Health psychology: Psychological adjustment to chronic disease. *Annual Reviews in Psychology, 58*, 565–592.

Stark, D., Keily, M., Smith, A., Velikova, G., House, A., & Selby, P. (2002). Anxiety disorders in cancer patients: Their nature, associations , and relation to quality of life. *Journal of Clinical Oncology, 20*, 3137–3148.

Steer, R. A., Ranieri, W. F., Beck, A. T., & Clark, D. A. (1993). Further evidence for the validity of the Beck Anxiety Inventory with psychiatric outpatients. *Journal of Anxiety Disorders, 7*, 195–205.

Stephens, T., J., & Joubert, N. (2001). The economic burden of mental health problems in Canada. *Chronic Diseases in Canada, 22*, 18–23.

Stern, M. J., Pascale, L., & Ackerman, A. (1977). Life adjustment postmyocardial infarction: Determining predictive variables. *Archives of Internal Medicine, 137*, 1680–1685.

Stewart, A. L., Ware, J., Sherbourne, C. D., & Willis, K. (1992). Psychological distress/well-being and cognitive function measures. In A. L. Stewart & J. Ware (Eds.), *Measuring functioning and psychological well-being: The medical outcomes approach* (pp. 102–142). New York: Rand.

Stokes, J., & Wilson, D. G. (1984). Inventory of socially supportive behaviors: Dimensionality, prediction, and gender differences. *American Journal of Community Psychology, 2*, 53–64.

Stommel, M., Given, B. A., Given, C. W., Kalaian, H. A., Schulz, R., & McCorkle, R. (1993). Gender bias in the measurement properties of the Center for Epidemiological Studies Depression Scale (CES-D). *Psychiatry Research, 49*, 239–250.

Strine, T. W., Hootman, J. M., Okoro, C. A., Balluz, L., Moriarty, D.G., Owens, M., et al. (2004). Frequent mental distress status among adults with arthritis age 45 years and older, 2001. *Arthritis Rheumatology, 51*, 533–537.

Strong, V., Waters, R., Hibberd, C., Murray, G., Wall, L., Walker, J., et al. (2008). Management of depression for people with cancer (SMaRT oncology 1): A randomised trial. *Lancet, 372*, 40–48.

Targ, E. F., & Levine, E. G. (2002). The efficacy of a mind-body-spirit group for women with breast cancer: A randomized controlled trial. *General Hospital Psychiatry, 24*, 238–248.

Taylor-Piliae, R. E., & Chair, S. Y. (2002). The effect of nursing interventions utilizing music therapy or sensory information on Chinese patients' anxiety prior to cardiac catheterization: A pilot study. *European Journal of Cardiovascular Nursing, 1*, 203–211.

Thomas, L. A. (2003). Clinical management of stressors perceived by patients on mechanical ventilation. *AACN Clinical Issues, 14*, 73–81.

Thompson, S., & Janigan, A. (1988). Life schemes: A framework for understanding the search for meaning. *Social and Clinical Psychology, 7*, 260–280.

Tomich, P. L., & Helgeson, V. S. (2004). Is finding something good in the bad always good? Benefit finding among women with breast cancer. *Health Psychology, 23*, 16–23.

Trask, P. C., Paterson, A., Riba, M., Brines, B., Griffith, K., Parker, P., et al. (2002). Assessment of psychological distress in prospective bone marrow transplant patients. *Bone Marrow Transplantation, 29*, 917–925.

Turner, J., & Kelly, B. (2000). Emotional dimensions of chronic disease. *Western Journal of Medicine, 172*, 124–188.

Twiss, E., Seaver, J., & McCaffrey, R. (2007). The effect of music listening on older adults undergoing cardiovascular surgery. *Nursing in Critical Care, 11*, 224–231.

Veach, T. A., Nicholas, D. R., & Barton, M. A. (2002). *Cancer and the family life cycle: A practitioner's guide.* New York: Brunner-Routledge.

Ward, S. E. (1993). The common sense model: An organizing framework for knowledge development in nursing. *Scholarly Inquiry in Nursing Practice, 7*(2), 79–84.

Ware, J. E., Jr., & Sherbourne, C. D. (1992) The MOS 36-item short-form health survey (SF-36): I. Conceptual framework and item selection. *Medical Care, 30,* 473–483.

Watson, M. (2001). Psychosocial issues in cancer. *Current Science, 81,* 566–570.

Watson, L. C., Lewis, C. L., Kistler, C. E., Amick, H. R., & Boustani, M. (2004). Can we trust depression screening instruments in healthy "old-old" adults? *International Journal of Geriatric Psychiatry, 19,* 278–285.

Weiss, I. K., Nagel, C. L., & Aronson, M. K. (1986). Applicability of depression scales to the old old person. *Journal of the American Geriatrics Society, 34,* 215–218.

Wells, K. B., & Sherbourne, C. D. (1999). Functioning and utility for current health of patients with depression on chronic medical conditions in managed primary care practices. *Archives of General Psychiatry, 56,* 897–904.

Wengstrom, Y., Haggmark, C., Strander, H., & Forsberg, C. (1999). Effects of a nursing intervention on subjective distress, side effects and quality of life of breast cancer patients receiving curative radiation therapy: A randomized study. *Acta Oncologica, 38,* 763–770.

Westlake, C., Dracup, K., Fonarow, G., & Hamilton, M. (2005). Depression in patients with heart failure. *Journal of Cardiac Failure, 11*(1), 30–35.

Williams, S. A., & Schreier, A. M. (2004). The effect of education in managing side effects in women receiving chemotherapy for treatment of breast cancer. *Oncology Nursing Forum, 31,* E16–E23.

Witchen, H. U. (1994). Reliability and validity studies of the WHO Composite International Diagnostic Interview (CIDI): A critical review. *Journal of Psychiatric Research, 28,* 57–84.

Wohlgemuth, E., & Betz, N. E. (1991). Gender as a moderator of the relationships of stress and social support to physical health in college students. *Journal of Counseling Psychology, 38,* 367–374.

Yesavage, J. A., Brink, T., Rose, T. L., Lum, O., Huang, V., Adey, M., et al. (1983). Development and validation of a geriatric depression screening scale: A preliminary report. *Journal of Psychiatric Research, 17,* 37–49.

Yin, P., & Fan, X. (2000). Assessing the reliability of Beck Depression Inventory Scores: Reliability generalization across studies. *Education and Psychological Measurement, 60,* 201–223.

Zabora, J. R. (1998). Screening procedures for psychosocial distress. In J. C. Holland (Ed.), *Psycho-Oncology* (pp. 653–661). New York: Oxford University Press.

Zigmond, A. S., & Snaith, R. P. (1983). The Hospital Anxiety and Depression Scale. *Acta Psychiatrica Scandinavica, 67,* 361–370.

Zung, W. W. K. (1965). A self-rating depression scale. *Archives of General Psychiatry, 12,* 60–78.

Zung, W. W. K. (1971). A rating instrument for anxiety disorders. *Psychosomatics, 12,* 371–379.

Zung, W. W. K. (1974). The measurement affects: Depression and anxiety. *Modern Problems of Pharmacopsychiatry, 7,* 170–188.

Zung, W. W. K. (1980). *How normal is anxiety?* Kalamazoo, MI: Upjohn Company.

Patient Satisfaction as a Nurse-Sensitive Outcome

Heather K. Spence Laschinger
Stephanie Gilbert
Lesley Smith

INTRODUCTION

Patient satisfaction with care is a key quality indicator in current healthcare settings (Titler, 2002; Tomlinson & Clifford, 2006; Zimmerman, 2001). Healthcare facilities are expected, and in some jurisdictions required, to report patient satisfaction levels in annual report cards available to the public (Tomlinson & Clifford). The American Nurses Association (ANA; 1996) identifies patient satisfaction with nursing care as a key nurse-sensitive outcome. Healthcare organizations collect patient satisfaction data for a variety of reasons: to market their organization to consumers, to provide incentives for units within organizations, and, most important, as a benchmark to monitor initiatives to improve quality. Given the importance placed on patient satisfaction and its influence on policy, reliable and valid measures are critical for evidence-based decision-making. Furthermore, because nursing care represents a major feature of the patient care experience, it is imperative that measures used to drive policy capture key aspects of nursing care quality. Although numerous measures of patient satisfaction with nursing care are available in the literature, there have been recent efforts to develop and test psychometrically strong instruments that are relevant to today's quality-conscious healthcare environment (Lynn, McMillen, & Sidani, 2007; Wagner & Bear, 2009).

Arguably, patient satisfaction has always been the goal of professional health care because health professionals are guided by, and required to maintain, standards of care thought to be necessary for optimal, high-quality, safe patient care. According to Donabedian (1988), patient satisfaction can be considered an element of health status and thus a fundamental component of any measure of quality. In response to calls for accountability for escalating healthcare costs over the past two decades, both healthcare funders and researchers have scrutinized patient satisfaction as a valued outcome of patient care quality.

The Total Quality Management (TQM) movement in the 1980s was a major initiative aimed at improving patient care processes to maximize effectiveness and efficiency in healthcare settings. The expected outcomes of the TQM approach were lower costs and more satisfied clients. At the same time, managed care approaches to healthcare delivery were becoming more prevalent. The competitive nature of these systems made patient satisfaction an important outcome to consider as healthcare businesses struggled for survival in the healthcare market. In the 1980s and 1990s, as the public gained greater access to previously difficult-to-obtain information regarding health and disease, a cadre of more knowledgeable and demanding healthcare consumers required healthcare providers to pay closer attention to their needs and opinions. Consequently, the notion of patient as healthcare consumer became prominent.

There are few well-developed conceptual descriptions of patient satisfaction in the literature (Sitzia & Wood, 1997; Thomas & Bond, 1996). Existing instruments have varying degrees of comprehensiveness, and in many cases, no known reliability and validity. Institutions wishing to evaluate patient satisfaction as part of their quality improvement programs often have developed measures locally. Consequently, studies replicating their use have not been conducted. As a result, research in this field has been disadvantaged by inconsistent conceptualization of the phenomenon and a lack of comparable results across settings.

Patient satisfaction has been conceptualized broadly as a patient's overall response to the total healthcare experience and in relationship to particular aspects of care, such as nursing and medical care or admission and discharge processes. A key component in these definitions has been the notion of a match between patients' expectations of care and what they actually received during the episode of care. When care fails to meet expectations, patients are dissatisfied with what they perceive to be poor-quality care (Ludwig-Beymer et al., 1993). Thus, patient satisfaction is one of several indicators of service quality, an important determinant of accreditation for healthcare institutions.

There are many conceptual and methodological problems in measuring patient satisfaction. K. Chang (1997) argued that current measures of patient satisfaction fail to capture key nursing actions and thus are poor indicators of nursing care quality. This makes it difficult to meaningfully link nursing actions to patients' perceptions of the quality of nursing care. Pascoe (1983) pointed out that patients often have difficulty differentiating nursing personnel from other healthcare workers in hospital environments, which confounds patients' ratings of satisfaction with nursing care. As a result, the measures have questionable reliability and validity. Patient satisfaction ratings are usually positively skewed with a constricted range of values. These data characteristics affect statistical analyses and make it difficult to determine true effects that may exist. As a result, policy changes cannot be justified based on high-quality evidence. Finally, there is no standardization of measures of satisfaction with nursing care, making it impossible to compare results across settings.

Several authors (Bond & Thomas, 1992; Lynn & Moore, 1997; Lynn et al., 2007) have pointed out that the majority of patient satisfaction measures reflect issues important to providers and do not include the patient's perspective. This is problematic because numerous studies have demonstrated provider/patient differences in importance ratings of various elements of satisfaction. More recently, researchers have begun to determine patient expectations of care and incorporate these perspectives into measures of patient satisfaction (Lynn & McMillen, 1999; Lynn et al.). Instruments that include both nurse and patient perspectives of good nursing care quality are more likely to yield meaningful results that can be used as a basis for quality improvement initiatives.

To summarize, there are several reasons for the intensified interest in measuring patient satisfaction with nursing and health care: (a) the demand for public accountability for healthcare outcomes and the need to provide evidence of quality; (b) incentives to tie government funding to standards of quality in healthcare delivery; (c) the TQM movement to monitor efforts to reduce costs and maintain quality; (d) a shift from the notion of patients as passive recipients of care to one of informed healthcare consumers who are willing and able to choose healthcare services based on their perceptions of quality provided; (e) the managed competition approach to healthcare delivery in the United States, with its associated market share implications; and (f) the changing mix of healthcare workers in acute care settings. As a result of these changes, patient satisfaction has emerged as an important indicator of healthcare quality that has implications for the survival of healthcare organizations and the well-being of patients under their care.

This chapter updates the available literature on patient satisfaction viewed as a concept reflecting an outcome of nursing care. The purposes of the review are to:
- Clarify the concept of patient satisfaction at the theoretical and empirical levels
- Identify instruments measuring patient satisfaction that demonstrated acceptable reliability, validity, and sensitivity to change
- Determine structural and process factors that influence patient satisfaction
- Determine the extent to which patient satisfaction is an outcome sensitive/responsive to nursing care

The methodology used to identify the relevant literature, as well as the criteria to select and systematically review it, was discussed in Chapter 1. A systematic search of the nursing and healthcare databases yielded a total of 400 sources that were either empirical or conceptual papers addressing patient satisfaction. A total of 160 of these met the preset inclusion and exclusion criteria and are reviewed in this chapter.

THEORETICAL BACKGROUND: DEFINITION OF THE CONCEPT

This section summarizes the results of a concept analysis that we conducted to clarify the concept of patient satisfaction at the theoretical and operational levels. The strategies we adopted involved the following:

- Carefully reading each article selected on the basis of the inclusion and exclusion criteria
- Abstracting the theoretical definitions of patient satisfaction that were provided in theoretical/conceptual sources and in the framework or literature review section of empirical sources
- Comparing and contrasting the essential attributes that define the concept of patient satisfaction, as comprised in the theoretical definitions
- Summarizing the essential attributes that are common and consistent across the definitions and the conceptualizations of patient satisfaction
- Identifying the antecedents and consequences of patient satisfaction

Definitions of Patient Satisfaction

Patient satisfaction is frequently defined as the extent to which patients' expectations of care matched the actual care received (Abramowitz, Cote, & Berry, 1987; Hill, 1997; Linder-Pelz, 1982; Ludwig-Beymer et al., 1993; Petersen, 1988; Risser, 1975; Swan, 1985). In a thorough concept analysis of patient satisfaction, Eriksen (1995) defined patient satisfaction with nursing care as "the patients' subjective evaluation of the cognitive-emotional response that results from the interaction of the patients' expectations of nursing care and their perception of actual nurse behaviors/characteristics" (p. 71). Cleary and McNeil (1988) proposed a similar definition in the health services literature. However, Williams (1994) noted that few studies have actually found empirical support for this conception of satisfaction. Many argue that patient satisfaction is a general affective response to the overall healthcare experience rather than a focused assessment of distinct aspects of the care episode (B. L. Chang, Uman, Lawrence, Ware, & Kane, 1984; Taylor, 1994; Williams, 1994). A more recent definition by Mrayyan (2006) provided a more holistic view of the concept, defining patient satisfaction as "the degree to which nursing care meets patients' expectations in terms of art of care, technical quality, physical environment, availability and continuity of care, and the efficacy/outcomes of care" (p. 226). Wagner and Bear (2009) identified the critical attributes of patient satisfaction as "affective support, health information, decisional control, and professional/technical competencies" (p. 695). Interestingly, although technical competence of nurses is included in most measures of patient satisfaction with nursing care, patients in Lynn et al.'s (2007) study did not identify this factor in their assessments of nursing care quality. According to Lynn et al., any measure of patient satisfaction must assess aspects of care identified as important by patients in order to be considered as a valid measure of the construct.

In the health services marketing literature, there is considerable debate about the importance of distinguishing between the concepts of patient satisfaction and patient perceptions of quality of care (Cronin & Taylor, 1992; Taylor, 1994). The argument is based on the notion that, although related, they are really distinct concepts and should be measured separately. Patient satisfaction is viewed as a mediator between patient perception of quality and future intentions to reuse the service or recommend the service to others (Woodside, Frey, & Daly, 1989). Taylor defined perceived quality as a long-term attitude developed over time. On the other hand, patient satisfaction is defined as a short-term response to a specific experience. According to Taylor, it is important to be able to measure the two concepts separately in order to enable healthcare marketers to determine which of their marketing strategies are most effective. This debate was not evident in the nursing literature reviewed, most likely because of a differing perspective on the goal of collecting patient satisfaction data. Nursing is more concerned with using the data to improve the patients' health status and less concerned about patients' future intentions to choose a particular healthcare setting or to recommend the organization to others (a logical interest of healthcare marketers).

Several researchers have found consistent differences in the importance ratings of aspects of care reported by nurses and patients, which suggests that nurses' and patients' definitions of satisfaction with patient care quality differ (Lynn & Moore, 1997). In several studies, nurses consistently overestimated the importance of emotional care for patients (Farrell, 1991; von Essen & Sjoden, 1991, 1995; Young, Minnick, & Marcantonio, 1996). However, patients gave higher ratings to the importance of technical care, such as monitoring and following through, and providing explanations regarding their condition and care. These findings are consistent with those of Kovner (1989) and Larson (1987). Kovner's results are important because she found that the less patients and nurses disagreed on desirability of outcomes, the more satisfied patients were with their care. These results, which led to a concern that what was being measured in these surveys reflected provider perspectives, provided the impetus for a variety of qualitative studies to ascertain patients' perspectives of high-quality care (Bond & Thomas, 1992; Lynn & Moore; Webb & Hope, 1995).

Determinants of Patient Satisfaction

Researchers have identified many factors that have an impact on patient satisfaction. Personal characteristics of patients, such as cultural background and availability of a supportive network, as well as patient age, sex, and education, have been shown to be related to patient satisfaction ratings in several studies (Bacon & Mark, 2009; Conbere, McGovern, Kochevar, & Widtfeldt, 1992). However, others have found no relationship between patient satisfaction and demographic variables (Rubin, Ware, & Hays, 1990). Patients' perceptions of the quality of their interactions with nurses are also important determinants of patient satisfaction. Among the many interpersonal factors identified are: (a) involving patients in decisions about their care and supporting their right to convey their thoughts or opinions about care options (Andaleeb, 1998; B. L. Chang et al., 1984; Cleary & McNeil, 1988; D. A. Forbes, 1996; Kovner, 1989; Krouse & Roberts, 1989); (b) providing information about patients' conditions and explanations of symptoms they may experience (Bowling, 1992; Cleary & McNeil; Cottle, 1989; Fosbinder, 1994; Mahon, 1996); (c) using a compassionate caring approach (Cleary & McNeil; Cottle; D. A. Forbes; Fosbinder; Lewis & Woodside, 1992); and (d) creating an equitable relationship that ensures fairness (Swan, 1985). Other important determinants of patients' satisfaction with care include prompt attention to patient concerns and efficient execution of therapeutic interventions (Cottle; Denton, 1989; Thompson, Yarnold, Williams, & Adams, 1996).

Several structural factors, including patients' perceptions of nurses' competency (Andaleeb, 1998; Cottle, 1989; Hanan & Karp, 1989) and the methods used to deliver nursing care, such as primary nursing, critical pathways, case management, and professional practice models, have been shown to affect patient satisfaction with nursing care (Goode, 1995; Hayes, 1992; Heinemann, Lengacher, Van Cott, Mabe, & Swymer, 1996; Mahon, 1996; Twardon & Gartner, 1991). Advanced practice nurses, such as nurse practitioners in nurse-led clinics and clinical nurse specialists in inpatient settings, have also been associated with positive patient satisfaction ratings (Baradell, 1995; Graveley & Littlefield, 1992; Hill, 1997; Knaus et al., 1997).

The impact of nurses' job satisfaction on patient satisfaction with nursing care has been demonstrated (Atkins, Marshall, & Javalgi, 1996; Kaldenberg & Regrut, 1999; Leiter, Harvie, & Frizzel, 1998; Weisman & Nathanson, 1985). However, methodological problems limit the generalizability of many of these studies. Numerous studies have failed to establish this relationship (Goodell & Van Ess Coeling, 1994; Niedz, 1998). Until recently, strong empirical evidence for the link between nurse job satisfaction and patient satisfaction did not exist (Kangas, Kee, & McKee-Waddle, 1999). Methodological difficulties and the complex nature of patient care quality may account for this situation. More recently, Sengin (2001) found that patients on units with high job satisfaction reported higher levels of overall satisfaction with care, as well as satisfaction with patient care quality. However, Larrabee et al. (2004) did not find a significant relationship between nurses' job satisfaction and patient satisfaction in her study in the southern United States.

Recent research has shown links between nursing work environment characteristics and patient satisfaction. This research emerged from the focus on nursing-sensitive outcomes that evolved following the downsizing of the 1990s. Nurse researchers set about to empirically document how nursing activities and working conditions of nurses affected patient care outcomes to provide evidence that supported the need to maintain high-quality work environments and adequate staffing levels.

Two main categories of nursing worklife have been found to influence patient satisfaction: (1) staffing levels and (2) nurses' perceptions of the quality of their work environments. Studies in Canada, the United States, and Finland all established significant relationships between nursing staffing levels, operationalized as hours of nursing care per patient day and number of nursing hours, and patient satisfaction (Clark, Leddy, Drain, & Kaldenberg, 2007; McGillis-Hall et al., 2003; Moore, Lynn, McMillen, & Evans, 1999; Potter, Barr, McSweeney, & Sledge, 2003; Sovie & Jowad, 2001; Tervo-Heikkinen, Partanen, Aalto, & Vehvilainen-Julkunen, 2008). These results support the importance of adequate staffing to the ability to meet patient needs.

Other studies have linked "Magnet hospital" characteristics in nursing work environments to patient satisfaction (Tervo-Heikkinen, Kvist, Partanen, Vehvilainen-Julkunen, & Aalto, 2008; Vahey, Aiken, Sloane, Clarke, & Vargas, 2004). Patient satisfaction has also been linked to other aspects of nursing worklife. Stumpf (2001) found that patients had higher satisfaction on units using a shared governance model. Donahue, Piazza, Griffin, Dykes, and Fitzpatrick (2008) found that nurses' perceptions of access to empowering work conditions were significantly related to patient satisfaction in a large acute care hospital in Connecticut. Bacon and Mark (2009) found that patients on units with higher levels of support services for nursing and greater work engagement among nurses were more likely to be satisfied with the quality of nursing care. Although more research is needed to support this important link between provider working conditions and patient outcomes, there is considerably more evidence to support this link than there was 5 years ago.

Several studies have examined the effects of specific nursing interventions on patient satisfaction. Yeakel, Maljanian, Bohannon, and Coulombe (2003) found that a multifaceted intervention designed to improve nursing caring behaviors resulted in greater patient satisfaction and patient ratings of nursing caring practices. Innis, Bikaunieks, Petryshen, Zellermeyer, and Ciccarelli (2004) found significant pain management satisfaction scores following an educational program for nurses related to effective pain management. Many small studies in the nursing literature include patient satisfaction as an outcome of topic-specific educational programs. However, the generalizability of these findings is limited because the studies occurred in single sites, the patient satisfaction measures were generally developed by institutions, and few details are available on the content and psychometric properties of these tools.

A few studies were found that evaluated the effect of structural and process changes in the nursing work environment on patient satisfaction. Kangas et al. (1999) found that patients in units that used primary nursing were more satisfied with nursing care than those that used team nursing or care management approaches. However, Barkell, Killinger, and Schultz (2002) found no significant difference in patient satisfaction following a change in care delivery model (team nursing vs total patient care). Goode (1995) observed higher patient satisfaction on units that used critical pathways for managing care.

Consequences of Patient Satisfaction with Nursing Care

Several health service researchers have studied the consequences of patient satisfaction with nursing care. Patient satisfaction with nursing care has been shown to be strongly related to overall satisfaction with the healthcare encounter in many studies (Abramowitz et al., 1987; Batalden & Nelson, 1990; Carey & Posavac, 1982; Hays, Nelson, Rubin, Ware, & Meterko, 1990; Laschinger, Hall, Pedersen, & Almost, 2005; Peterson, Charles, DiCenso, & Sword, 2005). Some researchers have identified adherence to medically prescribed regimens as an outcome of patient satisfaction with nursing care (Lynn et al., 2007; Swan & Carroll, 1980; Weisman & Nathanson, 1985). Davidow and Uttal (1989) argued that more satisfied patients are more cooperative with their caregivers, although this claim was not supported by empirical evidence. Finally, there is evidence to support the relationships among patient satisfaction with nursing care, patients' intentions to use a service in the future, and their likelihood of recommending the service to others (Abramowitz et al.; Laschinger et al.; Otani & Kurz, 2004; Rubin et al., 1988). This outcome is particularly important in U.S. managed care settings but is less salient in the Canadian healthcare context.

In nursing, Doran, Sidani, Keatings, and Doidge (2002) found that patients who reported higher levels of patient satisfaction also reported higher levels of functional status, self-care ability, and emotional health at discharge. Laschinger et al. (2005) found that higher levels of patient satisfaction were positively related to overall satisfaction with quality of care during the hospital stay and their intentions to recommend the hospital to family and friends. Lynn et al. (2007) found similar results; they found that patients with high satisfaction scores reported greater adherence to discharge orders. These results highlight the importance of patient satisfaction with nursing care for client health after discharge.

Conceptual/Theoretical Models of Patient Satisfaction

Few systematic attempts have been made to develop explanatory models of patient satisfaction (Abramowitz et al., 1987). Particularly in early studies, the concept seems to have been seen as self-explanatory; consequently, numerous idiosyncratic tools were developed locally to measure it. The models that have been proposed have not been widely tested. By far the most common model found in the literature is the discrepancy model—that is, the degree of match/mismatch between expectations for care and perceptions of care received. However, conceptual notions of the phenomenon are also implied by the content of the instruments themselves. The elements of these models vary based on their developer's orientation.

Linder-Pelz (1982) developed a model of patient satisfaction that suggested that patients' expectations of care, healthcare values, sense of entitlement, and interpersonal comparisons of care were antecedents of positive evaluations of care. However, when tested in a primary care setting, these variables explained only 8% of the variance in patient satisfaction levels. Greeneich (1993) proposed a model describing nurse, patient, and organizational characteristics that influence patient satisfaction. She also posited the notion of a critical nursing event, usually in relation to meeting or not meeting an important patient need that has a lasting salient effect on a patient's satisfaction with care. This model has not been tested.

Comley and Beard (1998) attempted to derive a theory of patient satisfaction from various job satisfaction models and a review of factors reported in the literature found to influence patient satisfaction. They suggested that patient satisfaction, like job satisfaction, is a function of personal intrinsic factors and extrinsic organizational factors and thus is not completely controllable by healthcare providers. Intrinsic factors include age, sex, socioeconomic status, ethnicity, occupation, diagnosis, and degree of illness. Extrinsic factors include type of nursing care delivery system, provider competence, promptness of service, comfort and cleanliness of the physical environment, and food quality. This model has not been empirically tested in a prospective study.

Pascoe (1983) described two models of consumer satisfaction based on the marketing literature. In the contrast model, clients compare service with previous experiences. Dissatisfaction results if there is a mismatch. In the assimilation model, clients attempt to resolve a sense of psychological dissonance created by the failure to have their expectations met by lowering those expectations. Thus, their satisfaction ratings are in relation to this lowered standard and are falsely high. Eriksen (1995) suggested that this explanation may account for the consistent findings of positively skewed patient satisfaction scores.

Wagner and Bear (2009) conducted a comprehensive concept analysis of patient satisfaction using a nursing model of client health behavior. Cox's (1982) model describes patient and nurse factors that combine to influence client outcomes—personal client resources and the nature of the client–provider interaction. Key components of patient satisfaction in this model are affective support, access to health information, decisional control, and professional competence. These components are consistent with most of the measures of patient satisfaction with nursing care that are available in the nursing literature. The authors provide empirical evidence from the nursing literature that supports the conceptualization of patient satisfaction within Cox's nursing model of client behavior. This model is conceptually consistent with the Doran et al. (2002) Nursing Effectiveness model, although the latter is more comprehensive in terms of organizational factors hypothesized to influence patient outcomes. On the other hand, the Cox model is more comprehensive in relation to patient attributes and processes that influence client behavior. Thus, there is merit in combining the two models to provide a more comprehensive model of patient satisfaction.

APPROACHES TO MEASUREMENT OF PATIENT SATISFACTION WITH NURSING CARE

The majority of patient satisfaction instruments in the literature are not based on theoretical models. However, the conceptualization of patient satisfaction is implied by the nature of the items in the questionnaires. Thirty-one instruments available in the nursing and health services literature were evaluated for their appropriateness as a nurse-sensitive outcome in this review. These instruments have varying degrees of reported psychometric data. The characteristics of these instruments are summarized in **TABLE 8-1** (Parts A and B). For each measure, the title and author are identified, as well as the sample in which it was developed. The measurement domains, number of items, response format, and method of administration are also identified. Finally, evidence for the instrument's reliability and validity is reported. The details of the studies in which these instruments were used are presented in **TABLE 8-2**.

Several criteria were used to assess the relative value of these tools. First, the tool's comprehensiveness was assessed with regard to factors identified in the literature as determinants of patient satisfaction with nursing care quality. Also, based on recommendations in the literature that measures of patient satisfaction should reflect both nurse and patient perspectives, these tools were further evaluated to determine the extent to which quality indicators that patients identified in the literature were included. Comparisons of selected instruments using these two sets of criteria are shown in **TABLE 8-3** and **TABLE 8-4**. In addition, the instruments were also evaluated in terms of availability of psychometric data, readability of items, length of the tool, ease of scoring, and sensitivity to actual nursing activities/responsibilities. Finally, the instruments were assessed to determine the extent to which the results of the responses to items on the questionnaire could

TABLE 8-1A Selected Measures of Patient Satisfaction with Nursing Care Developed by Nursing Researchers

Instrument (author)	Target population	Domains (number of items and response format)	Method of administration	Reliability	Validity	Sensitivity to nursing care
Patient's Assessment of Quality Scale-Acute Care Version (PAQS-ACV) (Lynn et al., 2007)	Patients in medical-surgical nursing units	45 items on five subscales: individualization, nurse characteristics, caring, environment, and responsiveness.	Self-administered	Cronbach's reliability for the subscales ranged from .68 to .94.	Content	No information available
Davis Consumer Emergency Care Satisfaction Scale (Davis et al., 2005)	Urgent and nonurgent patients discharged from the emergency department (ED) (n = 113)	19 items scored on a 5-point Likert-type scale: Two dimensions of nursing care are discharge teaching and caring.	Self-administered	Cronbach's reliability for the discharge teaching scale had an alpha coefficient of 0.88, whereas the caring scale had an alpha coefficient of 0.97.	Construct	Nurses and others measuring patient satisfaction with nursing care in the ED can use the CECSS knowing that it has had repeated testing and supported validity.
Patient Satisfaction with Nursing Care Quality Questionnaire (Laschinger et al., 2005)	Patients discharged from medical-surgical units in April, May, and June of 2002	19 items plus 3 additional questions designed to tap satisfaction with the overall quality of care during the hospital stay, overall quality of nursing care, and intention to recommend the hospital to family and friends (5-point Likert scale was used for each item).	Self-administered	Cronbach's alpha reliability of .97 for total scale.	Construct	Nurse managers can utilize this instrument as a way to evaluate the contribution of nurses to the patient care process.
Patients' Judgments of Nursing Care (Larrabee et al., 2004)	Medical, surgical, and intensive care step-down patients	9 items with a 5-point Likert scale response format.	Self-administered	Cronbach's alpha reliability of 0.94 for total scale.	Content	Patient-perceived nurse caring is a major predictor of patient satisfaction with nurse–physician (RN/MD) collaboration as the only other direct predictor.
Penn State Inpatient Psychiatry Satisfaction Survey (PSIPSS) (Woodring et al., 2004)	Psychiatric patients discharged from inpatient care	15 items related to staff attributes, efficiency of care, environment, explanations of treatments, involvement in care, and appropriateness of the length of hospitalization.	Self-administered	Cronbach's alpha reliability of 0.94 for total scale	Content, construct	No information available
Schmidt Perception of Nursing Care Survey (Schmidt, 2003)	Patients discharged from medical-surgical units	4 subscales: seeing the individual patient (five items), explaining (three items), responding (three items), and watching over (four items).	Self-administered	Cronbach's alpha reliability of 0.96 for total scale.	No information available	No information available

(continues)

TABLE 8-1A Selected Measures of Patient Satisfaction with Nursing Care Developed by Nursing Researchers (continued)

Instrument (author)	Target population	Domains (number of items and response format)	Method of administration	Reliability	Validity	Sensitivity to nursing care
Patient Satisfaction Instrument (Yellen et al., 2002)	Ambulatory surgery patients scheduled for a minimally invasive surgery	30 items with a 4-point rating scale; the higher the total score, the greater the satisfaction	Self-administered	Cronbach's alpha reliability of 0.86 for total scale.	Construct	Three components contribute to patient satisfaction with nursing care: Professionally competent nursing care, interpersonal relationship with the nurse involving availability, and interpersonal relationship with the nurse involving humaneness.
Patient Satisfaction Tool (Benkert et al., 2002)	Patients who have visited a nurse-managed center	17 items: 3 components (patient perceptions of clinic care, patient perceptions of phone contact, likelihood to return or recommend the nurse-managed centers)	Self-administered	Cronbach's alpha reliability of 0.94 for total scale	No information available	Professional responsiveness and respect and courtesy from nurse practitioners were rated high on the composite satisfaction levels from a heterogeneous sample of consumers.
Patient Satisfaction with Health Care Provider Scale (Marsh, 1999)	Patients of nurse practitioners and physicians	Access, humaneness, quality, and general satisfaction; 18 items rated on 5-point scale	Self-administered	Cronbach's alpha reliability of .93 for total scale	Content	No information available
Patients' Perceptions of Quality Scale-Acute Care Version (Lynn & Moore, 1997)	Medical/surgical inpatients	Professional demeanor, treats me like an individual, mindfulness, and responsiveness; 54 items rated on a 5-point scale	Self-administered	Cronbach's alpha reliabilities for the subscales of .80 to .94 (Lynn & Moore, 1997) and .62 to .96 (Moore et al., 1999)	Content	Percentage of RNs on unit and total nursing care hours per patient day were positive predictors of patient satisfaction (Moore et al., 1999).
Newcastle Satisfaction with Nursing Scale (McColl, Thomas, & Bond, 1996)	Inpatient hospital setting	Two scales: patient's experiences of nursing (manner, attentiveness, availability, reassurance, individual treatment, information, professionalism, knowledge, openness, informality) and satisfaction with that care (ward organization, ward environment); 45 items rated on 5- and 7-point scales	Self-administered	No information available	Content	No information available

Instrument	Setting/Population	Description	Administration	Reliability	Validity	Comments
Patient Satisfaction Questionnaire (M. L. Forbes & Brown, 1995)	Outpatient surgery centre	Caring, continuity of care, competence of nurses, and education of patients and family members; 21 items rated on a 5-point scale	Self-administered	Cronbach's alpha reliability of .83; test-retest reliability assessed.	Content	No information available
Satisfaction with Nursing Care Questionnaire (Nash et al., 1994) *Adaptation of Eriksen's (1987) tool	Inpatient hospital setting	Particular concerns and rating scale for evaluation of care; 16 items rated on a 3-point scale	Self-administered	No information available	Content	No information available
SERVQUAL for Patient Satisfaction with Nursing (Scardina, 1994)	Postoperative cardiothoracic patients	Expectations vs perceptions: Domains include tangibles, reliability, responsiveness, assurance, and empathy; 44 items with 22 pairs of matching expectation/perception.	Self-administered	Cronbach's alpha reliability of .74 to .98, with the exception of empathy perception (.40).	Content	No information available
SERVQUAL for Quality Disconfirmation in Nursing (Scardina, 1994)	Patients in medical-surgical units	22 items based on five dimensions; demographic variables, overall satisfaction with hospital service, overall satisfaction with nursing care, patients' intent to return to hospital for future care, and patient intent to recommend hospital to others	Self-administered	Cronbach's alpha reliability of .845 to .894	Content, construct	Reliability is the most significant dimension in predicting a subject's overall satisfaction with nursing care and intent to return.
Care/Satisfaction Questionnaire (Larson & Ferketich, 1993)	Inpatient hospital setting	Nursing behaviors that denoted caring to nurses and patient: accessibility, anticipation, comfort, trusting relationship, explaining and facilitating, and monitoring/following through. Domains include benign neglect, enabling, and assistive; 29 items rated by marking an "X" on a line indicating how much the patient agrees or disagrees (1–10).	Self-administered	Cronbach's alpha reliability of .94 for total scale	Content, construct	No information available
Quality of Multidisciplinary Care Scale (Blegen & Goode, 1993)	Maternity patients	Technical, communication, interpersonal, outcome, participation, general satisfaction, and maternity care; 31 items rated on a 5-point scale	Self-administered	Cronbach's alpha reliability of .94 for total scale	No information available	Patient satisfaction with nursing care was significantly higher following implementation of a critical pathway system (Goode, 1995).

(continues)

TABLE 8-1A   Selected Measures of Patient Satisfaction with Nursing Care Developed by Nursing Researchers (continued)

Instrument (author)	Target population	Domains (number of items and response format)	Method of administration	Reliability	Validity	Sensitivity to nursing care
Critical Care Patient Satisfaction Survey (Megivern, Halm, & Jones, 1992)	Critical care setting	Art of care, technical quality of care, physical environment, availability, continuity of care, efficacy/outcomes of care, recognition of individual qualities and needs, reassuring presence, promotion of patient autonomy, and patient/family education: 43 items rated on a 5-point scale with open-ended questions	Self-administered	Interrater reliability	Content	No information available
Patient Satisfaction with Nursing Care Questionnaire (Eriksen, 1987, 1995)	Inpatient hospital setting	Art of care, technical quality of care, physical environment, availability, continuity of care, and efficacy/outcomes of care; original 35 items, revised 34 items rated on a magnitude estimation scale	Self-administered	No information available	Construct, content	No information available
La Monica-Oberst Patient Satisfaction Scale (La Monica et al., 1986); adapted by Munro et al. (1994). *Adaptation of Risser's (1975) tool.	Oncology patients (La Monica et al., 1986); C-section non-oncologic hysterectomy patients; and women with gestational diabetes (Munro et al., 1994)	Patients' ratings of the extent to which they have experienced nurse behaviors during their hospital stay; domains include technical/professional, trusting relationship, education, dissatisfaction, interpersonal support, and good impression; original 41 items revised to 28 by Munro et al. (1994); five- or seven-item scales	Self-administered	Cronbach's alpha reliability of .92 to .97 for total scale; .80 to .96 for subscales	Construct, content	Patient satisfaction with nursing care and patients' perceptions of organizational climate for service were each positively related to patients' perception of service quality (La Monica et al., 1986).

Patient Satisfaction Instrument (Hinshaw & Atwood, 1982) *Adaptation of Risser's (1975) tool.	Medical/surgical inpatients and outpatients	Technical/professional, education, and trusting relationship; 25 items rated on a 5-point scale	Self-administered	Cronbach's alpha reliability of .44 to .97 for subscales	Construct, concurrent	Nursing care delivery model and patient length of time on the unit were significant predictors of patient satisfaction with nursing care (Kangas et al., 1999); higher satisfaction scores reported by patients cared for by RNs working in a unit with shared governance, as opposed to units with traditional governance (Stumpf, 2001).
Patient Satisfaction Scale (Risser, 1975)	Ambulatory setting	Degree of congruency between patients' expectations of ideal nursing care and their perception of the real nursing care they receive; domains included technical/professional, education, and trusting relationship; 25 items rated on a 5-point scale.	Self-administered	Cronbach's alpha reliabilities of .91 for total scale; .63 to .89 for subscales	Construct, content	Collaboration between RN/NA resulted in two areas of increased patient satisfaction: trust in the nurse, and feeling cared about by the nurse (Hayes, 1992).

TABLE 8-1B   Selected Measures of Patient Satisfaction with Nursing Care Developed by Health Services Researchers

Instrument (author)	Target population	Domains (number of items and response format)	Method of administration	Reliability	Validity	Sensitivity to nursing care
Quality of End-of-Life Care and Satisfaction with Treatment (QUEST) scale; adapted by Sulmasy, McIlvane, Pasley, & Rahn (2002)	Medical inpatients	9 items regarding the quality of the interpersonal aspects of care; 6 items regarding patients' satisfaction with care; 5-point scale to assess how often particular behaviors or styles of care were true of physicians or nurses	Self-administered	Cronbach's alpha scores of 0.83 for patient ratings of physician quality and 0.88 for nurse quality	Content	This scale is useful in assessing quality and satisfaction with the care rendered by physicians and nurses to hospitalized patients at the end of life.
Inpatient Nursing Service Quality (Koerner, 2000)	Inpatient hospital setting	Close relationship, uncertainly reduction, individualized care, compassion, and reliability; 14 items, number of items varies for each subscale.	Self-administered	Cronbach's alpha reliabilities of .74 to .91 for subscales	Content	No information available
Press Ganey Satisfaction Measurement (Kaldenberg & Regrut, 1999)	Inpatient emergency, and ambulatory care	Registration/access, lab/x-ray, nurses/staff, physicians, center/building; 26–32 items; number of items varies for each subscale.	Self-administered	Cronbach's alpha reliabilities of .86 to .92 for subscales	Content	A study reported in their own publication found a strong correlation between nurse job satisfaction and patient satisfaction and patient satisfaction when the Press Ganey inpatient satisfaction instrument was used.
Quality of Care Monitors (Carey & Seibert, 1993)	Inpatient, emergency; and ambulatory care	Different aspects of hospital experience: admission/billing, courtesy, nursing care, physician care, religious care, medical outcomes, food services, comfort and cleanliness, overall quality of care, and willingness to return and recommend; number of items varies; response format: 5-point Likert scale.	Self-administered	Cronbach's alpha reliabilities of .44 to .92 for subscales; test-retest reliability showed a kappa value of more than 60% (Charles et al., 1994).	Content, construct (Charles et al., 1994)	The nursing scale had the highest correlation with overall patient care ratings, with 59% of the variance in patient satisfaction explained by the nursing care subscale, courtesy subscale, comfort/cleanliness subscale, and physician care subscale.
Modified SERVQUAL (Babakus & Mangold, 1992)	Inpatient hospital setting	Reliability, responsiveness, assurance, empathy, and tangibles; 15 pairs of matching expectation/perception items rated on 5-point scales	Self-administered	Cronbach's alpha reliabilities of .49 to .90 for subscales	Construct, content	No information available

Instrument	Setting	Description	Administration	Reliability	Validity	Comments
Picker-Commonwealth Survey of Patient-Centered Care (Cleary et al., 1991)	Hospitals, ambulatory care	Respect for patients; values preferences and expressed needs; coordination of care and integration of services; information, communication, and education; physical comfort; emotional support and alleviation of fear and anxiety; involvement of family and friends; transition and continuity; item number varies.	Self-administered	Test-retest reliability assessed	Content	A strong predictor of patient satisfaction with hospitalization was the interunit working relationships and hours per patient day (Sovie & Jawad, 2001).
Patient Judgments of Hospital Quality Questionnaire (Meterko et al., 1990)	Inpatient hospital setting	Nursing and daily care, hospital environment and ancillary staff, medical care, information admissions, discharge and billing, overall quality of care and services, recommendations and intentions and overall health outcomes; 106 items used in pilot study; various forms available. Response format is 5-point Likert scale.	Self-administered	Cronbach's alpha reliabilities for subscales ranged from .66 to .94; test-retest reliability assessed	Construct, content	Nursing subscale was the strongest predictor of overall rating of hospital quality and behavioral intentions (intention to return to the hospital if necessary and intention to recommend the hospital to others). Patients' perceptions of the overall quality of care were significantly related to the degree of emotional exhaustion that nurses experience (Leiter et al., 1998).
Patient Questionnaire (Abramowitz et al., 1987)	Inpatient hospital setting	Attribute satisfaction for 9 sets of services (admission, attending physicians, housing staff, nurses, nurses' aides, housekeeping, food services, escort services, and other staff); three outcome measures: overall satisfaction, intent to return to hospital, and intent to recommend hospital to others; 37 items; Likert-response format.	Self-administered	Internal consistency reliability ranged from .51 to .95.	Construct content	Patient satisfaction with nursing care was the only service related to overall satisfaction with hospital stay.
Patient Satisfaction Questionnaire (Guzman et al., 1988)	Inpatient hospital setting	Nursing care, admission process, other hospital services, information-giving and interpersonal skills: 30 items rated on a 3-point and a 5-point scale.	Self-administered	None reported	None reported	No information available

TABLE 8-2 Studies Investigating the Relation Between Nursing Variables and Patient Satisfaction

Author/date	Design of study	Characteristics of the sample, response rate, and setting	Patient satisfaction outcome	Intervention being evaluated/nursing variable being evaluated	Major results	Limitations
Shen, Sherwood, McNeill, & Li (2008)	Cross-sectional survey	Randomized sample of four to seven surgery wards within five randomly selected tertiary hospitals; $n = 974$; ($RR = 31\%$)	Houston Patient Outcome Instrument (HPOI) (McNeill et al., 2003)	To describe pain management outcomes and determine relationships between patient satisfaction and other clinical pain outcomes	Patients reported higher ratings of satisfaction with care from the doctor than from the nurse. The majority of participants reported high overall satisfaction despite high pain ratings.	Low response rate (31%)
Tervo-Heikkinen, Partanen, et al. (2008)	Cross-sectional survey	34 inpatient wards at four Finnish university hospitals; patients ($n = 4045$; $RR = 43\%$); head nurses ($n = 34$; $RR = 100\%$); registered nurses ($n = 664$; $RR = 68\%$)	Patient Satisfaction Survey	To assess patient satisfaction and analyze its relationship to nurse staffing levels	RN hours per patient load had a statistically significant positive correlation with patient satisfaction ($R^2 = 31.9\%$); when RN hours per patient load increased, satisfaction also increased.	No limitations noted
Tervo-Heikkinen, Kvist et al. (2008)	Cross-sectional survey	664 registered nurses on 34 acute care inpatient hospital wards ($RR = 68\%$); patient data ($n = 4045$)	Nursing Work Index-Revised (NWI-R) (Kramer & Hafner, 1989)	To assess the interrelationships between nurses' work environment and patient outcomes	When RN evaluations on standards of professional nursing increased ($R^2 = 17.5\%$), staffing adequacy was also evaluated positively ($R^2 = 16.7\%$), nursing respect and relationships were high ($R^2 = 13.0\%$), and patients' level of satisfaction increased.	Indicators of frequency of adverse events are subject (potential for bias) to varying response rate across different wards.
Clark et al. (2007)	Descriptive, correlational	827,430 patients, 733 hospitals, and 25 states participated in this study.	Patient Satisfaction Instrument (Hinshaw & Atwood, 1982); Hospital Care Quality Information from the Consumer Perspective (HCAHP)	To explore the relationship between nursing shortages and patient satisfaction	Strong significant correlation between RN supply and patients' satisfaction with the experience of nursing care ($r = 0.54$)	Study does not possess data from all 50 states.

Author	Design	Sample	Instrument	Purpose	Findings	Comments
Kee et al. (2005)	Descriptive, correlational, and comparative quantitative design	Data were collected from 138 patients (RR = 33%) and 103 nurses (RR = 56%) in four medical-surgical units and four ICUs in two Army Medical Centers.	Patient Satisfaction Instrument (Hinshaw & Atwood, 1982), Nursing Work Index-Revised (Kramer & Hafner, 1989)	To identify differences in patient satisfaction outcomes between mixed medical-surgical bed and specialty intensive care units (ICUs)	Satisfaction with nursing care was higher for patients in the ICUs (intensive care units $M = 103.50$, $SD = 14.71$) as compared with medical-surgical units ($M = 99.40$, $SD = 12.40$).	Differences in military patients vs civilian patients, exclusion of patients who were sickest and most acutely ill.
Innis et al. (2004)	Longitudinal survey	50 patients were surveyed during Time 1, and 50 different patients were surveyed during Time 2 (RR = 100%).	American Pain Society's Pain Satisfaction Questionnaire in Hospitalized Patients with Acute Pain or Chronic Pain	To explore the impact of pain education for nurses on patient satisfaction with pain management	Pain education has an impact on patient satisfaction with pain management: Time 1 (62%), Time 2 (82%); ($2 = 6.151$, $df = 2$, $p = .046$).	Patients did not experience less pain, despite being more satisfied.
Lageson (2004)	Descriptive cross-sectional survey	53 non-ICU nursing units; nurse managers, RNs, other nursing personnel (LPNs and nursing assistants), and physicians (RR = 47%). Patient data were collected as part of a quarterly standardized survey distributed by the hospital.	Quality of Care Monitor	To examine the relationship between the quality focus of the first-line nurse manager and patient satisfaction, job satisfaction of the nursing personnel, unit effectiveness, staff perceptions of quality, and nursing personnel turnover.	Quality focus was found to be a significant predictor variable only for staff nurse job satisfaction. Overall patient satisfaction ($R^2 = 0.020$) proved to be insignificant when related to quality focus.	Convenience sampling; results across units may not be comparable; timing of retrieval; complicated recruitment.
Larrabee et al. (2004)	Predictive, nonexperimental study, retrospective	Academic medical center in north-central West Virginia. Convenience samples of patients ($N = 362$) and RNs ($N = 90$) were recruited from two medical units, two surgical units, and three intensive care step-down units.	Work Quality Index (Whitley & Putzier, 1994); Patient's Judgments of Nursing Care Questionnaire (Larrabee et al., 2004)	To investigate the influence of RN job satisfaction on patient satisfaction	RN job satisfaction is not a significant predictor of patient satisfaction ($r = .04$, $p > .05$).	Homogenous sample, did not consider rules about aggregation of individual data to units.
Otani & Kurz (2004)	Cross-sectional study	Stratified random sampling; patients ($n = 6,000$) selected from the four participating hospitals between 1997 and 1998.	Survey instrument not specified	To investigate which health-care attributes are significantly related to patient satisfaction and how they affect overall patient satisfaction and behavioral intentions	Improving the nursing care attribute is the most effective manner for enhancing patient satisfaction and behavioral intentions (patient overall satisfaction, $R^2 = 0.66$; behavioral intentions, $R^2 = 0.63$).	Cross-sectional study; nonrespondents and missing values; sampling distribution of predictor and dependent variables were not normal.

(continues)

TABLE 8-2   Studies Investigating the Relation Between Nursing Variables and Patient Satisfaction (continued)

Author/date	Design of study	Characteristics of the sample, response rate, and setting	Patient satisfaction outcome	Intervention being evaluated/nursing variable being evaluated	Major results	Limitations
Vahey et al. (2004)	Cross-sectional study	Sample consisted of nurses ($n = 820$; $RR = 86\%$) and patients ($n = 722$; $RR = 86\%$) from 40 units in 20 urban hospitals across the United States.	La Monica-Oberst Patient Satisfaction Scale (La Monica et al., 1986)	The effect of the nurse work environment on nurse burn-out, and the effects of the nurse work environment and nurse burnout on patients' satisfaction with their nursing care	Patients on units with positive environments are 1.49 times as likely as those on average units and $1.49^2 = 2.2$ times as likely as those on negative units (in which nurses display emotional exhaustion, depersonalization, and intend to leave within the next year) to be highly satisfied with their nursing care.	Information not available
Yen & Lo (2004)	Cross-sectional survey	Adult hospitalized patients with medical or surgical diagnosis in southern Taiwan, ROC (Republic of China); ($n = 755$; $RR = 75\%$)	Patient Assessment of Hospital Care (Picker Institute, 1988)	To explore the relationship between and among structure, process, and outcome variables with respect to patient perceptions of care and patient satisfaction	Perceived nursing care quality had a moderate positive effect on comfort ($r = 0.22$) and overall satisfaction ($r = 0.24$). Process variables, patient-perceived continuity, and quality of care positively influenced patient comfort and patient satisfaction. Furthermore, higher coordination of care resulted in shorter length of stay.	Extraneous variables related to health status; need to consider additional process factors and additional outcomes.
McGillis Hall et al. (2003)	Repeated-measures study	Sample comprised 19 teaching hospitals in Ontario, Canada (adult medical-surgical and obstetric inpatients); $n = 1875$	Patient Judgment of Hospital Quality Questionnaire (Meterko et al., 1990).	To evaluate the impact of different nurse staffing models on the patient outcomes of functional status, pain control, and patient satisfaction with nursing care.	Patients were more highly satisfied with obstetric nursing care when there was a higher proportion of regulated staff. No nurse staffing variables or professional mix variables were related to patient satisfaction in medical-surgical patients.	Response rate (patient attrition could have resulted in some types of patients not participating in the study).

Author (Year)	Design	Sample	Instrument	Purpose	Findings	Notes
Yeakel et al. (2003)	Quasi-experimental design	Patients discharged from general surgery units; preintervention period (*n* = 172), postintervention period (*n* = 181)	Hartford Hospital Patient Satisfaction Survey	The intervention, aimed at improving nurse caring behaviors, is composed of five facets: the provision of a formal education session, staff identification of goals, peer reinforcement, incorporation of goals into performance management, and posting of examples of caring behaviors. This was implemented to measure the effect of improved nurse caring behaviors on patient satisfaction.	A multifaceted intervention involving all nursing unit staff is able to improve patients' ratings of nurse caring ($Z = -2.14$, $p = .032$) and satisfaction ($Z = -2.86$, $p = .004$). Furthermore, there is a positive and significant correlation between nurse caring and patient satisfaction ($r = 0.791$).	Findings are not generalizable (the study took place on one unit of a single hospital).
Barkell et al. (2002)	Descriptive comparison	$N = 139$ prechange group; $n = 108$ posttest group; inpatient surgical unit in a Midwest community-based teaching hospital.	Parkside Patient Satisfaction Survey	Effects of a change in care delivery model (team nursing to total patient care) on patient satisfaction	No significant differences between the groups in overall patient satisfaction	Cronbach's alpha reliabilities not reported
Burney, Purden, & McVey (2002)	Mixed methods	384 patients who had been discharged from a hospital's cardiology step-down unit (*RR = 42%*)	System to Evaluate the Quality of Care and the Users' Satisfaction (SEQUS, Version 2, 1998)	To evaluate patients' satisfaction in relation to the quality of care they receive during discharge	Overall, 52% of patients were satisfied with how their discharge needs were met.	No information available
Doran et al. (2002)	Cross-sectional survey	372 patients (RR = 73%) and 254 nurses (RR = 35%) from 26 general medical-surgical and cardiac units in a southern Ontario tertiary hospital	Patient Judgments of Hospital Quality-Nursing Subscale (Meterko et al., 1990).	The impact of nurse, unit, and patient structural variables on patient outcomes, and nurses' and patients' perceptions of nurses' role performance	Patient satisfaction with nursing care was higher on units where nurses reported good communication among the healthcare team members; patient satisfaction with nursing care was related to functional status, self-care ability, and emotional health at discharge.	Low nursing response rate (39%)
Johansson, Oleni, & Fridlund (2002)	Literature review of patient satisfaction with nursing care	30 studies published between 1987 and 1999 were found. The majority of the articles were statistically analyzed observation studies, which were carried out in the United Kingdom, Sweden, and the United States.	N/A	To explore patient satisfaction with nursing care in the context of health care	Patients' expectations regarding health care are a key factor when it comes to satisfaction with nursing care	The literature study primarily illuminates patient satisfaction from a Western world perspective; the scientific articles originate from the United Kingdom, Sweden, and the United States.

(continues)

TABLE 8-2　Studies Investigating the Relation Between Nursing Variables and Patient Satisfaction (continued)

Author/date	Design of study	Characteristics of the sample, response rate, and setting	Patient satisfaction outcome	Intervention being evaluated/nursing variable being evaluated	Major results	Limitations
Tzeng, Ketefian, & Redman (2002)	Exploratory study	17 patient care units from a tertiary healthcare organization in the Midwest; 520 nurses ($RR = 28\%$) and 345 patients ($RR = 36\%$) participated in this study.	Nurse Assessment Survey (Braskamp & Maehr, 1985); the Nursing Services Inpatient Satisfaction Survey (Ketefian, Redman, Nash, & Bogue, 1997)	Self-administered questionnaires were used to test the relationship between nurses' job satisfaction and patient satisfaction with nursing care.	Nurses' job satisfaction predicted inpatient satisfaction significantly and positively; path coefficient based on simple regression analysis revealed an indirect effect of .38.	Small sample size, low response rate, timing of data collection
Tzeng & Ketefian (2002)	Exploratory study	Data were collected from six inpatient units at a teaching hospital located in southern Taiwan. Patients ($n = 59$) and nurses ($n = 103$) participated in this study; $RR = 91\%$.	The Patient Satisfaction Questionnaire with Quality of Nursing Care; the Nurses' Job Satisfaction Questionnaire	To test the relationship between nurses' job satisfaction and inpatient satisfaction with quality of nursing care in Taiwan.	General job satisfaction was significantly correlated with inpatient satisfaction, particularly with pain management and discomfort ($p = 0.866$).	Small sample size, study design
Sengin (2001)	Secondary analysis	95 units located within 21 hospitals; 6,440 patients and 1,228 nurses participated in this study.	The Inpatient Satisfaction Survey (Regrut, 1997); the Employee Satisfaction survey (Press, 2000), Press Ganey Patient Satisfaction Survey.	Correlational and multilevel regression models were used to examine the relationship between RN job satisfaction and patient satisfaction in acute care hospitals.	RN job satisfaction has a significant effect on patient satisfaction with nursing care ($t = 2.14$, $p = 0.03$) and overall patient satisfaction ($t = 2.17$, $p = 0.034$). In addition, patient satisfaction with nursing care had a significant effect on RN job satisfaction ($t = 2.28$, $p = 0.024$).	Data set did not include any demographic information regarding the patients or nurses in the sample; differences in nursing composition data can only be generalized to acute care hospitals.

Author (year)	Design; setting	Sample	Instrument	Purpose	Findings	Limitations
Sovie & Jawad (2001)	3-year longitudinal study; two acute care adult inpatient units from 29 U.S. university teaching hospitals	N ranged from 12 to 26 per unit; RR not reported	Combination of the Picker Institute and Press Ganey Patient Satisfaction surveys	3-year study of restructuring collected data on nurse full-time equivalents (FTEs), skill mix, and hours worked per patient day (HPPD)	Patient satisfaction increased to mid-80% range when HPPD increased from the 4- to 4.5-hour to the 5- to 6-hour range; interunit working relationships and HPPD were strong predictors of patient satisfaction with hospitalization; patient satisfaction with pain management was positively related to the HPPD and was influenced by physician-related factors on medical units and nurse-related factors on surgical units.	Variety of methods used to complete questionnaires—mail, telephone, and interviews; Cronbach's alpha reliability estimates not reported.
Stumpf (2001)	Ex post facto, correlational; five hospitals in southwestern Pennsylvania (three metropolitan, two rural)	16 units in five hospitals: 8 traditional/8 shared governance, N = 120 patients	Patients' Opinion of Nursing Care (Hinshaw & Atwood, 1982)	Influence of unit governance type (shared governance vs bureaucratic model) on culture, work satisfaction, nurse retention, and patient satisfaction.	There was a significant difference in the mean total scores for satisfaction with nursing care in a shared governance model vs a traditional governance model ($p < .05$), with patients in a shared governance model scoring higher.	Statistical details not reported.
Kaldenberg & Becker (1999)	Descriptive, correlational; multi-site	36,078 patients from 275 ambulatory surgery center across the United States	Press Ganey Satisfaction Measurement (Kaldenberg & Regrut, 1999)	Patient satisfaction with nurses/staff, physicians, center/building, registration/access, and lab/x-ray.	Highest mean ratings to friendliness of the nurse (95%), nurses' concern for comfort (92.6%), and information given by nurses before surgery (92.7%); nurses/staff and building/center factors strongest predictors of the likelihood to recommend.	Cronbach's alpha not reported.
Kangas et al. (1999)	Descriptive, correlational; multi-site	Three hospitals, 92 nurses, and 90 patients from medical-surgical and ICU units	Patient Satisfaction with Nursing Care (Hinshaw & Atwood, 1982).	RNs' job satisfaction, three nursing care delivery models (team nursing, case management, and primary nursing), organizational structures and culture, and controlling for patient characteristics	Nursing care delivery model and patient length of time on the unit were significant predictors of patient satisfaction with nursing care ($R^2 = .10$); patients receiving care in the primary nursing delivery model were more satisfied.	Relatively small explained variance ($R^2 = 10\%$)
Lynn & McMillen (1999)	Descriptive	350 nurses and 448 patients from 40 medical-surgical units in seven hospitals in the southern United States	Patients' Perceptions of Quality Scale– Acute Care Version (PPQS-AV)	Evaluation of the extent of agreement between nurses and patients on the importance of various elements of quality of nursing care	Patients ranked the physical environment, psychological aspects of care, and professionalism higher, whereas nurses ranked trust, empathy, competence, examinations, and explanations higher.	No limitations noted

(continues)

TABLE 8-2 Studies Investigating the Relation Between Nursing Variables and Patient Satisfaction (continued)

Author/date	Design of study	Characteristics of the sample, response rate, and setting	Patient satisfaction outcome	Intervention being evaluated/nursing variable being evaluated	Major results	Limitations
Moore et al. (1999)	Prospective and retrospective descriptive design	Patients and nurses from 16 medical-surgical units in a southeastern U.S. academic medical center	Patients' Perception of Quality Scale-Acute Care Version	ANA Nursing Quality Indicators	Percentage of RNs on the unit and total nursing care hours per patient day were predictors of patient satisfaction.	Small sample size following data aggregation (16 units)
Lynn & Moore (1997)	Retrospective correlational; survey completed 24 hours prior to discharge	Patients and nurses from 16 medical-surgical units in an academic medical center in the southwestern United States	Patients' Perceptions of Quality Scale-Acute Care Version (PPQS-AV); Nurses' Perceptions of Quality Scale-Acute Care Version (NPQS-AV)	Relationships between the patients' perceptions of care received, the nurses' perceptions of care delivered, and traditional measures of nursing care quality (volume, acuity, and risk management indicators)	Neither patients' nor nurses' perceptions of care quality were strong predictors of "traditional" measures of patient care quality; of all possible subscale correlations, only those of the NPQS-ACV were significantly related to any of the traditional quality indicators.	Small sample size following data aggregation (16 units)
Goode (1995)	Experimental	Postpartum units in a large acute care tertiary university-affiliated hospital in the midwestern United States; overall $RR = 69\%$. Experimental group: $n = 107$, data collection over 7.5 months; control group: $n = 100$, data collection over 6.5 months; no data collected during a 2-month phase-in period	Quality of Multidisciplinary Care Scale (Blegen & Goode, 1993)	Evaluated impact of multidisciplinary critical path with nurse case managers on patient satisfaction, staff job satisfaction, collaboration, and autonomy	Patients receiving care under the critical pathway system were significantly more satisfied than patients who received care under the old system (total patient care); participation in decisions was the only significantly different subscale between the two groups.	Cronbach's alpha reliabilities for subscales ranged from .66 to .86.
Larrabee et al. (1995)	Descriptive, correlational data collected at admission and discharge	Two medical-surgical units in a 455-bed urban hospital; 199 patients ($RR = 71\%$)	Patients' Judgments of Hospital Quality-Nursing Subscale (Meterko et al., 1990).	Testing a patient-focused model of quality by identifying predictors of patient perceptions of nursing care quality.	Pain severity at discharge and patient goal achievement were significant predictors of overall quality of care; nurses' perceptions of quality of care and goal achievement were not predictors of patient satisfaction.	No limitations noted

Study	Design	Sample	Instrument	Purpose	Findings	Limitations
Charles et al. (1994)	Cross-sectional survey	Stratified random sample of 57 public acute care hospitals in two provinces ($RR = 79\%$); 4,599 medical/surgical patients participated ($RR = 69\%$).	Modified version of the Picker Institute Patient Satisfaction Survey	Satisfaction with provider–patient communication, respect for preferences, attentiveness to physical needs, education, relationship between patient and physician, education and communication with family, pain management, and hospital discharge planning	61% of patients reported problems, with fewer than 5 of 39 specific care processes evaluated; patients who were dissatisfied with the postdischarge instructions by doctors and nurses reported significantly more problems.	No information on patient diagnosis or severity of illness for the episode of care
Goodell & Van Ess Coeling (1994)	Pilot study	Random sample of 33 matched pairs of nurses/patients in an urban midwestern U.S. teaching hospital	Patient Satisfaction Instrument (Hinshaw & Atwood, 1982)	Tested the relationship between patient satisfaction with nursing care and nurses' job satisfaction	Six subscales of nurses' job satisfaction were not significantly related to three subscales of patient satisfaction with nursing care All correlations were between $r = -.29$ and $.06$, $p > .05$ in all cases.	Small sample size
Hayes (1992)	Experimental design; control and experimental groups on six general medical/surgical units; data collected at beginning, middle, and end of project	444 patients and 118 RNs from a large urban teaching center	Patient Satisfaction with Nursing Care (Risser, 1975)	Evaluation of a professional practice model that included head nurses' involvement in restructuring the RN/NA working relationship, consistent assignments, clarification of the RN/NA relationship and responsibility, and team building.	RN/NA collaboration was significant with respect to two areas of increased patient satisfaction: trust in the nurse and feeling cared about by the nurse.	No information on instrument or psychometric properties
Abramowitz et al. (1987)	Descriptive, correlational	841 patients from several units in a large New York teaching hospital ($RR = 91.3\%$)	Patient Questionnaire (Abramowitz et al., 1987)	Patient assessments of 10 services, including nursing	Patient satisfaction with nursing care was the only service related to overall satisfaction with hospital stay; satisfaction with nursing care and expectations for hospital care accounted for 24% of the variance in overall satisfaction; overall satisfaction strongly related to paying attention to patients' concerns ($r = .65$).	No limitations noted

TABLE 8-3 Comparison of 10 Patient Satisfaction Instruments Using Quality Indicators Identified in the Literature

Identified quality indicators	CARE/SAT (Larson & Ferketich, 1993)	Satisfaction with nursing care (Eriksen, 1995)	La Monica-Oberst Patient Satisfaction Scale (Munro et al., 1994)	SERVQUAL for Patient Satisfaction with Nursing (Scardina, 1994)	Patient Judgments of Hospital Quality ± (Meterko et al., 1990)	Picker-Commonwealth Survey of Patient-Centred Care ± (Cleary et al., 1991)	Press Ganey Patient Satisfaction Survey ± (Kaldenberg & Regrut, 1999)	Patients' Judgements of Nursing Care ± (Larrabee et al., 2004)	Patient Satisfaction with Nursing Care Quality Questionnaire ± (Laschinger, et al. 2005)	Patient's Assessment of Quality Scale-Acute Care Version ± (Lynn et al., 2007)
Met expectations	*	****	****	**					*	
Caring style	**	****	******	****	*			*	**	******
Friendliness/ courtesy	*	****	****	**	*	***	**	*	*	**
Attention to patient concerns	*******	*******	***	**	****	****	*	**	***	*
Information sharing	****	*	*******	*	***	****	**	*	*****	
Communication and interpersonal skills	****	*	***	**	**	***	*	*	*	**
Competence/ skill	****	*	**	***	*	*	*	*	*	*
Goal achievement	**	****			**	***	*			
Professional practice/ care delivery models			*		*	**			*	
Organizational factors				*****	**	*	**			
Overall healthcare experience					*	**	*	*	*	**
TOTAL ITEMS	29	34	28	22	28	30	11	9	19	45

* Each asterisk represents an item on the questionnaire.
± Items relevant to nursing.

TABLE 8-4 Comparison of Ten Patient Satisfaction Instruments Using Patient-Identified Quality Indicators

Identified quality indicators	CARE/SAT (Larson & Ferketich, 1993)	Satisfaction with nursing care (Eriksen, 1995)	La Monica-Oberst Patient Satisfaction Scale (Munro et al., 1994)	SERVQUAL for Patient Satisfaction with Nursing (Scardina, 1994)	Patient Judgments of Hospital Quality ± (Meterko et al., 1990)	Picker-Commonwealth Survey of Patient-Centred Care ± (Cleary et al., 1991)	Press Ganey Patient Satisfaction Survey ± (Kaldenberg & Regrut, 1999)	Patients' Judgements of Nursing Care ± (Larrabee et al., 2004)	Patient Satisfaction with Nursing Care Quality Questionnaire ± (Laschinger et al., 2005)	Patient's Assessment of Quality Scale- Acute Care Version ± (Lynn et al., 2007)
Caring style	**	****	****	****	*			**	*	******
Respectful manner	*	**	***	*	*	***	**		*	**
Attention to patient concerns	*******	*******	***	**	****	****	*	**	*	*
Participation in care	***	*	*		**	**			**	
Availability/ timeliness of care	***	*	****	*****	**	****	*	*	***	*
Information sharing/ interpretation of symptoms	****	*	******		***	****	**	*	***	
Competence/ skill	****	*	**	***	*	*	*	*	*	*
Pain control	*	*	**		*	**				
Physical care	*	*	*							
Communication with other providers	**	*			**	***		*	**	
Education/ preparation for discharge	*	*			**	****	*		**	*
Pleasant physical environment	*	*		****	*		*		*	**
Overall healthcare experience			*		*	**	*	*		
TOTAL ITEMS	29	34	28	22	28	30	11	9	19	45

* Each asterisk represents an item on the questionnaire.
± Items relevant to nursing.

be used by nursing administrators to improve the patient care process. Few of the instruments addressed all the factors found in the literature.

Instruments Developed by Nursing Researchers

Numerous measures of patient satisfaction have been developed by nursing researchers. In this section, well established tools are described, as well as newer tools published in the past 5 years. All measures reported here have undergone vigorous psychometric analysis and address factors shown to be important by both patients and nurses in judging nursing care quality.

Risser (1975), who was the first nurse researcher to implicitly propose a model of patient satisfaction, created a standardized measure of patient satisfaction by using a match between expectations and care received as a definition of satisfaction. Satisfaction consisted of three dimensions: (a) technical/professional behaviors (i.e., nursing knowledge and techniques required for competent nursing care); (b) a trusting relationship (i.e., communication and interpersonal skills required to create a healing climate); and (c) an educational relationship (i.e., information-sharing about patient condition and care processes). This measure has served as the basis for other instruments developed over the years by nurse researchers. Hinshaw and Atwood (1982) modified this tool to make it more suitable to inpatient settings, but they maintained the same underlying dimensions. The Patient Satisfaction Instrument (PSI) continues to be used in nursing research and has shown respectable psychometric properties. Recently, Yellen, Davis, and Ricard (2002) adapted the PSI for use in ambulatory care and found it to be a valid and reliable measure in that setting. In developing the La Monica-Oberst Patient Satisfaction Scale (LOPSS), La Monica, Oberst, Madea, and Wolf (1986) added items related to physical and comfort care and obtained three categories of factors in an exploratory factor analysis: patient dissatisfaction, interpersonal support, and good impression. In La Monica et al.'s study, patient satisfaction with nursing care and patients' perceptions of the organizational climate for service were each positively related to patients' perceptions of service quality ($r = .74$, $p < .001$, and $r = .71$, $p < .001$, respectively). In 1994, Munro, Jacobsen, and Brooten modified the LOPSS and found two factors in a series of factor analyses: interpersonal support (14 items) and patient dissatisfaction (14 items).

In 1993, Larson and Ferketich developed the CARE/SAT, a 29-item measure of patient satisfaction with regard to nurses' caring behaviors. This tool was derived from the CARE-Q, a 50-item measure of nursing caring behaviors with well-established psychometric characteristics. The modified tool was designed to be easier to use in a clinical setting than the CARE-Q in that it contained fewer items and employed a visual analogue for easy scoring by patients. The CARE/SAT total scale and subscales all had acceptable internal consistency and strong correlations with the Risser (1975) patient satisfaction measure ($r = .80$), providing evidence of construct validity. Andrews, Daniels, and Hall (1996) found the CARE/SAT to require the shortest completion time (6 minutes) of several instruments tested in their study. In a recently published compendium of tools measuring caring in nursing, Watson (2009) included the CARE/SAT as a valid measure of caring effectiveness by nurses.

Eriksen (1995) revised the Patient Satisfaction with Nursing Care Questionnaire (PSNCQ) following an extensive concept analysis and literature review. She deleted items pertaining to the technical quality of nursing care, based on the belief that patients are not sufficiently qualified to evaluate professional standards of care (Oberst, 1984). Besides rewording items to more adequately reflect nursing care behaviors, she added new items, but no information is available in the published literature regarding their content. The revised instrument will require further testing to ascertain its psychometric properties. According to Pierce (1997), this tool is based on the clearest conceptualization of patient satisfaction available in the nursing literature. Nash et al. (1994) adapted this tool to evaluate the impact of a new professional practice model, shortening it from 34 items to 16 items and converting the scale to a yes/no/not applicable format to facilitate patient use. No results or psychometric properties were reported. However, patients reported having difficulty using the original scaling format and preferred the three-category response format previously described.

Mrayyan (2006) used a version of Eriksen's (1995) tool to study the relationships between Jordanian nurses' ($n = 200$) job satisfaction and patient satisfaction ($n = 510$). Patients rated their satisfaction with six aspects of nursing care on a 5-point Likert scale (1 = *very dissatisfied*, 5 = *very satisfied*). The Cronbach reliability for the total scale was .88. Patients reported moderate satisfaction on the six subscales: nurse availability, continuity of care, technical quality of care, art of care, efficacy of care, and physical environment (range 3.51–4.01). Nurses' job satisfaction was significantly and positively related to patient satisfaction ($r = .29$, $p = .01$). These results add further support for the psychometric properties of the PSNCQ and initial support for its use in countries outside North America.

Lynn and Moore (1997) sought to address criticisms in the literature that current patient satisfaction instruments reflected the provider's perspective to a greater extent than the patient's. Lynn and Sidani (1991) believed that any definition of patient satisfaction or description of quality must include the perspective of all parties involved in the care. Using both qualitative and quantitative methods, they elicited patients' perceptions of high-quality care in one-on-one interviews and developed a 54-item instrument, the Patient Perceptions of Quality Care-Acute Care Version (PPQC-ACV), to reflect attributes patients identified. A total of four factors were obtained in a factor analysis: professional demeanor, treating the patient like an individual, mindfulness, and responsiveness. They used a similar approach to create a 56-item tool to measure nurses' perceptions of the quality of care delivered to patients (Nurses' Perceptions of Quality Scale-Acute

Care Version [NPQS-ACV]). This tool consisted of five factors: developing a relationship, science of nursing, unit collaboration, the environment, and resources. Both tools were found to have good internal consistency and construct validity.

As the researchers predicted, neither the PPQC-ACV nor the NPQS-ACV was a strong predictor of traditional measures of patient care quality (volume, acuity, and risk management indicators), which supported the authors' contention that their traditional outcome measures are not valid nurse-sensitive quality indicators. Of all possible subscale correlations, only those of the NPQS-ACV were significantly related to any of the traditional quality indicators. Interestingly, all NPQS-ACV subscales were related to volume indicators such as the number of admissions and number of patient days. That is, nurses' perceptions of patient care quality were negatively related to workload factors, which suggested that the increasingly higher volume of patients to care for with the same or fewer resources was perceived to have a negative impact on patient care quality. These measures are of value because they represent patient and nurse perceptions of quality care elicited within the context of massive healthcare restructuring in the 1990s.

In a related study, Moore et al. (1999) examined the relationship between a modified version of the PPQC-ACV and the American Nurses Association Nursing Quality Indicators (ANA, 1996). Two structural quality indicators were significantly related to patient satisfaction with nursing care. The percentage of RNs on the unit was the most consistent predictor of patient satisfaction with nursing care, pain management, education, and overall care. The total number of nursing care hours provided per patient day was also a positive predictor of patient satisfaction with pain management and education. Internal consistency estimates for the factors ranged from 0.62 to 0.96.

In 2007, Lynn and colleagues reported the results of further development of the original PPQC-ACV. The title was changed to the Patient's Assessment of Quality Scale-Acute Care Version (PAQS-ACV). The sample for testing the PAQS-ACV included patients from 43 medical-surgical units who were 18 years of age or older, hospitalized for at least 48 hours, predicted to be discharged within 24 hours, and able to read and speak English, and who did not have an overt psychiatric disorder. The final sample consisted of 1,470 patients. Ten percent of the study participants were readministered the PAQS-ACV two weeks after discharge to assess test-retest reliability. Five additional items were included in the second mailing that asked about participants' healthcare experience. The same participants were also called 1 week later to ascertain the extent to which they were following their discharge orders, which were copied from their charts at the time of discharge. Each participant was assigned a score ranging from 1 to 4 based on the percentage adherence to discharge orders (ranging from < 25% to > 75%).

Construct validity was established by conducting a principal axis factor analysis with oblique rotation. Contrary to the original work with this measure that yielded four factors, this analysis supported a five-factor solution. Factors were: (1) individualization, (2) nurse characteristics, (3) caring, (4) environment, and (5) responsiveness, which were represented by 45 items on five factors that accounted for 54% of the variance. Cronbach's alpha for the five subscales ranged from .68 to .94, and correlations among the five subscales ranged from .26 to .70, satisfying the criteria for the uniqueness of each factor (Pedhazur & Schmelkin, 1991). Further construct validity was established by strong significant correlations between the PAQS-ACV and positive outcomes of patient care-patient's compliance with their prescribed regimen, their intention to return to the same facility for future care, and overall quality of care during their hospitalization. Interestingly, patients with lower perceived health status had significantly lower scores on all five PAQS-ACV factors, suggesting that the need to control for this variable when investigating patient satisfaction is warranted. Finally, patients who complied with 50% or more of their discharge orders had significantly higher PAQS-ACV scores (all factors) than did patients with less than 50% compliance or no compliance with their prescribed orders. The PAQS-ACV addresses all the patient-identified nursing care quality factors reported in the literature, with the exception of nursing competence. When Lynn and Moore (1997) conducted interviews with patients to obtain their views on important aspects of nursing care quality, competence was not an issue for patients. Rather, patients assumed that nurses employed in the hospital were technically competent. Thus, this dimension was not included in the measure.

Nursing researchers have also modified existing measures of patient care quality to focus specifically on nursing care. We found two measures that adapted a commonly used measure of patient care quality in health services research: the Patient Judgment of Hospital Quality (PJHQ) (Meterko et al., 1990).

Larrabee, Engle, and Tolley (1995) modified the Nursing and Daily Care subscale (NDCS) of the PJHQ (Meterko et al., 1990) to create a measure of patient satisfaction with nursing care quality. The scale consists of nine items with a 5-point Likert scale response format from 1 (*poor*) to 5 (*excellent*), with one item reflecting overall patient satisfaction. Scores for the first eight items are summed and averaged to yield a total patient satisfaction score. The Cronbach's alpha value for the total patient-perceived quality total scale was 0.94 in this study. The modified measure of patient satisfaction with aspects of nursing care quality was significantly related to patients' global assessment of nursing care ($r = 0.60$, $p < .01$), providing evidence of construct validity for this scale.

In a follow-up study, Larrabee et al. (2004) used a modified version of the NDCS, renamed the Patients' Judgment of Nursing Care (PJNC) scale, to test a theoretical model of patient satisfaction. A predictive nonexperimental survey design was used to collect data from 362 patients and 90 RNs in medical, surgical, and intensive care step-down units in a 450-bed academic medical center. Eligible patient participants were at least 18 years of age, were able to speak and read English, did not have a psychiatric diagnosis, and were admitted to one of the study units for at least 24 hours. Eligible nurse participants were employed on the study units for at least 3 months prior to completing the questionnaire. RN data were matched to patient participants for whom they had provided care during the study period. The Cronbach's alpha value for the PJNC was 0.94.

The PJNC assessed patient satisfaction with nursing care, self-reported health status, quality of life, and patient reading ability. The RN questionnaire assessed nurse job satisfaction, nurse manager leadership style, nurse–physician collaboration, and unit turbulence and staffing. Patients' perceptions of nurses' caring, as measured by the Caring Behaviors Inventory (Wolf et al., 1998), were a significant predictor of patient satisfaction with nursing care quality ($ß = 0.72, p < .001$). Nurses' ratings of nurse–physician (RN/MD) collaboration was the only nursing worklife predictor of patient satisfaction (PJNC) ($ß = 0.14, p = .003$). Age was an indirect predictor through patient-perceived nurse caring. The final model had a good fit to the data (chi square = 46.25, $df = 32$, $p = .049$, CFI = .98, TLI = .97, RMSEA = .04).

The Patient Satisfaction with Nursing Care Quality Questionnaire (PSNCQQ) is another measure of nursing care quality developed by Laschinger et al. (2005) and was derived from Meterko et al.'s (1990) PJHQ questionnaire. Following an extensive review of the literature on patient satisfaction with nursing care, selected items from the nine subscales of the original PJHQ were adapted to reflect satisfaction with components of nursing care. The PSNCQQ contains 19 items, with an additional 3 items designed for construct validity purposes measuring overall quality of care during hospital stay, overall quality of nursing care, and intention to recommend the hospital to family and friends. Each item was measured on a 5-point Likert scale ranging from *poor* to *excellent*. Prior to administering the new questionnaire, focus groups were conducted with nurse stakeholders to obtain feedback on the new instrument. The results established construct validity for the PSNCQQ based on agreement among the experts that the new instrument clearly and accurately reflected what nurses do. This study used a descriptive survey design and a random sample of 14 hospitals in Ontario, Canada, with a total of 1,041 participants. Patient satisfaction scores were high and similar across different hospital types, with means ranging from $M = 3.81$ ($SD = 0.89$) to $M = 4.30$ ($SD = 1.08$). The Cronbach's alpha reliability estimate was excellent ($α = .97$) for all hospital categories, suggesting that patients in different hospital systems interpreted items in a consistent manner. Construct validity was established through exploratory factor analysis, which suggested a one-factor solution, was confirmed in a confirmatory factor analysis. Further construct validity was established through testing its ability to predict generic measures of patient care quality used in health services research. After adjusting for length of stay, gender, age, and self-rated health, the PSNCQQ explained significant amounts of the variance in the overall quality of care and services (64%), overall quality of nursing care (73%), and intent to recommend the hospital to family and friends

(55%). To measure the sensitivity of the PSNCQQ, the overall satisfaction with care measure was dichotomized into excellent/very good and poor/fair responses. The PSNCQQ was found to discriminate between high and low levels of overall satisfaction of patients with the care they received during their hospital stay, adding further support for the construct validity of the instrument. The results of this study provided initial support for the reliability and validity of the PSNCQQ.

Because of the recency of the publication of the PSNCQQ, there have been few published reports of its use in the nursing literature. In a doctoral study of 604 patients from 26 general hospital wards in Taiwan, Chiu and Chung (2008) found that, contrary to the analysis in Laschinger et al.'s (2005) study, a three-factor model solution for the PSNCQQ was a good fit to the data. The factors obtained in the initial exploratory factor analysis were: (1) information offered, (2) daily care, and (3) environment. These factors were confirmed in a subsequent CFA. Cronbach's alpha reliabilities for each of the three factors ranged from .87 to .95. Scores for this study were similar to those in Laschinger et al.'s study, with factor means ranging from $M = 4.13$ $(SD = 0.69)$ to $M = 4.22$ $(SD = .064)$.

Further construct validity was established in Chiu and Chung's (2008) study through strong significant correlations between the PSNCQQ subscales, and overall satisfaction with hospital care quality and intentions to recommend the hospital to family and friends. Information offered, daily care, and environment all correlated highly with overall satisfaction ($r = .75, p < .001; r = .77, p < .001; r = .75, p < .001$, respectively). After controlling for number of hospital stays, information (ß $= .30, p < .001$), daily care (ß $= 0.29, p < .001$), and environment (ß $= 0.24, p < .001$) were significant independent predictors of total patient satisfaction, accounting for 64% of the variance in total patient satisfaction. Also, after controlling for number of hospital stays, the information (ß $= .41, p < .001$) and daily care (ß $= .24$, p $< .001$) PSNCQQ subscales were significant predictors of the patients' willingness to return to the hospital facility and to recommend it to friends and family ($R2 = .537$). Environment was not a significant predictor (ß $= .11, p = .065$). It should be noted that the two items related to discharge planning—discharge instructions and coordination of care after discharge—were excluded given that patients were asked to fill out the questionnaire during their hospital stay. The results of this study provide further support for the PSNCQQ as a valid measure of patient satisfaction with nursing care and validates its use in an Asian population.

The measures developed by Larrabee et al. (2004) and Laschinger et al. (2005) appear to have similar predictive power of global quality indicators. The PSNCQQ and the PJNC share similar items (although the PSNCQQ items include more detail on each item) and use the same 5-point rating scale, from *excellent* to *poor* (the PJNC also includes a *don't know* option). Both tools assess individualization of care, concern and caring by nurses, skill and competence of nurses, collaboration among nursing staff, provision of comfort, responsiveness of nurses, information provided by nurses, and a separate item measuring overall quality of nursing care. The PSNCQQ contains more items related to information needs, such as information provided about tests and treatments, instructions, ease of getting information, and more items related to discharge instructions and coordination of care after discharge. Both tools have the advantage of being relatively short and easy for patients to use. The PSNCQQ provides more detailed information on aspects of nursing amenable to change and would be more appropriately administered following discharge, given the items related to discharge planning and follow-up. Furthermore, both tools have the advantage of containing items similar to a patient satisfaction with quality of care measure widely used in the health services literature, which makes the results somewhat amenable to comparisons with more general hospital quality measures. Both tools contain items related to patient-identified quality indicators reported in the nursing literature and health services literature.

Instruments Developed by Health Services Researchers

In health services research, Ware, Davies-Avery, and Stewart (1978) were leaders in patient satisfaction research as part of their work to measure patient care quality outcomes. Ware et al.'s (1978) model, derived from interviews with both patients and providers, consisted of eight dimensions thought to be considered by patients when they evaluated their healthcare experience: the art of care, technical care quality, accessibility/convenience, payment method, physical environment, availability of providers, continuity of care, and efficacy/outcomes (K. Chang, 1997). The Patient Satisfaction Questionnaires I and II are used to operationalize components of the model. However, the tool is clearly oriented toward assessing aspects of medical care, not nursing care. Ware et al.'s (1978) model has been adapted by nurse researchers to develop taxonomies to analyze patient satisfaction with nursing care (Chang; Greeneich, Long, & Miller, 1992).

More recently, Ware and his associates (Rubin et al., 1990) developed another tool to operationalize a service quality evaluation model, the PJHQ. The model suggests that patients evaluate distinct categories of hospital care: (a) nursing and daily care, (b) hospital environment and ancillary staff, (c) medical care, (d) information, (e) the admissions process, and (f) discharge and billing. This tool contains five specific items—nurses' skill and competence, nurses' attention to the patient's condition, nursing staff response to calls, nurses demonstrating a concerned and caring attitude, and information provided by nursing—evaluating nursing care included in the NDCS. Nelson and Niederberger (1990) captured similar facets in their model: access to care, administrative management, clinical management, interpersonal management, continuity of care, and general satisfaction. A tool very similar to the PJHQ, the Patient Judgment Systems, is used to operationalize this model. The PJHQ was found to have sound psychometric properties and has been used extensively in health services research. Demographic characteristics were found to have little effect on patient ratings. Interestingly, the nursing subscale was the strongest predictor of overall rating of hospital quality and behavioral intentions (intention to return to the hospital if necessary and intention to recommend the hospital to others). Atkins et al. (1996) found that two items—concern and caring attitude, and information provided by nurses—were strongly related to overall quality ($r = 0.69$ and $r = 0.71, p < 0.005$, respectively). In a study by Doran et al. (2002), patients reported higher levels of satisfaction with nursing care on units where nurses reported good communication among the healthcare team members (b = .14). Patient satisfaction with nursing care was also related to functional status (b = .11), self-care ability (b = .15), and emotional health at discharge (b =−.18). Leiter et al. (1998) found that patients' perceptions of the overall quality of care were significantly related to the degree of emotional exhaustion that nurses experienced. Patients on units where nurses found their work meaningful were more satisfied with all aspects of their hospital stay ($r = 0.79, p < 0.01$). Likewise, patients were less satisfied with their care on units where nursing staff more frequently expressed the intention to quit ($r = 20.53, p < 0.05$) and where nurses expressed cynicism ($r = 20.53, p < 0.05$). More recently, Meterko, Mohr, and Young (2004) found that patient satisfaction was higher in hospitals with a culture of teamwork than in hospitals with a strong bureaucratic culture.

Parasuraman, Zeithaml, and Berry (1985) developed a marketing model of patient satisfaction from the business quality literature, using the SERVQUAL instrument to operationalize the model. The five general categories of quality are: (a) assurance, or the knowledge and courtesy of employees and their ability to inspire confidence, including competence, communication, credibility, courtesy, and security; (b) reliability, or the ability to perform the promised service reliably and accurately; (c) empathy, or the provision of caring, individualized attention to customers; (d) responsiveness, or the willingness to help customers and provide prompt service; and (e) tangibles, or the physical environment, equipment, and appearance of personnel. This tool contains items tapping both patients' expectations of various aspects of care and patients' perceptions of the extent to which they received the care. However, support for this model in healthcare settings has been equivocal, raising questions about its generalizability and comprehensiveness for health care. The model has been criticized for its relative lack of attention to the emotional and interpersonal aspects of quality (Bowers, Swan, & Koehler, 1994; Gummesson, 1991; Koerner, 2000). It has also been criticized for its use of different scores in operationalizing patient satisfaction, given the well-known reliability problems with such measures (Edwards, 1994; Nunnally & Bernstein, 1994). Babakus and Mangold (1992) established convergent validity of a modified version of this tool, which consisted only of perceived care received (SERVPERF).

They found strong correlations between this scale, a single-item measure of overall perceived quality, and a measure of intention to repeat use of the hospital's services if needed (.83 and .76, respectively). Niedz (1998) used the SERVPERF and found that items tapping patient perceptions of actual care received were significantly related to overall patient perception of satisfaction with nursing care. In her study, expectation scores did not contribute to the prediction of these outcomes beyond that contributed by actual perceptions of care received. This finding is consistent with those of Taylor and Cronin (1994).

Scardina (1994) adapted the SERVQUAL for use in evaluating nursing care. In a pilot study of 10 patients, the tool was found to have adequate content validity. A translated version of the SERVQUAL was found to have excellent psychometric qualities in a recent study in Spain (Gonzalez-Valentin, Padin-Lopez, & de Ramon-Garrido, 2005). Cronbach's alpha for the total scale was excellent (.90), and subscale alphas were mostly acceptable. The subscale differential scores were significantly related to patients' satisfaction with overall quality of care and satisfaction with nursing care during their hospital stay. These results support the construct validity of this measure in a large European sample.

Others have suggested the need to use service-specific measures of quality in healthcare settings and to add other attributes, such as caring and communication (Bowers et al., 1994). In a well-designed mixed methods study, Koerner (2000) added items to the SERVQUAL to reflect aspects of compassionate care described in patient interviews. However, in her final analysis, very few of the original SERVQUAL items were found to have construct validity. As a result, the new tool, Inpatient Nursing Service Quality Scale (INSQS), was developed as a more valid measure of satisfaction with nursing care. The INSQS consists of five dimensions: compassion, individualized care, reliability, close relationships, and uncertainty reduction. Compassion and reliability were the strongest predictors of overall satisfaction with quality and intention to recommend the hospital to others.

The Parkside organization designed another market research-based tool, the Quality of Care Monitor, to measure both inpatient and outpatient perceptions of quality. This tool taps eight dimensions of patient care and contains nine items related to nursing care quality, including those that nurse researchers have identified, such as competence, interpersonal relationships, and information sharing, among others. The nursing scale had high internal consistency (.88) and achieved the highest correlation with overall patient care ratings (Carey & Seibert, 1993). Carey and Seibert also found that 59% of the variance in patient satisfaction was explained by the nursing care subscale, courtesy subscale, comfort/cleanliness subscale, and physician care subscale.

Other commercially available measures, such as those developed by the Picker Institute and Press Ganey Associates, are commonly used by hospitals as part of their measurement of patient care quality. The Picker instrument consists of seven categories: (a) patient preferences, (b) coordination of care, (c) information and education, (d) physical comfort, (e) emotional support, (f) involvement family and friends, and (g) continuity and transition. This instrument has been widely used in Canada. Charles et al. (1994) adapted this tool in a national survey of adult medical-surgical patients to identify common sources of patient satisfaction across 57 hospitals in six Canadian provinces. Over 90% of patients surveyed were satisfied with their relationship with their physician and with the degree of participation in decision-making. Problem areas identified were pain management, expectations for tests and procedures, knowledge of medications, and home management of their condition.

The Press Ganey tool includes items relating to comfort, pain management, patient explanations/education, promotions, caring relationships, and courtesy. This organization has recently acquired the Parkside group. In a study reported in their own publication (Kaldenberg & Regrut, 1999), a strong correlation was found between nurse job satisfaction and patient satisfaction when their inpatient satisfaction instrument was used ($r = .84$). It is difficult to ascertain from the brief report exactly how the analysis was conducted. However, because the highest correlations found were between nurses' satisfaction with variables commonly associated with empowering work environments, and patient satisfaction, replication of this study seems warranted.

One of the positive attributes of these commercially available tools is that most were developed from data obtained in focus groups with both patients and providers, thereby overcoming some of the criticisms of earlier measures. In addition, these commercial enterprises provide data on the psychometric analyses conducted on these instruments and maintain large publicly accessible normative databases for various patient populations. However, many have been criticized for not tapping important aspects of nursing care and for being too global in nature. Thus, it is very important for nursing experts to be consulted in the process of choosing a tool for evaluating patient satisfaction with hospital care to ensure that satisfaction with nursing care will be adequately evaluated.

ISSUES IN MEASURING PATIENT SATISFACTION

Several issues are associated with the assessment of patient satisfaction. Although patient satisfaction with nursing care has been shown to be the most critical determinant of patients' overall satisfaction with hospital care, K. Chang (1997) maintained that many instruments commonly used in large patient satisfaction surveys do not adequately capture important nursing activities, thereby limiting their utility as valid nurse-sensitive outcome measures. This is a problem when researchers attempt to link nursing activities and other factors, such as redesign of nursing care delivery systems (e.g., changes in staff mix and staffing ratios), to patient satisfaction. The wide range of healthcare personnel in hospital settings also makes it difficult for patients to differentiate nurses from nonnurses, thus threatening the reliability and validity of measurements of satisfaction with nursing care (Pascoe, 1983). Another issue relates to the positive skewness and lack of variability of most patient satisfaction ratings. These data characteristics create problems in determining the true effects of the phenomenon and can have a negative impact on the statistical comparisons and relationships being studied. As a result, policy changes are difficult to justify based on empirical evidence. Finally, there is no standardization of measures of satisfaction with nursing care, making it impossible to compare across settings. Various authors have suggested that this issue may be a direct result of a lack of conceptual clarity in the definition of patient satisfaction. Al-Mailam (2005) suggested that this may be related to conceptual ambiguity, thus leading to the creation of inadequate measures, particularly when single-item scales are used to measure this complex phenomenon. Unfortunately, it stands to reason that the elusive nature of the concept, along with the high degree of subjectivity in determining an operational definition, may negate future attempts to standardize such a measure despite one's aspirations.

Lin (1996) summarized a variety of factors shown to have an influence on patient satisfaction ratings. Several relate to methodological issues, whereas others have to do with patient demographic characteristics and attitudes, and nursing process variables. For instance, the timing of the survey has been found to affect patient satisfaction ratings. Although return rates tended to be better when patients were surveyed at discharge, the ratings were lower than when surveys were conducted several weeks postdischarge. Furthermore, ratings were higher when patients were surveyed several months postdischarge, in comparison with several weeks following discharge (Ley, Kinsey, & Atherton, 1976). Response rates were low (30%) when surveyed at several months postdischarge and several weeks following discharge. Opinions differ about the reasons for this. Ley et al. suggested that less satisfied patients may be less likely to return questionnaires, whereas Ware, Snyder, Wright, and Allison (1983) argued that more satisfied patients may be less likely to return questionnaires. More research is needed to address this issue if patient satisfaction data are to be of use to hospital administrators. Research has shown that using a response format that allows the patient to rate items on an excellent/poor rating scale (rather than agree/disagree) and including a neutral point on the scale both help to increase the variance of the score (Ware & Hays, 1988). This scaling method helps to address the problem of skewed data typically obtained in patient satisfaction surveys.

Several patient demographic variables, such as gender, age, education, and race, have been inconsistently associated with patient satisfaction with nursing care. Pascoe (1983), as well as Bacon and Mark (2009), found that older patients tended to report higher satisfaction with nursing care, whereas other studies have not supported this finding (Bader, 1988). Women have been found to be more satisfied with care than men in some studies (Pascoe; Ware et al., 1978), whereas other studies have found no gender effect (Doering, 1983; Hall & Dornan, 1990; Sitzia & Wood, 1997). Patient expectations also have been found to influence satisfaction ratings. Swan (1985) reported that patients with lower expectations and less knowledge of services available were more satisfied with their nursing care. In addition, patient health status has been shown to influence satisfaction ratings. That is, patients with good health status postdischarge report greater satisfaction than those with poor health status (Cleary et al., 1991; Cleary, Keroy, Karapanos, & McMullen, 1989).

Finally, patients' perceptions of the nature of the nursing care process they experience during hospitalization have been shown to influence patient satisfaction ratings. Patients' perceptions of the competence of nurses caring for them and the manner in which care was delivered, including the nurses' interpersonal manner, communication skills, friendliness, and attentiveness to specific patient needs, have been associated with higher satisfaction (Cleary & McNeil, 1988; Sitzia & Wood, 1997).

Lin's (1996) review of the literature shows little evidence of measures derived from extant theoretical frameworks, inconsistent conceptualizations of the concept, limited reporting of validity information across studies, and a general lack of sensitivity of the measures due to highly positively skewed scores on rating scales. In addition, she found few examples of replicated studies or models attempting to explain mechanisms by which patient satisfaction is developed. Her conclusions are consistent with other reviews of patient satisfaction measures. Another problem noted by several researchers has to do with the difficulty that many patients had distinguishing among the different categories of nursing personnel in hospital settings (Abramowitz et al., 1987; Moritz, 1991). This problem raises issues about the reliability of measures of satisfaction with nursing care.

DISCUSSION AND RECOMMENDATIONS

This update of the patient satisfaction literature revealed that considerable research has been conducted in the area of patient satisfaction with nursing care quality in the past 5 years. The literature on patient satisfaction is indeed extensive and varied in both nursing and health services research. The empirical research linking antecedents and consequences of patient satisfaction is of varying levels of quality, although this is improving. The majority of the research reported is related to instrument development. Single-site studies with sampling problems are common, and the lack of consistent measurement of the concept across settings does not allow for comparisons. Much of the research has been correlational in nature and atheoretical. However, the growing body of work that identifies antecedents and consequences of patient satisfaction can be used as a basis for developing models to be tested. Researchers in both nursing and health services have recognized the need to develop conceptual frameworks that clarify the nature of the concept. There are a few systematic concept analyses of patient satisfaction in the literature. However, these models should be tested empirically. There has been some progress in this area, and the results of studies situating patient satisfaction with nursing care within plausible explanatory frameworks are beginning to appear in the literature. However, more work is needed in this area to provide health administrators with evidence-based theory-driven strategies for monitoring and improving nursing care that is valued by clients.

There appears to be consensus in the literature that patient satisfaction is a multidimensional concept and that efforts should continue to clarify the concept to ensure that it is measured accurately. In response to criticisms that many patient satisfaction measures tap primarily the provider's conception of aspects of quality that influence patient satisfaction, recent efforts have incorporated the patient's perspective in the concept's measurement. Several nursing researchers have shown that nurses' and patients' perceptions of what is satisfying in relation to patient care are different. Consistent pleas have arisen for the development and testing of sensitive instruments that are conceptually based and that have undergone extensive psychometric development and testing. Although many instruments exist in the literature, only recently have concerted efforts been made to assure adequate conceptualization, reliability, and validity. For example, several researchers have studied the impact of different methods of data collection on patient satisfaction ratings.

The most consistent substantive finding in the literature continues to be that satisfaction with nursing care is the strongest predictor of overall satisfaction with the healthcare experience. The quality of interpersonal relationships between nurses and patients has been shown to be one of the most important aspects of nursing behavior that influence patient satisfaction. Although there is debate in the literature regarding the extent to which patients are capable of evaluating the competence of health professionals such as nurses and physicians, patients' perceptions of their competence have nonetheless been linked to patients' satisfaction with their care in numerous studies. Patient satisfaction ratings are typically high, purportedly because of social desirability and feelings of vulnerability. This situation has resulted in a lack of sensitivity in statistical analyses.

There is still a paucity of controlled studies that examine patient satisfaction with nursing care as an outcome of specific nursing interventions. Patient satisfaction with nursing care was found to be significantly higher following implementation of a critical pathway system in a postpartum unit (Goode, 1995) and following a hospital restructuring process (Sovie & Jawad, 2001). Kangas et al. (1999) found that patients cared for in a primary nursing model reported higher satisfaction with nursing care than did those in traditional nursing care delivery models, such as team nursing. Stumpf (2001) reported that patient satisfaction with nursing care was higher for patients cared for by nurses working in a unit with shared governance. Several studies reporting a significant impact of organizational interventions on patient satisfaction with nursing care did not specifically identify the instrument used to measure patient satisfaction. Many used their hospitals' existing patient satisfaction measures. Thus, information was insufficient to evaluate these studies. Other factors, such as nurses' job satisfaction, burnout, and staffing variables, appear to indirectly influence patient satisfaction with nursing care (Atkins et al., 1996; Kaldenberg & Regrut, 1999; Leiter et al., 1998; Moore et al., 1999; Sengin, 2001; Sovie & Jowad). Evidence to support the links among nursing worklife factors has increased in the past 5 years in light of the increase in the number of studies on nursing-sensitive outcomes.

The increased interest in patient satisfaction as a quality indicator in U.S. managed care environments has stimulated greater attention to developing standardized measures of the concept with adequate psychometric properties. With the change to a market orientation, healthcare marketers and consulting firms have become involved in the development and administration of patient satisfaction measures. These tools have been exported to Canada and other countries such as the United Kingdom and other European countries. Many of these measures have been developed without the input of healthcare professionals and have been criticized, in particular, for not capturing the essence of nursing activities related to patient care. However, more collaboration between nursing and health services researchers in the past decade has resulted in a mutual enrichment of the field. Several authors emphasized the importance of including nursing representatives in the process of selecting a commercially available patient satisfaction measure to assure that appropriate aspects of nursing care are contained in the instrument. Given the integral role of nursing services in the patient care experience and the consistent link between satisfaction with nursing care and overall patient satisfaction, this practice is crucial to obtaining meaningful data.

Based on this updated review of the literature relating to patient satisfaction with nursing care, several recommendations are offered:

- Continue efforts to clarify and define the nature of patient satisfaction. Develop and test theoretical models that articulate the mechanisms that affect changes in satisfaction over time. Ensure that both patients' and providers' viewpoints are represented. Use both qualitative and quantitative approaches to develop and validate these models.
- Develop and refine reliable and valid measures of satisfaction based on conceptually sound theoretical models. Avoid broad measures of patient satisfaction and develop multidimensional measures of quality that include both affective and instrumental components of satisfaction with nursing care. Use both closed- and open-ended items to maximize information. Test innovative approaches to measuring the concept in order to optimize sensitivity and usability of instruments (e.g., item design, scoring procedures).

- Use well-designed measures available in the literature to allow comparability of findings across studies and samples. Establish norms for these measures in various patient populations and create an online repository of commonly used instruments available to researchers and healthcare organizations.
- Integrate measures of nursing care quality with measures of interdisciplinary teamwork and quality of care to obtain measures of interdisciplinary care.
- Develop and implement strong designs (e.g., multisite, longitudinal studies) to empirically test models of patient satisfaction. Employ sophisticated data analysis techniques to evaluate models of satisfaction (e.g., structural equation modeling, hierarchical linear modeling, time series analyses). Replicate studies to increase generalizability of findings.
- Publish information about patient satisfaction measures, including dimensions, sample items, and scoring procedures, as well as psychometric data and research results, in accessible sources, such as the World Wide Web, journals, Publish Ahead of Print opportunities.
- Increase collaboration between nurse researchers and health services researchers to further develop the body of knowledge related to patients' satisfaction with nursing care quality.

REFERENCES

Abramowitz, S., Cote, A. A., & Berry, E. (1987). Analyzing patient satisfaction: A multianalytic approach. *Quality Review Bulletin, 13,* 122–130.

Al-Mailam, F. F. (2005). The effect of nursing care on overall patient satisfaction and its predictive value on return-to-provider behavior: A survey study. *Quality Management in Healthcare, 14(2),* 116–120.

American Nurses Association. (1996). *Nursing quality indicators: A guide for implementation.* Washington, DC: American Nurses Publishing.

Andaleeb, S. S. (1998). Determinants of customer satisfaction with hospitals: A managerial model. *International Journal of Health Care Quality Assurance, 11,* 181–187.

Andrews, L. W., Daniels, P., & Hall, A. G. (1996). Nurse caring behaviors: Comparing five tools to define perceptions. *Ostomy Wound Management, 42(5),* 28–37.

Atkins, P. M., Marshall, B. S., & Javalgi, R. G. (1996). Happy employees lead to loyal patients. *Journal of Health Care Marketing, 16(4),* 15–23.

Babakus, E., & Mangold, W. G. (1992). Adapting the SERVQUAL scale to hospital services: An empirical investigation. *Health Services Research, 26,* 767–786.

Bader, M. M. (1988). Nursing care behaviors that predict patient satisfaction. *Journal of Nursing Quality Assurance, 2,* 11–17.

Bacon, C. T., & Mark, B. (2009). Organizational effects on patient satisfaction in hospital medical-surgical units. *Journal of Nursing Administration, 39,* 220–227.

Baradell, J. G. (1995). Clinical outcomes and satisfaction of patients of clinical nurse specialists in psychiatric-mental health nursing. *Archives of Psychiatric Nursing, 9,* 240–250.

Barkell, N. P., Killinger, K. A., & Schultz, S. D. (2002). The relationship between nurse staffing models and patient outcomes: A descriptive study. *Outcomes Management, 6*(1), 27–33.

Batalden, P. B., & Nelson, E. C. (1990). Hospital quality: Patient, physician, and employee judgments. *International Journal of Health Care Quality Assurance, 3,* 7–17.

Benkert, R., Barkauskas, V., Pohl, J., Corser, W., Tanner, C., Wells, M., et al. (2002). Patient satisfaction outcomes in nurse-managed centers. *Outcomes Management, 6,* 174–181.

Blegen, M. A., & Goode, C. J. (1993, November). *Measuring the quality of multidisciplinary care.* Paper presented at the ANA Council of Nurse Researchers meeting, Washington, DC.

Bond, S., & Thomas, L. (1992). Measuring patients' satisfaction with nursing care. *Journal of Advanced Nursing, 17,* 52–63.

Bowers, M. R., Swan, J. E., & Koehler, W. F. (1994). What attributes determine quality and satisfaction with health care delivery? *Health Care Manager Review, 19*(4), 49–55.

Bowling, A. (1992). Assessing health needs and measuring patient satisfaction. *Nursing Times, 88*(31), 31–33.

Braskamp, L. A., & Maehr, M. L. (1985). *Spectrum: An Organizational Development Tool.* Champaign, IL: MetriTech.

Burney, M., Purden, M., & McVey, L. (2002). Patient satisfaction and nurses' perceptions of quality in an inpatient cardiology population. *Journal of Nursing Care Quality, 16*(4), 56–67.

Carey, R. G., & Posavac, E. J. (1982). Using patient information to identify areas for service improvement. *Healthcare Management Review, 7*(2), 43–48.

Carey, R. G., & Seibert, J. H. (1993). A patient survey system to measure quality improvement questionnaire reliability and validity. *Medical Care, 31,* 834–845.

Chang, B. L., Uman, G. C., Lawrence, L. S., Ware, J. E., & Kane, R. L. (1984). The effect of systematically varying components of nursing care satisfaction in elderly ambulatory women. *Western Journal of Nursing Research, 6,* 366–379.

Chang, K. (1997). Dimensions and indicators of patients' perceived nursing care quality in the hospital setting. *Journal of Nursing Care Quality, 11*(6), 26–37.

Charles, C., Gauld, M., Chambers, L., O'Brien, B., Haynes, B., & LaBelle, R. (1994). How was your hospital stay? Patients' reports about their care in Canadian hospitals. *Canadian Medical Association Journal, 150,* 1813–1822.

Chiu, E., & Chung, R. (2008). *The influence of team empowerment climate and self-leadership ability on service performance and medical service satisfaction: The mediator of job satisfaction.* Unpublished doctoral dissertation, National Changhua University of Education, Changhua, Taiwan.

Clark, P. A., Leddy, K., Drain, M., & Kaldenberg, D. (2007). State nursing shortages and patient satisfaction: more RNS—better patient experiences. *Journal of Nursing Care Quality, 22*(2), 119–127.

Cleary, P. D., Edgman-Levitan, S., Roberts, M., Moloney, T. W., McMullen, W., Walker, J. D., et al. (1991). Patients evaluate their hospital care: A national survey. *Health Affairs, 10,* 254–267.

Cleary, P. D., Keroy, L., Karapanos, G., & McMullen, W. (1989). Patient assessments of hospital care. *Quality Review Bulletin, 15,* 172–179.

Cleary, P. D., & McNeil, B. J. (1988). Patient satisfaction as an indicator of quality care. *Inquiry, 25,* 25–36.

Comley, A. L., & Beard, M. T. (1998). Toward a derived theory of patient satisfaction. *Journal of Theory Construction and Testing, 2*(2), 44–50.

Conbere, P. C., McGovern, P., Kochevar, L., & Widtfeldt, A. (1992). Measuring satisfaction with medical case management: A quality improvement tool. *American Association of Occupational Health Nurses Journal, 40,* 333–341, 358–360.

Cottle, D. W. (1989). *Client-centered service: How to keep them coming back for more.* New York: Wiley.

Cox, C. L. (1982). An interaction model of client health behavior: Theoretical prescription for nursing. *Advances in Nursing Science, 5,* 41–56.

Cronin, J. J., & Taylor, S. A. (1992). Measuring service quality: A reexamination and extension. *Journal of Marketing, 56*(3), 55.

Davidow, W. A., & Uttal, B. (1989). *Total customer service.* New York: Harper and Row.

Davis, B. A., Kiesel, C. K., McFarland, J., Collard, A., Coston, K., & Keeton, A. (2005). Evaluating instruments for quality: Testing convergent validity of the consumer emergency care satisfaction scale. *Journal of Nursing Care Quality, 20*(4), 364–368.

Denton, D. K. (1989). *Quality service.* Houston, TX: Gulf.

Doering, E. R. (1983). Factors influencing inpatient satisfaction with care. *Quality Review Bulletin, 9,* 291–299.

Donabedian, A. (1988). Quality assessment and assurance: Unity of purpose, diversity of means. *Inquiry, 25,* 173–219.

Donahue, M. O., Piazza, I. M., Griffin, M. Q., Dykes, P. C., & Fitzpatrick, J. J. (2008). The relationship between nurses' perceptions of empowerment and patient satisfaction. *Applied Nursing Research, 21,* 2–7.

Doran, D. M., Sidani, S., Keatings, M., & Doidge, D. (2002). An empirical test of the Nursing Role Effectiveness model. *Journal of Advanced Nursing, 38,* 29–39.

Edwards, J. R. (1994). The study of congruence in organizational behavior research: Critique and a proposed alternative. *Organizational Behavior and Human Decision Processes, 58, 51–100 (erratum, 58, 323–325).*

Eriksen, L. R. (1987). Patient satisfaction: An indicator of nursing care quality? *Nursing Management, 18*(7), 31–35.

Eriksen, L. R. (1995). Patient satisfaction with nursing care: Concept satisfaction. *Journal of Nursing Measurement, 3,* 59–76.

Farrell, G. A. (1991). How accurately do nurses perceive patients' needs? A comparison of general and psychiatric settings. *Journal of Advanced Nursing, 16,* 1062–1070.

Forbes, D. A. (1996). Clarification of the constructs of satisfaction and dissatisfaction with home care. *Public Health Nursing, 13,* 377–385.

Forbes, M. L., & Brown, H. N. (1995). Developing an instrument for measuring patient satisfaction. *Association of Operating Room Nurses Journal, 61,* 737–743.

Fosbinder, D. (1994). Patient perceptions of nursing care: An emerging theory of interpersonal competence. *Journal of Advanced Nursing, 20,* 1085–1093.

Gonzalez-Valentin, A., Padin-Lopez, S., & de Ramon-Garrido, E. (2005). Patient satisfaction with nursing care in a regional university hospital in southern Spain. *Journal of Nursing Care Quality, 20(1),* 63–72.

Goode, C. J. (1995). Impact of a CareMap and case management on patient satisfaction and staff satisfaction, collaboration, and autonomy. *Nursing Economics, 13,* 337–348.

Goodell, T., & Van Ess Coeling, H. (1994). Outcomes of nurses' job satisfaction. *Journal of Nursing Administration, 24*(11), 36–41.

Graveley, E., & Littlefield, J. (1992). A cost-effectiveness analysis of three staffing models for the delivery of low-risk prenatal care. *American Journal of Public Health, 82,* 180–184.

Greeneich, D. (1993). The link between new and return business and quality of care: Patient satisfaction. *Advances in Nursing Science, 16,* 62–67.

Greeneich, D. S., Long, C. O., & Miller, B. K. (1992). Patient satisfaction update: Research applied to practice. *Applied Nursing Research, 5*(1), 43–48.

Gummesson, E. (1991). Service quality: A holistic view. In S. W. Brown, E. Gummesson, B. B., Edvardsson, & B. Gustavsson (Eds.), *Service quality: Multidisciplinary and multinational perspectives* (pp. 3–22). Lexington, MA: Lexington Books.

Guzman, P. M., Sliepcevich, E. M., Lacey, E. P., Vitello, E. M., Matten, M. R., Woehlke, P. L., et al. (1988). Tapping patient satisfaction: A strategy for quality assessment. *Patient Education and Counseling, 12,* 225–233.

Hall, J. A., & Dornan, M. C. (1990). Patient sociodemographic characteristics as predictors of satisfaction with medical care: A meta-analysis. *Social Science and Medicine, 30,* 811–818.

Hanan, M., & Karp, P. (1989). *Customer satisfaction.* New York: American Management Association.

Hayes, P. (1992). Evaluation of a professional practice model. *Nursing Administration Quarterly, 16*(4), 57–64.

Hays, R. D., Nelson, E. C., Rubin, H. R., Ware, J. E., & Meterko, M. (1990). Further evaluations of the PJHQ scales. *Medical Care, 28*(Suppl. 9), S29–S39.

Heinemann, D., Lengacher, C. A., van Cott, M. L., Mabe, P., & Swymer, S. (1996). Partners in patient care: Measuring the effects on patient satisfaction and other quality indicators. *Nursing Economics, 14,* 276–285.

Hill, J. (1997). Patient satisfaction in a nurse-led rheumatology clinic. *Journal of Advanced Nursing, 25,* 347–354.

Hinshaw, A., & Atwood, J. (1982). A patient satisfaction instrument: Precision by replication. *Nursing Research, 31,* 170–175.

Innis, J., Bikaunieks, N., Petryshen, P., Zellermeyer, V., & Ciccarelli, L. (2004). Patient satisfaction and pain management: An educational approach. *Journal of Nursing Care Quality, 19*(4), 322–327.

Johansson, P., Oleni, M., & Fridlund, B. (2002). Patient satisfaction with nursing care in the context of health care: A literature study. *Scandinavian Journal of Caring Sciences, 16,* 337–344.

Kaldenberg, D. O., & Becker, B. W. (1999). Evaluations of care by ambulatory surgery patients. *Health Care Management Review, 24*(3), 73–81.

Kaldenberg, D. O., & Regrut, B. A. (1999). Do satisfied patients depend on satisfied employees? Or, do satisfied employees depend on satisfied patients? In *The Satisfaction Report Newsletter* (Vol. 3, pp. 1–4). South Bend, IN: Press, Ganey Associates.

Kangas, S., Kee, C. C., & McKee-Waddle, R. (1999). Organizational factors, nurses' job satisfaction, and patient satisfaction with nursing care. *Journal of Nursing Administration, 29,* 32–42.

Kee, C. C., Foley, B. J., Dudley, W. N., Jennings, B. M., Minick, P., & Harvey, S. S. (2005). Nursing structure, processes, and patient outcomes in Army medical centers. *Western Journal of Nursing Research, 27,* 1040–1058.

Ketefian, S., Redman, R., Nash, M. G., & Bogue, E. (1997). Inpatient and ambulatory patient satisfaction with nursing care. *Quality Management in Health Care, 5,* 66–75.

Knaus, V. L., Felten, S., Burton, S., Fobes, P., & Davis, K. (1997). The use of nurse practitioners in the acute care setting. *Journal of Nursing Administration, 27*(2), 20–27.

Koerner, M. M. (2000). The conceptual domain of service quality for inpatient nursing services. *Journal of Business Research, 48,* 267–283.

Kovner, C. (1989). Nurse-patient agreement and outcomes after surgery. *Western Journal of Nursing Research, 11,* 7–17.

Kramer, M., & Hafner, L.P. (1989). Shared values: Impact on staff nurse job satisfaction and perceived productivity. *Nursing Research, 38,* 172–177.

Krouse, H., & Roberts, S. (1989). Nurse-patient interactive styles: Power, control and satisfaction. *Western Journal of Nursing Research, 11,* 717–725.

La Monica, E. L., Oberst, M. T., Madea, A. R., & Wolf, R. M. (1986). Development of a patient satisfaction scale. *Research in Nursing and Health, 9,* 43–50.

Lageson, C. (2004). Quality focus of the first line nurse manager and relationship to unit outcomes. *Journal of Nursing Care Quality, 19*(4), 336–342.

Larrabee, J. H., Engle, V. F., & Tolley, E. A. (1995). Predictors of patient-perceived quality. *Scandinavian Journal of Caring Science, 9,* 153–164.

Larrabee, J. H., Ostrow, C. L., Withrow, M. L., Janney, M. A., Hobbs, G. R., & Burant, C. (2004). Predictors of patient satisfaction with inpatient hospital nursing care. *Research in Nursing and Health, 27,* 254–268.

Larson, P. J. (1987). Comparison of cancer patients' and professional nurses' perceptions of important nurse caring behaviors. *Heart and Lung, 16,* 187–193.

Larson, P. J., & Ferketich, S. L. (1993). Patients' satisfaction with nurses' caring during hospitalization. *Western Journal of Nursing Research, 15,* 690–707.

Laschinger, H. S., Hall, L. M., Pedersen, C., & Almost, J. (2005). A psychometric analysis of the patient satisfaction with nursing care quality questionnaire: An actionable approach to measuring patient satisfaction. *Journal of Nursing Care Quality, 20*(3), 220–230.

Leiter, M. P., Harvie, P., & Frizzel, C. (1998). The correspondence of patient satisfaction and nurse burnout. *Social Science and Medicine, 47,* 1611–1617.

Lewis, K., & Woodside, R. (1992). Patient satisfaction with care in the emergency department. *Journal of Advanced Nursing, 17,* 959–964.

Ley, P. J., Kinsey, S. T., & Atherton, B. (1976). Increasing patients' satisfaction with communication. *British Journal of Social and Clinical Psychology, 15,* 403–413.

Lin, C. (1996). Patient satisfaction with nursing care as an outcome variable: Dilemmas for nursing evaluation researchers. *Journal of Professional Nursing, 12,* 207–216.

Linder-Pelz, S. (1982). Toward a theory of patient satisfaction. *Social Science and Medicine, 16,* 577–582.

Ludwig-Beymer, P., Ryan, C. J., Johnson, N. J., Hennessey, K. A., Gattuso, M. C., & Epsom, R. (1993). Using patient perceptions to improve quality care. *Journal of Nursing Care Quality, 7*(2), 42–51.

Lynn, M. R., & McMillen, B. J. (1999). Do nurses know what patients think is important in nursing care? *Journal of Nursing Care Quality, 13*(5), 65–74.

Lynn, M. R., McMillen, B. J., & Sidani, S. (2007). Understanding and measuring patients' assessment of the quality of nursing care. *Nursing Research, 56,* 159–166.

Lynn, M. R., & Moore, K. (1997). Relationship between traditional quality indicators and perceptions of care. *Seminars for Nurse Managers, 5,* 187–193.

Lynn, M. R., & Sidani, S. (1991). *The next step: The patient's perception of quality scale.* Paper presented at the 24th Annual WSRN Communicating Nursing Research Conference, Albuquerque, New Mexico.

Mahon, P. Y. (1996). An analysis of the concept patient satisfaction as it relates to contemporary nursing. *Journal of Advanced Nursing, 24,* 1241–1248.

Marsh, G. W. (1999). Measuring patient satisfaction outcomes across provider disciplines. *Journal of Nursing Measurement, 7*(1), 47–62.

McColl, E., Thomas, L., & Bond, S. (1996). A study to determine patient satisfaction with nursing care. *Nursing Standard, 10,* 34–38.

McGillis-Hall, L. M., Doran, D., Baker, G. R., Pink, G. H., Sidani, S., O'Brien-Pallas, L., et al. (2003). Nurse staffing models as predictors of patient outcomes. *Medical Care, 41,* 1096–1109.

McNeill, J., Sherwood, G., Starck, P., Disnard, G., Rodriquez, T., & Palos, G. (2003). Design strategies in pain management research with Hispanics. *Hispanic Health Care International, 2*(2), 73–80.

Megivern, K., Halm, M. A., & Jones, G. (1992). Measuring patient satisfaction as an outcome of nursing care. *Journal of Nursing Care Quality, 6*(4), 9–24.

Meterko, M., Mohr, D., & Young, G. (2004). Teamwork culture and patient satisfaction in hospitals, *Medical Care, 42,* 492–498.

Meterko, M., Nelson, E. C., Rubin, H. R., Batalden, P., Berwick, D. M., Hays, R. D., et al. (1990). Patients' judgment of hospital quality: A report on a pilot study. *Medical Care, 28*(Supplement), S1–S56.

Moore, K., Lynn, M. R., McMillen, B. J., & Evans, S. (1999). Implementation of the ANA report card. *Journal of Nursing Administration, 29(6),* 48–54.

Moritz, P. (1991). Innovative nursing practice models and patient outcomes. *Nursing Outlook, 39,* 111–114.

Mrayyan, M. T. (2006). Jordanian nurses' job satisfaction, patients' satisfaction and quality of nursing care. *International Nursing Review, 53,* 224–230.

Munro, B., Jacobsen, B. S., & Brooten, D. A. (1994). Re-examination of the psychometric characteristics of the La Monica-Oberst Patient Satisfaction Scale. *Research in Nursing and Health, 17,* 119–125.

Nash, M. G., Blackwood, D., Boone, E. B., Klar, R., Lewis, E., MacInnis, K., et al. (1994). Managing expectations between patient and nurse. *Journal of Nursing Administration, 24*(11), 49–55.

Nelson, C. W., & Niederberger, J. (1990). Patient satisfaction surveys: An opportunity for total quality improvement. *Hospital and Health Services Administration, 35,* 409–427.

Niedz, B. A. (1998). Correlates of hospitalized patients' perceptions of service quality. *Research in Nursing and Health, 21,* 339–349.

Nunnally, J. C., & Bernstein, I. H. (1994). *Psychometric theory* (3rd ed.). New York: McGraw-Hill.

Oberst, M. T. (1984). Patient's perceptions of care. *Cancer, 53,* 2366–2375.

Otani, K., & Kurz, R. S. (2004). The impact of nursing care and other healthcare attributes on hospitalized patient satisfaction and behavioral intentions. *Journal of Healthcare Management, 49,* 181–196.

Parasuraman, A., Zeithaml, V., & Berry, L. (1985). A conceptual model of service quality and its implications for future research. *Journal of Marketing, 49,* 41–50.

Pascoe, G. C. (1983). Patient satisfaction in primary health care: A literature review and analysis. *Evaluation and Program Planning, 6,* 185–210.

Pedhazur, E. J., & Schmelkin, L. P. (1991). *Measurement, design, and analysis: An integrated approach.* Hillsdale, NJ: Erlbaum.

Petersen, M. (1988). Measuring patient satisfaction: Collecting useful data. *Journal of Nursing Quality Assurance, 2*(3), 25–35.

Peterson, W., Charles, C., DiCenso, A. & Sword, W. (2005). The Newcastle satisfaction with nursing scales: A valid measure of maternal satisfaction with inpatient postpartum nursing care. *Journal of Advanced Nursing, 52,* 672–681.

The Picker Institute. (1988). *Patient Assessment of Hospital Care.* Boston, MA: The Picker Institute.

Pierce, S. F. (1997). Nurse-sensitive health care outcomes in acute care settings: An integrative analysis of the literature. *Journal of Nursing Care Quality, 11*(4), 60–72.

Potter, P., Barr, N., McSweeney, M., & Sledge, J. (2003). Identifying nurse staffing and patient outcome relationships: A guide for change in care delivery, *Nursing Economics, 21,* 158–166.

Press, G. (2000). *Client reference manual.* South Bend, IN: Press, Ganey Associates.

Regrut, B. (Ed.). (1997). Press, Ganey revised inpatient survey. *The Satisfaction Monitor,* 7–9.

Risser, N. (1975). Development of an instrument to measure patient satisfaction with nurses and nursing care in primary care settings. *Nursing Research, 24,* 45–52.

Rubin, H. R., Gandeck, B., Rogers, W. H., Kosinski, M., McHorney, C. A., & Ware, J. E. (1988). Patients' ratings of outpatient visits in different practice settings: Results from the medical outcomes study. *Journal of the American Medical Association, 270,* 835–840.

Rubin, H. R., Ware, J. E., & Hays, R. D. (1990). The PJHQ questionnaire: Exploratory factor analysis and empirical scale construction. *Medical Care, 28*(Suppl. 9), S22–S29.

Scardina, S. A. (1994). SERVQUAL: A tool for evaluating patient satisfaction with nursing care. *Journal of Nursing Care Quality, 8*(2), 38–46.

Schmidt, L. A. (2003) Patients' perceptions of nursing care in the hospital setting. *Journal of Advanced Nursing, 44,* 393–399.

Sengin, K. K. (2001). *The relationship between job satisfaction of registered nurses and patient satisfaction with nursing care in acute care hospitals* (Paper AAI3003692). Unpublished doctoral dissertation, University of Pennsylvania. Retrieved June 12, 2009, from http://repository.upenn.edu/dissertations/AAI3003692

SEQUS Version 2.0. (1998). Computer software. Montreal, Quebec, Canada: Andromed.

Shen, Q., Sherwood, G. D., McNeill, J. A., & Li, Z. (2008). Postoperative pain management outcome in Chinese inpatients. *Western Journal of Nursing Research, 30,* 975–990.

Sitzia, J., & Wood, N. (1997). Patient satisfaction: A review of issues and concepts. *Social Science and Medicine, 45,* 1829–1843.

Sovie, M. D., & Jawad, A. F. (2001). Hospital restructuring and its impact on outcomes: Nursing staff regulations are premature. *Journal of Nursing Administration, 31,* 588–600.

Stumpf, L. R. (2001). A comparison of governance types and patient satisfaction outcomes. *Journal of Nursing Administration, 31,* 196–202.

Sulmasy, D. P., McIlvane, J. M., Pasley, P. M., & Rahn, M. (2002). A scale of measuring patient perceptions of the quality of end-of-life care and satisfaction with treatment: The reliability and validity of QUEST. *Journal of Pain and Symptom Management, 23,* 458–470.

Swan, J. (1985). Deepening the understanding of hospital patient satisfaction: Fulfillment and equity of effects. *Journal of Health Care Marketing, 5*(3), 14.

Swan, J. E., & Carroll, M. G. (1980). Patient satisfaction and overview of research—1965 to 1978. In H. K. Hunt & R. L. Day (Eds.), *Refining concepts and measures of consumer satisfaction and complaining behavior* (pp. 112–118). Bloomington: Indiana University, Foundation for the School of Business.

Taylor, S. A. (1994). Distinguishing service quality from patient satisfaction in developing health care marketing strategies. *Hospital and Health Services Administration, 39,* 221–236.

Taylor, S., & Cronin, J. (1994). Modeling patient satisfaction and service quality. *Journal of Health Care Marketing, 14*(1), 34.

Tervo-Heikkinen, T., Kvist, T., Partanen, P., Vehvilainen-Julkunen, K., & Aalto, P. (2008). Patient satisfaction as a positive nursing outcome. *Journal of Nursing Care Quality, 23*(1), 58–65.

Tervo-Heikkinen, T., Partanen, P., Aalto, P., & Vehvilainen-Julkunen, K. (2008). Nurses' work environment and nursing outcomes: A survey study among Finnish university hospital registered nurses. *International Journal of Nursing Practice, 14,* 357–365.

Thomas, L. H., & Bond, S. (1996). Measuring patients' satisfaction with nursing: 1990–1994. *Journal of Advanced Nursing, 23,* 747–756.

Thompson, D. A., Yarnold, P. R., Williams, D. R., & Adams, S. L. (1996). Effects of actual waiting time, perceived waiting time, information delivery and expressive quality on patient satisfaction in the emergency department. *Annals of Emergency Medicine, 28,* 657–665.

Titler, M. G. (2002). Use of research in practice. In G. LoBiondo-Wood & J. Haber (Eds.), *Nursing research* (pp. 411–444). St. Louis: Mosby-Year Book.

Tomlinson, J. S., & Clifford, Y. K. (2006). Patient satisfaction: An increasingly important measure of quality. *Annals of Surgical Oncology, 13(6),* 764–765.

Twardon, C., & Gartner, M. (1991). Empowering nurses: Patient satisfaction with primary nursing in home health. *Journal of Nursing Administration, 21*(11), 39–43.

Tzeng, H., & Ketefian, S. (2002). The relationship between nurses' job satisfaction and inpatient satisfaction: An exploratory study in a Taiwan teaching hospital. *Journal of Nursing Care Quality, 16*(2), 39–49.

Tzeng, H. M., Ketefian, S., & Redman, R. W. (2002). Relationship of nurses' assessment of organizational culture, job satisfaction, and patient satisfaction with nursing care. *International Journal of Nursing Studies, 39,* 79–84.

Vahey, D. C., Aiken, L. H., Sloane, D. M., Clarke, S. P., & Vargas, D. (2004). Nurse burnout and patient satisfaction. *Medical Care, 42*(2 Suppl.), II57–II66.

von Essen, L., & Sjoden, P. O. (1991). Patient and staff perceptions of caring: Review and replication. *Journal of Advanced Nursing, 16,* 1363–1374.

von Essen, L., & Sjoden, P. (1995). Perceived occurrence and importance of caring behaviors among patients and staff in psychiatric, medical, and surgical care. *Journal of Advanced Nursing, 21,* 266–276.

Wagner, D., & Bear, M. (2009). Patient satisfaction with nursing care: A concept analysis within a nursing framework. *Journal of Advanced Nursing, 65,* 692–701.

Ware, J., Jr., Davies-Avery, A., & Stewart, A. (1978). The measurement and meaning of patient satisfaction. *Health and Medical Care Services Review, 1,* 1.

Ware, J. E., & Hays, R. D. (1988). Methods for measuring patient satisfaction with specific medical encounters. *Medical Care, 26,* 393–401.

Ware, J. E., Snyder, M. K., Wright, W. R., & Allison, R. D. (1983). Defining and measuring patient satisfaction with medical care. *Evaluation and Program Planning, 6,* 247–263.

Watson, J. (2009). *Assessing and measuring caring in nursing and health sciences* (2nd ed.). New York: Springer.

Webb, C., & Hope, K. (1995). What kind of nurses do patients want? *Journal of Clinical Nursing, 4,* 101–108.

Weisman, C. S., & Nathanson, C. A. (1985). Professional satisfaction and client outcomes: A comparative organizational analysis. *Medical Care, 23,* 1179–1192.

Whitley, M. P., & Putzier, D. J. (1994). Measuring nurses' satisfaction with the quality of their work and work environment. *Journal of Nursing Care Quality, 8*(3), 43–51.

Williams, B. (1994). Patient satisfaction: A valid concept? *Social Science and Medicine, 38,* 509–516.

Wolf, Z. R., Colahan, M., Costello, A., Warwick, F., Ambrose, M. S., & Giardino, E. R. (1998). Research utilization: Relationship between nurse caring and patient satisfaction. *MEDSURG Nursing, 7,* 99–105.

Woodring, S., Polomano, R. C., Haagen, B. F., Haack, M. M., Nunn, R. R., Miller, G. L., et al. (2004). Development and testing of patient satisfaction measure for inpatient psychiatry care. *Journal of Nursing Care Quality, 19*(2), 137–148.

Woodside, A. G., Frey, L. L., & Daly, R. T. (1989). Linking service quality, customer satisfaction, and behavioral intention. *Journal of Health Care Marketing, 9*(4), 5–17.

Yeakel, S., Maljanian, R., Bohannon, R. W., & Coulombe, K. H. (2003). Nurse caring behaviors and patient satisfaction: Improvement after a multifaceted staff intervention. *Journal of Nursing Administration, 33,* 434–436.

Yellen, E., Davis, G. C., & Ricard, R. (2002). The measurement of patient satisfaction. *Journal of Nursing Care Quality, 16*(4), 23–29.

Yen, M., & Lo, L. (2004). A model for testing the relationship of nursing care and patient outcomes. *Nursing Economics, 22*(2), 75–80.

Young, W. B., Minnick, A. F., & Marcantonio, R. (1996). How wide is the gap in defining quality care? Comparison of patient and nurse perceptions of important aspects of patient care. *Journal of Nursing Administration, 26,* 15–20.

Zimmerman, P. (2001). The problems with healthcare customer satisfaction surveys. In J. M. Dochterman & H. K. Grace (Eds.), *Current issues in nursing* (6th ed., pp. 255–260). St. Louis, MO: Mosby.

Mortality Rate as a Nurse-Sensitive Outcome

Ann E. Tourangeau

INTRODUCTION

Mortality rate is an important quality indicator in a variety of healthcare sectors for many groups of healthcare recipients (referred to as patients). The most important rationale establishing the mortality rate as a quality of care indicator is the existence of wide variation in risk- and case-mix-adjusted mortality rates for homogenous groups of patients. There are three known sources of variation in mortality rates: patients' own characteristics, structures and processes of health care, and random sources (Silber, Rosenbaum, & Ross, 1995). Patients' own characteristics (e.g., comorbid conditions, age) have been shown to have the greatest impact on mortality (Silber & Rosenbaum, 1997). To isolate and understand the impact of the structures and processes of health care on mortality rates, the impact of patients' own characteristics must be identified and controlled using risk-adjustment methods (Iezzoni, 2003a). Furthermore, because there may be significant variation in crude (unadjusted) mortality rates for different populations or subpopulations of patients, mortality outcome research should also adjust or account for differences in the mix of patients within healthcare organizational settings. For example, if one healthcare organization cares for a much larger proportion of patients known to have higher mortality rates, this healthcare setting will have higher mortality rates because of the mix of patients rather than the structures and processes of health care in that organization. Once the impact or risk of patients' own characteristics on mortality and the mix of patients within a healthcare organization are accounted for, it is reasonable to assume that much

409

of the remaining variation in mortality rates is influenced by the structures and processes of health care. Because nursing care accounts for much of the structures and processes of health care in most healthcare organizations, it is reasonable to suspect that the structures and processes of nursing care have an impact on mortality rates (Tourangeau, 2007). Mortality outcome research aims to account for the impact of patients' characteristics on mortality so that the impact of the structures and processes of care can be examined and quantified.

If we understand what structures and processes of care influence mortality rates, we can modify those structures and processes of care to reduce mortality rates and prevent unnecessary patient death. Understanding what structures and processes of health care impact mortality facilitates redesign of nursing care delivery to minimize unnecessary patient death. It is important to note that for some healthcare recipients, death is an expected outcome. Therefore, in settings such as palliative care, mortality rates should not be considered as a quality-of-care outcome.

LITERATURE SEARCH STRATEGY

To gather the most current knowledge related to mortality as a nursing-sensitive outcome, the research and theoretical published literature was searched over the 10-year period from 1999 to 2009 in the following databases: CINAHL, EBSCO, MEDLINE, and PubMed. The following terms were used to locate relevant publications: *mortality*, *hospital mortality*, *medical errors* (e.g., mortality), or *failure to rescue* AND *quality of nursing care*, *personnel staffing and scheduling*, *RN mix*, *patient safety*, *quality of healthcare*, or *nursing*. A total of 194 manuscripts were identified. Manuscripts were included that met the following six criteria: (1) the manuscript was a primary report of research that included at least one nursing-related structure or process of care indicator as a potential determinant of mortality; (2) the manuscript included methodological details related to calculation of the mortality rate outcome and nursing-related predictors of mortality; (3) the manuscript included a description of the method used to risk-adjust for the influence of patients' own characteristics on the mortality rate outcome; (4) the study of mortality rates and nursing-related determinants was a primary study objective rather than a casual consequence; (5) the manuscript was written in English; and (6) the manuscript was published between 1999 and 2009. A total of 17 manuscripts met the inclusion criteria and are included in this review of mortality rate as a nursing-sensitive outcome.

Because the literature search was restricted to the period between 1999 and 2009, several landmark studies establishing mortality as a nursing-sensitive outcome were not included. For example, Knaus, Draper, Wagner, and Zimmerman (1986) demonstrated that lower intensive care unit (ICU) mortality rates were associated with the existence of comprehensive clinical nursing education programs and more effective nurse–physician collaboration. Mitchell, Armstrong, Simpson, and Lentz (1989) reported that higher nurse–physician collaboration was associated with lower mortality rates in ICUs. In their landmark study of magnet and nonmagnet hospitals, Aiken, Smith, and Lake (1994) found that magnet hospitals characterized as having higher registered nurse status, more nurse autonomy, and more control over the practice setting also had significantly lower mortality rates. These and other earlier studies laid the foundation for more recent research examining nursing and other determinants of patient mortality rates.

OVERVIEW OF MORTALITY RATE RESEARCH LITERATURE

All 17 published manuscripts examined factors that influence mortality rates after an acute care hospitalization event. Interestingly, no studies were located that examined factors influencing mortality rates for recipients of health care outside of an acute care hospital. Two studies focused exclusively on pediatric or neonatal patient populations (Hamilton, Redshaw, & Tarnow-Mordi, 2007; Mark, Harless, & Berman, 2007). Eight of 17 studies examined mortality rates after hospitalization for patients cared for in U.S. hospitals (Aiken, Clarke, Cheung, Sloane, & Silber, 2003; Aiken, Clarke, Sloane, Lake, & Cheney, 2008; Aiken, Clarke, Sloane, Sochalski, & Silber, 2002; Halm et al., 2005; Mark et al., 2007; Needleman, Buerhaus, Mattke, Steward, & Zelevinsky, 2002; Person et al., 2004; Stone et al., 2007). Three studies examined factors that influence mortality rates after hospitalization for patients cared for in Canadian hospitals (Estabrooks, Midodzi, Cummings, Ricker, & Giovannetti, 2005; Tourangeau, Doran, et al., 2006; Tourangeau, Giovannetti, Tu, & Wood, 2002). Three studies examined mortality rates for United Kingdom hospitalized patients (Hamilton et al., 2007; Rafferty et al., 2007; Tarnow-Mordi, Hau, Warden, & Shearer, 2000). One study focused on hospitalized patients in Greece (Kiekkas et al., 2008), one studied patients in Thailand hospitals (Sasichay-Akkadechanunt, Scalzi, & Jawad, 2003), and one studied mortality rates for patients in Korean hospitals (Cho, Hwang, & Kim, 2008). The unit of analysis was the hospital in 13 of 17 studies, and four studies examined mortality rates at the patient care unit or individual patient levels.

DEFINITIONS OF THE CONCEPT MORTALITY RATE

Although mortality, in its simplest meaning, reflects death, mortality can be conceptualized and then operationally defined in a variety of ways. When referring to an individual patient, death is a dichotomous variable (death or survival). However, when examining death as a quality-of-care outcome, rates of death are examined for specific patient samples or populations. The most common operational definition used in quality and research activities is a rate that is calculated as a percentage or proportion of those who die within a defined setting, with specified health conditions, and over a specified period of time. Mortality rates may reflect the proportion of patients who die within a particular healthcare facility (e.g., in-hospital death) or after receiving healthcare services within a particular patient care unit (e.g., death within intensive care units); the proportion of patients who die with specific health conditions (e.g., post–acute myocardial infarction death rate); or the proportion of patients who die after receiving a medical intervention (e.g., death rates for surgical patients). Mortality-rate measurement also includes specified time periods related to the healthcare episode. For example, mortality rates may be measured for in-hospital time periods; 30 days after admission to the hospital; or for longer periods after the initial healthcare service interface, such as 60 days after admission to the hospital. The time period for observing mortality rates depends on the purposes and objectives of the research study and practical concerns related to accessibility of mortality event data both inside and outside healthcare settings. Generally, the standard for measuring mortality as an outcome is 30 days after admission to the hospital, or 30 days after a specified healthcare event (Person et al., 2004). The rationale is that the full impact of hospitalization or a healthcare event is usually realized within 30 days without the introduction of too many competing risks that might occur with longer time periods (Jencks, Williams, & Kay, 1988; Silber, Williams, Krakauer, & Schwartz, 1992).

More recently, some scholars have developed variations on the concept of mortality rates, such as failure-to-rescue (FTR) rates (Clarke & Aiken, 2003; Schmid, Hoffman, Happ, Wolf, & DeVita, 2007). The concept of FTR was originally developed by Silber and colleagues (1992) and is defined as death after a complication (Silber et al., 2007). FTR, a variation of the concept of mortality, is built on the assumption that complication rates alone are not ideal or appropriate outcome measures because they usually reflect patient severity rather than the quality of hospital or healthcare organization care. These scholars advocate that hospital quality is better reflected and understood by knowing how well a patient with an existing complication is rescued or saved from death. The rationale is that healthcare organizations with better quality are those that quickly identify patients with complications and provide aggressive treatment. It is hypothesized that effective and quick assessment and intervention result in lower FTR rates. Studies that examine FTR rates as a mortality outcome only include patient cases that have experienced one or more of a specified list of complications. Variations in methods of measurement of FTR have been reported (Silber et al., 2007). These variations in FTR measurement primarily differ by which complications are selected for inclusion of patients in the calculation of the FTR rate. Strong evidence of both reliability and validity of FTR rates has been reported (Silber et al.,

2007). Silber and colleagues reported (2007) that the advantage of examining FTR rates over traditional mortality rates is that mortality rates are largely determined by patient characteristics, whereas FTR rates are influenced by both patient and healthcare organization characteristics (Silber et al., 1992). For those who study or use mortality rates as a measure of care quality, this claim further underscores the imperative to implement effective strategies to adjust for the impact of patients' own characteristics in mortality rate outcome research.

THEORETICAL PERSPECTIVES: RELATIONSHIP BETWEEN MORTALITY RATE, AND NURSING STRUCTURES AND PROCESSES OF CARE

Although examination of relationships between mortality rates and nursing care dates back at least to British healthcare reforms made around the time of the Crimean War under Florence Nightingale's leadership (Cohen, 1984), the earliest modern and prominent theoretical perspective explaining the relationship between mortality rates for patients who have received healthcare services and the organizational structures and processes of nursing care was postulated and tested by Aiken and colleagues (Aiken, Sochalski, & Lake, 1997; Aiken et al., 1994). The underlying rationale for postulating and studying these relationships centers on the surveillance role that nurses have as the professional healthcare providers within hospitals. Nurses provide 24-hour care to hospitalized patients, and what nurses do or fail to do is hypothesized to be directly related to outcomes, including mortality rates. Furthermore, it is the exercise of professional judgment by nurses—which includes timely and accurate assessment, communication, and intervention—that results in prevention of adverse events such as unnecessary patient death. Aiken and colleagues (Aiken et al., 1994; Aiken, Sochalski, & Lake, 1997) further hypothesized that organizational characteristics and practices impact what nurses do and do not do. They hypothesized that hospitals with work environments that facilitate nurse autonomy, nurse control over nursing practice, and good relationships between nurses and physicians will be the hospitals in which nurses effectively and routinely exercise their professional judgment. This exercise of effective judgment and subsequent assessment, communication, and intervention activities are postulated to lead to better quality patient outcomes such as lower mortality rates.

Tourangeau and colleagues (Tourangeau, 2003, 2005; Tourangeau, Giovannetti, & Wood, 2002) extended the work of Aiken and colleagues (Aiken et al., 1994; Aiken, Sochalski, & Lake, 1997) and continued development of a theoretical perspective hypothesizing relationships between nursing structures and processes of care with mortality rates. The hypothesized model (Tourangeau,

2005) suggests that, in addition to the direct impact that patients' own characteristics have on mortality rates, a number of other healthcare organizational characteristics related to delivery of nursing services both directly and indirectly influence mortality rates. These hospital characteristics include amount or dose of nurse staffing, nurse staffing skill mix (proportion of registered nurses), amount of professional role support available to support nurses and nursing practice, continuity of nursing care provider, nurse experience, nurse capacity to work (e.g., nurse health or number of hours of missed work), condition of the nursing practice work environment, and nurse responses to their work (e.g., burnout and overall job satisfaction).

OVERVIEW OF EMPIRICAL EVIDENCE OF RELATIONSHIPS BETWEEN MORTALITY RATES, AND NURSING-RELATED ORGANIZATIONAL STRUCTURES AND PROCESSES OF CARE

Across the 17 studies, 23 mortality outcomes were measured: 9 measuring in-hospital mortality rates; 8 measuring 30-day (after admission to hospital) mortality rates; 3 measuring 30-day (after admission to hospital) FTR rates; and 3 measuring in-hospital FTR rates. For each of these 17 studies, **TABLE 9-1** outlines how mortality rate outcomes were defined and provides a brief summary of each study report.

Review of these 17 studies revealed that five categories of nursing-related organizational structures and processes of care have been examined to test relationships with, and impact on, mortality rates. These five categories were: nurse staffing structures of care; characteristics of the work environment and work relationships; nurse responses to work and work environments; nurse professional characteristics (educational preparation and experience); and processes of delivering and managing care.

Nurse Staffing Structures of Care

Each of the 17 studies included at least one indicator of nurse staffing as a potential determinant of mortality rates. In all studies, nurse staffing was estimated for each patient, patient care unit, or hospital (depending on study unit of analysis) from at least one of three general sources of information: study-specific nurse surveys, large administrative databases, and study-specific organizational administrative record surveys. In some studies, such as that by Tourangeau, Doran, et al. (2006), more than one source of data was used.

In five studies, a nurse staffing or nursing workload variable (assigned patients per nurse) was calculated from questions asked in a nurse survey related to the number of patients assigned to various categories of nursing personnel on respondents' last worked shift (Aiken et al., 2002, 2003, 2008; Estabrooks et al., 2005;

TABLE 9-1 Study Summaries Investigating Relationships Among Nursing Structural Variables, Nursing Process Variables, and Mortality Rates

Author(s) (Date)	Design	Setting/subjects	Definition of the outcome concept	Nurse structural variables	Nurse process variable	Results
Aiken et al. (2008)	Retrospective design using cross-sectional analyses. Secondary sources of data from the American Hospital Association Annual Survey 1998–1999 and Pennsylvania Department of Health Hospital Questionnaire, and a 1999 study-specific nurse survey. Unit of analysis = hospital.	232,342 general surgical patients discharged from 168 Pennsylvania acute care hospitals (1998–1999). Study-specific survey of a 50% random sample of nurses working in the 168 Pennsylvania hospitals (response rate = 52%).	30-day mortality: Patient death within 30 days after admission to hospital. 30-day failure-to-rescue: Patient death within 30 days after admission among patients with selected complications.	1. RN staffing— mean number of patients assigned to each staff nurse as reported on nurse survey. 2. Nurse education— % of staff nurses holding baccalaureate or higher degrees as reported on nurse surveys. 3. Care environment— composite score of *better, mixed,* or *poor* environment for each hospital based on hospital-level medians of three subscales of the practice environment scale of the Nursing Work Index (foundations for quality care; nurse manager ability, leadership and support; collegial nurse-physician relationships).	None included	30-day mortality rate for general surgical patients reported as 19.5 per 1,000 admissions (1.95%). 30-day failure-to-rescue rate reported as 84.4 patients per 1,000 admissions (8.4%). Impact of nursing structural variables on mortality and failure-to-rescue rate examined using logistic regression models that adjusted for patient clinical characteristics (133 variables including age, sex, type of admission, surgery type, comorbid conditions) and hospital characteristics. Better care environments (OR = .91; 95% CI = .85–.98), nurse staffing (OR = 1.08; 95% CI = 1.03–1.13), and higher nurse education levels (OR = .94; 95% CI = .90–.97) were all found to be associated with lower 30-day mortality ($p < .01$). Better care environments, more nurse staffing, and higher nurse education levels (OR=.93; 95% CI = .89–.97) were all found to be associated with lower 30-day failure-to-rescue ($p < .01$).

(continues)

CI = confidence interval; FTR = failure-to-rescue; ICU = intensive care unit; OR = odds ratio.

TABLE 9-1   Study Summaries Investigating Relationships Among Nursing Structural Variables, Nursing Process Variables, and Mortality Rates (continued)

Author(s) (Date)	Design	Setting/subjects	Definition of the outcome concept	Nurse structural variables	Nurse process variable	Results
Aiken et al. (2003)	Retrospective design with cross-sectional analyses. Secondary sources of data from the American Hospital Association Annual Survey 1998–1999 and Pennsylvania Department of Health Hospital Questionnaire, as well as a 1999 study-specific nurse survey. Unit of analysis = hospital.	232,342 general surgical patients discharged from 168 Pennsylvania acute care hospitals (1998–1999). Study specific survey of a 50% random sample of nurses working in 168 Pennsylvania hospitals (response rate = 52%).	30-day mortality: Patient death within 30 days after admission to hospital. 30-day failure-to-rescue: Patient death within 30 days after admission among patients with selected complications.	1. Registered nurse education level (% with baccalaureate or higher education). 2. Nursing workload (mean number of patients assigned last shift worked). 3. Years (mean) of nurse experience as a RN.	None included	Mean hospital 30-day mortality rate was 2.0 (not risk-adjusted). Mean hospital failure-to-rescue rate was 8.4% (not risk-adjusted). Using logistic regression modeling found that: 1. Higher proportion of baccalaureate-educated nurses and lower nurse workload both were associated with lower risk-adjusted 30-day mortality rates. 2. Higher proportion of baccalaureate educated nurses and lower nurse workload were both associated with lower risk-adjusted failure-to- rescue rates.
Aiken et al. (2002)	Retrospective design using cross-sectional analyses. Secondary sources of data from the American Hospital Association Annual Survey 1998–1999 and Pennsylvania Department of Health Hospital Questionnaire, as well as a 1999 study-specific nurse survey. Unit of analysis = hospital.	232,342 general surgical patients discharged from 168 Pennsylvania acute care hospitals (1998–1999). Study-specific survey of a 50% random sample of nurses working in 168 Pennsylvania hospitals (response rate = 52%).	30-day mortality: Patient death within 30 days after admission to hospital. 30-day failure-to-rescue: Patient death within 30 days after admission among patients with selected complications.	RN staffing (patient-to-nurse ratio on last shift) as reported by nurses on study-specific nurse survey.	None included	Mean 30-day mortality rate reported as 1.95% and mean 30-day failure-to-rescue rate reported as 8.4%. Impact of hospital nurse staffing on 30-day mortality and failure-to-rescue rate examined using logistic regression modeling while controlling for impact of patient's clinical characteristics, hospital characteristics, and clustering of patients within hospitals: 1. Higher patient-to-nurse ratio found to be associated with higher 30-day mortality ($p < .001$). Odds of patient death increased by 7% for every additional patient in nurse workload. 2. Higher patient-to-nurse ratio found to be associated with higher 30-day failure-to-rescue ($p < .001$). Odds of patient death after complication increased by 7% for every additional patient in nurse workload.

Study	Design	Sample	Outcome Definition	Nurse Variables		Findings
Cho et al. (2008)	Retrospective design using cross-sectional analysis. Three data sources: • ICU survey data • Medical claims • Korean National Health Insurance enrollee database. Unit of analysis = hospital.	27,372 ICU patients discharged from 236 Korean hospitals.	Mortality defined as deaths that occurred in hospital or on date of discharge.	1. Mean years of ICU nurse experience. 2. RN staffing (ratio of average daily census to total number of full-time equivalent RNs in the ICU (estimated over a 3-month period).	None included	Mean crude mortality rate was 17% in tertiary hospitals and 22% in secondary hospitals. Using logistic regression modeling found that every additional assigned patient per RN in secondary hospitals was associated with a 9% increase in odds of dying. Nurse experience not found to be associated with patient mortality.
Estabrooks et al. (2005)	Retrospective design using cross-sectional analyses. Accessed secondary sources of large administrative/clinical databases and a study-specific nurse survey. Unit of analysis = hospital.	18,142 patients discharged from 49 Alberta, Canada, acute care hospitals with an acute medical diagnosis of acute myocardial infarction, congestive heart failure, chronic obstructive pulmonary disease, pneumonia, or stroke during fiscal year 1998–1999. 39 small hospitals (150 beds or fewer) and 10 large hospitals (more than 150 beds). Included nurse-reported study-specific data for sample of 4,799 nurses working in these hospitals (response rate = 52.8%).	Mortality defined as death within 30 days after admission (as identified in the Alberta Health Care Insurance Plan Registry).	1. Nurse education level (baccalaureate or higher). 2. Skill mix (% RN to total nursing staff). 3. Nurse employment status (permanent, temporary, casual). 4. Nurse perception of staffing adequacy. 5. Nurse perceptions of unmet patient needs. 6. Amount of nonnursing activities performed by nurses. 7. Nurse job satisfaction. 8. Nurse support for float policy. 9. Nurse-reported autonomy. 10. Nurse–physician relationship. 11. Frequency of emotional abuse experience by nurses.	None included	Used hierarchical linear modeling techniques to partition variance into 2 components: patient level and hospital level that adjusted for patient characteristics before examining impact of hospital characteristics. Found 4 nurse variables significantly associated with lower 30-day mortality rates: 1. Higher proportion of baccalaureate prepared nurses. 2. Higher proportion of RNs in nursing staff mix. 3. Higher proportion of permanent RNs. 4. Higher reported nurse-physician collaboration.

(continues)

CI = confidence interval; FTR = failure-to-rescue; ICU = intensive care unit; OR = odds ratio.

TABLE 9-1　Study Summaries Investigating Relationships Among Nursing Structural Variables, Nursing Process Variables, and Mortality Rates (continued)

Author(s) (Date)	Design	Setting/subjects	Definition of the outcome concept	Nurse structural variables	Nurse process variable	Results
Halm et al. (2005)	Cross-sectional correlation design Patient data accessed through hospital databases. Unit of analysis = individual units in one hospital. Number of units included in study not reported, though likely very low (e.g., approximately 5 units).	Included 2,709 general-surgical patients and 140 staff RNs in one large midwestern U.S. acute care hospital.	30-day mortality (death within 30 days after admission to hospital). In hospital failure-to-rescue (in hospital death for those experienced a set of complications).	RN staffing: Unit-level nurse-to-patient ratio calculated using staffing data and daily unit census data over a 1-year period.	None included	Crude 30-day mortality rate reported as 1.2%. Crude inpatient failure-to-rescue rate reported as 3.7% (authors noted that mortality data may have been incomplete). Explored impact of nurse staffing levels on 30-day mortality and inpatient failure-to-rescue rates on unspecified number of units at one hospital. Using logistic regression modeling and controlling for a small number of patient characteristics found that nurse staffing was not associated with 30-day mortality or inpatient failure-to-rescue.
Hamilton et al. (2007)	Prospective design including patients in 54 U.K. neonatal ICUs. Patient data accessed from U.K. Neonatal Staffing Study (1998–1999). Staffing data from 35,651 shift records of staffing and infants over a 1-year period (1998–1999). Unit of analysis = neonatal ICU.	2,636 low birth weight or preterm infants (inclusion criteria: birth weight less than or equal to 1,500 grams and/or gestation less than or equal to 3 weeks) in 54 U.K. neonatal ICUs.	Observed mortality defined as in-hospital death or death when discharged home to die.	1. Total number of RNs per shift (applied to each patient). 2. Nursing provision ratio per shift. 3. Specialist nursing provision ratio per shift (index of nurses with neonatal specialist qualification).	None included	Observed morality rate was 10.4%. Explored impact of three nurse study variables in preterm/low birth weight neonatal patients, while adjusting for patient characteristics using a "predicted mortality" score based on diagnostic information collected at 12 hours after birth (gestation, size, sex, mode of delivery, etc.). Using stepwise multivariate logistic analysis, lower risk-adjusted observed mortality rates were associated with higher specialist nursing provision.

	Study design	Sample	Outcome	Variables	Controls	Findings
Kiekkas et al. (2008)	Observational single-center prospective study. Collected study-specific data. Unit of analysis = patient.	Convenience sampling of 396 patients admitted to a general tertiary 14-bed academic Greek hospital between October 2005 and September 2006.	Mortality defined as observed death while in ICU.	Daily nursing workload calculated by dividing the total daily patient therapeutic intervention scores by the number of nurses that worked over the 24-hour period—then calculated workload exposure as one of three values for each study day and attributed to each study patient for that day of stay.	None included	Used binary logistic regression (enter method) to evaluate association between ICU mortality and median patient exposure to workload (categorized as low, medium, and high while adjusting for patient clinical severity using the Acute Physiology and Chronic Health Evaluation II (APACHE II) scores. Overall mortality rates not reported. No statistically significant associations were found in risk-adjusted ICU mortality regardless of the category of level of patient exposure to nursing workload.
Mark et al. (2007)	Retrospective study using secondary data sources. Accessed patient and hospital information from the California Office of Statewide Health Planning and Development patient discharge data and annual hospital disclosure reports. Unit of analysis = hospital.	Large sample of pediatric patients aged 1–14 years (total unspecified but likely greater than 1 million) who were discharged from 169 general acute care and children's hospitals in California between 1996 and 2001.	In hospital mortality—deaths during hospitalization.	1. RN staffing—hours of RN care provided per patient day (risk-adjusted for patient requirements for care using the Medstat resource demand scale). 2. Licensed vocational nurse (LVN) staffing— hours of LVN care provided per patient per day (risk adjusted as per above). 3. Unlicensed hours of care provided per patient day (risk adjusted as above).	None included	Observed in-hospital mortality rate for sample hospitals across a period of 6 years was 10% and ranged from 6.7 to 19.6%. Using a fixed-effects Poisson model to examine relationships between nurse staffing for pediatric patients and mortality rates while controlling for hospital characteristics and risk-adjusting for patients' characteristics using Medstat's disease-staging methodology found no relationship between in-hospital pediatric death and nurse staffing for hospitalized California pediatric patients.

CI = confidence interval; FTR = failure-to-rescue; ICU = intensive care unit; OR = odds ratio.

(continues)

TABLE 9-1 Study Summaries Investigating Relationships Among Nursing Structural Variables, Nursing Process Variables, and Mortality Rates (continued)

Author(s) (Date)	Design	Setting/subjects	Definition of the outcome concept	Nurse structural variables	Nurse process variable	Results
Needleman et al. (2002)	Retrospective study. Accessed secondary sources data retrieved from the American Hospital Association's Annual Survey of Hospitals (few details included). Unit of analysis = hospital.	Included medical and surgical patient discharges from 799 hospitals in 11 U.S. states over the calendar year 1997.	Mortality defined as rate of in-hospital death. Failure-to-rescue defined as rate of in-hospital death for patients with hospital-acquired pneumonia, shock or cardiac arrest, upper gastrointestinal bleeding, sepsis, or deep venous thrombosis.	Calculated following eight nurse staffing indicators for each hospital as the weighted average of staffing in the 1997 and 1998 fiscal years: 1. Number of RN hours of nursing care per patient day. 2. Number of licensed practical nurse hours per patient day. 3. Number of aid hours of care per patient day. 4. Total hours of nursing care per patient day. 5. Proportion of RN hours of all hours of nursing care. 6. Proportion of licensed practical nurse hours of all hours of nursing care. 7. Number of hours of care provided by licensed nurses (RN + practical nurse) per patient day. 8. RN hours as a proportion of licensed nurse hours.	None included	Mean in-hospital mortality across hospitals for medical patients was 3.2% and for surgical patients, 1.6%. Mean in-hospital failure-to-rescue rate for medical patients was 18.6% and for surgical patients, 19.7%. Both in-hospital mortality and in-hospital failure-to-rescue rates were risk-adjusted for patient characteristics using estimates of predicted death for each patient. Using negative binomial regression modeling, no statistically significant relationships were found between in-hospital mortality rates and nurse staffing indicators. Using negative binomial regression modeling, the following two statistically significant relationships were found between lower hospital failure-to-rescue rates and nurse staffing: 1. For medical patients, a higher proportion of hours of care provided by RNs. 2. For surgical patients, a greater number of hours of care provided by RNs.
Person et al. (2004)	Retrospective study. Patient data accessed through the cooperative cardiovascular project data set and hospital data	Study of 118,940 acute myocardial infarction (AMI) patients from 4,401 U.S. hospitals in 1994–1995.	Mortality defined as within-hospital death rate for those admitted for AMI.	1. Ratio of full-time equivalent RNs to average daily census. 2. Ratio of full-time equivalent licensed practical and	None included	No crude or risk-adjusted in-hospital mortality rates reported. Reported mortality rates for quartiles of hospitals' RN staffing (range = 17.4–20.1%) and quartiles of licensed practical and vocational nursing staff (17.2– 20.1%).

						Findings
	accessed from the American Hospital Assessment Survey of Hospital Characteristics (1994–1995). Unit of analysis = hospital.			vocational nurses per average daily census. • Part-time nursing staff estimated as 0.5 full-time equivalent.		In-hospital mortality rates adjusted for teaching status, volume, and location, as well as patient characteristics (age, sex, race, and comorbidities). Multivariate logistical regression modeling used to examine relationships between in-hospital mortality for AMI patients and nurse staffing. The following two significant relationships were found: 1. Lower in-hospital mortality rates were associated with higher RN staffing in hospitals. 2. Higher in-hospital mortality rates were associated with higher licensed vocational/practical staffing in hospitals.
Rafferty et al. (2007)	Cross-sectional retrospective study. Accessed secondary sources of large clinical/administrative databases and a study-specific nurse survey. Unit of analysis = hospital.	Included a sample of 118,752 surgical patients in 30 U.K. acute trusts in 1998. Surveyed a sample of 3,984 nurses (mostly RNs) working in the 30 study trusts in 1999 (49.4% response rate).	Mortality defined as inpatient death. Failure-to-rescue defined as inpatient death among patients who experienced complications. (Complications data were difficult to obtain, so length of stay longer than 1.25 times the median for each healthcare resource group of patients was used as a proxy for complications.)	Mean hospital patient–nurse ratio derived from survey of nurses (related to number of patients on last worked shift).	None included	Mean crude input mortality rate for surgical patients was 2.3%, and mean failure-to-rescue rate for the 35.9% of patients who experienced complication (length of stay longer than 1.25 times median) was 6.4%. Logistic regression analyses were used to estimate effects of nurse staffing on inpatient mortality and failure-to-rescue rates. Mortality and failure-to-rescue rates were risk-adjusted using logistic regression modeling (to determine each patient's odds of dying) using age, diagnosis procedures received, and interaction terms. Findings: Patients cared for in hospital with the highest patient-to-nurse ratios had 26% higher mortality rates and 29% higher failure-to-rescue rates than those in the lowest quartile of patient-to-nurse ratios.

CI = confidence interval; FTR = failure-to-rescue; ICU = intensive care unit; OR = odds ratio.

(continues)

TABLE 9-1   Study Summaries Investigating Relationships Among Nursing Structural Variables, Nursing Process Variables, and Mortality Rates (continued)

Author(s) (Date)	Design	Setting/subjects	Definition of the outcome concept	Nurse structural variables	Nurse process variable	Results
Sasichay-Akkadecha-nunt et al. (2003)	Retrospective cross-sectional observational design. Patient data accessed from patient charts. Nurse staffing data accessed from nursing service department databases. Unit of analysis = inpatient unit.	Studied 2,531 medical-surgical patients from 17 inpatient units in one Thailand university hospital with principal diagnoses in following groups: diseases of the heart, malignant neoplasms, hypertension, cerebrovascular diseases, and pneumonia/other lung diseases.	In-hospital mortality rate (proportion of deaths in each study unit).	1. Ratio of total nursing staff to patients. 2. Proportion of RN to total nursing staff. 3. Mean years RN experience. 4. Percentage of baccalaureate-educated nurses.	None included	Using multivariate logistic regression and controlling for the impact of patient characteristics on inpatient mortality with Acute Physiology and Chronic Health Evaluation III (APACHE III) scores and seven additional patient indicators (e.g., sex, diagnosis, type of admission), they found that a higher nurse–patient ratio was significantly associated with lower inpatient unit mortality rates.
Stone et al. (2007)	Observational study. Patient data accessed through Medicare files. Hospital characteristic data accessed through the American Hospital Association Survey of Hospital data. Study-specific nurse survey used to collect nurse data. Unit of analysis = individual ICU (not explicitly stated).	Convenience sample of 15,846 ICU patients in 51 ICUs in 31 U.S. hospitals. Surveyed ICU RNs to assess organizational climate (number of nurses not identified).	30-day mortality defined as death within 30 days after admission to hospital.	1. Nursing staffing measured by RN hours per patient day in the ICU. 2. Overtime use measured as proportion of overtime to regular hours. 3. Organizational climate in ICU measured as composite score of Perception of Nurse Work Environment (Choi et al., 2004).	None included	Mean 30-day mortality rate reported as 22%. Multivariate logistic regression modeling used to examine relationship between dependent nursing variables and 30-day mortality for ICU patients. Thirty-day mortality outcomes risk-adjusted for patient's own characteristics (age, gender, SES, etc.). Findings: Patients admitted to ICUs with more RN hours per patient day had significantly lower 30-day mortality. No significant relationships were observed with either overtime use or ICU organizational climate and 30-day mortality.

	Design	Sample	Outcome	Variables		Findings
Tarnow-Mordi et al. (2000)	Retrospective study. Both patient and nurse workload data collected as part of previous study. Unit of analysis = patient episode of care.	Sample of 1,050 patient episodes in one medical-surgical ICU in a Scottish hospital between 1992 and 1995.	In-hospital mortality (death during hospitalization in or outside ICU).	Nursing workload calculated as nursing requirement per ICU shift, defined as the highest number of nurses required for the ICU for each shift (as per recommendation by U.K. Intensive Care Society). Average and peak values of nursing requirements per ICU shift were calculated for each patient's day of stay in the ICU.	None included	Hospital mortality (in and outside ICU) was reported as 32%. Used multiple logistic regression analyses to examine relationship between nursing workload and inpatient mortality in one ICU. Mortality rate was risk-adjusted using Acute Physiology and Chronic Health Evaluation II scores (APACHE II) to calculate estimated probability of death. Findings: Higher hospital mortality was significantly associated with patients' exposure to high versus moderate overall ICU workload.
Tourangeau, Doran, et al. (2006)	Retrospective design using cross-sectional analysis. Secondary data accessed from large clinical and administrative databases (2002–2003). Nurse data collected from a 2004 study-specific nurse survey. Unit of analysis = hospital.	49,993 patients discharged from 75 Ontario, Canada, teaching and community acute care hospitals in 2002–2003 with a most responsible diagnosis in one of four acute medical diagnostic categories: acute myocardial infarction, stroke, pneumonia, or septicemia. Nurse survey (2003) sent to population of 5,980 nurses (RNs and registered practical nurses) working in these 75 Ontario hospitals and who worked in medical or combined medical-surgical areas (response rate = 65%; N=3,886).	Risk-adjusted 30-day mortality rate: Ratio of observed deaths divided by number of expected deaths for each hospital.	1. Nursing staff mix (proportion of RNs in nursing staff). 2. Nursing staff dose. 3. Percentage of full time nursing staff. 4. Years experience on unit. 5. Percentage of nurses with baccalaureate or higher. 6. Overall nurse health level. 7. Hours of missed work in preceding 3 months. 8. Quality of nurse–physician relationships. 9. Nurse-rated manager ability and support. 10. Nurse-rated adequacy of staffing and resources. 11. Amount of teamwork. 12. Overall nurse job satisfaction.	Frequency of use of care maps/protocols to guide patient care (one nurse survey item with 5-point frequency response option).	Mean risk-adjusted 30-day mortality rate reported as 17.4% and ranged from 9.9 to 28.3%. Calculated risk-adjusted standard mortality rates for each hospital using the general formula of observed deaths divided by expected deaths in each hospital. First, calculated expected probability of death for each patient through four logistic regression models (one for each of the four diagnostic groups of patients) and summed the probabilities of death within each hospital to determine the expected number of deaths for each hospital. Then, using the standard mortality rates in backward regression modeling, explained 45% variance ($p < .0001$) with eight predictors. Lower 30-day mortality rates found to be associated with: 1. Higher proportion of registered nursing staff 2. Higher proportion of baccalaureate-educated nurses 3. Lower total dose of all categories of nursing staff 4. Higher nurse-reported adequacy of staffing and resources

CI = confidence interval; FTR = failure-to-rescue; ICU = intensive care unit; OR = odds ratio.

(continues)

TABLE 9-1   Study Summaries Investigating Relationships Among Nursing Structural Variables, Nursing Process Variables, and Mortality Rates (continued)

Author(s) (Date)	Design	Setting/subjects	Definition of the outcome concept	Nurse structural variables	Nurse process variable	Results
Tourangeau, Doran, et al. (2006) *(continued)*				13. Nurse-reported quality of care. 14. Nurse burnout. 15. Amount of professional role support available for nursing staff.		5. Higher use of care maps/protocols 6. Higher nurse-reported quality of care 7. Lower nurse-reported manager ability and support 8. Higher nurse burnout
Tourangeau et al. (2002)	Retrospective design using cross-sectional analysis. Secondary data accessed from 1998–1999 large clinical and administrative databases. Nurse data collected from a 1999 study-specific nurse survey. Unit of analysis = hospital.	49,941 patients discharged from 75 Ontario, Canada, teaching and community acute care hospitals with a most responsible diagnosis in one of four acute medical diagnostic categories: acute myocardial infarction, stroke, pneumonia, or septicemia in 1998–1999. Modified random sample of 3,988 RNs working in medical units in the 75 study hospitals (response rate = 57%) who completed a nurse survey in 1999.	Risk-adjusted 30-day mortality rate: Ratio of observed deaths divided by expected number of deaths for each hospital.	1. Nurse staffing dose. 2. Nursing skill mix (proportion of RNs of all nursing staff). 3. Availability of professional role support. 4. Years experience in clinical unit. 5. Nurse capacity to work (number of shifts missed in preceding 3 months). 6. Condition of nursing practice environment (measured with a one factor score of the Revised Nursing Index). 7. Continuity of RN care.		Mean risk-adjusted mortality rate reported as 15.03% and ranged from 10.5 to 21.5%. Calculated risk-adjusted standard mortality rates for each hospital using the general formula of observed deaths divided by expected deaths in each hospital. First, calculated expected probability of death for each patient through four logistic regression models (one for each of the four diagnostic groups of patients) and summed the probabilities of death within each hospital to determine the expected number of deaths for each hospital. Then, using the standard mortality rates in stepwise regression modeling, explained 32% of variance ($p = .0004$) in risk-adjusted hospital mortality rates with three predictors. Lower 30-day mortality was found to be significantly associated with: 1. Higher proportions of RN staffing 2. More years of nurse experience on the clinical unit 3. Higher number of shifts missed by nurses in the preceding 3 months

CI = confidence interval; FTR = failure-to-rescue; ICU = intensive care unit; OR = odds ratio.

Rafferty et al., 2007; Tourangeau, Doran, et al., 2006). These primary sources of data were used to calculate nurse staffing variables such as the mean number of patients assigned to nurses on their last shift (nurse–patient ratio), or to calculate the proportion of each category of nursing personnel on the last shift worked. In two of these studies, employment status variables (proportion of temporary and casual nursing staff and proportion of full-time nursing staff) were calculated to determine their impact on mortality rates (Estabrooks et al.; Tourangeau, Doran, et al.).

In six studies, data to calculate nurse staffing variables were accessed through large administrative databases such as the American Hospital Association Annual Survey and the Canadian Discharge Abstract Database (Mark et al., 2007; Needleman et al., 2002; Person et al., 2004; Stone et al., 2007; Tourangeau, Doran, et al., 2006; Tourangeau et al., 2002). These secondary sources of data were accessed to calculate nurse staffing variables such as the proportion of hours of nursing care provided by registered nurses (frequently referred to as skill mix) or amount (hours) of nursing care provided for some denominator unit of measure (e.g., per patient day, per weighted case, per average daily census). Most often, nurse staffing variables calculated from large administrative data sets were variables at the hospital organizational level.

The third source of nurse staffing data, study-specific organizational administrative record surveys, was used to calculate nurse staffing variables in six studies (Cho et al., 2008; Halm et al., 2005; Hamilton et al., 2007; Kiekkas et al., 2008; Sasichay-Akkadechanunt et al., 2003; Tarnow-Mordi et al., 2000). These study-specific primary sources of data collected through administrative record survey were used to calculate unit- or patient-level nurse staffing variables such as nurse-to-patient ratios, proportion of specific categories of nurses of all nursing personnel (staff mix), or the amount (hours) of specialist nurse care per shift.

Overall, 14 of 17 studies found a statistically significant direct relationship between one or more nurse staffing variables and mortality rates. The following nurse staffing variables were found to be associated with lower mortality rates (mortality rate defined in each study):

- Fewer assigned patients on the last worked shift and higher nurse-to-patient ratios (Aiken et al., 2002, 2003, 2008; Cho et al., 2008; Rafferty et al., 2007; Sasichay-Akkadechanunt et al., 2003; Tarnow-Mordi et al., 2000)
- Higher proportion of registered nurses in the nursing staff mix (Estabrooks et al., 2005; Needleman et al., 2002; Person et al., 2004; Tourangeau, Doran, et al., 2006; Tourangeau et al., 2002)
- Higher registered nurse hours per patient day (Needleman et al., 2002; Stone et al., 2007)
- Lower proportion of casual or temporary nursing staff (Estabrooks et al., 2005)
- Higher nurse specialist hours per patient day (Hamilton et al., 2007).

Many studies included clear interpretations of the impact of nurse staffing on mortality rates. For example, Aiken et al. (2002) concluded that for a large sample of 232,342 surgical patients in the United States, each additional patient assigned to a nurse was associated with a 7% increase in the likelihood of dying within 30 days after admission, and a 7% increase in the odds of FTR. Tourangeau, Doran, et al. (2006) concluded that for a large sample of almost 47,000 Canadian acute medical patients, a 10% increase in the proportion of registered nurses in the nurse staff mix was associated with 6 fewer deaths for every 1,000 patients discharged from hospital.

No association was found between mortality rates and nurse staffing in 3 of 17 studies (Halm et al., 2005; Kiekkas et al., 2008; Mark et al., 2007). Given the similarity in findings across the world, it is reasonable to conclude that both the amount and type of nurse staffing in hospitals are related to mortality rates.

Characteristics of the Nurse Work Environment and Work Relationships

Five of 17 studies tested relationships between various aspects of the nurse work environment and mortality rates (Aiken et al., 2008; Estabrooks et al., 2005; Stone et al., 2007; Tourangeau, Doran, et al., 2006; Tourangeau et al., 2002). In each of these studies, the work environment was measured through questions on a nurse survey. In three studies, composite scores were calculated to measure the following overall conditions of the work environment:
- Organizational climate in intensive care units (Stone et al., 2007) was measured using a composite score of the Perceptions of Nurse Work Environments scale (Choi, Bakken, Larson, Du, & Stone, 2004).
- Nurse care work environments characterized by foundations for quality care, nurse manager ability and support, and the quality of nurse–physician relationships (Aiken et al., 2008) was measured using a composite score of three subscales of the Practice Environment Scale of the Nursing Work Index (Lake, 2002).
- Overall condition of the work environment (Tourangeau et al., 2002) was measured using the Canadian Practice Environment instrument (Estabrooks et al., 2002) to assess amount of nurse autonomy and control over practice, quality of leadership, quality of relationship between nurses and physicians, and adequacy of staffing and resources.

All three instruments share many common items.

Two studies examining relationships between nurse work environments and mortality rates measured discrete aspects of the work environment to determine their relationships with mortality. Estabrooks et al. (2005) used individual items from a nurse survey to assess six aspects of the hospital work environment:

adequacy of staffing, amount of nonnursing activities performed by nurses, support for a nurse float policy, nurse autonomy, quality of nurse–physician relationships, and frequency of emotional abuse. Tourangeau, Doran, et al. (2006) used individual nurse survey items and subscales of the Revised Nursing Work Index (Estabrooks et al., 2002; Lake, 2002) to assess five aspects of hospital work environments: quality of nurse–physician relationships, manager ability and support, adequacy of staffing, amount of teamwork among nurses, and availability of professional role support resources.

Across these five studies were mixed findings of relationships between nurse work environments and mortality rates (mortality was defined in each study). The statistically significant relationships found between nurse work environment and lower mortality rates were:

- Higher rated overall nurse care environments (Aiken et al., 2008)
- Better relationships between nurses and physicians (Estabrooks et al., 2005)
- Less nurse manager ability and support (Tourangeau, Doran, et al., 2006)
- More adequate staffing and resources (Tourangeau, Doran, et al., 2006)

Some study reports included interpretations of the impact of nurse work environments on mortality rates. Aiken et al. (2008) reported that the likelihood of surgical patients dying within 30 days after admission was 14% lower in hospitals with better nurse-reported care environments. Tourangeau, Doran, et al. (2006) reported that for a large sample of Canadian medical patients, a 10% increase in nurse-reported adequacy of staffing and resources was associated with 17 fewer patient deaths for every 1,000 discharged patients. However, the inconsistency in findings related to relationships between nurse work environments and mortality rates suggests that further research should be implemented to explore such relationships and that there should be more consistent use of similar operational definition to measure work environments.

Nurse Responses to Work and Work Environments

In 3 of 17 studies, relationships between nurse responses to work environments and mortality rates were examined (Estabrooks et al., 2005; Tourangeau, Doran, et al., 2006; Tourangeau et al., 2002). All three were Canadian studies. Estabrooks et al. and Tourangeau, Doran, et al. examined the relationship between nurse job satisfaction and 30-day mortality. Estabrooks et al. (2005) calculated job satisfaction using a single item from a nurse survey, whereas Tourangeau, Doran, et al. used a composite job satisfaction score using the McCloskey Mueller Job Satisfaction Scale (Tourangeau, McGillis Hall, Doran, & Petch, 2006) Two studies examined the relationship between missed shifts or hours and mortality (Tourangeau, Doran, et al.; Tourangeau et al., 2002). Both studies used a single item in a nurse survey to calculate the number of missed shifts by each nurse over the preceding 3-month period. Tourangeau, Doran, et al. also explored relationships between mortality rates and three additional nurse responses to work and work environments: overall health, evaluation of quality of care on the unit, and nurse burnout. Overall nurse health and quality of care were assessed using single items in a nurse survey. Nurse burnout levels were assessed using the nine-item emotional exhaustion subscale of the Maslach Burnout Inventory (Maslach, Jackson, & Leiter, 1996).

Across these three studies, three statistically significant relationships were found with lower mortality rates (mortality defined in each study):

- Higher ratings of care quality on the unit (Tourangeau, Doran, et al., 2006)
- Higher levels of nurse burnout (Tourangeau, Doran, et al., 2006)
- Higher number of missed shifts in the preceding 3-month period (Tourangeau et al., 2002)

Tourangeau, Doran, et al. (2006) found that a 10% increase in nurse-reported quality of care was associated with 21 fewer deaths for every 1,000 discharged patients. They interpreted the unexpected finding of the negative relationship between nurse burnout and mortality rates as higher burnout (moderate and higher levels) possibly acting as motivation that enables nurses to detect and intervene promptly with patients experiencing serious complications that may lead to unnecessary death if left unattended or detected too late. The inconsistency in findings related to relationships between nurse responses to work and work environments and mortality rates suggests that further research should be implemented to explore such relationships.

Nurse Professional Characteristics: Educational Preparation and Experience

Seven of 17 studies examined relationships between nurse professional characteristics (educational preparation and/or experience) and mortality rates (Aiken et al., 2003, 2008; Cho et al., 2008; Estabrooks et al., 2005; Sasichay-Akkadechanunt et al., 2003; Tourangeau, Doran, et al., 2006; Tourangeau et al., 2002). Five examined the impact of nurse educational preparation on mortality rates. In all five studies, this variable was calculated as the proportion of nurses who reported being educated at the baccalaureate level or higher using a single nurse survey item (Aiken et al., 2003, 2008; Estabrooks et al.; Sasichay-Akkadechanunt et al.; Tourangeau, Doran, et al.). Five studies examined relationships between nurse experience (as a registered nurse or on the clinical unit) and mortality rates (Aiken et al., 2003; Cho et al.; Sasichay-Akkadechanunt et al.; Tourangeau, Doran, et al.; Tourangeau et al., 2002).

Across these seven studies, the following statistically significant relationships were found with lower mortality rates (mortality defined in each study):

- Higher proportions of baccalaureate-educated nurses (Aiken et al., 2003, 2008; Estabrooks et al., 2005; Tourangeau, Doran, et al., 2006)
- More years of nurse experience (Tourangeau et al., 2002)

Interpretations of the impact of nurse education preparation on mortality rates were provided within several study reports. For example, Aiken and colleagues (2003) reported that a 10% increase in the proportion of nurses educated at the baccalaureate or higher level was associated with a 5% decrease in both 30-day mortality and 30-day FTR rates for surgical patients. Tourangeau, Doran et al. (2006) reported that a 10% increase in the proportion of nurses with a baccalaureate degree or higher was associated with 9 fewer deaths for every 1,000 discharged acute medical patients in Ontario, Canada, hospitals. These findings suggest that there is considerable evidence supporting the impact that higher proportions of baccalaureate-educated nurses have on lower mortality rates. However, the evidence related to the impact of nurse experience on mortality rates is inconsistent and weak.

Processes of Nursing Care

Of all 17 studies, only one examined the relationship between mortality rates and processes of care. Tourangeau, Doran, et al. (2006) examined the relationship between use of care maps or protocols and mortality rates. To calculate this variable, nurses were asked in a single item to identify how frequently they used care maps or protocols to guide patient care using a 5-point response option scale. Using backward regression, a statistically significant relationship was found between use of care maps or protocols and 30-day mortality for a sample of acute medical patients cared for in Ontario, Canada, hospitals. They found that a 10% increase in nurse-reported use of care maps or protocols was associated with 10 fewer deaths for every 1,000 acute medicine discharged patients. This finding suggests that more research is required to investigate the relationship between use of care maps or protocols and mortality rates.

Conclusions Based on the Empirical Evidence

Over the past 10 years, there has been considerable research investigating relationships between the structures and processes of nursing care and the quality outcome of mortality rates. The focus of these studies has been on investigation of relationships between nurse staffing and mortality rates. There is convincing evidence that higher proportions of registered nurses in the mix of nursing staff and higher amounts of registered nurse staffing are both related to lower mortality rates.

Research investigating relationships between the nurse work environment and nurse responses to their work and work environments is conflicting and still in developmental stages. Some studies have reported finding significant relationships, whereas others have found no relationships among work environments and mortality rates or between nurse responses to their work environments and mortality rates.

Considerable evidence supports the existence of relationships between higher proportions of baccalaureate-educated nurses and lower mortality rates but much less evidence supporting the existence of relationships between nurse experience and mortality rates. Finally, only one study examined relationships between nursing care processes and mortality rates. Little is known about processes of care that impact mortality rates.

MEASUREMENT/CALCULATION OF MORTALITY RATES

Overall, three general methods were used to calculate mortality rates: direct standardization methods, indirect standardization methods, and multistep methods such as hierarchical linear modeling. Unfortunately, most study reports did not contain sufficient details of the calculation of the mortality rate outcomes to easily allow replication. This may be because calculation of a mortality rate is very complex, particularly in relation to risk-adjustment procedures that adjust for the impact of patients' own characteristics on their mortality or survival and for the mix of patient types within a sample.

The most common methodology used to calculate mortality rates was the direct standardization method, which includes all potential predictors, both patient level and organizational level (patient or unit as appropriate), in the analytic model (Aiken et al., 2002, 2003, 2008; Cho et al., 2008; Halm et al., 2005; Hamilton et al., 2007; Kiekkas et al., 2008; Stone et al., 2007). The mortality rate is calculated as the proportion of deaths divided by the number of patients in the whole sample. The outcome is risk-adjusted by including indicators of patient characteristics that are suspected of contributing to patient death.

A second common method used to calculate mortality rates is an indirect standardization method (Mark et al., 2007; Needleman et al., 2002; Person et al., 2004; Rafferty et al., 2007; Tarnow-Mordi et al., 2000; Tourangeau, Doran, et al., 2006; Tourangeau et al., 2002). This method usually involves a two step process—the first to calculate risk-adjusted standard mortality rates using the general formula of actual observed number of deaths divided by expected number of deaths (Bland, 1999; Shwartz & Ash, 2003; Tourangeau, 2006a; Tourangeau & Tu, 2003). The expected number of deaths for each unit of analysis (e.g., patient care unit, hospital) is the sum of all the probabilities of death for the entire group of patients within each unit of analysis. The expected probability of death is usually calculated using logistic regression models that include patient characteristics suspected of contributing to or preventing death. In several studies, adjustments were also made at this stage of the calculation to adjust for the mix of patients within facilities (Tourangeau, Doran, et al.; Tourangeau et al., 2002). The second step involves testing the relationships between the risk-adjusted standard mortality rate and the structures and processes of care within analytic models using procedures such as multiple regression.

A third method used to calculate mortality rates is hierarchical generalized linear modeling (Estabrooks et al., 2005). Estabrooks and colleagues implemented a multistage procedure to partition the variance in mortality rates into two components—patient and hospital levels (Raudenbush & Bryk, 2002). The effects of patient characteristics were accounted for in the first modeling stage, and the second stage involved simultaneous testing of the effects of all hospital nursing-related variables on 30-day mortality rates for a sample of Alberta, Canada, hospitals. Such modeling techniques have been used over the past three decades by social scientists and are now being increasingly used in health services research to analyze data characterized by intercluster units such as patient-level, nurse-level, or hospital-level units of cluster (Estabrooks et al.).

DATA ISSUES IN MORTALITY RATE RESEARCH

Three key data issues are associated with calculation of mortality rates: access to and source of mortality data; data quality (reliability); and adequacy of risk-adjustment procedures. One of the most challenging issues in mortality rate outcome research is securing access to mortality and patient characteristic data that are required to implement risk and case-mix-adjustment strategies (Iezzoni, 2003b, 2003c, 2003d). Across the 17 studies, two general sources of data were used to calculate mortality rates: study-specific primary data (5 studies) and secondary-source large administrative and clinical databases (12 studies). Both sources were used to identify patient death or survival and to identify patient characteristic data. Studies that collected study-specific mortality rate data generally included smaller sample hospital or patient care unit sizes (Halm et al., 2005; Kiekkas et al., 2008; Hamilton et al., 2007; Sasichay-Akkadechanunt et al., 2003; Tarnow-Mordi et al., 2000), whereas studies that accessed large administrative or clinical databases to calculate mortality rates tended to have much larger sample sizes or even included entire populations (Aiken et al., 2002, 2003, 2008; Cho et al., 2008; Estabrooks et al., 2005; Mark et al., 2007; Needleman et al., 2002; Person et al., 2004; Rafferty et al., 2007; Stone et al., 2007; Tourangeau, Doran, et al., 2006; Tourangeau et al., 2002). Although it is generally accepted that 30-day mortality rates are most appropriate to examine care quality (Jencks et al., 1988; Silber et al., 1992; Tourangeau et al., 2002), many studies included analyses using in-hospital mortality rates. This may reflect challenges in accessing death data outside a hospital or healthcare facility. In some jurisdictions, vital statistics data that include birth and death dates may or may not be accessible to identify whether a patient died outside a hospital within a specified time period after hospital admission. If available, these data must be linked with patient hospitalization data to calculate the dichotomous variable of patient death or survival within a specified period of time. Unfortunately, linkage of these data sets may be compromised by lack of access to a patient-level variable common in both data sets.

A second serious issue in mortality rate outcome research involves the quality of data used to calculate mortality rates (Tourangeau & Tu, 2003). This threat exists regardless of whether study-specific primary data or secondary data sources from large administrative or clinical databases are used. Both sources of data may be vulnerable to measurement error and questionable accuracy because of errors in extracting patient hospitalization records, incomplete or missing data, and so on (Daley, Ash, & Iezzoni, 2003; Tourangeau & Tu). Mortality rate outcome research should report on reliability of data used to calculate risk-adjusted mortality rates, regardless of the source of these data.

A third issue in mortality rate outcome research is the adequacy of risk-adjustment procedures to account for the impact of patient characteristics on mortality (Shwartz & Ash, 2003). Effective risk-adjustment procedures should demonstrate strong predictive validity. Risk-adjustment procedures should accurately predict patient death or survival based on patient characteristics. Unless the impact of patient characteristics is effectively accounted for, it may not be possible to accurately identify the influence of healthcare structures and processes of care on mortality rates. Credible mortality outcome research should include some estimation of the adequacy and effectiveness of the methods used in risk adjustment. As in all research, study results are only as credible as the data used. Mortality rate outcome research that does not include evidence of the predictive validity of the risk-adjustment strategy should be considered to have considerable potential for unreliability. Shwartz and Ash have outlined multiple strategies to evaluate the predictive validity of risk-adjustment models in outcome research.

The issue of risk-adjustment procedure adequacy is further complicated because patient characteristics that put patients at risk for death may be different from patient characteristics that predict other important healthcare quality outcomes. Furthermore, for different diagnostic groups of patients, different patient characteristics will contribute to their death. For example, Tourangeau and Tu (2003) completed separate risk-adjustment models for four distinct homogeneous groups of Canadian patients with acute medical conditions. They reported that different patient characteristics predicted 30-day mortality across the four groups of patients.

A variety of methods have been used to measure risk of patient death or survival. In five studies (Estabrooks et al., 2005; Rafferty et al., 2007; Stone et al.,

2007; Tourangeau, Doran, et al., 2006; Tourangeau et al., 2002), well-established risk-adjustment strategies, such as adaptions of the Charlson Comorbidity Index (Charlson, Pompei, Ales, & MacKenzie, 1987; Deyo, Cherkin, & Ciol, 1992) and the Elixhauser method (Elixhauser, Steiner, Harris, & Coffey, 1998), were used to guide choice of patient characteristics included in risk-adjustment models to predict patient death or survival. In four studies (Kiekkas et al., 2008; Sasichay-Akkadechanunt et al., 2003; Tarnow-Mordi et al., 2000), well-established scoring systems, such as the Acute Physiology Score and Chronic Health Evaluation (APACHE) scoring system (Adomat & Hewison, 2004; Knaus, Zimmerman, Wagner, Draper, & Lawrence, 1981; Zimmerman et al., 1998) or the Medstat Disease Staging methodology (Gonnella, Hornbrook, & Louis, 1984), were used to calculate a measure of clinical severity for use in risk-adjustment modeling (Kiekkas et al.; Sasichay-Akkadechanunt et al.; Tarnow-Mordi et al.). The remaining eight study reports did not identify a specific method used to guide their risk-adjustment modeling.

RECOMMENDATIONS AND DIRECTIONS FOR FUTURE RESEARCH

In hospitals, nursing and nurse staffing are inextricably linked to patient safety outcomes such as mortality (Collins Sharp & Clancy, 2008). Although there is a strong evidence-based link between nurse staffing and mortality rates, there is an urgent need to continue to provide evidence of these links while exploring relationships between other organizational characteristics and mortality rates, including nurse work and work environments, nurse responses to their work and work environments, and nurse professional characteristics. If the goal of mortality rate outcome research is to develop knowledge to assist nurse and healthcare leaders and clinicians to improve mortality rates and prevent unnecessary patient death, we must move beyond the existing focus of examining the impact of nurse staffing on mortality rates. This foundation could be used to broaden research that examines those other nursing-related healthcare organization factors that may also impact mortality rates.

Researchers must continue to develop evidence-based knowledge of relationships between mortality rates and nursing-related organizational structures and processes of care, and theoretical models explaining these relationships should be developed, tested and refined. An integrated theory-driven approach would facilitate examination of patient, nurse, and other organizational factors that influence mortality rates (Sidani & Braden, 1998). A more complete body of knowledge could then be developed. Continuing to examine the impact of nurse staffing alone on mortality rates would present an incomplete picture of the relationships between mortality rates and healthcare organizational structures and processes of care. This recommendation has cost implications for researchers because including examination of multiple factors in mortality rate outcome research would involve considerable additional data collection burden from multiple primary and secondary sources. Nonetheless, this is an important consideration to advance knowledge of the determinants of mortality rates.

The variety of risk-adjustment procedures and the lack of detail describing these methods in many of the study reports suggest that there is considerable opportunity to develop, test, and refine risk-adjustment procedures useful in mortality rate outcome research. Given the beginning evidence of the impact of patient characteristics on distinct subpopulations of healthcare recipients, it is likely that no single formula can be used to account for the risk that patients' own characteristics have on death or survival (Tourangeau, 2006a; Tourangeau & Tu, 2003). This suggests that further research is required to explore those factors that influence the various subpopulations of patients who access healthcare services. Further research is required to evaluate the effectiveness of various analytical approaches used in risk-adjustment procedures in mortality rate outcome research. For example, an important methodological question would involve addressing the variations in results when different analytical approaches are implemented in mortality rate outcome research.

Finally, nurse researchers need to further develop and disseminate their knowledge and skills in accessing and linking large administrative and clinical databases to advance knowledge of determinants of mortality rates. These data are accessible in most jurisdictions, but there are few opportunities in nursing education programs for novice nurse researchers to learn the knowledge and skills required to access and link these valuable sources of information (Tourangeau, 2006b). Consequently, nurse researchers may rely on others, such as analysts, to access and link these databases. This may result in less effective use of these data because analysts do not necessarily understand or explore the theoretical and practical utility of these data sources.

REFERENCES

Adomat, R., & Hewison, A. (2004). Assessing patient category/dependence systems for determining the nurse/patient ration in ICU and HDU: A review of approaches. *Journal of Nursing Management, 12,* 299–308.

Aiken, L. H., Clarke, S. P., Cheung, R. B., Sloane, D. M., & Silber, J. H. (2003). Education levels of hospital nurses and surgical patient mortality. *Journal of the American Medical Association, 290,* 1617–1623.

Aiken, L. H., Clarke, S. P., Sloane, D. M., Lake, E. T., & Cheney, T. (2008). Effects of hospital care environment on patient mortality and nurse outcomes. *Journal of Nursing Administration, 38*(5), 223–229.

Aiken, L. H., Clarke, S. P., Sloane, D. M., Sochalski, J., & Silber, J. H. (2002). Hospital nurse staffing and patient mortality, nurse burnout, and job dissatisfaction. *Journal of the American Medical Association, 288,* 1987–1993.

Aiken, L. H. Smith, H. L., & Lake, E. T. (1994). Lower Medicare mortality among a set of hospitals known for good nursing care. *Medical Care, 32,* 771–787.

Aiken, L. H., Sochalski, J., & Lake, E. (1997). Studying outcomes of organizational change in health services. *Medical Care, 35*(11), NS6–NS18.

Bland, M. (1999). *An introduction to medical statistics.* Oxford, England: Oxford University Press.

Charlson, M. E., Pompei, P., Ales, K. L., & MacKenzie, C. R. (1987). A new method of classifying prognostic comorbidity in longitudinal studies: Development and validation. *Journal of Chronic Disease, 40,* 373–383.

Cho, S., Hwang, J. H., & Kim, J. (2008). Nurse staffing and patient mortality in intensive care units. *Nursing Research, 57,* 322–330.

Choi, J., Bakken, S., Larson, E., Du, Y., & Stone, P. W. (2004). Perceived nursing work environment. *Nursing Research, 53,* 370–378.

Clarke, S. P, & Aiken, L. H. (2003). Failure to rescue. *American Journal of Nursing. 103*(10), 42–47.

Cohen, I. B. (1984). Florence Nightingale. *Scientific American, 250*(3), 128–137.

Collins Sharp, B. A., & Clancy, C. M. (2008). Limiting nurse overtime, and promoting other good working conditions, influences patient safety. *Journal of Nursing Care Quality, 23*(2), 97–100.

Daley, J., Ash, A. S., & Iezzoni, L. I. (2003). Validity and reliability of risk adjusters. In L. I. Iezzoni (Ed.), *Risk adjustment for measuring health care outcomes* (3rd ed., pp. 207–230). Chicago: Health Administration Press.

Deyo, R. A., Cherkin, D. C., & Ciol, M. A. (1992). Adapting a clinical comorbidity index for use with ICD-9-CM administrative databases. *Journal of Clinical Epidemiology, 45,* 613–619.

Elixhauser, A., Steiner, C. Harris, D. R., & Coffey, R. M. (1998). Co-morbidity measures for use with administrative data. *Medical Care, 36,* 8–27.

Estabrooks, C. A., Midodzi, W. K., Cummings, G. G., Ricker, K. L., & Giovannetti, P. (2005). The impact of hospital nursing characteristics on 30-day mortality. *Nursing Research, 54*(2), 74–84.

Estabrooks, C. A., Tourangeau, A. E., Humphrey, C. K., Hesketh, K. L., Giovannetti, P. Thomson, D., et al. (2002). Measuring the hospital practice environment: A Canadian perspective. *Research in Nursing and Health, 25,* 256–268.

Gonnella, J. S., Hornbrook, M. C., & Louis, D. Z. (1984). Staging of disease: A case-mix measurement. *Journal of the American Medical Association, 251,* 637–644.

Halm, M., Kandels, M., Blalock, M., Gryczman, A., Krisko-Hagel, K., Lemay, D., et al. (2005). *Clinical Nurse Specialist, 19,* 241–251.

Hamilton, K. E., Redshaw, M. E., & Tarnow-Mordi, W. (2007). Nurse staffing in relation to risk-adjusted mortality in neonatal care. *Archives of Disease in Childhood Fetal and Neonatal Edition, 92*(2), 99–103.

Iezzoni, L. I. (2003a). Reasons for risk adjustment. In L. I. Iezzoni (Ed.), *Risk adjustment for measuring health care outcomes* (3rd ed., pp. 1–16). Chicago: Health Administration Press.

Iezzoni, L. I. (2003b). Coded data from administrative sources. In L. I. Iezzoni (Ed.), *Risk adjustment for measuring health care outcomes* (3rd ed., pp. 83–138). Chicago: Health Administration Press.

Iezzoni, L. I. (2003c). Clinical data from medical records or providers. In L. I. Iezzoni (Ed.), *Risk adjustment for measuring health care outcomes* (3rd ed., pp. 139–162). Chicago: Health Administration Press.

Iezzoni, L. I. (2003d). Data from surveys or asking patients. In L. I. Iezzoni (Ed.), *Risk adjustment for measuring health care outcomes* (3rd ed., pp. 163–177). Chicago: Health Administration Press.

Jencks, S. F., Williams, D. K., & Kay, T. L. (1988). Assessing hospital-associated deaths from discharge data: The role of length of stay and comorbidities. *Journal of the American Medical Association, 260,* 2240–2246.

Kiekkas, P., Sakellaropoulos, G. C., Brokalaki, H., Manolis, E., Samios, A., Skartsani, C., et al. (2008). Association between nursing workload and mortality of intensive care unit patients. *Journal of Nursing Scholarship, 40,* 385–390.

Knaus, W. A., Draper, E. A., Wagner, D. P., & Zimmerman, J. E. (1986). An evaluation of outcome from intensive care in major medical centers. *Annals of Internal Medicine, 104,* 410–418.

Knaus, W. A., Zimmerman, J. E., Wagner, D. P., Draper, E. A., & Lawrence, D. E. (1981). APACHE—acute physiology and chronic health evaluation: A physiologically based classification system. *Critical Care Medicine, 9,* 591–597.

Lake, E. T. (2002). Development of the practice environment scale of the nursing work index. *Research in Nursing and Health, 25,* 176–188.

Mark, B. A., Harless, D. W., & Berman, W. F. (2007). Nurse staffing and adverse events in hospitalized children. *Policy, Politics, and Nursing Practice, 8*(2), 93–92.

Maslach, C., Jackson, S., & Leiter, M. (1996). *Maslach Burnout Inventory manual* (3rd ed.). Palo Alto, CA: Consulting Psychologists Press.

Mitchell, P. H., Armstrong, S., Simpson, T. F., & Lentz, M. (1989). American association of critical care nurses demonstration project: Profile of excellence in critical care nursing. *Heart and Lung, 18,* 219–237.

Needleman, J., Buerhaus, P., Mattke, S., Steward, M., & Zelevinsky, K. (2002). Nurse-staffing levels and the quality of care in hospitals. *New England Journal of Medicine, 346,* 1715–1722.

Person, S. D., Allison, J. J., Kiefe, C. I., Weaver, M. T., Williams, O. D., Centor, R. M., et al. (2004). Nurse staffing and mortality for Medicare patients with acute myocardial infarction. *Medical Care, 42*(1), 4–12.

Rafferty, A. M., Clarke, S. P., Coles, J., Ball, J., James, P., McKee, M., et al. (2007). Outcomes of variation in hospital nurse staffing in English hospitals: Cross-sectional analysis of survey data and discharge records. *International Journal of Nursing Studies, 44,* 175–182.

Raudenbush, S. W., & Bryk, A. S. (2002). *Hierarchical linear models: Applications and data analysis methods* (2nd ed.). London: Sage.

Sasichay-Akkadechanunt, T., Scalzi, C. C., & Jawad, A. F. (2003). The relationship between nurse staffing and patient outcomes. *Journal of Nursing Administration, 33,* 479–485.

Schmid, A., Hoffman, L., Happ, M. B., Wolf, G. A., & DeVita, M. (2007). Failure to rescue: A literature review. *Journal of Nursing Administration, 37,* 188–198.

Shwartz, M., & Ash, A. S. (2003). Evaluating risk-adjustment models empirically In L. I. Iezzoni (Ed.), *Risk adjustment for measuring health care outcomes* (3rd ed., pp. 231–273). Chicago: Health Administration Press.

Sidani, S., & Braden, C. J. (1998). *Evaluating nursing interventions: A theory-driven approach.* Thousand Oaks, CA: Sage.

Silber, J. H., Romano, P. S., Rosen, A. K., Wang, Y., Even-Shoshan, O., & Volpp, K. G. (2007). Failure-to-rescue: Comparing definitions to measure quality of care. *Medical Care, 45,* 918–925.

Silber, J. H., & Rosenbaum, P. R. (1997). A spurious correlation between hospital mortality and complication rates. *Medical Care, 30,* OS77–OS92.

Silber, J. H., Rosenbaum, P. R., & Ross, R. N. (1995). Comparing the contributions of groups of predictors: Which outcomes vary with hospital rather than with patient characteristics? *Journal of the American Statistical Association, 90*(429), 7–18.

Silber, J. H., Williams, S. V., Krakauer, H., & Schwartz, J. S. (1992). Hospital and patient charac-teristics associated with death after surgery: A study of adverse occurrence and failure-to-rescue. *Medical Care, 30,* 615–629.

Stone, P. W., Mooney-Kane, C., Larson, E. L., Horan, T., Glance, L. G., Zwanziger, J., et al. (2007). Nurse working conditions and patient safety outcomes. *Medical Care, 45,* 571–578.

Tarnow-Mordi, W. O., Hau, C., Warden, A., & Shearer, A. J. (2000). Hospital mortality in rela-tion to staff workload: A 4-year study in an adult intensive-care unit. *The Lancet, 356,* 185–189.

Tourangeau, A. E. (2003). Modeling the determinants of mortality for hospitalized patients. *International Nursing Perspectives, 3*(1), 37–48.

Tourangeau, A. E. (2005). A theoretical model of the determinants of mortality. *Advances in Nursing Science, 28*(1), 58–69.

Tourangeau, A. E. (2006a). Taux de mortalité a 30 jours ajustes sur le risque et sur le diagnostic [30-day mortality rates risk adjusted by diagnosis group]. *Risques & Qualite, 3*(1), 25–31.

Tourangeau, A. E. (2006b). Nursing information and outcomes. In J. M. Hibberd & D. L. Smith (Eds.), *Nursing leadership and management in Canada* (3rd ed., pp. 461–479). Toronto, Ontario, Canada: Elsevier Mosby.

Tourangeau, A. E. (2007). Choices and tradeoffs: Decreasing costs or improving hospital mortal-ity rates. *Healthcare Quarterly, 11*(1), 21–22.

Tourangeau, A. E., Doran, D. M., McGillis Hall, L., O'Brien Pallas, L., Pringle, D., Tu, J. V., et al. (2006). Impact of hospital nursing care on 30-day mortality for acute medical patients. *Journal of Advanced Nursing, 57*(1), 32–44.

Tourangeau, A. E., Giovannetti, P., Tu, J. V., & Wood, M. (2002). Nursing-related determinants of 30-day mortality for hospitalized patients. *Canadian Journal of Nursing Research, 33*(4), 71–88.

Tourangeau, A. E., McGillis Hall, L., Doran, D. M., & Petch, T. (2006). Measurement of nurse satisfaction using the McCloskey Mueller Satisfaction Scale. *Nursing Research, 55,* 128–136.

Tourangeau, A. E., & Tu, J. V. (2003). Developing risk-adjusted 30-day mortality rates. *Research in Nursing and Health, 26,* 483–496.

Zimmerman, J. E., Wagner, D. P., Draper, E. A., Wright, L., Alzola, C., & Knaus, W. A. (1998). Evaluation of acute physiology and chronic health evaluation III predictions of hospital mor-tality in an independent database. *Critical Care Medicine, 26,* 1317–1326.

Healthcare Utilization

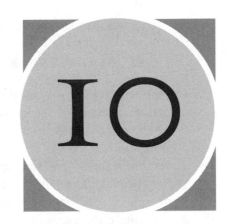

Sean P. Clarke

INTRODUCTION

Nearly every healthcare system in the industrialized world is facing exploding costs. The culprits are not only inflation, population growth, and aging, but also a tendency to deliver more care and a greater number of expensive services to the population, sometimes with questionable returns on investment in terms of patient health. Nurses' roles both in the delivery of safe, effective, and efficient hospital care and in health promotion and chronic disease management are well-recognized. Not surprisingly, over the years, many inside and outside the nursing profession have discussed potential cost savings that might result from greater investments in nurses and nursing services. For a number of years, researchers in nursing have incorporated healthcare utilization variables in a variety of study designs, especially as secondary outcomes in evaluations of the effectiveness of interventions.

In this chapter, research addressing the contention that factors related to nurses, nursing services, and nursing interventions affect clients' healthcare utilization will be explored. More specifically, research that investigates the possibility that nursing factors or nursing care can decrease service utilization or costs will be the focus. There are two basic methods of decreasing healthcare costs. One is to reduce the number of patient-provider or patient-system contacts, perhaps by keeping patients physically and mentally healthier. A second approach is to somehow decrease costs associated with the contacts themselves—that is, to keep contacts short and avoid unnecessary deviations and detours in care. The literature reviewed here will discuss research addressing both of these pathways.

A few precisions regarding the scope of this review are in order. First, the studies described here do not include those in which increased use of appropriate services is considered a desirable outcome. Some healthcare services tend to be underused by at least some clients (Persily, 2003; Spenceley, 2005). Patients/clients or providers may be uninformed regarding available services or are, for some reason, reluctant to make use of them. In such circumstances, nurses can increase awareness of options and raise utilization and visits to clinics or other interventions (with a possible beneficial downstream impact on health outcomes). Thus, in some instances, effective nursing actions could lead to increases in "appropriate" healthcare utilization—that is, the heightened use of services that can reasonably be expected to benefit patients, such as screening and other provider-delivered preventive measures, as well as closer follow-up of patients' conditions. (For an example of this type of study, see Jones, Jones, & Katz, 1989).

A second narrowing of the studies and articles reviewed related to the types of nurses or nursing under study. This review excluded studies of nurses engaged primarily in delivering services customarily provided by physicians. It is sometimes argued that advanced practice nurses (APNs) can decrease per-contact or per-care-day costs because their salaries are often lower than those of the physicians and other providers they work alongside, and yet they provide selected types of care at a comparable, if not superior, level of quality. The reader is referred to reviews elsewhere of the methodologically diverse evaluation literature on the safety and cost-effectiveness of APNs in models of care involving physician replacement (Horrocks, Anderson, & Salisbury, 2002; Hughes, Clarke, Sampson, Fairman, & Sullivan-Marx, 2003).

Research reports and scholarly articles dealing with healthcare utilization, hospital length of stay, hospitalizations (or rehospitalizations), emergency department (ED) visits or repeat visits, and total healthcare costs in connection with nurses or nursing were sought in MEDLINE, CINAHL, and the ISI Web of Science from 1996 to 2009 using various keyword combinations. If an article did not report results involving one or more of these outcomes or if it did not deal with potential associations between nursing variables and healthcare utilization, it was not included in this review. Although many researchers in nursing have examined complications that can prolong length of stay, and make an economic argument for increased investments to reduce complication-driven costs, such articles have not been reviewed here. An additional search was conducted for research dealing with patient-level predictors of rehospitalizations and ED visits. Reference lists for the articles were reviewed for "classic" references of potential relevance. The research reviewed here deals for the most part with services provided by generalist (staff) nurses. A number of studies also deal with outcomes of interventions by APNs whose roles do not chiefly involve replacement of physicians.

Because healthcare delivery and social conditions differ markedly across countries, patterns of care and "best practices" are not necessarily comparable across healthcare systems. Therefore, for simplicity's sake, this review is confined to studies conducted in Canada and the United States. This is because the majority of research in this area of the literature has taken place in these two systems and is not intended to imply any value judgments about these systems. Furthermore, because practice patterns change over time, the time frames of studies are particularly important in reading this literature. For instance, patient preferences and healthcare system-level financial considerations over the past decade in North America have led managers and clinicians to engineer reductions in length of stay. We have therefore restricted our attention primarily to empirical literature reported over the past two decades. The reader is cautioned to bear in mind both time and place of the data collections, especially when reflecting on the generalizability of the findings.

THEORETICAL BACKGROUND: DEFINITION OF THE CONCEPT

Healthcare utilization can be thought of as the sum or aggregate of services consumed by patients in their attempts to maintain or regain a level of health status, along with the costs of these services (see, for instance, Bernstein et al., 2003). In other words, healthcare utilization measures address how many services or how much money and other resources are consumed in dealing with patients' health-related needs. Healthcare utilization can be considered at the societal or healthcare-system-wide level (per capita costs), although this is not normally the focus in clinical research. More commonly, the resources consumed by particular patients or clinical populations for narrow or broad segments of their care trajectories are analyzed. For instance, some evaluation research considers lifelong costs or average annual costs of care, and other studies examine costs associated with a single hospitalization. On occasion, the types of care received across settings received by a patient over an episode of care are calculated—for example, in hip replacement surgery, the costs associated with office or clinic preoperative visits, inpatient care, rehabilitation, and longer-term follow-up.

THEORETICAL BACKGROUND: PROCESSES

Most healthcare utilization is triggered by perceptions by patients or their caregivers of a need for care. The resources consumed are, of course, affected by the availability of services both at the point of initial contact and through the various encounters that follow. Once care is under way, a host of factors influence consumption. Most prominent among these are the severity or complexity of the patient's health conditions, and patient and provider preferences. Cascades of further service use tend to arise when difficulties in coordination of care and complications of treatment or care emerge. Phillips, Morrison, Andersen, and Aday (1998) reviewed a model that primarily considers contextual factors and provider- and patient-level factors that influence service use and evidence supporting the framework to date.

Healthcare utilization is a social psychological phenomenon involving multiple actors. For instance, regarding ED use, Padgett and Brodsky (1992) discussed three stages of a help-seeking process: (1) problem recognition; (2) a decision to seek help; and (3) the decision to use the ED. There is one stage, of course, that comes before help-seeking arises—the appearance of symptoms or signs that may either be indications of a worsening condition, or "normal" sensations that patients interpret as potentially serious. Likewise, a provider's decision to admit a patient to the hospital is the result of a chain of events and reflects a perception that the patient's condition or his or her situation at home is unsuited to managing his or her condition in the community. Nurses do not make decisions to admit patients, nor to discharge them (these actions do not fall under the normal purview of generalist nurses), nor do nurses directly influence many of the resource allocation decisions made by patients and families about where and when to present for care. Nurses' involvement in the pathways that lead to the use of health care is usually indirect: through their influence on patient and family health status and, to some extent, as facilitators of an appropriate path through care via their actions or communication with others.

The mechanisms through which nurses or nursing care potentially decrease healthcare costs are often implicit, rather than overtly stated in scholarly papers. Nonetheless, there are two major categories of potential routes whereby nurses might influence utilization. Higher-quality nursing care might reduce disease exacerbations or complications of illnesses and their treatments that require extra time and resources to address. Meticulous physical nursing care while patients are in the hospital, risk reduction for issues such as falls or skin breakdown, and close surveillance of patients at risk of complications, accompanied by quick intervention at the earliest signs of deterioration are examples. Avoiding downturns, or exacerbations caught and reversed early, might prevent the need for some services altogether (i.e., a prevented visit or hospitalization) or decrease the resources associated with a unit of service (for instance, length of hospital stay). Specific interventions in the community that nurses commonly carry out include patient and family teaching to improve patient and family management of immediate postdischarge or postprocedural care in the short term, and chronic disease management in the longer term.

A second potential mechanism through which nurses might decrease healthcare utilization is through coordination of care and facilitation of communication among members of the healthcare team—which of course includes not only healthcare workers but also patients and families. Putting more nurses in place, ensuring that they are educated for these responsibilities, and assigning specific nurses to coordination roles may improve patient flow through systems of care, lead the best health care provider(s) to address emerging situations to be chosen early, and avoid unnecessary delays in treatments or in discharging patients. All these actions might save costs for at least some types of care.

CONCEPTUAL DEFINITION

For the purposes of this chapter, healthcare utilization refers to the quantity (total or partial) of healthcare services consumed intended to improve clients' health. Implicit in this definition is an assumption that more time or expense spent on care may not be necessary or wise for either the client or society. Four commonly used indices of healthcare utilization are the focus.

Consistently high *lengths of hospital stay* are sometimes thought of as a proxy for inefficient resource use—the failure either to move patients effectively through care systems or to stabilize patients' situations rapidly, whether in connection with preventable or treatable clinical deterioration or not. *Rehospitalizations* tend to reflect serious downturns in a patient's condition that may or may not have been foreseeable or preventable. They may reflect low quality of predischarge care and/or premature discharge. In the latter case, inadequate stabilization of the patient's medical condition, a failure to investigate and remedy possible problems with the patient's ability to care for himself or herself before returning to the community, or both may be involved. Various changes in healthcare delivery have resulted in relatively few patients being admitted to hospitals, with more and more receiving treatment in outpatient or ED settings without any inpatient admissions. Readmission rates are under increasing discussion as a potential indicator of quality of care. The public reporting of these rates and potentially tying performance on them to reimbursement levels are being raised, particularly in the United States. Furthermore, in the United States, there is talk of health insurance plans withholding reimbursement for readmissions judged preventable (Healy, 2009). However, because the threshold for admissions is already quite high and not all clinical deteriorations are avoidable, the preventability of many rehospitalizations is a matter of vigorous debate (Ashton & Wray, 1992; Benbassat & Taragin, 2000; Clarke, 2004). *Emergency department visits* are sometimes the result of destabilizations of patients' conditions that may have been prevented by more careful management and follow-up in the community, and/or a failure to identify and remedy problems that patients may have in complying with self-care. In some nonemergent situations, ED visits will be at the discretion of patients.

Total costs, aggregating some combination of inpatient, outpatient, and community services, are often intended to capture the package of expenses incurred in caring for a patient population. Often in clinical research, total costs are examined to investigate the possibility that care management models may add supplemental costs to treatment on one side but can alter the trajectory of illness or the types of services required on the other, to yield a net cost savings. Formal economic analyses involve a consideration of the costs and benefits of care provided in several different scenarios, with a careful review of whom the costs and benefits accrue to, as well as an attempt to account for less obvious costs and benefits (Drummond, Sculpher, Torrance, O'Brien, & Stoddart, 2005; Stone, Curran, & Bakken, 2002).

CONTROVERSIES AND ISSUES IN ASSESSING HEALTHCARE UTILIZATION

What Is Preventable (or Avoidable) versus Appropriate Care?

A starting point for any discussion or research addressing a nursing role in curbing healthcare utilization is the idea that at least some needs for service and/or actual care-seeking are potentially preventable through specific clinical actions. However, the converse is also true: Many patients come to clinics or the emergency department for logical reasons, mostly involving a new or worsening problem they believe might be treatable. Furthermore, at least some patients' clinical conditions deteriorate despite the best efforts of both clinicians and of patients and their families. Whereas appropriateness of utilization is often discussed in relation to avoidable service use, discussions of the appropriateness of specific forms of medical treatment frequently relate distinctions regarding whether patients are receiving treatments that are not indicated for their conditions according to the state of the science (Brook, 2009; Chassin et al., 1986; Kahn et al., 1988). This is not a distinction that nurse leaders and researchers tend to make at the present time.

It can be quite difficult to make objective judgments regarding the preventability of patients' clinical states that trigger a visit or an admission. Even if it is felt that patient or family uncertainty about the significance of a particular sign or symptom, rather than an actual physiological or serious psychological injury or disturbance, was the major cause of a visit, appropriateness can be difficult to judge. Similarly, it can be challenging to make general statements about the preventability of longer hospital stays for specific patients without knowing quite a bit about their care and their clinical evolution. Many patients who have vulnerabilities of various types will be at high risk for complications, regardless of whether care is competent (Silber, Rosenbaum, Schwartz, Ross, & Williams, 1995; Silber, Williams, Krakauer, & Schwartz, 1992). The distinction between the preventable and appropriate or unavoidable care has implications that not only are important for framing research questions, but have clinical and policy consequences as well.

Any judgments regarding the appropriateness of utilization, whether made by providers, patients, or researchers, will often be made on the basis of facts or documentation known only after the fact, and by necessity, these judgments will be imbued with assumptions and biases (Maharaj, Hsu & Beadman, 2006). However, some researchers attempt to make their assumptions explicit in reviewing cases and records by constructing review algorithms; readers must then assess how reasonable and biased these determinations are likely to be. The appropriateness and/ or preventability of healthcare consumption is less of an issue when service consumption or costs are being compared across groups of patients to estimate general costs associated with a specific pattern of patient management than when risks for individual patients of consuming resources or being readmitted under specific circumstances are under study. Often, researchers do not attempt to make any distinctions between service use or days of stay in terms of how avoidable they were.

A different approach to the dilemma of avoidable versus unavoidable healthcare consumption is to attempt to take into account non-service-related factors (i.e., the clinical, psychological, and social characteristics of individual patients, discussed in a later section) by measuring and/or controlling for them statistically so that "uncontrollable" influences on health status or healthcare-seeking from the point of view of healthcare providers are somehow handled by the research design. This approach is often called "risk adjustment" (Iezzoni, 1999).

It should also be noted that high-quality nursing care may not always be associated with lower healthcare utilization. As we stated at the outset, some nursing interventions are designed to explicitly increase use of services. Furthermore, competent patient/family teaching always involves explaining the circumstances under which return visits or other service consumption are expected or necessary. Certainly, making patients and families very hesitant to contact or visit providers could lead to needless and potentially dangerous and costly treatment delays.

Nursing assessments can help clinicians identify patients at high risk for difficulties, lead them to initiate additional preventive measures, or push nurses to intervene quickly to reverse clinical problems so that fewer resources are needed in the end. However, in some cases, more thorough nursing assessments identify patients who are not ready for discharge (i.e., patients who are not clinically stable or who will be discharged into a situation not suited to their care needs). Such patients might be vulnerable for deterioration in the community and at high risk for readmission. Thus, in selected instances, nurses' assessments and advocacy for patients might lengthen hospital stays for some patients (a different healthcare utilization measure), yet few would argue against the appropriateness of these added costs.

Trends toward shorter hospital lengths of stay and placing more responsibility for care and its follow-up outside hospitals or other covered services are controversial. Clearly, if the timing of hospital discharges is not driven by patient stability and needs, the consequences for patients and families can be severe. It is also worthwhile to note that encouraging families and patients to reduce their healthcare consumption may translate into placing more responsibility for care in their hands. The advisability of this is a question of values as much as it is one of facts; shifting some of the burden or the costs of care from one segment of the healthcare system to another or from healthcare providers to family members or other caregivers can be thought of as wise or as cruel, depending on the circumstances and the values of the beholder.

DATA SOURCES: SELF-REPORTS AND SECONDARY DATA

Three basic data collection approaches for measuring healthcare utilization exist: (1) asking patients where and when they have sought care; (2) observing healthcare consumption concurrently in some way (i.e., somehow monitoring who is presenting for care at facilities or in clinics on an ongoing basis); and (3) consulting secondary databases that track encounters or billings. The second of these options is usually considered overly cumbersome and expensive for most applications, so researchers generally rely on the first or the third method.

In a self-report approach, patients and/or their families and partners are asked either to track their use of health care prospectively (for instance, to record all healthcare contacts in a special diary) or, more commonly, to answer questions retrospectively regarding office/clinic visits, hospitalizations, or ED visits during a specified period of time. Prospective data collection by patients or families is unlikely to work particularly well unless contacts are frequent, and the individuals involved are highly motivated to record data. Self-report of service use brings with it all the validity issues that accompany asking individuals to report any behavior. The potential for over- or underreporting because of errors in memory is obvious, particularly if the time periods in question are long, yet many researchers stress the high quality of data that can be obtained at reasonable expense this way (see, for instance, Lubeck & Hubert, 2005; Schweikert, Hahmann , & Leidl, 2008; van den Brink et al., 2005).

The third approach, the use of secondary data (usually from administrative databases), is quite common in both large-scale analyses of healthcare utilization variables and in smaller-scale clinical research. Secondary analysis involves the use of data gathered for distinctly different purposes to address new research questions. In exchange for savings of time and energy involved, there are usually certain trade-offs in terms of validity. Many researchers seek access to databases that track patient contacts with hospitals, EDs, or other providers and are maintained by a government authority in a particular state, province, or country.

The use of secondary data is often convenient but has some drawbacks. The primary purpose of carrying out the abstraction and data entry for many of these data sources is billing health plans. Those responsible for the quality of the data are often most concerned about administrative monitoring of costs. In perhaps the most comprehensive discussion of secondary analysis issues confronted by users of healthcare administrative data, Iezzoni (1999) discussed some of the major concerns. The motivations of the coders or institutions relate to maximizing reimbursements, not recording clinical details that have relatively minor significance for reimbursement to maintain absolute accuracy in record-keeping. Lags and lapses in providers submitting data about visits or encounters by clinicians or facilities will obviously reduce both the reliability and validity of these data. There will occasionally be circumstances in which encounters cannot be tied to specific patients because of data entry errors, as well as errors in which encounters are attributed to the wrong patients. Finally, there are often considerable delays between healthcare encounters, the inclusion of records of the encounters in databases, and eventual release to researchers of the databases—frequently at least 6 months and sometimes several years or longer—which can create problems for research studies with limited funding.

When examining hospital readmissions and ED visits, some researchers have confined their operational definitions to revisits or readmissions to a single institution, reflected in a single facility's databases, to avoid the expenses and delays involved in using administrative data sets. Depending on the size of the community and the type of conditions being studied, this may provide underestimates of utilization, because a variety of circumstances may push patients to seek care from providers (hospitals or clinics) other than the ones responsible for their initial or "index" admissions.

Finally, it should be mentioned that across healthcare systems, attention to privacy concerns is leading to increasingly tight regulation of the research use of health records or data sets containing fields that identify individual patients. Although researchers can sometimes arrange for permission to access records without asking for the explicit consent of the patients involved, in most cases, inclusion of patients in research on healthcare utilization variables will require obtaining formal consent; this can incorporate serious selection biases into research projects.

EVIDENCE CONCERNING FACTORS INFLUENCING HEALTHCARE UTILIZATION

The literature assembled in **TABLE 10-1** (6 review articles, 37 research papers) points to several different categories of patient variables linked with healthcare utilization. A first major category is clinical variables. One of the major groups of variables consists of markers of either physical or psychiatric disease severity. Clinical severity of disease can be measured objectively in terms of the degree of organ impairment (e.g., cardiac ejection fraction); in terms of the presence, absence, or severity of signs or symptoms; or by proxy (for instance, the presence or absence of specific forms of drug therapy in a patient record can be a proxy for clinician ratings of seriousness). Presumably more severe disease will often produce a greater number of more severe disease manifestations (signs and

TABLE 10-1 Patient-Level Predictors of Healthcare Utilization

Author and date	Study design	Characteristics of sample, and setting	Healthcare utilization variables studied	Major results	Limitations/comments
REVIEW ARTICLES					
Bahadori & FitzGerald (2007)	Systematic review	PubMed, MEDLINE (1966–October 2006), EMBASE (1988–October 2006), BIOSIS, CINAHL, PsycINFO, and Cochrane databases searched for cohort, retrospective and prospective, cross-sectional and case control studies regarding predictors of hospital use in COPD patients. 17 (of 1,500) articles included. Patient populations studied: 61+ years of age and older, mostly male.	Hospitalizations and rehospitalizations	Increased PaCO$_2$, long-term use of oxygen therapy, oral and inhaled corticosteroids, severe dyspnea predictive of increased hospitalizations.	
de Boer, Wijker, & de Haes (1997)	Literature review	53 studies of chronically ill patients. Published 1966–1997.	ED visits, hospitalization rates, and physician visits	Disease severity, symptom severity, and complications associated with higher health care utilization; no association with disease duration and comorbidities. Depression and psychological distress were among the strongest predictors of hospitalizations and physician visits.	
Gerolamo (2004)	Systematic literature review	Medline, CINAHL, HealthSTAR and PsycINFO searched for articles examining client outcomes after treatment in acute care inpatient psychiatric hospitals and psychiatric units of general hospitals. Published 1991–2004. $N = 47$ studies met inclusion criteria.	Readmission to a psychiatric ward	Previous hospital admissions a dominant predictor of readmission.	Questionable reliability and validity of clients' psychiatric diagnoses and statistical analysis issues identified.
Padgett & Brodsky (1992)	Literature review	70 articles dealing with psychosocial factors and their influence on nonurgent ED use. Mix of U.S. and Sweden studies.	ED visits	The most common reason for nonurgent ED use was "other care not available" (such as absence of primary care provider); other factors include socioeconomic stress, psychiatric comorbidities, and lack of social support.	No discussion of ethnicity

Ross et al. (2008)	Systematic literature review	Databases: MEDLINE, Scopus, PsycINFO, and four Ovid Evidence-Based Medicine Reviews from January 1, 1950 to November 19, 2007 reviewed for research on predictors of hospital readmissions for heart failure. 117 articles met inclusion criteria; majority of studies examined patient characteristics associated with readmission, 5 involved development and validation of risk adjustment models	Hospital readmissions	Age, sex, and non–heart failure comorbidities such as diabetes and hypertension were inconsistently associated with readmission. A number of heart severity variables were frequently studied but inconsistently associated with readmissions: notably systolic ejection fraction and New York Heart Association class.	
Zolnierek (2009)	Literature review	CINAHL and PubMed searched for articles on severely mentally ill patients hospitalized in general medical-surgical settings for nonpsychiatric conditions (1998–2008). 12 studies met inclusion criteria (peer-reviewed and investigated patient outcome).	Hospital LOS, cost of care, and use of services (e.g., outpatient services).	All 12 studies showed increased resource use for patients with concurrent psychiatric illness.	
ARTICLES					
Bartlett et al. (2001)	Prospective cohort study	Baseline and 6-month surveys were administered to 177 mothers with asthma in inner-city Baltimore, Maryland, and Washington, D.C.	ED use Center for Epidemiological Studies Depression (CES-D) Scale.	Mothers with high depressive symptoms were 40% more likely to report taking their child to the ED.	Self-report of ED access
Blank et al. (2005)	Retrospective descriptive pilot study	Setting: 600-bed academic urban tertiary-care facility in Massachusetts; October 1, 2002, to September 30, 2003, to describe and compare 234 high users (12+ visits/annually) and low/moderate users: 62,886 low (1–3 visits) / 3,432 medium (4–11 visits).	ED use	High frequency users more likely to have insurance (84 vs 72%) and primary care providers (93 vs 76%); also more likely to have chronic illnesses in general (asthma, sickle cell anemia, etc.).	Single institution study
Dendukuri, McCusker, & Belzile (2004)	Tool validation study	Setting: Four university-affiliated hospitals in Montreal. Two cohorts of patients aged 65 and older who were to be released from an ED ($n = 1,122$; $n = 1,889$).	ED visits over 5 months after the index visit	Identification of Seniors at Risk (ISAR) tool described detecting severe functional impairment and depression and predicting likelihood of increased utilization of health services. Predictive validity for increased depressive symptoms and high utilization of health services ranged from 0.61 to 0.71.	Self-report of disability and depression

COPD = chronic obstructive pulmonary disease; ED = emergency department; LOS = length of stay; $PaCO_2$ = partial pressure of carbon dioxide in the blood (an indicator of gas exchange and acid-base balance); U.S. = United States; USD = United States dollars.

(continues)

TABLE 10-1 Patient-Level Predictors of Healthcare Utilization (continued)

Author and date	Study design	Characteristics of sample, and setting	Healthcare utilization variables studied	Major results	Limitations/ comments
Friedmann et al. (2001)	Prospective cohort study	Patients 65 years or older at single ED; location not specified (U.S.). N = 463 completed the study.	ED revisit, hospital admission, or death 30 or 90 days after discharge from index ED visit. Katz Index of Activities of Daily Living (ADL) and Short-Form 36 Health Survey, Mini-Mental Status Exams.	Physical functioning, number of hospitalizations in the 6 months before the index ED visit, and ADL and cognitive deficits were predictors of rehospitalizations or death.	Single-site study; self-report of health and functional status, use of a composite outcomes indicator.
Gajic et al. (2008)	Prospective cohort study	Setting: Medical-surgical ICU of University of Amsterdam, Netherlands, and the medical ICU at St. Mary's Hospital, Mayo Clinic, Rochester, Minnesota (from June to December 2005 at both hospitals). N = 1,131 medical ICU patients.	Unplanned ICU readmission	Logistic regression analysis showed predictors of readmission were ICU admission source, ICU LOS, and day-of-discharge neurologic (Glasgow Coma Scale) and respiratory impairment. Similar pattern in North American and European ICUs; latter less consistent.	
Gifford et al. (2000)	Cross-sectional interview study to determine whether HIV patients (adults) seek care in the ED or with primary health provider.	Patients in care in the 48 contiguous United States studied 1996–1997. N = 2,864 adults were interviewed (1,616 advanced stage of HIV vs 1,248 subjects at early stage) by CD4 count.	ED visits	ED users were more likely to be African American or Hispanic, to be poor, and to report lower psychological well-being.	
Gordon, An, Hayward, & Williams (1998)	Retrospective observational study	Study population: All patients with two or more visits to the University of Michigan ED (1995–1996). Early-return population (n = 1,422), and early-return population admitted to the hospital ("return-admit," n = 313).	ED repeat visits and hospitalizations	Dehydration was the most common diagnosis in the general, early-return, and return-admit populations.	
Han, Ospina, Blitz, Strome, & Rowe (2007)	Retrospective cohort	2 EDs in Edmonton, Alberta, Canada: Patients 17 years of age and older in 2004. N = 894	ED visits	61% of patients reported seeking alternative care before ED visits. Alternative care included mainly contacting primary care physician (56% of study population).	Selection and report biases

Study	Design	Sample	Measures	Findings	Limitations
				89 of the patients who attempted alternative access before the ED visit felt that the ED was their best care option. Multivariate logistic regression analysis showed that injury presentation, living arrangements, smoking status, and having a family practitioner were predictors for seeking alternative care prior to ED visit.	
Hastings, George, et al. (2008)	Secondary analysis of a longitudinal, prospective data set	$N = 1,662$ ED patients, mean age 77.3 years of age. Setting: Five-county area in North Carolina; four waves of data collection (1986/1987, 1989/1990, 1992/1993, and 1996/1997).	ED visits. Duke Social Support Index for type and level of social support patient received.	Subjects who lived alone were 60% more likely to visit the ED than those who lived with their spouse. Neither type nor level of social support predicted ED use. Other indicators of poor physical health (prior hospitalization, poorer self-rated health, and functional disability) were predictors of ED visits.	Data on severity of illnesses leading to initial ED visits were not tracked.
Hastings, Oddone, Fillenbaum, Sloane, & Schmader (2008)	Secondary analysis of data from the (U.S.) Medicare Current Beneficiary Survey	$N = 1,851$ community-dwelling Medicare fee-for-service enrollees, 65 years of age or older discharged from the ED, 2000–2002.	Outpatient ED visit, hospital readmission, nursing home admission or death within 90 days of the index ED visit.	Patients who were older, who had more chronic health conditions, and who had concurrent insurance indicative of special vulnerability, as well as prior health care use and recent ED or hospital use, were at particularly high risk for repeat ED visits.	
Ionescu-Irtu et al. (2007)	Secondary analysis of cross-sectional administrative data	Random sample of 95,173 people aged 65 years or older from Quebec, Canada; 2000–2001.	ED visits. Continuity of care measured through claims data.	After adjusting for age, sex, and comorbidity, the study found that an increased rate of ED use was associated with lack of a primary physician and low or medium (vs high) levels of continuity of care with a primary physician.	
Janson-Bjerklie, Ferketich, & Benner (1993)	Prospective cohort study (questionnaires and follow-up interviews)	$N = 95$ asthmatic adult patients, U.S.	ED visits	ED visits related to feelings of panic/fear; perceived severity of asthmatic episodes and perceived danger.	Relatively small sample size, self-report of utilization

COPD = chronic obstructive pulmonary disease; ED = emergency department; LOS = length of stay; $PaCO_2$ = partial pressure of carbon dioxide in the blood (an indicator of gas exchange and acid-base balance); U.S. = United States; USD = United States dollars.

(continues)

TABLE 10-1 Patient-Level Predictors of Healthcare Utilization (continued)

Author and date	Study design	Characteristics of sample, and setting	Healthcare utilization variables studied	Major results	Limitations/comments
LeDuc, Rosebrook, Rannie, & Gao (2006)	Comparative study using chart reviews and telephone interviews.	Children's Hospital, Denver, Colorado, 1997/1998. N = 100.	Repeat ED visits within 3 months or within 48 hours	Predictive factors for return to ED include age (patients younger than 1 year twice as likely to have return ED visits); some organ system diseases more connected to repeat visits than others.	Single-hospital study. Small number of cases.
Lyons et al. (1997)	Prospective cohort study	Setting: Chicago, 1994-1995. N = 255 patients consecutively admitted to any of seven psychiatric hospitals in a regional managed care program.	Readmission within 30 days or within 6 months	Greater impairment in self-care, higher symptom severity, and less family support in patients with 30-day readmissions.	
McCusker, Cardin, Bellavance, & Belzile (2000)	Observational cohort study	N = 1,122 ED patients aged 65 years and older presenting during the daytime hours on weekdays during a 3-month period in 1996. Setting: Four urban university-affiliated hospitals in Montreal, Quebec, Canada.	Return ED within 6 months of an index visit	Hospitalization during the previous 6 months, functional impairment, visual impairment, and multiple medications (3+), age over 85 years, poor self-reported health and living alone were predictive of return ED visits	Choosing patients presenting to ED on weekdays likely to have produced selection biases
McCusker, Healey Bellavance, & Connolly (1997)	Prospective study of a convenience sample of ED patients aged 75 or older to determine factors associated with repeat visits (within 90 days of initial visit).	N = 167 ED patients aged 75 years and over. Setting: 400-bed university-affiliated acute care community hospital in Montreal.	Repeat ED visits	Factors associated with repeated ED visits included moderate to severe cognitive impairment, past ED visits, and functional status problems.	Single-institution study. Exclusion of patients aged 65–74 years and those who visited the ED at night.
Miller, Larkin, & Jimenez (2005)	Prospective cross-sectional ED survey.	1,168 patients surveyed. Criteria: ED patients (> 18 years) taking chronic medications for congestive heart failure, diabetes, and/or hypertension. Study conducted for 6 weeks to interview patient who visited the ED and determine if it was for medication refill. Setting: ED in Texas.	Medication refill-seeking behavior in the ED	Lack of knowledge about refill or pharmacy numbers on the medication bottle was the main reason for ED visit. Univariate predictors included age younger than 50 years, non-Hispanic ethnicity, low income (< $5,000 USD per year), self-paying status.	

Nouwen, Freeston Labbé, & Boulet (1999)	Matched cohort study	60 asthmatic patients: N = 30 frequent ED users, N = 30 matched nonfrequent ED users. Patients recruited from six university-affiliated hospitals in Quebec, Canada.	ED visits	High attenders reported more panic/fear symptoms, lower self-efficacy, and more perceived illness interference.	Self-report
Ortega et al. (2001)	Retrospective cohort study with home interviews	1,002 families with child with asthma selected, 1996–1998, a convenience sample from seven New England hospitals. (n = 804).	ED use	Medicaid versus private insurance predicted increased ED use. Black children receiving Medicaid were less likely to have had multiple routine primary care visits for asthma in the previous year than Black privately insured children. White children on Medicaid were 2.5 times more likely to use the ED for asthma than privately insured White children.	Use of a convenience sampling frame, reliance on subject recall.
Parboosingh & Larsen (1987)	Prospective cohort	A random sample of 75 noninstitutionalized persons aged 65 years and older in a large city in Alberta, Canada.	ED visits over a 3-month period	Number of hospital admissions, sources of health care, and attitude toward health care use were important predictors of ED use. Patients with more hospital admissions, more than one source of care, and a positive attitude about health services used ED more. Younger patients and those with more hospital admissions more likely to show appropriate use.	Small study group, questionable generalizability.
Pines & Buford (2006)	Retrospective cohort study	N = 1,799 self-described asthmatics in the Philadelphia Health Management Corporation's Southeastern Pennsylvania Household Health Survey in 2004 (response rate was 30%).	ED use	Predictors of frequent ED use were: prescription for asthma medications, Medicaid or Medical Assistance (health insurance coverage for low-income families), number of children living in the house with a high school education or less, living in the most heavily urban part of the region, number of clinic and office visits.	Self-report biases, low response rate in parent survey.

COPD = chronic obstructive pulmonary disease; ED = emergency department; LOS = length of stay; $PaCO_2$ = partial pressure of carbon dioxide in the blood (an indicator of gas exchange and acid-base balance); U.S. = United States; USD = United States dollars.

(continues)

TABLE 10-1 Patient-Level Predictors of Healthcare Utilization (continued)

Author and date	Study design	Characteristics of sample, and setting	Healthcare utilization variables studied	Major results	Limitations/comments
Polivka et al. (2000)	Cross-sectional study	Low-income women ($N = 474$) with a child 6 years or younger completed a structured face-to-face interview at human service offices or Women, Infants, and Children (WIC) clinics in four central Ohio counties, 1995–1996.	ED visits and hospitalizations for children	Hospitalization of children was related to maternal hospitalization the previous year; child younger than 1 year old and more than two chronic conditions. Maternal ED use in last year, Medicaid fee for service plan, and rural residence were predictive of ED use.	
Proctor, Morrow-Howell, Li, & Dore (2000)	Prospective observational study	Setting: Elderly congestive heart failure patients from a large urban midwestern hospital, 1990–1991. $N = 253$.	Hospital readmission within 14 weeks of discharge. Adequate home care assistance (formal or informal) as perceived by the patient.	By 14 weeks postdischarge, 42% of the patients readmitted to hospitals. Patient ratings of adequacy of care arrangement were significantly related to readmission.	Small sample size, selection biases, single location, and self-report biases.
Rask, Williams, McNagny, Parker, & Baker (1998)	Cohort study	Random sample of $N = 351$ adults initially surveyed in the ED in May 1992 and followed for 2 years. Setting: A public hospital in Atlanta, Georgia.	ED visits	High rates of ED use associated with multiple chronic medical conditions, or a chronic medical condition complicated by a psychiatric diagnosis or substance abuse.	
Reuben et al. (2002)	Retrospective cohort study, model development/validation	Setting: Elderly patients from three communities: East Boston, Iowa, and New Haven; data source 1981–1992 from established Populations for Epidemiologic Studies of the Elderly (EPESE). $N = 3,742$.	Hospital days and hospital costs (defined as 11 or more hospital days during the next 3 years) and overall Part A Medicare hospital costs during the next 3 years.	Independent predictors included hospitalizations in prior 2 years, male gender, fair/poor self-rated health, not working, infrequent religious participation, needing help bathing, being unable to walk ½ mile, diabetes, taking loop diuretics, low serum albumin, and low serum iron.	
Rosenblatt et al. (2000)	Retrospective cross-sectional study with secondary data	Setting: Data collected from Medicare patients older than 65 years in Washington State during 1994. Total visits: 105,647.	ED visits over a 1 year period	Patients with a primary care physician were less than half as likely to have an ED visit within the study year	Secondary claims data limitations
Schatz et al. (2004)	Retrospective cohort study, development/validation of risk stratification scheme	Predictors from 1999 date of ED care for asthma in 2000 were evaluated in 2 groups in California.	ED visits during study year	Factors predictive of asthma-related ED visits included ED visit/hospitalization history; use	

Study	Design	Sample/Setting	Outcome measures	Findings	Limitations
Schatz, Zeiger, Mosen, & Vollmer (2008)	Prospective cohort	Training set (n = 8,789; 2,000 emergency hospital care = 5.5%) in San Diego and a testing set (n = 6104; 2000 emergency hospital care = 7.9%) in Fontana. N = 1,006 HMO patients with active asthma completed surveys (mini-AQLQ and prior-year history of acute episodes included in survey). Setting: Kaiser Permanente managed care adult members aged 18–56 years from the Northern California and Northwest region.	ED visits. Mini-AQLQ (Asthma Quality of Life Questionnaire).	of oral corticosteroids and heavy use of beta-agonists. Low quality of life or a history of prior acute episodes provided high sensitivity (90.4%) and identified a group nearly 6 times more likely to require emergency hospital care.	
Schonwetter et al. (2008)	Retrospective comparative (chart review-based)	145 cardiac hospice patients who visited the ED and a comparison who died at home; Temple Terrace, Florida, 2006.	End-of-life ED visits	Peripheral vascular disease and diabetes predicted increased ED visits. Presence of caregiver, hospice emergency kit, patient on morphine, compliance with medications, being Caucasian, and frequent nursing visits decreased ED visits.	
Schwarz & Elman (2003)	Prospective cohort design	Setting: Heart failure patients from two community hospitals in northeastern Ohio with their caregivers. Initially there were 156 patient-caregiver dyads, but only 128 patient-caregiver dyads completed the study; all patients were interviewed 7–10 days after discharge.	Hospital readmission	Hospital readmission significantly predicted by interaction of severity of cardiac illness and functional status, and interaction of caregiver stress and depression predicted risk of hospital readmission.	Selection biases (patient and caregiver both required to provide consent); self-report biases.
Shah, Rathouz, & Chin (2001)	Retrospective, exploratory study; cross-sectional study	Data collected from 1993 Medicare Current Beneficiary Survey, a database on a random cross-section survey of elderly Medicare beneficiaries. N = 9,784 in the study population, patient 65 years of age or older.	ED visits	ED users were older, were less educated, were more likely to live alone, had lower income and higher Charlson Comorbidity Index scores, and were less satisfied with their ability to access care as compared with nonusers.	Secondary data
Sharma et al. (2000)	Retrospective population cohort study involving record linkage between birth registry and service database	Administrative data set 1995 birth cohort in the State of Missouri. N = 70,043.	ED visits, urgent vs nonurgent (assessed using a classification for diagnosis codes).	Total and nonurgent ED visits linked with Medicaid (health insurance for very low-income families), self-pay/uninsured, Black race, rural region, presence of birth defects, and a nursery stay of > 2 days.	

COPD = chronic obstructive pulmonary disease; ED = emergency department; LOS = length of stay; $PaCO_2$ = partial pressure of carbon dioxide in the blood (an indicator of gas exchange and acid-base balance); U.S. = United States; USD = United States dollars.

(continues)

TABLE 10-1   Patient-Level Predictors of Healthcare Utilization (continued)

Author and date	Study design	Characteristics of sample, and setting	Healthcare utilization variables studied	Major results	Limitations/ comments
Shelton, Sager, & Schraeder (2000)	Cohort study using secondary administrative (claims) data/ risk model development/ validation	1,054 community-dwelling elderly patients enrolled in a U.S. Medicare demonstration project	Hospitalizations and ED visits	Having two or more chronic illnesses, taking five or more prescription medications, and having had a hospitalization or ED encounter in the previous 12 months were associated service utilization.	
Shiber, Longley, & Brewer (2009)	Retrospective cohort study	Convenience sample of Central Florida teaching hospital ED patients, 2004. Cohort (n = 49) of individuals with 35 or more visits over a 4 year period was compared with a randomly selected group of non-high-use patients (n = 50).	ED use	Frequent users more likely to have cardiovascular, genitourinary, or psychiatric disease and present with psychiatric, substance abuse, and pulmonary chief complaints.	Small sample from a single institution.
White-Means, Thornton, & Yeo (1989)	Prospective cohort study (secondary analysis of interview data)	Data source: National Medical Care Utilization and Expenditure Survey (NMCUES), a national sample of the noninstitutionalized civilian U.S. population interviewed five times in 14 months, 1980–1981; subsets of the sample: N = 1,258 Blacks and Hispanics who reported health conditions were selected.	ED use for nonurgent medical conditions	Within this sample, Blacks, 18- to 34-year-olds, patients with digestive disorders and those with physical impairments were more likely to seek ED care..	Small sample size relative to the population that used the ED; self-report biases.
Wisnivesky, Leventhal, & Halm (2006)	Prospective cohort, interviewed patients	198 adults hospitalized for asthma in an inner-city hospital over a period of 1 year were interviewed. The mean age of patients was 49.9 ±17.4 years, 78% were women, and 97% were non-White.	Health outcomes focused on were quality of life and health-care utilization (ED visits) information obtained through interview.	Asthma severity: Patients with a physician in charge of their asthma care had lower odds of resource utilization (odds ratio, 0.4; $p = .03$). Conversely, a self-reported history of cockroach allergy was associated with greater utilization (odds ratio, 2.3; $p = .05$).	Self-report biases
Yamada, Korman, & Hughes (2000)	Prospective cohort study	Setting: United States N = 163 subjects with severe mental illness followed for 37–54 months after index hospitalization.	Hospital readmission	Number of previous hospitalizations and White race were predictors of readmissions; White race was the only independent risk factor after factoring in residential and case management program enrollment.	

COPD = chronic obstructive pulmonary disease; ED = emergency department; LOS = length of stay; $PaCO_2$ = partial pressure of carbon dioxide in the blood (an indicator of gas exchange and acid-base balance); U.S. = United States; USD = United States dollars.

symptoms) requiring more intense treatment. Co-occurring medical conditions, sometimes called comorbidities, complicate treatment and impose more serious burdens on patients and families in terms of self-care and also tend to raise health-care consumption. Similarly, patients with worse impairment in functional status tend to show more healthcare utilization, perhaps because functional impairment reflects the impact of the totality of medical conditions such patients face or serves as a marker for the personal intrinsic resources patients have to manage their care.

Past use of healthcare services frequently predicts future use (see, for instance, Hastings, George, et al., 2008; Hastings, Oddone, Fillenbaum, Sloane, & Schmader, 2008). Two mechanisms are likely responsible. The first is that ED, hospital, and clinic use may reflect more severe or complicated disease. A second is that past behavior is often a predictor of future behavior. In the case of healthcare utilization, previous service use likely reflects psychological and social factors that influence patient/family decisions to seek out care. Examples of the types of mechanisms likely involved include coping styles and dispositions.

Psychological distress and psychiatric diagnoses, particularly depression, emerge in multiple studies as predictors of high healthcare utilization. This is a persistent pattern that has been seen for many decades in the literature and continues to be replicated (Kurdyak, Gnam, Goering, Chong, & Alter, 2008). There is a tremendous range of patient coping with illnesses even of the same apparent "objective" severity. Furthermore, psychological distress or disorder can predate or follow the development of physical or psychiatric health problems. Therefore, it is not always clear whether these associations are seen because psychological distress (1) is partly related to illness severity and impact, (2) interferes with self-management of illness, and/or (3) increases perceptions of signs and symptoms and lowers the threshold for seeking help. All three pathways are likely involved at least some of the time. Patients who experience more disease-related interference with quality of life tend to consume more health resources, and the web of causal factors involved is similarly complex and understudied.

Age tends to be associated with utilization, probably for a variety of reasons—not only the association of age with more disease and worse disease, but also the likelihood that at least some older patients have thinner resources to deal with crises and are likely to have a lower threshold for help-seeking. The contexts of patients' lives in the community also appear to be important. Patients under social and economic stress, such as those who are poorer, who are from disadvantaged backgrounds, who do not live with a spouse, or who have home care arrangements they believe to be inadequate appear to consume more health care, probably because of fewer actual or perceived resources they have for coping with health downturns.

Access to healthcare services also predicts utilization, although not always in the directions one might expect. Patients without primary care providers appear to come to EDs more often, as do those who have limited other options for dealing with immediate healthcare concerns. Patients without health insurance may or may not differentially seek some venues of care over others. The pattern of findings regarding access and utilization tend to vary somewhat across studies, probably because of patient population and health system differences.

These factors have a number of implications. One is that specific types of patients appear to be at high risk for deterioration that may require intense use of healthcare services, at high risk for feeling overwhelmed by the demands of their illnesses, or both. These patient groups may merit special study and/or targeting with interventions. Second, specific characteristics linked with healthcare utilization may also suggest mechanisms that are responsible for high service use and thus inform the design of systems or processes of care. Third, they show that analyses of healthcare utilization data must take at least some clinical and psychosocial risk factors into account to be interpretable and for comparisons between groups to be meaningful. Many research papers and evaluations present limited data about patient characteristics that might inform readers whether the population studied was at high or low risk for heavy service consumption, such that crude (unadjusted) utilization rates may not be particularly useful. Furthermore, it is often unclear whether controlling for risk factors and clinical background characteristics would change the interpretation of results or illuminate new relationships or differences.

EVIDENCE CONCERNING THE RELATIONSHIP BETWEEN NURSING AND HEALTHCARE UTILIZATION: NURSING STRUCTURAL VARIABLES

Nursing structural variables, reflecting the resources and settings where nursing care is provided, have been most frequently studied in relation to length of stay in hospitals and healthcare costs (see Dall, Chen, Seifert, Maddox, & Hogan, 2009; Estabrooks et al., 2009; Kane, Shamliyan, Mueller, Duval, & Wilt, 2007; Thungjaroenkul, Cummings, & Embleton, 2007; and 13 individual articles in **TABLE 10-2**). Notably, higher levels of hospital nurse staffing, particularly registered-nurse-to-patient ratios, are consistently linked with lower lengths of stay. This is probably the most robust finding in this literature. Another structural variable that may have links to length and costs of care is shift length. One early set of study results suggests that length of stay may be reduced when nurses work longer shifts, which may be due to a possible link with better coordination of care. Similarly, some results suggest that admission to a nursing unit specializing in the care of a particular patient population, the use of rapid rounding to assess care coordination needs, competency-based (goal-directed) nursing care, and clinical pathways all appear to reduce length of stay for specific populations in isolated studies. Interestingly, the mechanisms at work are generally not clear, although again, two major contenders are prevention of complications and more

TABLE 10-2   Nursing Structural Variables and Healthcare Utilization

Author and date	Study design	Characteristics of sample, and response rate and setting	Healthcare utilization variables studied	Nursing intervention being evaluated/ nursing factors	Major results	Limitations
REVIEW ARTICLES						
Dall et al. (2009)	Literature review and extrapolation of effect size to U.S. national sample	Findings from 27 articles on the relationship between RN staffing levels and nursing-sensitive patient outcomes in acute care hospitals were used to generate economic models, and then used to analyze 5.4 million discharges from 610 hospitals; hospital discharge data were from the 2005 Nationwide Inpatient Sample (U.S.).	LOS and costs	RN staffing in hospitals	Increased nurse staffing levels are associated with decreased risk of nosocomial infections and decreased LOS. Economic value of increasing the RN workforce to set RN hours per patient day staffing in all U.S. hospitals to the 75th percentile for 2005: $1,700 net annual savings to health care system per RN hired.	
Estabrooks et al. (2009)	Literature review	12 articles that examined the effect of shift length (8-h vs 12-h shifts) on quality of patient care and judged to be of adequate methodological quality.	LOS	Length of the shifts (hours) worked by hospital nurses	One study reported decreased patient complications and LOS with longer shifts.	Further study is needed.
Kane et al. (2007)	Systematic review and meta-analysis	MEDLINE, CINAHL, Cochrane databases, BioMed Central, federal reports, American Nurses Association, and Digital Dissertations in 2006 to identify studies conducted in the United States and Canada that investigated the association between nurse staffing and patient outcomes. 28 studies used 17 cohort, 7 cross-sectional, and 4 case-control studies.	LOS	RN staffing per patient day	An increase of 1 RN full-time equivalent per patient day was associated with a 34% shorter length of stay in ICUs and 31% in surgical patients.	
Thungjaroenkul et al. (2007)	Systematic review	Five databases—MEDLINE, CINAHL, HealthSTAR, Cochrane, and ABI/Inform—searched for studies from 1990 to 2006 on nurse staffing in relation to LOS and hospital costs. 17 articles selected.	LOS and costs	Nursing-staff-to-patient ratio	Of the 17 studies, 10 suggested that increased nurse-to-patient ratios were related to lowered hospital resource use.	
ARTICLES						
Amaravadi et al. (2000)	Retrospective observational cohort study, secondary administrative data regarding patients.	Setting: 52 nonfederal acute care hospitals in Maryland from 1994 to 1998. N = 353 esophagectomy patients	LOS and hospital costs	Night-RN-to-patient ratios greater than or less than 1:2 in the ICU.	A 39% increase in in-hospital LOS and decreased costs for patients where ratios more favorable.	

ED = emergency department; ICU = intensive care unit; LOS = length of stay; RN = registered nurse; U.S.=United States; USD=United States Dollars.

(continues)

TABLE 10-2   Nursing Structural Variables and Healthcare Utilization (continued)

Author and date	Study design	Characteristics of sample, and response rate and setting	Healthcare utilization variables studied	Nursing intervention being evaluated/ nursing factors	Major results	Limitations
Cho, Ketefian, Barkaus-kas, & Smith (2003)	Retrospective cohort study; sec-ondary administra-tive data	$N = 124,204$ patients in 20 surgical diagnosis-related groups treated in 232 California acute care hospitals	LOS, costs	Nurse-to-staff ratio	Lower nurse staffing levels were linked to pneumonia and pres-sure ulcers.	
Czaplinski & Diers (1998)	Retrospective cohort study	$N = 11,316$ admitted to Yale New Haven Hospital in 16 diagnosis-related groups (DRGs) from 1987 to 1993.	LOS	Patient treatment on specialty-specific units	9 of the 16 DRG patients cared for on specialized nursing units had shorter LOSs. Specialized units that had decreased LOS on specialized units were chest pain, angina pec-toris, major bowel procedure, total and partial mastectomy, and transurethral prostatectomy.	
Decker (2008)	Retrospective study; cross-sectional	Data on short-stay $N = 4,086$ dis-charges from facilities in 1997–1999 in the National Nursing Home Survey.	LOS	Nurse staffing levels	Higher levels of RN staffing were associated with shorter LOS among recovered/stabilized dis-charged patients. (Increase of physical thera-pist hours also associated with showed decreased LOS.)	
Geary, Cale, Quinn, & Winchell (2009)	Comparative time-series	Setting: Sutter Medical Center, Sacramento, California. Rapid rounding implemented on medical-surgical and telemetry areas.	LOS	Rapid rounding team consists of two nursing directors, two case managers, a staff nurse, and clinical nurse spe-cialists; the meet-ings were short and encouraged com-munication with the nursing staff.	After implementation of rapid rounds in 2007, there was a decrease in LOS (mean 3 days to mean 2 days).	Single-institution study

Citation	Design	Setting/Sample	Outcome	Nursing variable	Findings	Comments
Jette, Warren, & Wirtalla (2004)	Cohort study; secondary analysis	$N = 6,897$ patients covered by Medicare + Choice plan and admitted to 68 skilled nursing facilities for rehabilitation.	Discharge to the community rather than long-term care facilities and LOS in skilled nursing.	Nursing staff level	Patients in facilities with a nursing staff level of 3.5 or more hrs of staffing per resident per day showed greater odds of being discharged to the community rather than another institution.	
Johnson et al. (2000)	Prospective cohort	Setting: Hospitals in Michigan Study group ($N = 705$): Women and newborns discharged during the first 5 months of the new program for postpartum care in 1996. Control group ($N = 722$): Women and newborns discharged during the last 5 months of the traditional standard of perinatal care in 1995–1996.	Postdischarge maternal and neonate ED visit and readmit to the hospital data were analyzed, and hospital cost was also measured.	Structured competency-based assessment and delivery of nursing care to postpartum patients	Postdischarge maternal ED visits and/or readmits did not increase. There was a marked reduction in hospital costs for mothers and newborns. Patient satisfaction remained high.	
Lee & Anderson (2007)	Pretest/ posttest design	Inpatient cases with primary diagnoses of chronic obstructive pulmonary disease, congestive heart failure, diabetes, myocardial infarction, and pneumonia from 1999 to 2003 in a rural hospital in a midwestern state.	LOS	Implementation of clinical pathways (treatment protocol to reduce variation of care for nurses and other healthcare providers)	Of the five pathways studied, only one (for myocardial infarction, $p < 0.01$) showed an association with a statistical significance in decreasing LOS.	
Lichtig, Knauf, & Milholland (1999)	Retrospective cohort study, secondary data	Setting: All California acute care facilities ($N = 462$) and all acute care hospitals in New York State ($N = 229$). From 1992 to 1994.	Hospital LOS	Nurse staffing level and the proportion of RNs in the skill mix of staff, adjusted for nursing intensity weights (NIW; estimates of the intensity of nursing care generally required by different case types).	Regression analysis revealed that more nursing hours per NIW and higher RN skill mix both are associated with reduced hospital LOS.	According to the researchers, many hospitals had to be excluded because of missing data; however, how many were excluded was not specified.
Needleman, Buerhaus, Stewart, Zelevinsky, & Mattke (2006)	Retrospective cohort study/ secondary analysis of staffing parameters and patient outcomes from administrative data sources	Data from 799 nonfederal acute care general hospitals in 11 U.S. states in 1997. Discharge abstracts and nurse staffing data were obtained from the states; data on hospital size, location, and teaching status were from the American Hospital Association annual survey; and cost-to-charge ratios were from Medicare cost reports.	LOS, system costs of care	RN hours per patient day, LPN hours per patient day	Models suggest that increasing both total licensed hours and RN skill mix to the 75th percentile would avoid 4,106,315 hospital days and 70,416 negative outcomes, for an avoided $6.707 billion and $224 million USD; however, the majority of these cost savings was attributable to increased skill mix.	Many assumptions in the models

(continues)

ED = emergency department; ICU = intensive care unit; LOS = length of stay; RN = registered nurse; U.S.=United States; USD=United States Dollars.

TABLE 10-2 Nursing Structural Variables and Healthcare Utilization (continued)

Author and date	Study design	Characteristics of sample, and response rate and setting	Healthcare utilization variables studied	Nursing intervention being evaluated/ nursing factors	Major results	Limitations
Titler et al. (2005)	Cohort	Setting: United States. Data collected between 1998 and 2002 as part of a larger study; 11,756 hospitalizations in 8,988 patients aged 60 or older.	Cost of care for patients at risk of falls	Nurse staffing level and nursing intervention costs	For each 20% decrease in nursing staff level, a $1,178 increase in patient care costs was observed, and a net return on costs of nursing interventions was observed.	
Titler et al. (2008)	Retrospective, exploratory analysis to determine the impact of patient characteristics, clinical conditions, hospital unit characteristics, and healthcare interventions on hospital cost of patients with heart failure	Administrative and clinical data from $n = 1,075$ heart failure patients 60 years of age or older from 1998 to 2002 at an 843-bed academic medical center in the midwestern U.S.	Hospitalization costs	RN staffing	Patients cared for under nurse staffing below institutional means experienced increased hospital costs.	Single-hospital study
Tschannen & Kalisch (2009)	Prospective, comparative study	Setting: Two hospitals—midwestern hospital (900-bed university medical center) and a 230-bed community hospital. A total of 135 nurses and 310 patients across two hospitals and four units with various levels of staffing, skill mix, and experience of the nurses. 5-week study involved collecting data from patients and nursing staff.	LOS	Staffing (hours per day) and skill mix (mix of RN, LPN and assistive personnel), nurses' level of experience	Increased hours of care per patient/day and higher skill mix associated with decreased LOS; increased nursing experience linked to increased LOS.	Covariation of staffing patterns and LOS with other factors is likely.

ED = emergency department; ICU = intensive care unit; LOS = length of stay; RN = registered nurse; U.S. = United States; USD = United States Dollars.

effective coordination of care, leading to timely progression and discharge. Patient and clinician characteristics that influence whether various structural factors play a role in healthcare consumption also merit further investigation.

EVIDENCE CONCERNING THE RELATIONSHIP BETWEEN NURSING AND HEALTHCARE UTILIZATION: NURSING INTERVENTIONS

TABLE 10-3 presents the results of seven review articles and 37 reports of individual studies of nursing interventions for a range of clienteles in which healthcare utilization was examined as an outcome. These interventions varied somewhat, but heavily represented in the studies reviewed were patient and family education to increase self-care ability; telephone or home interventions and clinical follow-up by nurses; case management, care coordination, and consistent follow-up by clinical specialists; and nursing involvement in the coordination of interdisciplinary teams. Reported studies often showed decreased utilization or a favorable cost-benefit ratio. However, most reviews describe findings of these studies as "mixed," and more than a few of the comparisons of healthcare utilization across groups failed to identify differences where they were expected. A recent set of U.S. trials of chronic disease patient teaching and care coordination by nurses for Medicare patients failed to show any net reductions or cost benefits, although some evidence of improved quality of care was found (Peikes, Chen, Schore, & Brown, 2009).

A number of trends are clear from a quick glance at the table. Interventions for some clienteles (for instance, asthma, diabetes, stroke, and heart failure patients) have been more extensively investigated than those for other conditions. ED visits and rehospitalizations dominated the health resource use outcomes investigated. The mechanisms responsible for the decreases in utiliz ation were generally not specified, nor in most cases were any specific patient subgroups that may have been more responsive to interventions identified.

On the latter points, which are enduring issues in all intervention research in nursing and related fields, recent work on specific clinical populations in which successive research projects have built on each other illuminates interesting patterns. For instance, Sochalski et al. (2009) reviewed literature on heart failure interventions that included a multidisciplinary and nursing component. The review highlighted the usefulness of multidisciplinary and face-to-face patient/ clinician interventions in reducing healthcare utilization. In general, however, although the nursing interventions described in the literature seem promising for reducing hospital and ED use, the components of observations that are most effective in reducing consumption of resources and which patients benefit most are unclear.

A number of studies—for instance, Lorig et al. (2001), in which a standardized intervention to increase self-management capacity in chronically ill patients

TABLE 10-3 Nursing Interventions and Healthcare Utilization

Study Date	Study type	Setting/sample	Healthcare utilization variables studied	Interventions	Major results	Limitations/comments
Bunn, Byrne, & Kendall (2005)	Systematic literature review	Cochrane collaboration analysis of RCTs, controlled studies, controlled before/after studies and interrupted time series of telephone consultation or triage in a general healthcare setting. Nine studies met criteria.	ED visits, physician consultations	Six studies compared telephone consultation for assessment and referral vs normal care (four by a nurse, one by a nurse, and one by a clinic clerk); two studies compared nurses with physicians; and one compared health assistants with doctors or nurses.	Mixed findings, but some support for reduction in ED and clinic visits and patient acceptability without increased risk of poor outcomes.	Further rigorous study of the interventions themselves, particularly their safety and cost, is needed.
Chiu & Newcomer (2007)	Systematic literature review	Systematic search of the PubMed database, 1996–2006, for articles on nurse-assisted case management intended to improve posthospital transitions for elderly patients. 15 clinical trials reviewed: full-text link, addressed elderly patients, and discharge transition.	Readmissions, LOS, and ED visits	All 15 articles examined nurse-directed case management (two studies involved interventions with physician collaborative care). Case management included home visit or over-the-phone follow-up, individualized discharge planning, education, and self-care promotion.	Seven of these studies showed statistically significant reductions in the number of hospital readmission days or LOS. Only three studies found significant reductions in presentations to ED.	Key limitations noted by authors included small samples (five studies had fewer than 100 participants in the control and intervention groups), high subject attrition, and inconsistencies in intervention implementation.
Coffman, Cabana, Halpin, & Yelin (2008)	Meta-analysis	Inclusion criteria included enrollment of children aged 2–17 years with a clinical diagnosis of asthma, resided in the U.S., RCT. 37 met the inclusion criteria; 27 compared educational interventions with usual care; and 10 compared different interventions.	Health outcome measures examined by the meta-analysis were ED visits and hospitalization.	Asthma educational programs	Patient education was associated with statistically significant decreases in mean hospitalizations and ED visits, and a trend toward lower odds of an ED visit.	

(continues)

Hastings & Heflin (2005)	Systematic review	27 studies reviewed that evaluated interventions designed to improve outcome for elders discharged from the ED: 6 RCT, 2 non-RCT, and 19 observational studies.	Rehospitalization	Nurses used in the majority of interventions involving discharge planning and home visits	Results were mixed; some studies documented reduced ED visits in intervention groups.
Langhorne et al. (2005)	Meta-analysis	Cochrane stroke group search; articles were from six countries: Australia, Canada, Norway, Sweden, Thailand, United Kingdom; two unpublished articles were from New Zealand and Australia.	LOS	Early supported discharge (ESD) for stroke patients with discharge planning and home care nursing interventions	The hospital stay was 8 days shorter for patients assigned ESD services than for those assigned conventional care ($p < 0.0001$).
Oeseburg, Wynia, Middel, & Reijneveld (2009)	Systematic review	Search for English-language, RCTs evaluating service use and costs of case management model for people with a chronic somatic disease or for impaired older people living in the community using keywords *case management, outcomes, costs, RCT, chronic disease, and older.* Eight relevant studies were identified.	Hospital readmissions and ED visits	In the eight studies reviewed, case management involved nurses specialized in either geriatric or public health. All studies had nurses intervention; patients were provided with an individualized care plan for home.	Patient advocacy case management led to decreased service use and to savings in costs.
Peikes et al. (2009)	15 RCTs summary	15 groups of patients in care coordination demonstration projects randomly assigned to treatment or control (usual care) status; U.S. 2002–2005. Total $N = 18,309$ ($n = 178$–$2,657$ per program)	Hospitalizations, monthly Medicare expenditures over at least 1 year	Nurses provided patient education and monitoring (mostly via telephone) to improve adherence and ability to communicate with physicians. Patients were contacted twice per month on average; frequency varied widely.	13 of 15 studies showed no significant differences in hospitalizations across study and control groups; 1 showed increased hospital use; 1 showed decreased hospital use. None of the trials showed cost savings in the intervention groups. Much variation in intervention design

APN = advanced practice nurse; ED = emergency department; LOS = length of stay; RCT = randomized controlled trial; U.S. = United States.

TABLE 10-3   Nursing Interventions and Healthcare Utilization (continued)

Study Date	Study type	Setting/sample	Healthcare utilization variables studied	Interventions	Major results	Limitations/comments
ARTICLES						
Aubert, Herman, & Waters (1998)	RCT	Setting: two large primary care clinics in Jacksonville, Florida; 128 patients with diabetes mellitus (111 type II diabetics).	ED visits and hospital admissions over 12 months	Nurse case managers provided interventions to the intervention group by following an algorithm for managing diabetes, which included teaching patients about diet and exercise, proper use of insulin, etc.	No significant changes/difference in ED use or hospitalizations (none of the ED visits or hospitalizations was diabetes-related).	
Berg & Wadhwa (2007)	Matched-cohort group observational design	1,220 elderly diabetic patients on Medicare+Choice program in Ohio, Kentucky, and Indiana	Hospitalizations, ED visits, physician evaluation and management visits, skilled nursing facility days over 24 months	A structured, evidence-based telephonic nursing intervention designed to provide patient education, counseling, and monitoring services	18% reduction in hospitalizations, 22% reduction in bed days, 12% increase in physician evaluation and management. Visits in intervention group.	
Berg & Wadhwa (2009)	Matched-cohort group observational design	980 diabetic patients on Medicaid program in Puerto Rico.	Hospitalization, ED visits, financial impacts	Telephonic nursing disease management involving a customized self-management intervention plan.	48% reduction in inpatient bed days in intervention group, return on investment 3.8:1.	
Berg, Wadhwa, & Johnson (2004)	Matched-cohort group observational design	1,066 elderly heart failure patients on Medicare + Choice program residing in Ohio, Kentucky, and Indiana.	Hospitalizations, ED visits, physician visits, skilled nursing facility (SNF) days, financial effect	Telephonic nursing intervention designed to provide patient education, counseling, and monitoring services	23% fewer hospitalizations, 26% fewer inpatient bed days, 22% fewer ED visits, 44% fewer heart failure hospitalizations, 70% fewer 30-day readmissions, and 45% fewer SNF bed days; return on investment was calculated to be 2.31:1.	

Brooten et al. (1986)	RCT	79 very low birth weight infants (less than or equal to 1500 g), U.S.	Rehospitalizations and acute care visits, hospital charges and physician charges	Infants in the control group (n = 40) were discharged according to routine nursery criteria, which included a weight of about 2200 g. In the early-discharge (intervention) group, instruction, counseling, home visits, and daily on-call availability of a hospital-based nurse specialist for 18 months.	No difference in rehospitalizations, but cost savings in intervention group for various categories of services, and overall after taking costs of intervention into account.
Brooten et al. (1994)	RCT	102 women with unplanned Caesarian deliveries, U.S.	Maternal and infant rehospitalizations to 8 weeks	Intervention group (discharged 30 h earlier on average) received comprehensive discharge planning, instruction, counseling, home visits, and daily on-call availability from nurse specialists.	Decreased maternal rehospitalizations, overall 29% reduction in healthcare charges in intervention group.
Brooten et al. (2001) Brooten et al. (2007)	RCT	173 women (and 194 infants) with high-risk pregnancies (gestational or pregestational diabetes mellitus, chronic hypertension, preterm labor, or high risk of preterm labor), U.S.	Prenatal and infant hospitalizations, hospital days and cost savings.	APN provided 8 weeks of health teaching, guidance, and counseling; treatments and procedures; case management. Postpartum care included teaching, counseling, telephone outreach, and daily telephone availability of the APNs with physician backup for intervention group.	Fewer preterm infants, more twin pregnancies carried to term, fewer prenatal hospitalizations, fewer infant rehospitalizations, and savings of total hospital days in intervention group.
Castro et al. (2003)	RCT	96 asthmatics, mainly young African American women, Washington, D.C., 1996–1999	Hospitalization, ED visits, costs over a 6-month period	Asthma nurse specialist worked with patients who were assigned to the intervention group.	60% reduction in total hospitalizations, with no significant change in ED visits in the intervention group. Readmissions for asthma were reduced by 54% in the intervention group.

APN = advanced practice nurse; ED = emergency department; LOS = length of stay; RCT = randomized controlled trial; U.S.=United States.

(continues)

TABLE 10-3   Nursing Interventions and Healthcare Utilization (continued)

Study Date	Study type	Setting/sample	Healthcare utilization variables studied	Interventions	Major results	Limitations/comments
Dansky, Vasey, & Bowles (2008)	RCT	N = 284 heart failure patients. 2004–2005. Setting: 10 home health agencies located in one mid-Atlantic state.	Health outcome determined by measuring ED visits and rehospitalization. Measure ED visits and rehospitalization at 60 days and 120 days after discharge.	Patients divided into three groups: telehomecare (telemonitoring video system; allows for nurse–patient interaction), one-way monitoring (info is provided by patient), and control group.	Compared with control group, telehomecare patients had a lower probability for hospitalization and ED visits compared with 60 days, but not 120 days, postdischarge.	
Davidson, Ansari, & Karlan (2007)	Single-group, pretest/posttest	N = 331 randomly selected diabetic patients from adult outpatient clinic in inner-city Los Angeles, California.	ED use over a 2-year period	Nurse-directed disease management program using treatment algorithms for glycemic control and recommended follow-up.	Preventable diabetic-related ED visits were reduced by 45% (p = 0.001). Costs of ED visits for the cohort prior to the program were $129,176, and $24,630 after.	
C. M. Dougherty; Thompson, & Lewis (2005)	RCT	N = 168 patients following implantation of an implantable defibrillator (ICD) (n = 83 usual care; n = 85 intervention), Pacific Northwest, U.S.	Rehospitalizations, ED visits at 6 months and 12 months	8-week educational telephone intervention directed by expert cardiovascular nurses, aiming to increase physical functioning, psychological adjustment, and self-efficacy in managing the challenges of recovery.	No significant differences	
G. Dougherty, Schiffrin, White, Soderstrom, & Sufrategui (1999)	RCT	63 newly diagnosed diabetic children, Montreal Children's Hospital, Montreal, Quebec, Canada.	ED visits and hospitalizations, costs; 2-year follow-up	Treating team for hospital and home-based groups was composed of the same three diabetologists, a psychologist, and a social worker. Hospital base treatment only received phone contacts. Intervention group received nurse visits once or twice daily to instruct and supervise treatment. The diabetes treatment nurse for the home-based group was expected to	No difference in adverse events requiring hospitalization. Overall increased health system costs of home-based intervention, but not in costs for families.	Use of different nurses for the two study groups

				spend more time with her patients, both initially and during follow-up.	Low participation rate
Dunagan et al. (2005)	RCT	Setting: Barnes-Jewish Hospital in St Louis, Missouri. N = 151 patients. Time period: 1999–2000	LOS and rehospitalization at 6 months and 1 year	Intervention group received call within 3 days after hospital discharge or program enrollment, and then at least weekly for 2 weeks. Nurse-administered, telephone-based disease intervention included promotion of self-management skills, appropriate diet, and adherence to guideline-based therapy prescribed by primary physicians.	Reduction in readmissions for intervention patients, ED, and rehospitalizations for heart failure and all causes.
Feldman et al. (2004)	RCT	N = 530 heart failure patients from home health agency; New York, 1996	Home visits by RNs, ED visits and rehospitalization	205 nurses provided skilled nursing visits to this population. Patients in special intervention group, Health Outcomes, Management and Evaluation (HOME) plan, received a special patient-oriented home care nursing plan.	Home health visits reduced in intervention group, no significant impact on ED visits.
Forster et al. (2005)	RCT with unblinded assignment	Setting: two teaching hospitals, Ottawa, Ontario, Canada, 2002. N = 620 sequentially admitted medical patients.	Postdischarge ED visits, hospital readmissions	Four clinical nurse specialists facilitated patient care by retrieving information collected by family physicians; arranging in-hospital imaging; facilitating patient discharge by arranging follow-up visits and providing patient education; and telephoning patients early after discharge from hospital.	Groups did not differ on postdischarge outcomes, including readmission.

APN = advanced practice nurse; ED = emergency department; LOS = length of stay; RCT = randomized controlled trial; U.S. = United States.

(continues)

TABLE 10-3   Nursing Interventions and Healthcare Utilization (continued)

Study Date	Study type	Setting/sample	Healthcare utilization variables studied	Interventions	Major results	Limitations/comments
Gagnon, Schein, McVey, & Bergman (1999)	RCT	A university hospital and two community health centers in Montreal. *N* = 427 frail older people (70 years of age or older and at risk for repeated hospital admissions) discharged home from the ED.	ED visit and LOS in hospital over the intervention period	Nursing intervention involved nurse case management of 10 months, including telephone follow-up health teaching.	No significant differences in healthcare utilization.	
Greineder, Loane, & Parks (1995)	Pretest/posttest (one group)	*N* = 53 asthmatic inner-city Boston ED patients, aged 1–17 years	ED visits and admissions and the cost to the healthcare system, two follow-ups	An asthma outreach nurse provided individualized care to the patients, including teaching around asthma management, triggers, and use of inhalers.	ED admissions were reduced 79% (from a rate of 72 visits per year to 15 visits per year, *p* < .0001), and hospital admissions were reduced 86% (from 35 per year to 5 per year, *p* < .001). The outreach nurse worked an average of 8 hours per week at an annualized cost of $11,115, for a cost savings of approximately $87,000.	
Guttman et al. (2005)	Time-series	Setting: Jewish General Hospital, Montreal, Quebec, Canada. 1999–2000. ED patients 75 years or older. *N* = 905 control. *N* = 819 intervention.	Unscheduled return to ED within 14 days after discharge	ED-based nurse discharge plan coordination intervention included patient education, coordination of appointments, and telephone follow-up with access to the nurse for up to 7 days postdischarge.	Unscheduled return visits reduced by 19–27% from 8 to 14 days postdischarge.	
Hickey et al. (2000)	RCT (block randomization by medical team)	Brigham and Women's Hospital, Boston, Massachusetts. 1994. *N* = 302 general medical patients.	Hospital LOS and deviation from planned LOS, and readmission/use of health services during the month after discharge	Case management (CM) was carried out by bachelor's-level nurse case managers who participated in physician daily rounds and telephoned patients 48 h after discharge.	No difference in LOS or other hospital use between groups. When patients were stratified by risk level, it revealed that for high-risk groups, CM hospital stay was 2.9 days shorter	Relatively small number of patients used medical services within 1 month of discharge. Incomplete data regarding high-, intermediate-, and low-risk patients.

		Patients were instructed to call their case manager after discharge with questions about medications, diet, activity progression, or symptom management.	than standard care ($p = 0.02$), but no differences were seen in the low- and intermediate-risk groups.	
Klinnert et al. (2005)	RCT	Low-income caregivers of infants aged 9–24 months with three or more physician-documented wheezing episodes. $N = 181$. Randomly assigned to environmental support intervention. Setting: Pediatric departments of local hospitals and clinics in the metropolitan Denver, Colorado.	Hospitalization and ED visits for 12 months	Nurse home visitors intervened for 1 year to decrease allergen and environmental tobacco smoke exposure and improve symptom perception and management.	Neither ED visits nor hospitalizations showed any reduction in the intervention group.	
Koniak-Griffin, Anderson, Verzemnieks, & Brecht (2000)	RCT	Setting: Southern California county; all pregnant adolescents were referred to the community health service division. $N = 121$ participants enrolled.	Hospitalizations through 6 weeks postpartum	Although both groups were visited by public health nurses, the early intervention program (EIP) group received approximately 17 structured pre- and post-partum home visits according to their determined need. including a variety of interventions in five major areas: health, sexuality and family planning, substance abuse, life skills and social support.	Infants in the EIP had significantly fewer total days of birth-related hospitalization and rehospitalization during the first 6 weeks of life than those receiving conventional follow-up.	A great deal of information was obtained through participant self-report.
Kurtz, Kurtz, Given, & Given (2006)	RCT	$N = 222$ cancer chemotherapy patients	ED visits and physician visits	10-contact, 20-week clinical nursing symptom control intervention involving patient education regarding specific strategies to be applied for controlling symptoms		Random effects regression model revealed that patients in the intervention group reported fewer ED visits.

APN = advanced practice nurse; ED = emergency department; LOS = length of stay; RCT = randomized controlled trial; U.S. = United States.

(continues)

TABLE 10-3 Nursing Interventions and Healthcare Utilization (continued)

Study Date	Study type	Setting/sample	Healthcare utilization variables studied	Interventions	Major results	Limitations/comments
Mayo et al. (2000)	RCT	Patients were randomized to either the home intervention group (n = 58) or the usual care group (n = 56).	LOS	Home group received a 4-week tailor-made home program of rehabilitation and nursing services. All patients in the intervention group received nursing visits, compared with only 52% in the control group. Nursing interventions.	Total LOS for the home group was, on average, 10 days—6 days shorter than that for the usual care group.	Unblinded study; the subjects knew what treatment they received, with the result that subjects in the intervention arm could have responded more favorably to the self-report measures.
Mayo et al. (2008)	RCT	Persons (n = 190) returning home directly from the acute care hospital following a first or recurrent stroke. Setting: Montreal, Quebec, Canada.	ED visits, hospitalizations within 6 months	Nurses involved in the 6-week intervention group were stroke care case managers. RNs provided home visits and coordinated care with the person's physician.	There were no differences between groups on health service utilization.	
Meng, Tiernan, Bernier, & Brooks (1998)	One-group pretest and posttest	N = 34. Patient 6–12 years of age with asthma. Setting: A local health club (Texas).	ED visits, hospitalization through parent self-report 1 year after camp	6-day summer camp. Multidisciplinary team including nurses provided health teaching about triggers, symptom management, and asthma pathology.	Reduction in ED visits and missed school days after intervention.	Sample size, design weaknesses
Mion et al. (2003)	RCT	N = 650 elderly patients discharged from the EDs of two academically affiliated U.S. hospitals. Patients separated into two groups—high risk (n = 291) and low risk (n = 35)—and separated into intervention and control groups.	Repeat ED visits, hospitalizations, or nursing home admissions, and healthcare costs at 30 and 120 days	Intervention consisted of comprehensive geriatric assessment in the ED by an APN (master's level) and subsequent referral to a community or social agency; primary care provider, and/or geriatric clinic for unmet health, social, and medical needs.	Intervention had no effect on overall service use rates at 30 or 120 days. Intervention was associated with lower nursing home admissions at 30 days; more effective in the high-risk group.	
Naylor et al. (1994)	RCT	Setting: Hospital of the University of Pennsylvania, Philadelphia.	Healthcare utilization is measured by health care cost, initial LOS, length of time between initial	Nurse specialists in gerontology executing comprehensive discharge planning protocol visited intervention group	Decreased readmissions during the first 6 weeks after discharge among medical patients receiving the interventions.	Potential selection biases: Only selected patients in one unit at one hospital, and limited to oriented, alert, English-speaking patients.

		276 patients enrolled, separated into medical group or surgical group based on admitting diagnosis.	hospital discharge and readmission, and rehospitalization rates. All patient assessed at 2, 6, and 12 weeks after discharge.	patients 48 hours after initial admission to work on discharge planning and also contacted caregiver. Individualized discharge planning including follow-up every 48 hours after the initial visit.	No differences in health-care utilization found between the surgical intervention and control groups during this period.	Potential selection biases: Only selected patients in one unit at one hospital, and limited to oriented, alert, English-speaking patients.
Naylor et al. (1994)	RCT	Setting: Hospital of the University of Pennsylvania, Philadelphia. 276 patients enrolled, separated into medical group or surgical group based on admitting diagnosis.	Healthcare utilization is measured by health care cost, initial LOS, length of time between initial hospital discharge and readmission, and rehospitalization rates. All patient assessed at 2, 6, and 12 weeks after discharge.	Nurse specialists in gerontology executing comprehensive discharge planning protocol visited intervention group patients 48 hours after initial admission to work on discharge planning and also contacted caregiver. Individualized discharge planning including follow-up every 48 hours after the initial visit.	Decreased readmissions during the first 6 weeks after discharge among medical patients receiving the interventions. No differences in health-care utilization found between the surgical intervention and control groups during this period.	
Naylor et al. (1999)	RCT	Setting: Two academic medical centers in Philadelphia, Pennsylvania. 1992–1996. N = 363 patients 65 years or older, hospitalized for one of several medical and surgical conditions.	Readmissions, time to first readmission, acute care visits after discharge, costs.	Intervention group patients received a comprehensive discharge planning and home follow-up protocol designed specifically for elders at risk for poor outcomes after discharge; implemented by APNs.	By week 24 after the index hospital discharge, intervention group patients were less likely to have been readmitted. Multiple readmissions were lower in the intervention group, as were total hospital days. Total Medicare reimbursements for health care were also lower.	
Naylor et al. (2004)	RCT	Setting: Six academic and community medical centers in Philadelphia, Pennsylvania. N = 239 patients aged 65 and older and hospitalized with heart failure.	Readmissions, total costs	Intervention group patients received a 3-month APN-directed discharge planning and home follow-up protocol.	Time to first readmission or death was longer in intervention patients. At 52 weeks, intervention group patients had fewer readmissions and lower mean total costs.	

APN = advanced practice nurse; ED = emergency department; LOS = length of stay; RCT = randomized controlled trial; U.S.=United States.

(continues)

TABLE 10-3   Nursing Interventions and Healthcare Utilization (continued)

Study/Date	Study type	Setting/sample	Healthcare utilization variables studied	Interventions	Major results	Limitations/comments
Rich et al. (1993)	RCT, pilot with patients assignment in 2:1 ratio in intervention vs usual care	Setting: Jewish Hospital at Washington University, a 550-bed secondary and tertiary care teaching hospital. N = 98 patients with heart failure, all 70 or older.	Readmission to hospital in 90 days and the LOS for those who were readmitted	Intensive inpatient teaching by a geriatric cardiac nurse for patients in intervention group; after discharge patients also received an assessment visit within 48 hours by a home care team	The 90-day readmission rate and mean number of days hospitalized were significantly lower in the intervention group.	
Riegel et al. (2002)	RCT, block randomization by treating physician	Heart failure patients were identified at hospitalization and assigned to receive 6 months of intervention (n = 130) vs. usual care (n = 228). Setting: Two Southern California hospitals.	Hospitalizations, readmissions, hospital days, days to first rehospitalization, multiple readmissions, ED visits, total inpatient costs.	Standardized nurse case management telephone intervention over 6 months.	The heart failure hospitalization rate at 3–6 months and inpatient costs were about 45% lower in the intervention group.	
Stout et al. (1998)	Pilot study; single-group pretest/posttest	N = 23 low-income children with asthma living in inner-city area. Data collected in 1994. Enrollment into program 1995. Setting: Children's Hospital and Medical Center, Washington, D.C.	Health outcomes measured by ED visits, hospitalization, unscheduled visit to health clinics.	Public health nurse involved in the community-based asthma care program.	A reduction in hospitalizations, ED visits, and unscheduled clinic visits, and an increase in follow-up clinic visits.	
Walsh, Barry, Scott, Lamorte, & Menzoian (2001)	Observational study	Setting: Boston Medical Center, a 600-bed facility in the South End of Boston. 1994–1996. N = 194 infrainguinal bypass surgery patients treated over evolution of the center's pathway/case management approach.	LOS	Nurse case managers/vascular nurse specialists were involved in management of patient care, including participating in daily rounds to reduce pathway deviations.	Use of a nurse case manager significantly reduced median postoperative LOS: from 7 days before the pathway was begun, to 6 days with the original pathway, and finally to 5 days after the introduction of a vascular nurse specialist.	Non-RCT; patients' medical charts selected based on when they were admitted to the hospital.

Weinberger, Oddone, & Henderson (1996)	RCT	Setting: Nine Veterans Affairs Medical Centers, United States. $N = 695$ patients in intervention group. $N = 701$ patients in control group. Patients who had chronic illness, such as diabetes type 2, chronic obstructive pulmonary disease, and congestive heart failure.	Readmission and ED visits over 6 months	Intervention involves having a nurse and primary care physician closely follow the patient before discharge and 6 months after; designed to increase access to primary care after discharge from the hospital.	Although the intervention group received more intensive primary care than the controls, patients in the intervention group had significantly higher rates of readmission and more days of rehospitalization The intervention group were more satisfied with their care ($p < 0.001$).	Uniqueness of population and treatment in veterans system
West et al. (1997)	Evaluative pretest/posttest design	Setting: Kaiser-Permanente medical center in Northern California. $N = 51$ heart failure patients.	ED visits, and rehospitalization	MULTIFIT, a physician-supervised, nurse-mediated home-based system. The nurse's role was to enhance dietary and pharmacologic adherence and to monitor clinical status through telephone contact.	Compared with the 6 months before enrollment and normalized for variable follow-up, the frequency of general medical and cardiology visits declined about 30%, ED visits for heart failure and for all causes declined about 60%, and hospitalization rates for heart failure and for all causes declined about 80% compared with the year before enrollment.	Small sample size and use of only one hospital/medical center questions the generalizability of this study.
Wheeler & Waterhouse (2006)	Pilot RCT	Setting: 40 heart failure patients treated by a home health care agency in the mid-Atlantic region in the United States. 12- to 14-week period of intervention.	Hospital readmission	Regular telephone interventions by fourth-year nursing students from a baccalaureate nursing program. Each student was paired with a community nursing staff member and assigned two heart failure patients to follow up via telephone calls for 12–14 weeks.	Patients who received telephone interventions had fewer hospital readmissions (13%) than the comparison group (35%).	Small sample size, relatively short period of study (one semester), only senior students used; junior-level students in the study may have different effects on the result; limited to one region, therefore questionable generalizability.

APN = advanced practice nurse; ED = emergency department; LOS = length of stay; RCT = randomized controlled trial; U.S. = United States.

(continues)

TABLE 10-3 Nursing Interventions and Healthcare Utilization (continued)

Study Date	Study type	Setting/sample	Healthcare utilization variables studied	Interventions	Major results	Limitations/comments
York et al. (1997)	RCT	Setting: United States. N = 96 American women seeking childbirth services with either diabetes or hypertension in pregnancy; English-speaking, had access to a telephone service.	Hospitalizations during pregnancy, postpartum hospital costs	Transitional home follow-up care provided by a nurse specialist. The nurse specialist contacted women in the intervention group soon after delivery to assist with preparation for early discharge. The intervention group received at least five home visits, and thereafter, three weekly telephone or clinic contacts until delivery; at least two scheduled home visits and 10 telephone calls during the 8-week follow-up period.	During pregnancy, the intervention group had significantly fewer hospitalizations than the control group. Postpartum hospital charges for the intervention group were also significantly lower than for the control group.	

APN = advanced practice nurse; ED = emergency department; LOS = length of stay; RCT = randomized controlled trial; U.S.=United States.

was tested—involved the types of interventions often carried out by nurses, but these were not reviewed here because they were either implemented by nonnurses, or those responsible for the intervention were not named. In the case of Lorig et al., relatively small decreases in healthcare consumption in terms of ED and physician visits were associated with the self-care intervention that nonetheless translated into cost savings of approximately $590 per participant when the intervention itself costs approximately $70 to $200 per person. The evaluation of this intervention, driven by a theoretical framework related to self-care that was previously tested in a number of settings, provides a good example of an approach that may prove useful in future work to control costs of chronic disease care, particularly in situations in which psychological and social factors are believed to play a key role in patient coping and help-seeking.

RECOMMENDATIONS AND DIRECTIONS FOR FUTURE RESEARCH

A number of trends emerged in this review. A range of patient clinical and psychosocial factors that appear to be related to healthcare utilization need to be kept in mind when designing research and interpreting findings. Lower nurse staffing in hospitals is consistently related to prolonged mean lengths of stay. In a number of contexts, notably chronic conditions characterized by frequent exacerbations, such as heart failure and asthma, the use of emergency department services appears sensitive to some nursing interventions. Close follow-up of certain clienteles by nurse specialists appears to be cost-effective in that it may reduce service utilization enough to exceed the costs of intervention. For many clienteles, nursing factors and interventions have not been studied in relation to service use. Even for patients with health conditions for which nursing interventions or factors have been linked to health care utilization, the mechanisms involved and the client subgroups whose utilization is most sensitive to nursing variables remain unknown.

A number of recommendations for next steps in research can be made. Whether observational studies or tests of interventions, careful attention should be paid in future studies to articulating the mechanisms through which healthcare service use or resource consumption is thought to be linked to the organization of nursing services or nursing interventions. Careful consideration should be given to the incorporation of patient clinical and sociodemographic characteristics in the data collection schemes and in analyses of any healthcare utilization in order to maximize the likelihood of meaningful conclusions. Finally, given the complexities and challenges involved, involving specialists in the use of data sets, outcomes researchers, and health economists in the conceptualization of studies and the design of the data-gathering schemes seems advisable in future research efforts.

It is a particularly important time in the history of the profession and of health care to be discussing healthcare utilization as a nurse-sensitive outcome.

Many in health policy circles are very open to the notion that nurses and nursing may offer partial answers to the dilemmas of optimizing access and quality while containing costs in health systems. It is therefore essential that the next generation of nursing organizational and intervention research studies contribute data to these discussions with rigorously collected healthcare utilization measures whose selection is guided by a coherent theoretical base.

REFERENCES

Amaravadi, R. K., Dimick, J. B., Pronovost, P. J, & Lipsett, P. A. (2000). ICU nurse-to-patient ratio is associated with complications and resource use after esophagectomy. *Intensive Care Medicine, 26,* 1857–1862.

Ashton, C. M., & Wray, N. P. (1992). A conceptual framework for the study of early readmission as an indicator of quality of care. *Social Science and Medicine, 43,* 1533–1541.

Aubert, R. E., Herman, W. H., & Waters, J. (1998). Nurse case management to improve glycemic control in diabetic patients in a health maintenance organization: A randomized, controlled trial. *Annals of Internal Medicine, 129,* 605–613.

Bahadori, K., & FitzGerald, J. M. (2007). Risk factors of hospitalization and readmission of patients with COPD exacerbation: Systematic review. *International Journal of COPD, 2,* 241–251.

Bartlett, S. J., Kolodner, K., Butz, A. M., Eggleston, P., Malveaux, F. J., & Rand, C. S. (2001). Maternal depressive symptoms and emergency department use among inner-city children with asthma. *Archives of Pediatrics and Adolescent Medicine. 155,* 347–453.

Benbassat, J., & Taragin, M. (2000). Hospital readmissions as a measure of quality of health care: Advantages and limitations. *Archives of Internal Medicine, 160,* 1074–1081.

Berg, G. D., & Wadhwa, S. (2007). Health services outcomes for a diabetes disease management program for the elderly. *Disease Management, 10,* 226–234.

Berg, G. D., & Wadhwa, S. (2009). Diabetes disease management results in Hispanic Medicaid patients. *Journal of Health Care for the Poor and Underserved, 20,* 432–443.

Berg, G. D., Wadhwa, S., & Johnson, A. E. (2004). A matched-cohort study of health services utilization and financial outcomes for a heart failure disease-management program in elderly patients. *Journal of the American Geriatrics Society, 52,* 1655–1661.

Bernstein, A. B., Hing, E., Moss, A. J., Allen, K. F., Siller, A. B., & Tiggle, R. B. (2003). *Health care in America: Trends in utilization.* Hyattsville, MD: National Center for Health Statistics. Retrieved September 28, 2009, from http://www.cdc.gov/nchs/data/misc/healthcare.pdf

Blank, F. S. J., Li, H., Henneman, P. L., Smithline, H., Santoro, J., Provost, D., et al. (2005). A descriptive study of heavy emergency department reveals heavy ED users have better access to care than average users. *Journal of Emergency Nursing, 31,* 139–144.

Brook, R. H. (2009). Assessing the appropriateness of care: Its time has come. *Journal of the American Medical Association, 302,* 997–998.

Brooten, D., Kumar, S., Brown, L. P., Butts, P., Finkler, S. A., Bakewell-Sachs, S., et al. (1986). A randomized clinical trial of early hospital discharge and home follow-up of very-low-birth-weight infants. *New England Journal of Medicine, 315,* 934–939.

Brooten, D., Roncoli, M., Finkler, S., Arnold, L., Cohen, A., & Mennuti, M. (1994). A randomized trial of early hospital discharge and home follow-up of women having caesarean birth. *Obstetrics and Gynecology, 84,* 832–838.

Brooten, D., Youngblut, J. M., Brown, L., Finkler, S. A., Neff, D. F., & Madigan, E. (2001). A randomized trial of nurse specialist home care for women with high-risk pregnancies: Outcomes and costs. *American Journal of Managed Care, 7,* 793–803.

Brooten, D., Youngblut, J. M., Donahue, D., Hamilton, M., Hannan, J., & Felber Neff, D. (2007). Women with high-risk pregnancies, problems, and APN interventions. *Journal of Nursing Scholarship, 39,* 349–357.

Bunn, F., Byrne, G., & Kendall, S. (2005). The effects of telephone consultation and triage on healthcare use and patient satisfaction: a systematic review. *British Journal of General Practice, 55,* 956–561.

Castro, M., Zimmermann, N. A., Crocker, S., Bradley, J., Leven, C., & Schechtman, K. B. (2003). Asthma intervention program prevents readmissions in high healthcare users. *American Journal of Respiratory and Critical Care Medicine, 168,*1095–1099.

Chassin, M. R., Brook, R. H., Park, R. E., Keesey, J., Fink, A., Kosecoff, J., et al. (1986). Variations in the use of medical and surgical services by the Medicare population. *New England Journal of Medicine, 314,* 285–290.

Chiu, W. K., & Newcomer, R. (2007). A systematic review of nurse-assisted case management to improve hospital discharge transition outcomes for the elderly. *Professional Case Management, 12,* 330–336.

Cho, S. H., Ketefian, S., Barkauskas, V. H., & Smith, D. G. (2003). The effects of nurse staffing on adverse events, morbidity, mortality, and medical costs. *Nursing Research, 52*(2), 71–79.

Clarke, A. (2004). Readmission to hospital: A measure of quality or outcome? *Quality and Safety in Health Care, 13*(1), 10–11.

Coffman, J. M., Cabana, M. D., Halpin, H. A., & Yelin, E. H. (2008). Effects of asthma education on children's use of acute care services: A meta-analysis. *Pediatrics, 121,* 575–586.

Czaplinski, C., & Diers, D. (1998). The effect of staffing nursing on length of stay and mortality. *Medical Care, 36,* 1626–1638.

Dall, T. M., Chen, Y. J., Seifert, R. F., Maddox, P. J., & Hogan, P. F. (2009). The economic value of professional nursing. *Medical Care, 47,* 97–104.

Dansky, K. H., Vasey, J., & Bowles, K. (2008). Impact of telehealth on clinical outcomes in patients with heart failure. *Clinical Nursing Research, 17,* 182–199.

Davidson, M. B., Ansari, A., & Karlan, V. J. (2007). Effect of a nurse-directed diabetes disease management program on urgent care/emergency room visits and hospitalizations in a minority population. *Diabetes Care, 30,* 224–227.

de Boer, A. G., Wijker, W., & de Haes, H. C. (1997). Predictors of health care utilization in the chronically ill: A review of the literature. *Health Policy, 42,* 101–115.

Decker, F. H. (2008). Outcomes and length of Medicare nursing home stays: The role of registered nurses and physical therapists. *American Journal of Medical Quality, 23,* 465–474.

Dendukuri, N., McCusker, J., & Belzile, E. (2004). The identification of seniors at risk screening tool: Further evidence of concurrent and predictive validity. *Journal of the American Geriatrics Society, 52,* 290–296.

Dougherty, C. M., Thompson, E. A., & Lewis, F. M. (2005). Long-term outcomes of a telephone intervention after an ICD. *Pacing and Clinical Electrophysiology, 28,* 1157–1167.

Dougherty, G., Schiffrin, A., White, D., Soderstrom, L., & Sufrategui, M. (1999). Home-based management can achieve intensification cost-effectively in type I diabetes. *Pediatrics, 103,* 122–128.

Drummond, M. F., Sculpher, M. J., Torrance, G. W., O'Brien, B. J., & Stoddart, G. L. (2005). *Methods for the economic evaluation of health care programmes* (3rd ed.) Oxford, England: Oxford University Press.

Dunagan, W. C., Littenberg, B., Ewald, G. A., Jones, C. A., Emery, V. B., Waterman, B. M., et al. (2005). Randomized trial of a nurse-administered, telephone-based disease management program for patients with heart failure. *Journal of Cardiac Failure, 11*, 358–365

Estabrooks, C. A., Cummings, G. G., Olivo, S. A., Squires, J. E., Giblin, C., & Simpson, N. (2009). Effect of shift length on quality of patient care and health provider outcome: Systematic review. *Quality and Safety in Health Care, 18*, 181–188.

Feldman, P. H., Peng, T. R., Murtaugh, C. M., Kelleher, C., Donelson, S. M., McCann, M. E., et al. (2004). A randomized intervention to improve heart failure outcomes in community-based home health care. *Home Health Care Service Quality, 23*, 1–23.

Forster, A. J., Clark, H. D., Menard, A., Dupuis, R., Chernish, N., Chandok, A., et al. (2005). Effect of a nurse team coordinator on outcomes for hospitalized medicine patients. *American Journal of Medicine, 118*, 1148–1153.

Friedmann, P. D., Jin, L., Karrison, T. G., Hayley, D. C., Mulliken, R., Walter, J., et al. (2001). Early revisit, hospitalization, or death among older persons discharged from the ED. *American Journal of Emergency Medicine, 19*,125–129.

Gagnon, A. J., Schein, C., McVey, L., & Bergman, H. (1999). Randomized controlled trial of nurse case management of frail older people. *Journal of American Geriatrics Society, 47*, 1118–1124.

Gajic, O., Malinchoc, M., Comfere, T. B., Harris, M. R., Achouiti, A., Yilmaz, M., et al (2008). The Stability and Workload Index for Transfer score predicts unplanned intensive care unit patient readmission: Initial development and validation. *Critical Care Medicine, 36*, 676–682.

Geary, S., Cale, D. D., Quinn, B., & Winchell, J. (2009). Daily rapid rounds: Decreasing length of stay and improving professional practice. *Journal of Nursing Administration, 39*, 293–298.

Gerolamo, A. M. (2004). State of the science: Outcomes of acute inpatient psychiatric care. *Archives of Psychiatric Nursing, 18*, 203–214.

Gifford, A. L., Collins, R., Timberlake, D., Schuster, M. A., Shapiro, M. F., Bozzette, S. A., et al. (2000). Propensity of HIV patients to seek urgent and emergent care. HIV Cost and Services Utilization Study Consortium. *Journal of General Internal Medicine. 15*, 833–840.

Gordon, J. A., An, L. C., Hayward, R. A., & Williams, B. C. (1998). Initial emergency department diagnosis and return visits: Risk versus perception. *Annals of Emergency Medicine, 32*, 569–573.

Greineder, D. K., Loane, K. C., & Parks, P. (1995). Reduction in resource utilization by an asthma outreach program. *Archives of Pediatrics and Adolescent Medicine, 149*, 415–420.

Guttman, A., Afilalo, M., Guttman, R., Colacone, A., Robitaille, C., Lang, E., et al. (2005). An emergency department-based nurse discharge coordinator for elder patients: Does it make a difference? *Academic Emergency Medicine, 11*, 1318–1327.

Han, A., Ospina, M., Blitz., S. B., Strome, T., & Rowe, B. H. (2007). Patients presenting to the emergency department: The use of other health care services and reasons for presentation. *Canadian Journal of Emergency Medicine, 9*, 428–434.

Hastings, S. N., & Heflin, M. T. (2005). A systematic review of interventions to improve outcomes for elders discharged from the emergency department. *Academic Emergency Medicine, 12*, 978–986.

Hastings, S. N., George, L. K., Fillenbaum, G. G., Park, R. S., Burchett, B., & Schmader, K. (2008). Does lack of social support lead to more ED visits for older adults? *American Journal of Emergency Medicine, 26*, 454–461.

Hastings, S. N., Oddone, E. Z., Fillenbaum, G., Sloane, R. J., & Schmader, K. E. (2008). Frequency and predictors of adverse health outcomes in older Medicare beneficiaries discharged from the emergency department. *Medical Care, 46*, 771–777.

Healy, B. (2009, May 1). *Health reform, too tough on hospital readmission*. Retrieved September 28, 2009, from http://health.usnews.com/blogs/heart-to-heart/2009/05/01/health-reform-too-tough-on-hospital-readmission.html

Hickey, M. L., Cook, E. F., Rossi, L. P., Conner, J., Dutkiewicz, C., Hassan, S. M., et al. (2000). Effect of case managers with a general medical patient population. *Journal of Evaluation in Clinical Practice, 6*, 23–29.

Horrocks, S., Anderson, E., & Salisbury, C. (2002). Systematic review of whether nurse practitioners working in primary care can provide equivalent care to doctors. *British Medical Journal, 324*, 819–823.

Hughes, F., Clarke, S. P., Sampson, D. A., Fairman, J., & Sullivan-Marx, E. M. (2003). Research on nurse practitioners. In M. D. Mezey, D. O. McGivern, & E. M. Sullivan-Marx (Eds.), *Nurses, nurse practitioners* (4th ed., pp. 85–107). New York: Springer.

Iezzoni, L. I. (1999). *Risk adjustment for measuring health care outcomes* (2nd ed.). Chicago: Health Administration Press.

Ionescu-Ittu, R., McCusker, J., Ciampi, A., Vadeboncoeur, A. M., Roberge, D., Larouche, D., et al. (2007). Continuity of primary care and emergency department utilization among elderly people. *Canadian Medical Association Journal, 177*, 1362–1368.

Janson-Bjerklie, S., Ferketich, S., & Benner, P. (1993). Predicting the outcomes of living with asthma. *Research in Nursing and Health, 16*, 241–250.

Jette, D. U., Warren, R. L., & Wirtalla, C. (2004). Effect of nursing staff level and therapy intensity on outcomes. *American Journal of Physical Medicine & Rehabilitation, 83*, 704–712.

Johnson, T. R., Zettelmaier, M. A., Warner, P. A., Hayashi, R. H., Avni, M., & Luke, B. (2000). A competency based approach to comprehensive pregnancy care. *Women's Health Issues, 10*, 240–247.

Jones, S. L., Jones, P. K., & Katz, J. (1989). A nursing intervention to increase compliance in otitis media (OM) patients. *Applied Nursing Research, 2*(2), 68–73.

Kahn, K. L., Kosecoff, J., Chassin, M. R., Flynn, M. F., Fink, A., Pattaphongse, N., et al. (1988). Measuring the clinical appropriateness of the use of a procedure. Can we do it? *Medical Care, 26*, 415–422.

Kane, R. L., Shamliyan, T. A., Mueller, C., Duval, S., Wilt, T. J. (2007). The association of registered nurse staffing levels and patient outcomes: Systematic review and meta-analysis. *Medical Care, 45*, 1195–1204.

Klinnert, M. D., Liu, A. H., Pearson, M. R., Ellison, M. C., Budhiraja, N., & Robinson, J. L. (2005). Short-term impact of a randomized multifaceted intervention for wheezing infants in low-income families. *Archives of Pediatrics and Adolescent Medicine, 159*, 75–82.

Koniak-Griffin, D., Anderson, N. L., Verzemnieks, I., & Brecht, M. L. (2000). A public health nursing early intervention program for adolescent mothers: Outcomes from pregnancy through 6 weeks postpartum. *Nursing Research, 49*, 130–138.

Kurdyak, P. A., Gnam, W. H., Goering, P., Chong, A., & Alter, D. A. (2008). The relationship between depressive symptoms, health service consumption, and prognosis after acute myocardial infarction: A prospective cohort study. *BMC Health Services Research, 8*, 200.

Kurtz, M. E., Kurtz, J. C., Given, C. W., & Given, B. (2006). Effects of a symptom control intervention on utilization of health care services among cancer patients. *Medical Science Monitor, 12*(7), CR319–CR324.

Langhorne, P., Taylor, G., Murray, G., Dennis, M., Anderson, C., Bautz-Holter, E., et al. (2005). Early supported discharge services for stroke patients: A meta-analysis of individual patients' data. *The Lancet, 365*(9458), 501–506.

LeDuc, K., Rosebrook, H., Rannie, M., & Gao, D. (2006). Pediatric emergency department recidivism: Demographic characteristics and diagnostic predictors. *Journal of Emergency Nursing, 32,* 131–138.

Lee, K. H., & Anderson, Y. M. (2007). The association between clinical pathways and hospital length of stay: A case study. *Journal of Medical Systems, 31*(1), 79–83.

Lichtig, L. K., Knauf, R. A., & Milholland, D. K. (1999). Some impacts of nursing on acute care hospital outcomes. *Journal of Nursing Administration, 29,* 25–33.

Lorig, K. R., Ritter, P., Stewart, A. L., Sobel, D. S., Brown, B. W., Jr., Bandura, A., et al., (2001). Chronic disease self-management program: 2-year health status and health care utilization outcomes. *Medical Care, 39,* 1217–1223.

Lubeck, D. P., & Hubert, H. B. (2005). Self-report was a viable method for obtaining health care utilization data in community-dwelling seniors. *Journal of Clinical Epidemiology, 58,* 286–290.

Lyons, J. S., O'Mahoney, M. T., Miller, S. I., Neme, J., Kabat, J., & Miller, F. (1997). Predicting readmission to the psychiatric hospital in a managed care environment: Implications for quality indicators. *American Journal of Psychiatry, 154,* 337–340.

Maharaj, V., Hsu, R., & Beadman, A.(2006). Preventing paediatric admissions for respiratory disease: A qualitative analysis of the views of health care professionals. *Journal of Evaluation in Clinical Practice, 12,* 515–522.

Mayo, N. E., Nadeau, L., Ahmed, S., White, C., Grad, R., Huang, A., et al. (2008). Bridging the gap: The effectiveness of teaming a stroke coordinator with patient's personal physician on the outcome of stroke. *Age and Ageing, 37*(1), 32–38.

Mayo, N. E., Wood-Dauphinee, S., Cote, R., Gayton, D., Carlton, J., Buttery, J., et al. (2000). There's no place like home: An evaluation of early supported discharge for stroke. *Stroke, 31,* 1016–1023.

McCusker, J., Cardin, S., Bellavance, F., & Belzile, E. (2000). Return to the emergency department among elders: Patterns and predictors. *Academic Emergency Medicine, 7,* 249–259.

McCusker, J., Healey, E., Bellavance, F., & Connolly, B. (1997). Predictors of repeat emergency department visits by elders. *Academic Emergency Medicine, 4,* 581–588.

Meng A., Tiernan, K., Bernier, M. J., & Brooks, E. G. (1998). Lessons from an evaluation of the effectiveness of an asthma day camp. *MCN: The American Journal of Maternal Child Nursing, 23,* 300–306

Miller, A. H., Larkin, G. L., & Jimenez, C. H. (2005). Predictors of medication refill-seeking behavior in the ED. *American Journal of Emergency Medicine, 23,* 423–428.

Mion, L. C., Palmer, R. M., Meldon, S. W., Bass, D. M., Singer, M. E., Payne, S. M., et al. (2003). Case finding and referral model for emergency department elders: A randomized clinical trial. *Annals of Emergency Medicine, 41,* 57–68.

Naylor, M. D., Brooten, D., Campbell, R., Jacobsen, B. S., Mezey, M. D., Pauly, M. V., et al. (1999). Comprehensive discharge planning and home follow-up of hospitalized elders: A randomized clinical trial. *Journal of the American Medical Association, 281,* 613–620.

Naylor, M. D., Brooten, D. A., Campbell, R. L., Maislin, G., McCauley, K. M., & Schwartz, J. S. (2004). Transitional care of older adults hospitalized with heart failure: A randomized, controlled trial. *Journal of the American Geriatrics Society, 52*(5), 675–684.

Naylor, M., Brooten, D., Jones, R., Lavizzo-Mourey, R., Mezey, M., & Pauly, M. (1994). Comprehensive discharge planning for the hospitalized elderly: A randomized clinical trial. *Annals of Internal Medicine, 120,* 999–1006.

Needleman, J., Buerhaus, P. I., Stewart, M., Zelevinsky, K., & Mattke, S. (2006). Nurse staffing in hospitals: Is there a business case for quality? *Health Affairs, 25,* 204–211.

Nouwen, A., Freeston, M. H., Labbé, R., & Boulet, L. P. (1999). Psychological factors associated with emergency room visits among asthmatic patients. *Behavior Modification, 23*, 217–233.

Oeseburg, B., Wynia, K., Middel, B., & Reijneveld, S. A. (2009). Effects of case management for frail older people or those with chronic illness: A systematic review. *Nursing Research, 58*, 201–210.

Ortega, A. N., Belanger, K. D., Paltiel, A. D., Horwitz, S. M., Bracken, M. B., & Leaderer, B. P. (2001). Use of health services by insurance status among children with asthma. *Medical Care, 39*, 1065–1074.

Padgett, D. K., & Brodsky, B. (1992). Psychosocial factors influencing non-urgent use of the emergency room: A review of the literature and recommendations for research and improved service delivery. *Social Science and Medicine, 35*, 1189–1197.

Parboosingh, E. J., & Larsen, D. E. (1987). Factors influencing frequency and appropriateness of utilization of the emergency room by the elderly. *Medical Care, 25*, 1139–1147.

Peikes, D., Chen, A., Schore, J., & Brown, R. (2009). Effects of care coordination on hospitalization, quality of care, and health care expenditures among Medicare beneficiaries: 15 randomized trials. *Journal of the American Medical Association, 301*, 603–618.

Persily, C. A. (2003). Lay home visiting may improve pregnancy outcomes. *Holistic Nursing Practice, 17*, 231–238.

Phillips, K. A, Morrison, K. R, Andersen, R., & Aday, L. A. (1998). Understanding the context of healthcare utilization: Assessing environmental and provider related variables in the behavioral model of utilization. *Health Services Research, 33*, 571–596.

Pines, J. M., & Buford, K. (2006). Predictors of frequent emergency department utilization in Southeastern Pennsylvania. *Journal of Asthma, 43*, 219–223.

Polivka, B. J., Nickel, J. T., Salsberry, P. J., Kuthy, R., Shapiro, N., & Slack, C. (2000). Hospital and emergency department use by young low-income children. *Nursing Research, 49*, 253–261.

Proctor, E. K., Morrow-Howell, N., Li, H., & Dore, P. (2000). Adequacy of home care and hospital readmission for elderly congestive heart failure patients. *Health and Social Work, 25*(2), 87–96.

Rask, K. J., Williams, M. V., McNagny, S. E., Parker, R. M., & Baker, D. W. (1998). Ambulatory health care use by patients in a public hospital emergency department. *Journal of General Internal Medicine, 13*, 614–620.

Reuben, D. B., Keeler, E., Seeman, T. E., Sewall, A., Hirsch, S. H., & Guralnik, J. M. (2002). Development of a method to identify seniors at high risk for high hospital utilization. *Medical Care, 40*, 782–793.

Rich, M. W., Vinson, J. M., Sperry, J. C., Shah, A. S., Spinner, L. R., Chung, M. K., et al., (1993). Prevention of readmission in elderly patients with congestive heart failure: Results of a prospective, randomized pilot study. *Journal of General Internal Medicine, 8*, 585–590.

Riegel, B., Carlson, B., Kopp, Z., LePetri, B., Glaser, D., & Unger, A. (2002). Effect of a standardized nurse case-management telephone intervention on resource use in patients with chronic heart failure. *Archives of Internal Medicine, 162*, 705–712.

Rosenblatt, R. A., Wright, G. E., Baldwin, L. M., Chan, L., Clitherow, P., Chen, F. M., et al. (2000). The effect of the doctor-patient relationship on emergency department use among the elderly. *American Journal of Public Health, 90*, 97–102.

Ross, J. S., Mulvey, G. K., Stauffer, B., Patlolla, V., Bernheim, S. M., Keenan P. S., & et al. (2008). Statistical models and patient predictors of readmission for heart failure: A systematic review. *Archives of Internal Medicine, 168*, 1371–1386.

Schatz, M., Nakahiro, R., Jones, C. H., Roth, R. M., Joshua, A., & Petitti, D. (2004). Asthma population management: Development and validation of a practical 3-level risk stratification scheme. *American Journal of Managed Care, 10*, 25–32.

Schatz, M., Zeiger, R. S., Mosen, D., & Vollmer, W. M. (2008). Asthma-specific quality of life and subsequent asthma emergency hospital care. *American Journal of Managed Care. 14*, 206–211.

Schonwetter, R. S., Clark, L. D., Leedy, S. A., Quinn, M. J., Azer, M., & Kim, S. (2008). Predicting emergency room visits and hospitalizations among hospice patients with cardiac disease. *Journal of Palliative Medicine, 11*, 1142–1150.

Schwarz, K. A., & Elman, C. S. (2003). Identification of factors predictive of hospital readmissions for patients with heart failure. *Heart and Lung, 32*, 88–99.

Schweikert, B., Hahmann, H., & Leidl, R. (2008). Development and first assessment of a questionnaire for health care utilization and costs for cardiac patients. *BMC Health Services Research, 8*, 187.

Shah, M. N., Rathouz, P. J., & Chin, M. H. (2001). Emergency department utilization by non institutionalized elders. *Academic Emergency Medicine, 8*, 267–273.

Sharma, V., Simon, S. D., Bakewell, J. M., Ellerbeck, E. F., Fox, M. H., & Wallace, D. D. (2000). Factors influencing infant visits to emergency departments. *Pediatrics, 106*, 1031–1039.

Shelton, P., Sager, M. A., & Schraeder, C. (2000). The community assessment risk screen (CARS): Identifying elderly persons at risk for hospitalization or emergency department visit. *American Journal of Managed Care, 6*, 925–933.

Shiber, J. R., Longley, M. B., & Brewer, K. L. (2009). Hyper-use of the ED. *American Journal of Emergency Medicine, 27*, 588–594.

Silber, J. H., Rosenbaum, P. R., Schwartz, J. S., Ross, R. N., & Williams, S. V. (1995). Evaluation of the complication rate as a measure of quality of care in coronary artery bypass graft surgery. *Journal of the American Medical Association, 274*, 317–323.

Silber, J. H., Williams, S. V., Krakauer, H., & Schwartz, J. S. (1992). Hospital and patient characteristics associated with death after surgery. A study of adverse occurrence and failure to rescue. *Medical Care, 30*, 615–629.

Sochalski, J., Jaarsma, T., Krumholz, H. M., Laramee, A., McMurray, J. J., Naylor, M. D., et al. (2009). What works in chronic care management: The case of heart failure. *Health Affairs, 28*, 179–189.

Spenceley, S. M. (2005). Access to health services by Canadians who are chronically ill. *Western Journal of Nursing Research, 27*, 465–486.

Stone, P. W., Curran, C. R., Bakken, S. (2002). Economic evidence for evidence-based practice. *Journal of Nursing Scholarship, 34*, 277–282.

Stout, J. W., White, L. C., Rogers, L. T., McRorie, T., Morray, B., Miller-Ratcliffe, M., et al. (1998). The Asthma Outreach Project: A promising approach to comprehensive asthma management. *Journal of Asthma, 35*, 119–127.

Thungjaroenkul, P., Cummings, G. G., & Embleton, A. (2007). The impact of nurse staffing on hospital costs and patient length of stay: A systematic review. *Nursing Economics, 25*, 255–266.

Titler, M., Dochterman, J., Picone, D. M., Everett, L., Xie, X. J., Kanak, M., et al. (2005). Cost of hospital care for elderly at risk of falling. *Nursing Economics, 23*, 290–306.

Titler, M. G., Jensen, G. A., Dochterman, J. M., Xie, X. J., Kanak, M., Reed. D., et al. (2008). Cost of hospital care for older adults with heart failure: Medical, pharmaceutical, and nursing costs. *Health Services Research, 43*, 635–655.

Tschannen, D., & Kalisch, B. J. (2009). The effect of variations in nurse staffing on patient length of stay in the acute care setting. *Western Journal of Nursing Research, 31*, 153–170.

van den Brink, M., van den Hout, W. B., Stiggelbout, A. M., Putter, H., van de Velde, C. J., & Kievit, J. (2005). Self-reports of health-care utilization: Diary or questionnaire? *International Journal of Technology Assessment in Health Care, 21*, 298–304.

Walsh, M. D., Barry, M., Scott, T. E., Lamorte, W. W., & Menzoian, J. O. (2001). The role of a nurse case manager in implementing a critical pathway for infrainguinal bypass surgery. *Joint Commission Journal on Quality Improvement, 27*, 230–238.

Weinberger, M., Oddone, E. Z., & Henderson, W. G. (1996). Does increased access to primary care reduce hospital readmissions? *New England Journal of Medicine, 334*, 1441–1447.

West, J. A., Miller, N. H., Parker, K. M., Senneca, D., Ghandour, G., Clark, M., et al. (1997). A comprehensive management system for heart failure improves clinical outcomes and reduces medical resource utilization. *American Journal of Cardiology, 79*, 58–63.

Wheeler, E. C., & Waterhouse, J. K. (2006). Telephone interventions by nursing students: Improving outcomes for heart failure patients in the community. *Journal of Community Health Nursing, 23*, 137–146.

White-Means, S. I., Thornton, M. C., & Yeo, J. S. (1989). Socio-demographic and health factors influencing black and Hispanic use of the hospital emergency room. *Journal of the National Medical Association, 81*, 72–80.

Wisnivesky, J. P., Leventhal, H., & Halm, E. A. (2006). Predictors of asthma-related health care utilization and quality of life among inner-city patients with asthma. *Journal of Allergy and Clinical Immunology, 116*, 636–642.

Yamada, M. M., Korman, M., & Hughes, C. W. (2000). Predicting rehospitalization of persons with severe mental illness. *Journal of Rehabilitation, 66*(2), 32–39.

York, R., Brown, L., Samuels, P., Finkler, S., Jacobsen, B., Persely, C., et al. (1997). A randomized trial of early discharge and nurse specialist transitional follow-up care of high-risk childbearing women. *Nursing Research, 46*, 254–261.

Zolnierek, C. D. (2009). Non-psychiatric hospitalization of people with mental illness: Systematic review. *Journal of Advanced Nursing, 65*, 1570–1583.

Nursing Minimum Data Sets

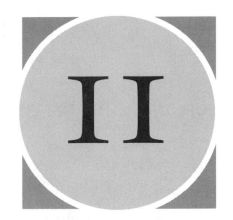

Manal Kleib
Anne Sales
Diane M. Doran
Claire Mallette
Deborah White

INTRODUCTION

Healthcare providers, as well as policy and decision makers, have identified the need for outcome data to evaluate the effectiveness and efficiency of healthcare systems (Canadian Nurses Association, 2000). A number of healthcare databases have been developed to record information about patients'/clients' healthcare utilization and health outcomes. These databases extract and record data such as length of stay, healthcare costs, admission and discharge dates, primary and secondary medical diagnoses, adverse occurrences, mortality, activities of daily living, and case mix (Delaney & Moorhead, 1995). This information can then be used to plan and evaluate services at the system level, develop report cards for accountability and benchmarking, and ultimately develop an accountability framework. The quality and validity of these databases are important because local, regional, and national policy makers use the information contained within these databases to make important decisions about our healthcare systems (Prophet & Delaney, 1998).

Unfortunately, much of the data needed to measure and evaluate nurses' contribution to patient care is largely absent from existing healthcare databases (Goossen et al., 1998). As a result, nurses' contributions to patient outcomes and health care remain, for the most part, invisible. To rectify this absence of meaningful information for evaluating nurses' contributions to health care, healthcare systems must have consistent data collection methods using standardized language to aggregate and compare data across programs, sectors, and jurisdictions (Blewitt & Jones, 1996). This chapter explores national and international initiatives to develop Nursing Minimum Data Sets (NMDSs). The overview includes a description of each database and its origin, stage of development, and level of testing for data quality and validity. An overview of similarities and differences, as well as strengths and limitations of NMDSs, is provided.

NURSING MINIMUM DATA SETS: HISTORICAL OVERVIEW

An NMDS approach has been adopted by a number of countries as a vehicle for documenting and aggregating nursing care data at the individual and group levels (Goossen et al., 1998; Mac Neela, Scott, Treacy, & Hyde, 2006). Early initiatives of data aggregation emerged in the early 1970s in the United States as a result of concerns about quality of care. This initiative lead to the development of a Uniform Minimum Health Data Set (UMHDS) by the U.S. National Committee on Vital and Health Statistics, which was primarily aimed at creating a consistent approach for collecting data from hospitals (Sermeus & Goossen, 2002). Soon after, and building on the UMHDS, the Uniform Hospital Discharge Data Set (UHDDS) was developed as a multipurpose tool to collect standardized data on all patients discharged from hospitals. Data collected through UHDDS included information related to clients' identity, the hospital, the physician involved, the diagnosis, the treatment, length of stay, the outcomes of hospitalization, and the expected source of payment (Sermeus & Goossen). Similar efforts were also evident in Europe in countries such as France, Great Britain, Norway, Belgium, Sweden, and the Netherlands (Goossen et al., 1998, 2006; Sermeus & Goossen). Neither the UMHDS nor the UHDDS contained data on nursing care delivered to hospitalized patients. NMDSs were developed in response to the lack of information about nursing care.

The development of an NMDS occurs in four stages. The first three stages are data driven and focus primarily on collection of multipurpose data (Mac Neela et al., 2006; Sermeus & Goossen, 2002). In the first stage, the focus is on the collection of data—identifying relevant variables and a language and coding scheme for these variables; the structure of the database; the unit of data collection (for example, the patient day); the frequency of data collection (for example, daily, at several points annually); the definition of sample size and design; the format for data collection (for example, paper based, electronic recording); and the collection of data itself. The second stage involves turning data into information—establishing data validity and reliability and designing a database for data storage and analysis. The third stage is the application—making use of the resulting data sets in local or strategic decision-making and in clinical, managerial, educational, or quality evaluation applications (Mac Neela et al., 2006; Sermeus & Goossen, 2002). The fourth stage has a more specific application focus, turning the data-information cycle to formulate information needs according to some decision-making problem (Sermeus & Goossen). A number of countries have invested in NMDS projects; some are already functional, some are in a development or piloting phase, and others are being explored.

NMDS INITIATIVES

··

United States: Nursing Minimum Data Sets

With the increased emphasis on cost-effectiveness and quality of care, a systematic approach for identifying and documenting nursing contributions to health care was seen as critical. The two primary approaches taken to achieve this goal were classification systems and NMDS (Mac Neela et al., 2006; Werley & Zorn, 1989). In the early 1980s and deriving from the general concept of UMHDS, Werley identified the need for a nursing-specific NMDS and defined it as "a minimum set of items of information with uniform definitions and categories concerning the specific dimension of professional nursing which meets the information needs of multiple data users in the health care system" (Werley, Devine, & Zorn, 1988, p. 7). In 1985, a national conference was held in Milwaukee, Wisconsin, where attendees were invited to deliberate the issues involved in the development, implementation, and evaluation of NMDSs and to generate an initial set of indicators (Werley, Lang, & Westlake, 1986a).

A recommendation of this conference was the development of a NMDS based on the UMHDS model, which included 16 elements that were categorized in three broad groups: (1) nursing care, (2) client demographics, and (3) service elements (Leske & Werley, 1992; Sermeus & Goossen, 2002; Werley et al., 1986a). The nursing care elements of the NMDS consisted of nursing diagnosis, nursing intervention, nursing outcome, and intensity of nursing care (Werley, Devine, Zorn, Ryan, & Westra, 1991). The patient demographics included five items, whereas the service elements included many aspects, such as (1) those related to the agency—unique service or agency number, unique health record number, and unique nurse identifier; (2) those related to the episode of care—episode or encounter date and discharge/termination date; (3) those related to resources; and (4) other aspects—disposition of patient and expected payer of the bills (Goossen et al., 1998, 2006).

The aim of the NMDS is to standardize, collect, store, and retrieve essential and comparable core nursing data (Leske & Werley, 1992; Werley et al., 1991). More specifically, the intent of the NMDS is to: (1) establish comparability of nursing data across clinical populations, setting, geographic areas, and time; (2) describe the nursing care of clients and their families in a variety of settings, both institutional and noninstitutional; (3) demonstrate or project trends regarding nursing care provided and allocation of nursing resources to clients according to their health problems and nursing diagnoses; (4) stimulate nursing research through links to the more detailed data existing in nursing information systems and other healthcare information systems; and (5) provide data about nursing care to facilitate and influence clinical, administrative, and health policy decision-making (Leske & Werley; Sermeus & Goossen, 2002). Expected or proposed outcomes of such a database were to document improved healthcare delivery, support the development of healthcare policy, and contribute to providing evidence about the impact of nursing care (Werley, Lang, & Westlake, 1986b). For example, when information about nurses' work is made available through NMDS, effective resource allocation can be made with respect to the use, effectiveness, and cost of nursing resources, potentially contributing to the overall effectiveness of healthcare delivery. Documenting and tracking nurses' contributions to health care could create compelling evidence on the effectiveness and value of nursing care, thus enabling nurses to effectively challenge decisions related to healthcare policy and resource allocation (Werley et al., 1986a, 1986b; Werley & Zorn, 1989).

Goossen and colleagues reported on the nature of research that has been carried out on NMDSs (Goossen et al., 1998, 2006; Sermeus & Goossen, 2002). With regard to data collection, sampling, aggregation, analysis, and feedback, they reported that both electronic and paper records could be used as a means of data collection, depending on inclusion criteria. The sample sizes ranged from 100 to more than 15,000 patients per study. Data analyses varied according to the type of questions explored and the type of data collected. Data aggregation in NMDSs is possible at the patient, unit, institution, and system levels. No national comparisons of data aggregated within these data sets have yet been attempted. Work on NMDSs has been reported and published at local, regional, national, and international levels, which has served to inform NMDS projects worldwide.

United States: Nursing Management Minimum Data Set (NMMDS)

The Nursing Management Minimum Data Set (NMMDS) project began in 1989 as a joint venture between the American Organization of Nurse Executives (AONE) and the University of Iowa to meet the needs of nurse executives (Huber & Delaney, 1997; Huber, Delaney, Crossley, Mehmert, & Ellerbe, 1992). It builds on basic concepts of NMDS proposed by Werley and Lang, the Donabedian quality model of structure, process, and outcome, and the Iowa Model of Nursing Administration (Huber, Schumacher, & Delaney, 1997). To allow for comparisons between different care settings, the NMMDS was designed to identify, define, and measure a clinically valid set of management data elements, defined for the particular context in which care was provided (Huber et al., 1992, 1997; Huber & Delaney). Initial phases of this multiphase research program yielded an 18-item list of acute care NMMDS elements. Subsequent research was aimed at piloting and validating these elements in other settings, including long-term care, ambulatory care, home healthcare, and occupational healthcare settings. To achieve a cross-settings consensus and refine the data set, an invitational working conference between the AONA and the research team was held; as a result,

17 elements with standardized definitions and measures were developed. These elements were grouped into three categories: environment, nurse resources, and financial resources (Huber et al., 1992, 1997; Huber & Delaney). The NMMDS is intended to facilitate managers' work through internal and external organizational benchmarking and evaluation of the care continuum (Huber et al., 1997).

United States: The Perioperative Nursing Data Set

In 1995 in collaboration with the Academy of Medical-Surgical Nurses (AMSN) and the National Association of Orthopedic Nurses (NAON), the Association of Operating Room Nurses (AORN) identified a need for developing a database unique to perioperative nursing (Grindel, 1996). The perioperative data set uses an NMDS approach by including nursing care elements and specifically focuses on establishing a classification system that describes and reflects nursing care aspects. The classification system is based on the North American Nursing Diagnoses Association System (NANDA) (diagnoses, interventions, patient outcomes), particularly in relation to nursing problems during the perioperative experience (Grindel; Seifert, 1999). The project was recognized by the American Nurses Association (ANA) as a step toward standardizing languages used in specialty areas such as the operating room. Few studies have been carried out to identify the commonly used nursing diagnoses among perioperative nurses and pilot the data set (Grindel; Seifert).

Nursing Outcomes Databases

In addition to its unique leadership in NMDS initiatives, the ANA also participated in a different type of NMDS: namely, nursing outcomes databases (NODs). The initial impetus behind NODs was research commissioned by the ANA in the early 1990s (ANA, 1999; Pierce, 1997; Rowell & Milholland, 1998) to identify patient outcomes that were sensitive to nursing care. The first set of nursing-sensitive indicators, focused on acute inpatient care, was published in the late 1990s. The ANA endorsed a quality and safety initiative that focused on identifying a group of quality indicators with a high probability of being associated predominantly with nursing care rather than other disciplines. Literature review and expert opinion were used to classify patient outcomes as nursing sensitive. Examples included rates of incident pressure ulcers (bed sores) incurred during hospitalization; incidence of patient falls; and several measures of patient satisfaction with care, specifically nursing care. In addition to these patient outcome indicators, other indicators focused on nurse staffing levels, as well as skill mix, which reflects the mix of different types of nursing providers used on a nursing unit. In the years following the ANA's work in this area, additional organizations have endorsed sets of nursing-sensitive indicators, including the National Quality

Forum, a semigovernment body in the United States, and the Joint Commission on the Accreditation of Healthcare Organizations, the primary quality accreditation organization for hospitals in the United States. The NODs are based primarily in the United States and comprise four main databases: (1) the National Database of Nursing Quality Indicators (NDNQI), (2) the California Nursing Outcomes Coalition (CalNOC), (3) the Military Nursing Outcomes Database (MilNOD), and (4) the Veterans Affairs Nursing Outcomes Database (VANOD).

The National Database of Nursing Quality Indicators (NDNQI)

Established by the ANA in 1998, the NDNQI is one of the early initiated nursing outcomes databases and the only national database that provides quarterly and annual reporting of structure, process, and outcome indicators to evaluate nursing care at the unit level (Montalvo, 2007). It is housed at the Midwest Research Institute (MRI) at Kansas City, Missouri, and is jointly managed by MRI and the University of Kansas School of Nursing (Alexander, 2007). Membership in this database is voluntary and requires payment of annual fees. At the end of 2006, more than 1,000 hospitals participated in NDNQI from within and outside the United States. NDNQI participation is required for hospitals and nursing services to achieve Magnet recognition through the American Nurses Credentialing Center. Because of this, NDNQI includes international participants. As of May 2007, 238 hospitals participated in the Magnet Recognition Program (http://www.nursecredentialing.org/Magnet/ProgramOverview.aspx). Magnet facilities represent about 20% of the facilities in the database. The remaining 80% of NDNQI participating facilities join because they believe in the value of evaluating the quality of nursing care and improving outcomes (Montalvo). The database is not available for public use (Alexander), although processes for permitting research access are under development.

The NDNQI aims to support patient safety and quality improvement efforts by providing research-based national comparative data on nursing care and the relationship of this care to patient outcomes (Montalvo, 2007). It promotes standardization of information submitted by hospitals across the United States on nursing quality and patient outcomes, which serves to eliminate duplication and promote collaboration with other developers of databases. **TABLE 11-1** shows a summary of indicators housed within the NDNQI. The NDNQI "provides options for others to submit data to them. Some believe, however, that because NDNQI membership is voluntary it is unlikely to ever provide a credible data source" (Alexander, 2007, p. 55S).

The California Nurse Outcomes Coalition Database Project (CalNOC)

This database was established in 1996 and is one of six initial American Nurses Association Nursing Quality Indicator Report Card Research and Development Projects (Alexander, 2007). It is a self-funded joint venture between the

TABLE 11-1   Indicators Housed Within Nursing Outcomes Databases

Database	Indicators
NDNQI	<ul><li>Nursing hours per patient day*<ul><li>RN hours per patient day</li><li>Licensed practical/vocational nurses (LPN/LVN) hours per patient day</li><li>Unlicensed assistive (UAP) hours per patient day</li></ul></li><li>Nursing turnover</li><li>Nosocomial infections*</li><li>Patient falls*</li><li>Patient falls with injury*<ul><li>Injury level</li></ul></li><li>Pressure ulcer rate<ul><li>Community-acquired</li><li>Hospital-acquired</li><li>Unit-acquired</li></ul></li><li>Pediatric pain assessment, intervention, reassessment (AIR) cycle</li><li>Pediatric peripheral intravenous infiltration</li><li>Psychiatric physical/sexual assault</li><li>RN education/certification</li><li>RN survey<ul><li>Job satisfaction scales</li><li>Practice environment scale (PES)*</li></ul></li><li>Restraints*</li><li>Staff mix *<ul><li>RN</li><li>LPN/LVNs</li><li>UAP</li><li>Percent agency staff</li></ul></li></ul>Additional data elements collected:<ul><li>Patient population—adult or pediatric</li><li>Hospital category, e.g. teaching, nonteaching, etc.</li><li>Type of unit (critical care, step-down, medical, surgical, combined med–surg, rehabilitation, and psychiatric).</li><li>Number of staffed beds designated by the hospital</li></ul>* Indicators endorsed by the National Quality Forum (NQF). *Source:* American Nurses Association. (2010). *Nursing-sensitive indicators.* Retrieved April 26, 2010, from http://www.nursingworld.org/MainMenuCategories/ThePracticeofProfessionalNursing/PatientSafetyQuality/Research-Measurement/The-National-Database/Nursing-Sensitive-Indicators_1.aspx
CalNOC	<ul><li>Nurse staffing—direct care hours, skill mix, patient days, nurse/patient ratios, and contracted staffing utilization, workload intensity (admissions, discharges, transfers), staff voluntary turnover, and use of sitters</li><li>RN education level, certification, and years of experience</li><li>Patient falls—risk, incidence (rate per 1000 pt. days) and consequences</li><li>Pressure ulcers—risk, prevalence, stage, and hospital acquired</li><li>Pressure ulcers—incidence of reportable hospital acquired pressure ulcers stage 3 and above (new indicator implemented in 2009 as part of CalNOC's Robert Wood Johnson Foundation-funded INQRI [Interdisciplinary Nursing Quality Research Initiative] project)</li><li>Restraint prevalence—type and clinical justification</li><li>PICC-CABSI—prevalence on medical–surgical units</li><li>Medication administration accuracy—observed prevalence of key safe practices and errors</li></ul>*Source:* The Center for Nursing Research & Innovation. (2009). *Collaborative Alliance for Nursing Outcomes.* Retrieved April 26, 2010, from http://nurseweb.ucsf.edu/conf/cripc/calnocov.htm

(continues)

TABLE 11-1   Indicators Housed Within Nursing Outcomes Databases (continued)

Database	Indicators
VANOD	• Nursing hours per patient day • Nursing hours and cost per outpatient encounter • Skill mix: NP, CNS, RN, LPN/LVN, UAP • Education and certification of RN, LPN, and NAs • Nursing staff injuries • Nursing staff turnover rates • RN job satisfaction • Patient falls • Patient satisfaction • Pressure ulcer data *Source:* Rick, C. (2009). *Nursing outcomes database (VANOD).* Retrieved April 26, 2010, from http://www.inqri.org/uploads/INQRIVANODPanel41309FINAL.ppt
MilNOD	Structural indicators: • Nursing care hours • Nursing skill mix • Nursing staff education, experience, and certification Outcomes indicators: • Job satisfaction • Needle stick injuries Explanatory variables: • Patient acuity • Patient turnover Contextual feature: • Nursing workforce environment attributes Patient outcomes indicators: • Patient ulcer prevalence • Restraint use prevalence • Falls Satisfaction with: • Care in general • Nursing care • Pain management • Education • Nurse medication administration errors *Source:* Loan, L.A., Brosch, L.R., McCarthy, M.S., & Patrician, P.A. (2005). Designing and implementing a national database depicting quality of nursing care. *Army Medical Department Journal.* PB 8-05-7/8/9 Jul/Aug/Sep.

Association of California Nurse Leaders and the ANA and is considered the nation's largest statewide nursing quality database (Alexander). It captures hospital-generated unit-level acute nurse staffing directly linked to patient outcome data, as well as factors associated with performance variations. Currently, it has a convenience sample of 175 hospitals. Membership in this database is voluntary. Current CalNOC nursing-sensitive measures include quality indicators based on the ANA Acute Care Indicators advanced for testing in 1995 (Table 11-1). CalNOC hospitals have the option to submit their data for inclusion in the ANA's NDNQI. Hospitals can compare themselves with like-sized hospitals, get detailed unit-specific information for each of their own units, or receive reports to compare hospitals within the same system. CalNOC provided methodological consultation in the establishment of MilNOD and VANOD, both of which largely replicated the CalNOC method (Alexander) and are described next.

The Veterans Affairs Nursing Outcomes Database (VANOD)

The Veterans Affairs Office of Nursing Services initiated VANOD in 2002. The VANOD provides an evidence base for evaluating nurse staffing and practice environments in relation to patient outcomes and will ultimately be useful for a variety of purposes, including quantifying the impact of patient care interventions, identifying successful nurse retention and recruitment strategies, and health policy decision-making (Haberfelde, Bedecarre, & Buffum, 2005). It provides unit- and hospital-level patient quality outcomes data that enable benchmarking within and among VA facilities (Alexander, 2007). It is capable of generating reports at the unit and hospital level. This database is available for research related to process, structure, and outcomes across the VA, beginning with acute care units. Both primary data and elements extracted from existing VA electronic data sources are collected on staffing, skill mix, falls, and pressure ulcers (Table 11-1). All analyses are at the unit level (Alexander, 2007).

The Military Nursing Outcome Database (MilNOD)

Established in 2002, this database collects data about nurse staffing and patient outcomes in the Department of Defense military treatment facilities (Army, Navy, and Air Force) for the purpose of benchmarking and comparison among these facilities. Table 11-1 shows a summary of indicators housed in this data set. It has been used to meet the requirements of the Joint Commission for assessing staffing effectiveness and patient outcomes (Alexander, 2007).

Reporting on NODs and Use of NOD Data

Use of NODs provides a viable approach to capturing critical data on how nursing factors, which account for critical resource consumption in healthcare systems, are associated with, and may be causally associated with, outcomes at the patient, provider, and system levels. However, to date, the empirical literature reporting on these databases is still small, although the output appears to have increased in recent years. Empirical studies exist primarily on NDNQI and CalNOC. Studies on NDNQI report mainly on two aspects: (1) staffing data and workforce characteristics in relation to patient outcomes (Dunton, Gajewski, Klaus, & Pierson, 2007; Dunton, Gajewski, Taunton, & Moore, 2004) and RN job satisfaction (Boyle, Miller, Gajewski, Hart, & Dunton, 2006), and (2) measurement of the validity and reliability of the NDNQI work satisfaction scale

(Taunton et al., 2004) and the NDNQI pressure ulcer prevalence indicator (Hart, Bergquist, Gajewski, & Dunton, 2006). Specific to NDNQI, there is an abundance of descriptive reports in the form of news releases, commentaries, and overviews that aim primarily at increasing awareness about this database and enhancing participation in it. For example, one paper was found that addressed continuing education needs of nurse managers regarding the use of the NDNQI reports (Dunton, 2008), and another paper reported on using NDNQI data to generate report cards and using them as a benchmark tool to implement new initiatives and improve care (Pierre, 2006).

A larger number of studies reporting data from the CalNOC database exist, perhaps because it was the first established database. Six studies addressed staffing in acute care hospitals in relation to patient outcomes (Aydin et al., 2004; Bolton, 2007; Bolton et al., 2001, 2003; Donaldson, Bolton, et al., 2005; Donaldson, Brown, Aydin, & Bolton, 2001), and two studies addressed the use of CalNOC data for benchmarking purposes, performance measurement, and quality improvement (Bolton & Goodenough, 2003; Donaldson, Brown, Aydin, Bolton, & Rutledge, 2005). There is considerable nonempirical literature available about NODs. This literature provides historical data about the inception of these databases and future plans about them. These include reports such as background material; overview of papers; news releases/commentaries; and discussion and/or commentary papers on related topics such as performance measurement in nursing, and nursing-sensitive outcomes/indicators.

To date, although the reports of empirical findings using these databases are interesting, there is not a sufficient body of literature exploring the same or similar outcomes across the databases to build strong evidence about nursing factors and how to organize and deliver care to optimize outcomes. Plans for analyses that provide views across the databases may be in process, but there is little evidence of systematic plans to link and analyze data across these databases. Each database has its own processes for data collection, management, and feedback to participating hospitals and facilities. These processes are not well described in the publicly available literature, making it difficult for individuals outside the teams that organize and develop the databases to plan research activities using these data. In addition, there are not clear processes in place for data access, limiting the opportunities for researchers outside the development teams. Priorities for using the data are not clear from the publicly available information about the four NODs. In fact, all four databases are fairly tightly controlled by the teams responsible for their development and maintenance, which may be a limiting factor in how much has been published out of them. In part because access to these databases has been complicated—with two held as proprietary databases controlled by the developers (CalNOC and NDNQI) and the other two limited by data access issues related to their healthcare systems (VANOD and MilNOD)—newer databases are being developed with minimal knowledge of or reference to the existing NODs. In addition, NODs outside the United States are not described in the literature, although some hospitals and healthcare systems outside the United States may be participating in NDNQI. This limits the amount of learning from these existing databases. Although it is likely that each new database of this type will require decisions about issues that are specific to different healthcare systems, unless there is some mechanism for discussions across the developer groups, and opportunities to use common standards and definitions, linking to and learning from the joint efforts of these initiatives will remain elusive.

Belgium: Nursing Minimum Data Set (Minimale Verpleegkundige Gegevens: MVG)

Similar to the United States' experience, healthcare information systems in Belgium began in the 1980s with a Hospital Discharge Data Set (HDDS) (Sermeus et al., 2004). Because of a lack of information related to nursing care in the HDDS, a project was initiated in 1988 to establish a national uniform NMDS. The NMDS was aimed at facilitating the description of nursing care and interventions in relation to nurse staffing in order to bridge the gap between nursing practice and policy-making (Boer & Delesie, 1998; Sermeus et al., 2004); describing health status; facilitating clinical research; determining costs and effectiveness of nursing care; determining the intensity of nursing care; determining hospital staffing and budgets; contributing to appropriate evaluation protocols; and producing care profiles per diagnosis-related groups (Goossen et al., 1998, 2006; Sermeus & Goossen, 2002).

The B-NMDS model used a unique approach to data collection by tracking variability of practice patterns, as opposed to a specific performance measurement indicator (e.g., length of stay). Data elements of the B-NMDS included three items related to patient demographics and the ICD-9-M as a method for aligning NMDS data to the hospital discharge data set. The nursing care elements included nursing interventions—a list of 23 nursing interventions and activities of daily living (ADL) (Boer & Delesie, 1998). Nursing diagnoses were not included; however, currently this aspect is being integrated into the new version of the B-NMDS (Goossen et al., 1998, 2006; Sermeus & Goossen, 2002). Service elements included several variables: (1) agency provider—unique hospital code, code specialty, code ward, and number of beds; (2) episode of care—admission date, length of stay, day of stay, and discharge date; and (3) resources—number of nursing hours available, number of nurses available, and qualification mix (Goossen et al., 1998, 2006).

With regard to data collection, several methods were used, including paper, bar code, or electronic surveys on 15 days four times a year. Graphics rather than numbers were used to represent nursing information in order to facilitate communication between nurses and management, as well as access to, and understanding of, information (Boer & Delesie, 1998; Goossen et al., 1998, 2006). The sample size was about 1.2 million nursing records per year. Currently, about

20 million nursing records have been collected since 1988 (Goossen et al., 1998, 2006). Several data analysis techniques were used, such as statistics for ordinal data and multivariate analysis, to address challenges related to the nature of patient care, which cannot be measured by one single indicator (Goossen et al., 2006). However, data analysis was cross-sectional rather than prospective or retrospective (Goossen et al., 1998, 2006). The aggregation level was a little more specific than in the U.S. data sets and included patient day, patient stay, patient, unit, hospital, and national levels (Goossen et al., 1998, 2006). Feedback reports and graphical presentations and fingerprints of data were shared with wards and at the institution level using electronic means such as CDs and Internet (Goossen et al., 1998, 2006).

The stability of this NMDS design and its ability to capture information at a national level allowed for comparisons, forecasting, and better resource utilization; however, it remained limited in its focus on budgets and workload calculations in hospitals (Goossen et al., 2000; Sermeus et al., 2004). The need to update the Belgian NMDS was identified in 2000 in response to several factors: limitations in the existing design, evolutions in health care, international developments of nursing languages and classifications, and a need for integration with the HDDS (Sermeus et al., 2005, 2006). In addition to these factors, it was also apparent that although the current system provided extensive data banks, it did not fully meet the needs of all users of data; therefore, mechanisms for enhancing the use of data were needed. A multiphase project set out to achieve this goal in four major phases: (1) the development of the conceptual framework based on literature review and secondary data analysis (the Nursing Interventions Classification [NIC] was selected as a framework for the revision of the NMDS); (2) language development with panels of clinical experts for six care programs (this phase led to an alpha version of the B-NMDS, which is an instrument based on the NIC framework); (3) data collection and validation of the instrument, the results of which would be the beta version of the B-NMDS and the integration of the revised tool with the HDDS; and (4) the development of information management applications (Sermeus, Delesie, & van den Heede, 2002; Sermeus et al., 2005, 2006).

Netherlands: Nursing Minimum Data Set

The primary goal of NMDSN was to design a data set that would describe the diversity of patient populations and the variability of nursing care for the purpose of enhancing decision-making related to resource allocation and planning of care and to allow the multiple use of the same data (Goossen et al., 2000, 2001). Based on a systematic review of NMDS projects worldwide, the research team involved in this research project concluded that the process of developing an NMDS involves a multistage approach that includes the identification of items to be included in the data set; testing of the method of data collection; analysis of collected data; and testing of the usefulness of the data set (Goossen et al., 2000).

The study used an exploratory, multimethod approach to identify and develop a set of items to be included in the data set (Goossen et al., 2000, 2001). These included five institution-related items, including type of institution and type of ward; six patient demographic items; seven medical condition items (medical diagnosis and medical condition items); and 10 items related to the use of the nursing process (Goossen et al., 2000, 2001). In addition, aspects of the nursing process included 24 nursing diagnoses, 32 nursing interventions, and 4 outcomes of nursing care—fixed list, and three additional items pertaining to the measurement of the complexity of care (Goossen, 2001). Other variables related to service elements included the episode of care—moment of stay (admission/discharge), and nursing's time for particular interventions (Goossen et al., 1998, 2006).

The NMDSN was tested in nine hospitals on 15 wards, and results indicated that the items identified reflect the diversity of the patient population and variations in nursing care (Goossen et al., 2001), and its validity and reliability have been explored in an intensive care ward, a nursing home, and a residential home (Goossen et al., 2003). In these tests, the Belgian MVG approach of graphic illustration was utilized.

Australia: Nursing Minimum Data Set

In Australia, the development of the Community Nursing Minimum Data Set (CNMDSA) began in 1990. Goossen et al. (1998) reported that the CNMDSA was developed to compare the performance of institutions, allocate resources, monitor and compare the health status of the population, and deliver information to decision makers and policy makers. Although the CNMDSA is used nationally, it is limited to community care settings. The indicators/items for the CNMDSA were identified based on consultations with 300 nurses working in the areas of field/community nursing, and middle and senior management; nonnurses with an interest in the CNMDSA; and nurses from hospitals, education, and other work settings. The consultations identified 66 possible items considered necessary for the practice of community nursing in Australia. A Delphi approach was used to prioritize the items, and a focus group was then conducted to determine the specific items and their operational definitions. The result was the 17-item CNMDSA. The nursing care data elements explored include nursing diagnosis, goals of nursing care (seven types), nursing intervention (eight types), client dependency, and discharge (four items). Patient demographic items included five items, and medical care items consisted of medical diagnoses (Goossen et al., 1998, 2006). With regard to service variables, several items were included: (1) agency provider (agency identifier and source of referral); (2) episode of care (date of first contact, date of referral, discharge date from hospital, date of first visit, discharge date, and date of last contact); (3) resources (resource utilization); and (4) information related to some support services (Goossen et al., 1998, 2006).

Data collection was primarily through electronic records, with data aggregation being at patient, institution, national, and international levels. Feedback reports go to the institution that participates, and others that have an interest. However, because no known reports of CNMDSA field testing have been published, it is not possible to comment on its validity and reliability in collecting data on nursing outcomes in the community setting, nor aspects related to sample size and approaches to data analysis (Goossen et al., 1998, 2000, 2006).

Canada: Nursing Minimum Data Set Health Information: Nursing Components

In Canada, the first step in developing a nursing minimum data set occurred in 1993 at the NMDS conference by the Canadian Nurses Association (Canadian Nurses Association, 2000). Leaders in the fields of information management, nursing research, and nursing classification systems participated in the conference. The overall objective was to develop an NMDS to ensure the availability and accessibility of nursing data in a standardized form. At the conclusion of the conference, participants proposed nursing-specific elements for inclusion in a national health data set (Canadian Nurses Association). The NMDS was given the name Health Information: Nursing Components (HI: NC) to reflect a focus on the patient and the patient's needs and outcomes rather than on individual healthcare professions (Goossen et al., 1998; Hannah & Anderson, 1994). The HI: NC can be used nationally and in all settings. It included:

- Eight patient demographic items
- Medical care items, such as medical diagnosis, procedures, and whether the patient is alive at the time of classification
- Nursing care elements, which describe the client status, nursing interventions, client outcomes, and nursing intensity
- Service elements, such as provincial/institutional chart number, doctor identifier, nurse identifier, and principal nurse provider
- Episode items, such as admission date and hour, discharge date and hour, and length of stay
- Other related data, such as the institution, main point of service, and payer (Canadian Nurses Association, 2000; Goossen et al., 1998).

An Ontario government-funded initiative, Health Outcomes for Better Information and Care (HOBIC), is establishing a minimum data set for nursing-sensitive outcomes. In April 2007, the Ministry of Health and Long-Term Care (MOHLTC) began funding healthcare organizations to collect data electronically on select patient outcomes sensitive to nursing care in acute care, home care, and complex continuing care settings. There are now 148 healthcare organizations from across the province engaged in HOBIC outcomes data collection, and this number will increase as the initiative is expanded throughout the province. Participation in HOBIC is voluntary. In addition, Canada Health Infoway has funded projects led by the Canadian Nurses Association that focus on HOBIC data collection with electronic health record integration in two other Canadian provinces (see http://www.cna-aiic.ca/c-hobic/about/default_e.aspx).

The HOBIC information system builds on the Canadian Institute of Health Information's Continuing Care Reporting System using standardized measures to assess health outcomes of care. The outcomes data, consisting of information on patients' functional health symptoms (pain, dyspnea, fatigue, nausea), pressure ulcers, falls, and therapeutic self-care, are collected electronically at the point of care, when nurses complete patient assessments. HOBIC introduces a systematic, structured language to admission. It includes admission and discharge assessments of patients receiving acute care to admission, quarterly (if condition changes) and admission/discharge assessments of patients receiving complex continuing care, long-term care, or home care. This language can be abstracted into provincial databases or electronic health records. The HOBIC system has been designed to benefit patients, decision makers, and researchers. Two databases exist, one live and accessible only by nurses and administrators, and one that contains deidentified data for researchers and policy makers and is housed at the Institute for Clinical and Evaluative Studies. For patients, HOBIC information is used by nurses to monitor the impact of care and ensure, for example, that patients are prepared for discharge. For managers and decision makers, HOBIC data are aggregated at the unit and institution level to inform quality improvement initiatives, performance monitoring, and resource allocation. For researchers, HOBIC data provide an opportunity to research the impact of health human resource utilization, quality work environments, and nursing practice on patient health outcomes. In Canada, HOBIC highlights the importance of patient outcomes data and is making it much more accessible to front-line providers of care (Hannah, White, Nagle, & Pringle, 2009; Pringle, 2004; White, Pringle, Doran, & Hall, 2005).

Switzerland: Nursing Minimum Data Set (CH-NMDS)

According to Junger and colleagues, some level of data collection exists in Switzerland in the form of CH-NMDS (Junger et al., 2004). This database registers relevant data at the most aggregate level to describe nursing care for statistical purposes. According to Junger et al., compared with initiatives in other countries, this level of data collection is not sufficient to comprehensively describe nursing care. Switzerland would benefit from a nationwide data collection similar to that of Belgium, for example. In 1998, it was decided that nursing data would be incorporated within the national data collection scheme. The NURSING data project aimed at creating: (1) a list of appropriate variables that represent the "why" and "how" of nursing care, (2) an accepted nursing classification system, and (3) a validated system for data analysis. To achieve these aims, the NURSING project utilized various models in the development of the database. Further information about the full NMDS draft can be found at http://www.chuv.ch.

Finland: Nursing Minimum Data Set

A minimum data set is being developed in Finland. The main goals of the Finnish NMDS are to (1) develop a nationally unified and standardized nursing documentation system, (2) use the standardized nursing data to manage and assess the quality of the nursing process, and (3) integrate the nursing documentation into multiprofessional patient records (Tanttu & Ikonen, 2006). The core data elements of the NMDS are based on the nursing process and include nursing diagnoses/needs, nursing interventions, nursing assessment and outcomes, patient care intensity classification, and nursing summary (Tanttu & Ikonen). The Finnish Nursing Classification System (FiCNI) utilized the Clinical Care Components developed in the United States, and the Oulu Patient Classification to measure patient care intensity. The classification for outcomes and the core data for nursing summary are still under development. Piloting of the NMDS was done in 23 healthcare organizations, including special care, primary care, and home care settings, during 2005–2007.

Thailand: Nursing Minimum Data Set

Initiatives are under way in Thailand to develop a nursing minimum data set. The project is in the initial phase of development. The framework of nursing process has been adopted; however, there is a need to identify, and link the data to, a unified nursing language such as International Classification of Nursing Practice (ICNP). Respondents to the initial surveys identified 10 items for inclusion in the NMDS (Phuphaibul, 2006).

Brazil: Nursing Minimum Data Set

Discussions on the need to develop an NMDS specific to the Brazilian healthcare system are in progress. Ribeiro and Marin (2006) proposed an NMDS for evaluating the health in home care elderly using domains from the American Nursing Minimum Data Set. The goal in this study was to stimulate discussion and research in the area of minimum data set development in Brazil.

Iceland: Nursing Minimum Data Set

Gudmundsdottir, Delaney, Thoroddsen, and Karlsson (2004) reported that the efforts toward standardization and documentation of nursing care have been ongoing since 1990 in Iceland. Initial efforts have aimed at translating into Icelandic and publishing the NANDA system and the labels and definitions of the NIC for the purpose of validating them in the Icelandic context (Gudmundsdottir et al.). The reliability of the Icelandic version of the Nursing Outcomes Classifications survey in acute care settings was acceptable; however its validation in other settings, such as primary health care and nursing homes, should be addressed in future research (Gudmundsdottir et al.). Other initiatives or reports on the progress of the development of NMDS in Iceland have not been reported in the literature.

Ireland: Nursing Minimum Data Set

Butler et al. (2006) reported on Irish initiatives toward developing an NMDS specific to Irish needs. The main goal for developing an Irish NMDS was to make nursing and the contributions of nurses in Ireland visible. In 2002, a 5-year research program funded by the Irish Health Research Board was initiated for the purpose of identifying patient problems, nursing interventions, and nursing outcomes to be included in the Irish NMDS. Using data from 11 focus group interviews with 59 registered nurses and a sample of 45 sets of nursing records, a range of patient problems, nursing interventions, and outcomes were identified. These will undergo further testing and validation (Butler et al.).

COMPARISONS OF NURSING MINIMUM DATA SETS

Goossen and colleagues examined the similarities and differences among national and international NMDS systems on several dimensions, including the scope of the NMDS, its data elements, methods of data management, analysis, feedback methods, and problems (Goossen et al., 1998, 2006). The comparisons revealed that NMDSs worldwide share many commonalities and differences; however, the goal should be to expand on these commonalities and eliminate differences (Goossen et al., 2006). In terms of the purposes of NMDSs, Goossen et al. (2006) reported that most NMDSs share an overarching goal of describing and comparing nursing care and that they serve to facilitate research and management and influence policy-making, specifically with regard to nursing care budgets and staff allocation. This area of commonality is significant and may contribute to the development of international initiatives related to NMDSs. However, several areas of differences do exist among NMDSs, primarily in relation to items identified in each NMDS, such as nursing care (e.g., nursing diagnosis, interventions, and outcomes) and demographic data (e.g., patient, nurse, and institution) items. Such differences pose challenges with regard to national and international comparisons. With regard to the methodology adopted in NMDSs, there are also differences in relation to approaches to data collection (e.g., paper vs electronic means), sample sizes, and approaches of data analysis, which are commonly project specific. However, most NMDS initiatives maintain some level of reporting in the literature in the form of research reports and conferences nationally and internationally.

STRENGTHS AND LIMITATIONS OF NURSING MINIMUM DATA SETS

In a comprehensive review of the NMDS movement worldwide, Goossen et al. offered a summary of the strengths and limitations of NMDSs in the context of evaluating their capacity to support nursing data needs at the national and international levels (Goossen et al., 1998, 2006). The major areas of strength in NMDSs pertain to their ability to: (1) enhance representation of nursing contributions to health care and, consequently, nursing visibility through means of consistent description of nursing care elements; (2) enable comparisons of nursing practice at different levels, which consequently promotes effective decision-making in relation to healthcare policy decisions; and (3) enable sharing of information among various key players in the healthcare system. According to Goossen et al. (2006) these strengths include:

1. Describe patient problems, nursing interventions, nurse-sensitive patient outcomes, and nursing resources across settings, clinical populations, geographic areas, and time.
2. Compare nursing practice at different levels, offer testimony on nursing issues, develop databases, assess the cost effectiveness of nursing interventions and the costs of nurse resources, and provide data to influence health policy makers.
3. Share data with various health providers and researchers. (p. 310)

In addition, Goossen et al. (1998, 2006) reported other strengths of NMDSs within the context of empirical evidence established to date on their relevance and effectiveness in informing decision-making and healthcare policy. Despite these strengths, NMDSs do have some limitations and problem areas. Next, we cite this list of limitations offered by Goossen et al.; we did not include citations of the studies that Goossen et al. quoted when they reported this list of limitations in their original paper. Readers are encouraged to locate the original work to view this information (Goossen et al., 2006, p. 311). As reported by Goossen et al., these are:

1. Lack of comparability of NMDS data items and inconsistent definitions.
2. Lack of relationships among nursing diagnoses, interventions, and outcomes in stored data.
3. Differences in the specificity and detail of vocabularies (Granularity).
4. The inability of one vocabulary to fit all purposes.
5. The inhibition of the use of standards because of the ownership of definitions.

6. The needs to address informed consent issues and to take measures to protect privacy.
7. The need to assess the reliability and validity of the database.
8. The expense of updating an NMDS and upgrading existing data collection; of changes in the methodology, instrument, or classification; of changes in information systems; and of the ongoing education of (new) users.
9. The paucity of electronic patient record systems that allow users to directly retrieve nursing minimal data

INTERNATIONAL MINIMUM DATA SET: INMDS

In the past decade, efforts have been concerted toward mobilizing national NMDSs to an international perspective. This project began in 1997 at the International Medical Informatics Association conference among experts working on NMDS projects worldwide (Goossen et al., 2006). Two international organizations cosponsor the iNMDS project: the International Council of Nurses (ICN) and the International Medical Informatics Association-Nursing Informatics Special Interest Group (IMIA-NI SIG). Planning and preparation for the piloting of the iNMDS took place in the period between 2000 and 2003. Results of the pilot and decisions regarding subsequent steps were reported at the Medinfo conference in 2004. The expansion of the scope of NMDS to an international scheme is timely because it responds to challenges currently imposed on the healthcare systems of many nations, such as limited resources and the need to justify cost of health care, the need for evidence to support care provided to more informed customers, and the expanded use of technology in health care—all of which require different approaches to data collection and use (Goossen et al., 2006).

The overarching goal of the iNMDS is to support the information needs in nursing, which is congruent with ICNP goals (Goossen et al., 2006). In addition, an iNMDS would serve to enhance data aggregation from the individual to group levels. The iNMDS uses the Nursing Information Reference Model developed by Goossen and colleagues in 1997 to identify information needs that support decision-making at different levels in health care. The first level addresses the needs for information by the individual practitioner in the primary care process. The second level involves the use of information to support clinical decision-making. The third level involves use of data at the institutional level to support nonclinical decisions such as staffing and resource allocation. The fourth level pertains to the national use of data to support health statistics and policy decisions. The iNMDS adds another level to this model by addressing information needs at the international level; in this context, such information helps international organizations such as ICN and the World Health Organization (WHO) to plan healthcare policy and facilitate standardization and regulation processes (Goossen et al., 2006).

The iNMDS pilot involved an extensive review of the literature to support a conceptual definition of iNMDS, and a survey design on the purposes, items, and possible methodologies of an iNMDS. In addition, a comprehensive data bank of all individuals in the different countries who were interested in participating in the project is under development (Goossen et al., 2006). The steering committee used convenience samples from four countries—Switzerland, The Netherlands, Belgium, and the United States—to conduct a retrospective analysis of data. Through this they identified methods for data collection, analysis, and potential variables for inclusion in the iNMDS using the ICNP classification system. These countries have some level of comparative data compared with other countries with NMDSs (Goossen et al., 2006). Despite the stability of these NMDSs and their comparability compared with NMDSs in other countries, the results of the pilot showed great variability in terms of the details of the data within each data set and in comparison with other data sets, and this impacted statistical analysis. Based on this, the research team decided to develop a beta version of the iNMDS and considered the use of prospective, as opposed to retrospective, design. Insights from the initial pilot helped the steering committee to redefine the purpose, variables, and future directions of the iNMDS.

In 2004, decisions regarding the conceptual framework were reached and included the specification of three areas for the data within iNMDS: (1) nursing care, (2) client, and (3) settings. In 2005, the ICN supported the iNMDS-Beta as a working data set (Goossen et al., 2006). Other specifications related to the data were set in order to enhance comparability of future data. In addition, data variables included considerations for aligning iNMDS goals with strategic goals of the ICN and the WHO. Based on the pilot, the steering committee proposed a clearer definition of the iNMDS and its purpose. An iNMDS was defined as "a minimum but essential data set of items of information with uniform definitions and categories concerning the specific dimension of nursing internationally that are maximally useful for different purposes, and which meets the information needs of multiple data users in the health care system worldwide" (Goossen et al., 2006, p. 317).

DISCUSSION

In the changing healthcare environment, there is an increasing need to identify, measure, and evaluate quality outcomes. The development of relevant quality outcomes requires partnerships among service providers, government, and the research community, as well as a common language to link them together (Hirdes & Carpenter, 1997). In the past, it has been difficult to develop evidence-based practice and policy because of ineffective communication mechanisms, limitations in knowledge, methodological issues, and a lack of data or the inability to access data (Hirdes & Carpenter). The use of databases such as an NMDSs and others may begin to resolve these issues.

Whichever database is chosen, it is important to recognize that the reliability and validity of databases are complex and often confused with the reliability and validity of the classification systems used within a minimum data set (Ryan & Delaney, 1995). Although the reliability and validity of the classification system will affect the reliability and validity of the data within a minimum data system, the reliability and validity of the actual data must also be considered. Incomplete records, unreliable or invalid coding, or missing variables may limit the value of the data (Ryan & Delaney). For the data to be reliable and valid, standardized classification systems must be used, and the reliability of the data needs to be monitored regularly (Ryan & Delaney).

All NMDS systems have the benefit of making nurses' work visible and providing evidence-based knowledge to guide both nursing practice and the decisions made by policy makers and healthcare providers. The information obtained through the use of an NMDS facilitates system-level planning and evaluation, as well as benchmarking within and against similar organizations. It also helps identify best practices. A growing body of evidence generated from NMDSs could provide the nursing profession with substantial benefits with respect to nursing effectiveness, quality assurance, mapping trends, and nursing research (Goossen et al., 1998, 2006). The challenge is to continue to implement clinical testing of the different components of an NMDS to determine their weaknesses, strengths, and applicability, and their validity and reliability in different clinical settings.

For NMDS systems to achieve their full potential, developers must address the issue of whether the same variables are being compared, and how to deal with differences in scope, population, sample, actual data, abstraction, and aggregation (Goossen et al., 1998, 2006). If the underlying structures of the data sets are incompatible, they cannot be compared. This raises the question of how to develop standardized data in different healthcare settings, countries, and healthcare delivery models. The issues of standardized language and classification systems continue to fuel the debate about whether there should be one acceptable classification system and, if so, which one it should be. One classification system would be advantageous, because everyone would be aware of the vocabulary and the classification and would have to utilize it (McCormick & Jones, 1998). The data would also be comparable across settings, place, and country. However, the assumption that all practicing nurses would embrace one classification system and learn to use it in a consistent manner is unrealistic. Data must be captured in a way that permits integration across levels and sites of care, delivery models, providers, and management domains (McCormick & Jones). The mapping of classification systems appears to be a feasible alternative to implementing one classification system. The work of the ICNP demonstrates potential in this area.

Goossen and colleagues raised the question of whether a specific NMDS still has relevance in today's healthcare environment (Goossen et al., 1998, 2006). This question is supported by the Cumulative Index to Nursing and Allied Health Literature (CINAHL) literature search, which revealed that most of the literature describing various nursing classification systems was published prior to 1997. The NOC system is the only NMDS that has published most of its work over the past 5 years. The cost of implementing and supporting minimum data sets within organizations, and the fact that client care is provided manly by multidisciplinary teams, suggests that the focus should be on developing multidisciplinary databases rather than discipline-specific ones.

Ideally, it would be advantageous to have a database that could capture clients' healthcare experiences as they move across the healthcare continuum. While the Resident Assessment Instrument (RAI/MDS) series holds the most promise of eventually providing this capability, it is not currently feasible for one classification system to cover all factors relevant to a client's care in all settings (Shaughnessy, Crisler, & Schlenker, 1998). Each database has been developed for a specific reason. For example, the NMDS systems were developed to capture and make nursing practice visible, the RAI was developed to deliver care to the elderly client, and the Outcome and Assessment Information Set is used in home care. The choice of which database to use depends on such factors as the type of clients, the purpose for measurement, the ease of data collection, the cost, and the degree of informatics technology within the organization. Regardless of this, the use of a minimum data set is necessary to identify best practices, nursing effectiveness, quality assurance, trends, and nursing research (Goossen et al., 1998, 2006). The challenge is to continue to identify methods of developing and using databases that are reliable and valid and that best reflect nursing practice.

REFERENCES

Alexander, G. R. (2007). Nursing sensitive databases: Their existence, challenges, and importance. *Medical Care Research and Review, 64*(Suppl. 2), 44S–63S.

American Nurses Association. (1999). *Nursing-sensitive quality indicators for acute care settings and ANA's safety and quality initiative.* Baltimore, MD: American Nurses Association.

Aydin, C. E., Bolton, L. B., Donaldson, N., Brown, D. S., Buffum, M., Elashoff, J. D., et al. (2004). Creating and analyzing a statewide nursing quality measurement database. *Journal of Nursing Scholarship, 36,* 371–378.

Blewitt, D. K., & Jones, K. R. (1996). Using elements of the nursing minimum data set for determining outcomes. *Journal of Nursing Administration, 26*(6), 48–56.

Boer, G. V., & Delesie, L. (1998). The federal nursing minimum basic data set and hospital management in Belgium: A case study of a nursing department. *European Journal of Operational Research, 105,* 317–331.

Bolton, L. B. (2007). Mandated nurse staffing ratios in California: A comparison of staffing and nursing-sensitive outcomes pre-and postregulation. *Policy, Politics, and Nursing Practice, 8*(4), 238–250.

Bolton, L. B., Aydin, C. E., Donaldson, N., Brown, D. S., Nelson, M. S., & Harms, D. (2003). Nurse staffing and patient perceptions of nursing care. *European Journal of Operational Research, 33*, 607–614.

Bolton, L. B., & Goodenough, A. (2003). A magnet nursing service approach to nursing's role in quality improvement. *Nursing Administration Quarterly, 27*, 344–354.

Bolton, L. B., Jones, D., Aydin, C. E., Donaldson, N., Brown, D. S., Lowe, M., et al. (2001). A response to California's mandated nursing ratios. *Journal of Nursing Scholarship, 33*, 179–184.

Boyle, D. K., Miller, P. A., Gajewski, B. J., Hart, S. E., & Dunton, N. (2006). Unit type differences in RN workgroup job satisfaction. *Western Journal of Nursing Research, 28*, 622–640.

Butler, M., Treacy, M., Scott, A., Hyde, A., Mac Neela, P., Irving, K., et al. (2006). Towards a nursing minimum data set for Ireland: Making Irish nursing visible. *Journal of Advanced Nursing, 55*, 364–375.

Canadian Nurses Association. (2000). *Collecting data to reflect nursing impact.* Ottawa, Ontario, Canada: Author.

Delaney, C., & Moorhead, S. (1995). The nursing minimum data set, standardized language, and health care quality. *Journal of Nursing Care Quality, 10*, 16–30.

Donaldson, N. E., Brown, D. S., Aydin, C. E., & Bolton, L. B. (2001). Nurse staffing in California hospitals 1998–2000: Findings from the California Nursing Outcomes Coalition Database Project. *Policy, Politics, and Nursing Practice, 2*, 19–28.

Donaldson, N., Brown, D. S., Aydin, C. E., Bolton, M. L. B., & Rutledge, D. N. (2005). Leveraging nurse-related dashboard benchmarks to expedite performance improvement and document excellence. *Journal of Nursing Administration, 35*, 163–172.

Donaldson, N., Bolton, L. B., Aydin, C., Brown, D., Elashoff, J. D., & Sandhu, M. (2005). Impact of California's licensed nurse-patient ratios on unit-level nurse staffing and patient outcomes. *Policy, Politics, and Nursing Practice, 6*, 198–210. doi:10.1177/1527154405280107

Dunton, N. E. (2008). Take a cue from the NDNQI. *Nursing Management, 39*(4), 20–23.

Dunton, N., Gajewski, B., Klaus, S., & Pierson, B. (2007). The relationship of nursing workforce characteristics to patient outcomes. *Online Journal of Issues in Nursing, 12*(3). Retrieved from http://www.nursingworld.org/MainMenuCategories/ANAMarketplace/ANAPeriodicals/OJIN/TableofContents/Volume122007/No3Sept07/NursingWorkforceCharacteristics.aspx

Dunton, N., Gajewski, B., Taunton, R. L., & Moore, J. (2004). Nurse staffing and patient falls on acute care hospital units. *Nursing Outlook, 52*, 53–59.

Goossen, W. T. (2001). Exploiting the nursing minimum data set for The Netherlands. *Studies in Health Technology and Informatics, 84*(Pt 2), 1334–1338.

Goossen, W. T. F., Delancy, C. W., Coenen, A., Saba, V. K., Sermeus, W., Warren, J. J., et al. (2006). The international nursing minimum data set (i-NMDS). In C. A. Weaver, C. W. Delaney, P. Weber, & R. L. Carr (Eds.), *Nursing and informatics for the 21st century: An international look at practice, trends and the future* (pp. 305–320). Chicago: Healthcare Information and Management Systems Society.

Goossen, W., Dassen, T., Dijkstra, A., Hasman, A., Tiesinga, L., & van den Heuvel, W. (2003). Validity and reliability of the nursing minimum data set for The Netherlands (NMDSN). *Scandinavian Journal of Caring Sciences, 17*, 19–29.

Goossen, W. T., Epping, P. J., Feuth, T., Dassen, T. W., Hasman, A., & van den Heuvel, W. J. (1998). A comparison of nursing minimal data sets. *Journal of the American Medical Informatics Association, 5*, 152–163.

Goossen, W. T., Epping, P. J., Feuth, T., van den Heuvel, W. J., Hasman, A., & Dassen, T. W. (2001). Using the Nursing Minimum Data Set for The Netherlands (NMDSN) to illustrate differences in patient populations and variations in nursing activities. *International Journal of Nursing Studies, 38*, 243–257.

Goossen, W. T., Epping, P. J., van den Heuvel, W. J., Feuth, T., Frederiks, C. M., & Hasman, A. (2000). Development of the Nursing Minimum Data Set for The Netherlands (NMDSN): Identification of categories and items. *Journal of Advanced Nursing, 31*, 536–547.

Grindel, C. G. (1996). Building nursing's minimum data set: The results of a pilot study. *Medsurg Nursing, 5*, 449–445.

Gudmundsdottir, E., Delaney, C., Thoroddsen, A., & Karlsson, T. (2004). Translation and validation of the nursing outcomes classification labels and definitions for acute care nursing in Iceland. *Journal of Advanced Nursing, 46*, 292–302.

Haberfelde, M., Bedecarre, D., & Buffum, M. (2005). Nurse-sensitive patient outcomes: An annotated bibliography. *Journal of Nursing Administration, 35*, 293–299.

Hannah, K. J., & Anderson, B. J. (1994). Management of nursing information. In J. M. Hibbered & M. E. Kyle (Eds.), *Nursing administration: A micro/macro approach for effective nurse executives* (pp. 533–561). Norwalk, CT: Appleton and Lange.

Hannah, K. J., White, P. A., Nagle, L. M., & Pringle, D. M. (2009). Standardizing nursing information in Canada for inclusion in electronic health records: C-HOBIC. *Journal of the American Medical Informatics Association, 16*(4), 524–530.

Hart, S., Bergquist, S., Gajewski, B., & Dunton, N. (2006). Reliability testing of the National Database of Nursing Quality Indicators pressure ulcer indicator. *Journal of Nursing Care Quality, 21*, 256–265.

Hirdes, J. P., & Carpenter, G. I. (1997). Health outcomes among the frail elderly in communities and institutions: Use of the minimum data set (MDS) to create effective linkages between research and policy. *Canadian Journal on Aging, 16*(Suppl.), 53–69.

Huber, D., & Delaney, C. (1997). The nursing management minimum data set. *Applied Nursing Research, 10*, 164–165.

Huber, D. G., Delaney, C., Crossley, J., Mehmert, M., & Ellerbe, S. (1992). A nursing management minimum data set: Significance and development. *Journal of Nursing Administration, 22*(7–8), 35–40.

Huber, D., Schumacher, L., & Delaney, C. (1997). Nursing management minimum data set (NMMDS). *Journal of Nursing Administration, 27*(4), 42–48.

Junger, A., Brenck, F., Hartmann, B., Klasen, J., Quinzio, L., Benson, M., et al. (2004). Automatic calculation of the nine equivalents of nursing manpower use score (NEMS) using a patient data management system. *Intensive Care Medicine, 30*, 1487–1490.

Leske, J. S., & Werley, H. H. (1992). Use of the nursing minimum data set. *Computers in Nursing, 10*, 259–263.

Mac Neela, P., Scott, P. A., Treacy, M. P., & Hyde, A. (2006). Nursing minimum data sets: A conceptual analysis and review. *Nursing Inquiry, 13*(1), 44–51. doi:10.1111/j.1440–1800.2006.00300.x

McCormick, K. A., & Jones, C. B. (1998). Is one taxonomy needed for health care vocabularies and classifications? *Online Journal of Issues in Nursing, 3*(2).

Montalvo, I. (2007). The National Database of Nursing Quality Indicators (NDNQI). *Online Journal of Issues in Nursing, 12*(3). Retrieved from http://www.nursingworld. org/MainMenuCategories/ANAMarketplace/ANAPeriodicals/OJIN/TableofContents/ Volume122007/No3Sept07/NursingQualityIndicators.aspx

Phuphaibul, R. (2006). Nursing data set development in Thailand. *Studies in Health Technology and Informatics, 122,* 991.

Pierce, S. F. (1997). Nurse-sensitive health care outcomes in acute care settings: An integrative analysis of the literature. *Journal of Nursing Care Quality, 11*(4), 60–72.

Pierre, J. S. (2006). Staff nurses' use of report card data for quality improvement: First steps. *Journal of Nursing Care Quality, 21*(1), 8–14.

Pringle, D. (2004). Nursing sensitive outcomes: Indicators for the Ontario database. Paper presented at the 15th International Nursing Research Congress, Dublin, Ireland. Abstract retrieved from http://www.nursinglibrary.org/Portal/main.aspx?pageid=4024&pid=4308

Prophet, C. M., & Delaney, C. W. (1998). Nursing outcomes classification: Implications for nursing information systems and the computer-based patient record. *Journal of Nursing Care Quality, 12*(5), 21–29.

Ribeiro, R. de Cassia, & Marin, H. de Fatima. (2006). Proposal for an essential nursing data set to evaluate the health in home care elderly persons. *Studies in Health Technology and Informatics, 122,* 790–791.

Rowell, P. A., & Milholland, D. K. (1998). Nursing and threats to patient and nurse safety and quality of patient care. *Journal of Nursing Care Quality, 12*(4), 9–13.

Ryan, P., & Delaney, C. (1995). Nursing minimum data set. *Annual Review of Nursing Research, 13,* 169–194.

Seifert, P. C. (1999). The perioperative nursing data set—power is knowledge. *AORN Journal, 70*(1), 8–11.

Sermeus, W., Delesie, L., & van den Heede, K. (2002). Updating the Belgian Nursing Minimum Data Set: Framework and methodology. *Studies in Health Technology and Informatics, 93,* 89–93.

Sermeus, W., & Goossen, W. (2002). A nursing minimum data set. *Studies in Health Technology and Informatics, 65,* 98–109.

Sermeus, W., van den Heede, K., Michiels, D., Delesie, L., Thonon, O., van Boven, C., et al. (2004). A nation-wide project for the revision of the Belgian Nursing Minimum Data Set: From concept to implementation. *Studies in Health Technology and Informatics, 110,* 21–26.

Sermeus, W., van den Heede, K., Michiels, D., Delesie, L., Thonon, O., van Boven, C., et al. (2005). Revising the Belgian Nursing Minimum Data Set: From concept to implementation. *International Journal of Medical Informatics, 74,* 946–951.

Sermeus, W., van den Heede, K., Michiels, D., van Herck, P., Delesie, L., Codognotto, J., et al. (2006). Revision of the Belgian Nursing Minimum Data Set: From data to information. *Studies in Health Technology and Informatics, 122,* 616–618.

Shaughnessy, P. W., Crisler, K. S., & Schlenker, R. E. (1998). Outcome-based quality improvement in home health care: The OASIS indicators. *Home Health Care Management and Practice, 10*(2), 11–19.

Tanttu, K., & Ikonen, H. (2006). Nationally standardized electronic nursing documentation in Finland by the year 2007. *Studies in Health Technology and Informatics, 122,* 540–541.

Taunton, R. L., Bott, M. J., Koehn, M. L., Miller, P., Rindner, E., Pace, K., et al. (2004). The NDNQI-adapted index of work satisfaction. *Journal of Nursing Measurement, 12,* 101–122.

Werley, H., Devine, E., & Zorn, C. (1988). *Nursing minimum data set data collection manual.* Milwaukee: School of Nursing, University of Wisconsin–Milwaukee.

Werley, H. H., Devine, E. C., Zorn, C. R., Ryan, P., & Westra, B. L. (1991). The nursing minimum data set: Abstraction tool for standardized, comparable, essential data. *American Journal of Public Health, 81,* 421–426.

Werley, H. H., Lang, N. M., & Westlake, S. K. (1986a). Brief summary of the nursing minimum data set conference. *Nursing Management., 17*(7), 42–45.

Werley, H. H., Lang, N. M., & Westlake, S. K. (1986b). The nursing minimum data set conference: Executive summary. *Journal of Professional Nursing, 2,* 217–224.

Werley, H. H., & Zorn, C. R. (1989). The nursing minimum data set and its relationship to classifications for nursing practice. *American Nurses Association Publications,* NP-74, 50–54.

White, P., Pringle, D., Doran, D., & Hall, L. M. (2005). The Nursing and Health Outcomes Project. *Canadian Nurse, 101*(9), 14–18.

Index

Figures and tables are indicated by *f* and *t* following page numbers.

A